THE BIG PICTURE

MEDICAL PHYSIOLOGY

THE BIG PICTURE

MEDICAL PHYSIOLOGY

Jonathan D. Kibble, PhD

Associate Professor
Faculty of Medicine
Memorial University
St. John's, Newfoundland,
Canada

Colby R. Halsey, MD

Resident
Internal Medicine
Washington University Barnes-Jewish Hospital
St. Louis, Missouri

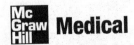 **Medical**

New York   Chicago   San Francisco   Lisbon   London   Madrid   Mexico City
New Delhi   San Juan   Seoul   Singapore   Sydney   Toronto

Medical Physiology: The Big Picture

1 2 3 4 5 6 7 8 9 0 CTP/CTP 12 11 10 9 8

ISBN 978-0-07-148567-8
MHID 0-07-148567-8

This book was set in Minion by Aptara®, Inc.
The editors were Michael Weitz, Susan Kelly, and Karen Davis.
The production supervisor was Catherine H. Saggese.
Production management was provided by Satvinder Kaur, Aptara, Inc.
The index was prepared by Alexandra Nickerson.
The text designer was Alan Barnett.
The cover designer was Elizabeth Pisacreta.

Cover image: Computer artwork of a nerve cell, also called a neuron. Neurons are responsible for passing information around the central nervous system (CNS) and from the CNS to the rest of the body. The nerve cell comprises a nerve cell body (center) surrounded by numerous extensions called dendrites, which collect information from other nerve cells or from sensory cells. Each neuron has one process called an axon through which information passes to other cells, including other nerve cells and muscle fibers.
Credit: Alfred Pasieka / Photo Researchers, Inc.

China Translation & Printing Services, Ltd., was printer and binder.
This book is printed on acid-free paper.

Library of Congress Cataloging-in-Publication Data

Kibble, Jonathan David.
  The big picture : medical physiology / by Jonathan David Kibble, Colby Ray Halsey.
      p. ; cm.
  ISBN-13: 978-0-07-148567-8 (pbk. : alk. paper)
  ISBN-10: 0-07-148567-8
 1. Human physiology. 2. Human physiology–Examinations, questions, etc. I. Halsey, Colby Ray. II. Title. III. Title: Medical physiology.
  [DNLM: 1. Physiological Processes–Examination Questions. QT 18.2 K46b 2009]
  QP34.5.K53 2009
  612–dc22

                                                                    2008039794

International Edition: ISBN 978-0-07-164005-3; MHID 0-07-164005-3
Copyright © 2009. Exclusive rights by The McGraw-Hill Companies, Inc., for manufacture and export. This book cannot be re-exported from the country to which it is consigned by McGraw-Hill. The International Edition is not available in North America.

DEDICATION

To my family for their love, support, and inspiration: my wife and soulmate,
Vicki, and our wonderful boys, Sam and Thomas; my mum and dad,
Sue and John; and my brother, Gary.
To my friend and mentor, Penny Hansen, for her wisdom; and to the students for
their amazing energy and enthusiasm.

—*Jonathan D. Kibble*

To my loving wife, Kathy, for her ever-present support and encouragement no matter
what challenge lies in front of us; to my daughter, Katie, for always bringing
sunshine and smiles to my life; to my mom and dad for leading by example;
and to my good friend and classmate, Terry, for being the best study partner ever.

—*Colby R. Halsey*

CONTENTS

PREFACE

The goal of this textbook is to help medical students efficiently learn and review physiology. The text offers a complete yet concise treatment of the major topics in medical physiology. Several design features are included to make the text easy to use.

- High-yield clinical pearls, see ▽ followed by ▼, are integrated throughout the text; clinical examples highlight the relevance and application of physiologic concepts.

- Approximately 450 four-color figures illustrate essential processes; explanatory figure legends allow figures to be used for review.

- *Key concepts* are highlighted in italics and **basic terms** are in bold when first mentioned.

- Bullets and numbers are used to break down complex processes.

- Study questions and answers are provided at the end of each chapter.

- A final examination is provided at the end of the book and is organized by body systems to allow either comprehensive testing or focused review.

The experiences of a seasoned medical physiology teacher and a new medical graduate have been combined to produce a text that is both accessible and relevant for students of medicine.

ACKNOWLEDGMENTS

Thank you to the excellent team assembled by McGraw-Hill to complete this textbook: to our development editor, Susan Kelly, for her rare mastery of the details and the Big Picture, all at the same time; to the artist, Matt Chansky, for turning our scribbles into real art and for being patient with all of our changes; and to Karen Davis and Michael Weitz for keeping us all on task. Particular thanks to our student reviewers James Thorburn, Aiden Brazil, and Brendan Sheehan for their excellent feedback, and to the Memorial University Medical School Class of 2011 for helping us to decide on which features to include in the book.

—*Jonathan D. Kibble*

—*Colby R. Halsey*

ABOUT THE AUTHORS

Jonathan David Kibble trained as a physiologist at the University of Manchester (UK) in the early 1990s. His previous academic positions have been at the University of Sheffield Medical School (UK) and at St. George's University (Grenada). Most recently he taught physiology at The Memorial University of Newfoundland (Canada), where, in addition to serving as the physiology course director, he did research in renal physiology and active learning methods. Currently he is helping to develop the medical curriculum at the University of Central Florida College of Medicine. He has taught physiology to over 4000 medical students from around the world.

Colby Ray Halsey received his undergraduate and graduate degrees from the University of Colorado at Boulder in Exercise Physiology and recently graduated from the University of Vermont College of Medicine, where he was elected into Alpha Omega Alpha Honor Medical Society and the Gold Humanism Honor Society. He was awarded the Ellsworth Amidon Award for outstanding proficiency in Internal Medicine. He is currently a resident in Internal Medicine at Washington University Barnes-Jewish Hospital in St. Louis. Colby worked on this project during his fourth year of medical school and offers a unique student/peer perspective to the clinical content of the book.

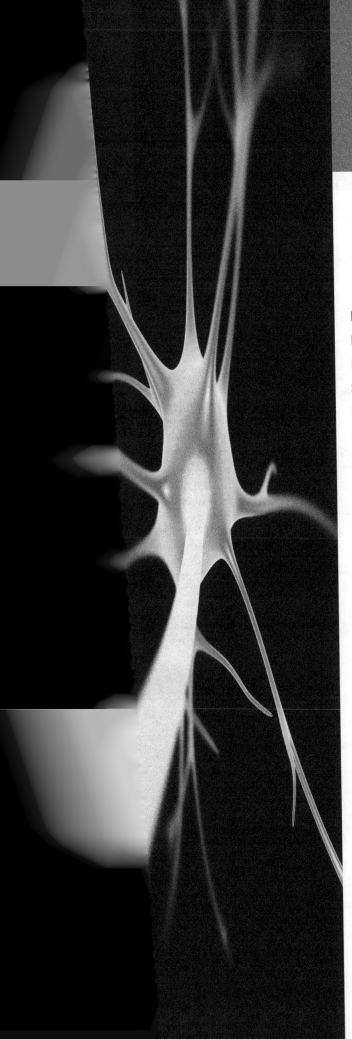

GENERAL PHYSIOLOGY

HOMEOSTASIS

Medical physiology is concerned with how a state of health and wellness is maintained in a person and, therefore, it takes a global view of how the body systems function and how they are controlled. There are 10 body systems, each with unique contributions to body function (Table 1-1). However, it is the integration of the body systems that allows the creation of a stable internal environment in which cells are able to function. For example, the maintenance of normal blood pressure requires the **integration of several organ systems:**

- The major determinants of blood pressure in the **cardiovascular system** are the rate of blood flow (cardiac output) and the vascular resistance.

- The volume of blood is a key determinant of blood pressure and is controlled by a balance between fluid and salt intake, via the **gastrointestinal system,** and their excretion via the **renal system.**

- Appetite and thirst are controlled by the **nervous system,** which, together with the **endocrine system,** integrates the body systems.

Such ability to *maintain* a stable internal environment is a central concept in physiology and is referred to as **homeostasis.**

TABLE 1-1. Major Components and Functions of the Body Systems

Body System	Component(s)	Major Function(s)
Cardiovascular	Heart, blood vessels, blood	Transport of materials throughout the body
Digestive	Gastrointestinal tract, liver, pancreas	Assimilation of nutrients; elimination of some wastes
Endocrine	Endocrine glands	Coordination of body functions through release of regulatory molecules
Immune	Thymus, spleen, lymphatic system, white blood cells	Defense against pathogens
Integumentary	Skin	Protection against external environment
Musculoskeletal	Skeletal muscle and bones	Movement and support
Nervous	Brain, spinal cord, peripheral nerves	Coordination of body functions through electrical signals and release of regulatory molecules; cognition
Reproductive	Gonads, penis, vagina, uterus	Procreation
Respiratory	Lungs	Oxygen and carbon dioxide exchange with external environment
Urinary	Kidneys, bladder	Homeostasis of ion concentrations in internal environment; elimination of wastes

NEGATIVE FEEDBACK CONTROL

The stability of the body's internal environment is defined by the maintenance of several **physiologic controlled variables** within narrow normal ranges (Table 1-2). The characteristic of minimal variation in a controlled variable is explained by the presence of negative feedback control mechanisms. **Negative feedback** is the initiation of responses that counter deviations of a controlled variable from its normal range and is *the major control process used to maintain a stable internal environment.* A negative feedback control system contains the following elements (Figure 1-1):

A **set point** value, which is at the center of the normal range and is treated by the control system as the target value.

Sensors that continuously monitor the controlled variable.

A **comparator,** which interprets input from the sensors to determine when deviations from the set point have occurred. The comparator initiates a counter response.

Effectors are the mechanisms that restore the set point to its normal level.

In the control of blood pressure, the controlled variable is **mean arterial blood pressure (MAP).** The normal set point for MAP is approximately 95 mm Hg. Pressure sensors are located

TABLE 1-2. Some Examples of Physiologic Controlled Variables

Controlled Variable (Arterial Blood Sample)	Typical Set Point Value
Arterial O_2 partial pressure	100 mm Hg
Arterial CO_2 partial pressure	40 mm Hg
Arterial blood pH	7.4
Glucose	90 mg/dL (5 mM)
Core body temperature	98.4°F (37°C)
Serum Na^+	140 mM/L
Serum K^+	4.0 mM/L
Serum Ca^{2+}	2.5 mM/L
Mean arterial blood pressure	90 mm Hg
Glomerular filtration rate	120 mL/min

in the carotid sinus and relay information to a comparator located in the central nervous system. If MAP suddenly changes, the activity of effectors (e.g., cardiac contractility, vascular tone, and urinary fluid excretion) is altered to restore normal blood pressure.

▽ Pathologic states occur when homeostasis is not maintained. For example, **diabetes mellitus** is a disease in which the blood glucose concentration (a controlled variable) is pathologically elevated. Diabetes is caused by dysregulation of the hormone insulin, which is the major effector in the control of blood glucose concentration. Virtually all hormones affect homeostasis and can therefore contribute to pathologic conditions when dysregulation occurs. ▽

THE INTERNAL ENVIRONMENT

The goal of homeostasis is to provide an optimal fluid environment for cellular function. The body fluids are divided into two major functional **compartments** (Figure 1-2):

1. The fluid inside cells, taken collectively, is the **intracellular fluid (ICF)** compartment.
2. The fluid outside cells is the **extracellular fluid (ECF)** compartment, which is subdivided into the **interstitial fluid** and the blood **plasma.**

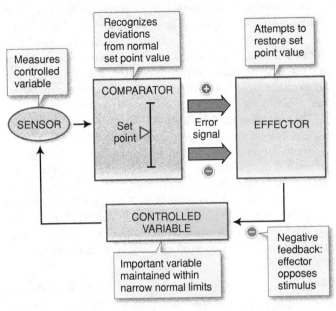

Figure 1-1: Components of a negative feedback control system.

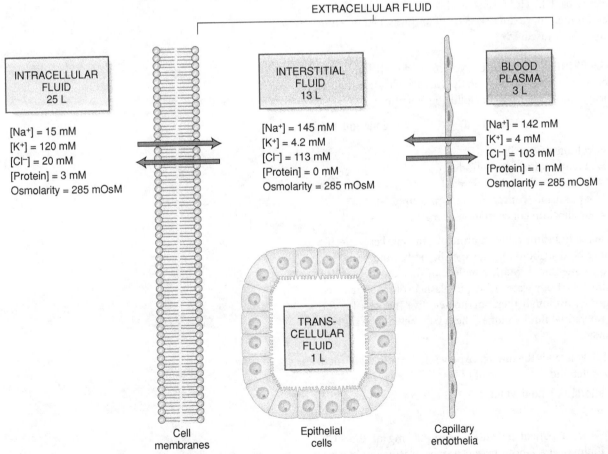

Figure 1-2: Body fluid compartments. Intracellular fluid (ICF) is separated from extracellular fluid (ECF) by cell membranes. ECF is composed of the interstitial fluid bathing cells and the blood plasma within the vascular system. Interstitial fluid is separated from plasma by capillary endothelia. Transcellular fluid is part of the ECF and includes epithelial secretions such as the cerebrospinal and extraocular fluids. ECF has a high [Na$^+$] and a low [K$^+$], whereas the opposite is true of ICF. All compartments have the same osmolarity at steady state.

The concept of an internal environment in the body correlates with the interstitial fluid bathing cells. There is free exchange of water and small solutes in the ECF between interstitial fluid and plasma across the blood capillaries. In contrast, the exchange of most substances between interstitial fluid and intracellular fluid is highly regulated and occurs across plasma cell membranes.

The volume of **total body water** is *approximately 60% of body weight in men and 50% in women.* About 60% of total body water is ICF and 40% is ECF. Approximately 80% of ECF is interstitial fluid and the remaining 20% is blood plasma, which is contained inside the vascular system. Figure 1-2 compares the basic compositions of body fluids. ECF is high in NaCl and low in K^+, whereas ICF is high in K^+ and low in NaCl. Interstitial fluid is similar in composition to plasma, except that interstitial fluid has almost no protein. Osmolarity is the same in all compartments.

▼ A large interstitial fluid volume is protective in the setting of **hemorrhage.** The capillary membrane that separates the intravascular space from the interstitial space is completely permeable to water, which allows the interstitial fluid to freely move into the intravascular space and helps to maintain adequate blood volume in a patient who is hemorrhaging. Because approximately 80% of the ECF is interstitial fluid and 20% is blood plasma, a hemorrhaging patient must lose about 5 L of ECF before the volume of the plasma volume is decreased by 1 L. The reverse is also true; to replace 1 L of plasma volume, approximately 5 L of intravascular isotonic saline must be infused. ▼

INDICATOR DILUTION PRINCIPLE The volume of a body fluid compartment can be determined from the volume of distribution of an indicator molecule using the following equation:

$$V = (Q - q) \div C \qquad \textbf{Equation 1-1}$$

V = Volume of distribution
Q = Quantity of marker introduced
q = Quantity of marker excreted or metabolized before equilibrium concentration is measured
C = Equilibrium concentration of marker

To use the indicator dilution principle, the marker molecule must only be distributed in the specific body fluid compartment to be measured. Marker molecules that can be used to determine total body water, ECF, and plasma volumes are listed in Table 1-3. Although there are no selective markers for the ICF or interstitial fluid volumes, these volumes can be derived as follows:

The **ICF volume** is the difference between the volume of total body water and the volume of ECF.

The **interstitial fluid volume** is the difference between the volume of ECF and the volume of plasma.

Example After a patient is infused with 400 mg of the ECF marker inulin over a 1-hour period, a stable plasma inulin concentration of 1 mg/dL is measured. During the infusion, 200 mg of inulin was excreted in the urine. Using Equation 1-1, the ECF volume is calculated as follows:

TABLE 1-3. Indicator Molecules for Body Fluid Compartments

Body Fluid Compartment	Indicator Molecule(s)
Total body water	Deuterium oxide (D_2O), antipyrine
Extracellular fluid	Inulin, mannitol
Plasma	^{125}I-labelled albumin

$$V = (Q - q) \div C$$
$$V = (400 \text{ mg} - 200 \text{ mg}) \div 1 \text{ mg/dL}$$
$$V = 200 \text{ dL} = 20 \text{ L}$$

MEMBRANE TRANSPORT MECHANISMS

OVERVIEW OF SOLUTE TRANSPORT

Cells constantly exchange solutes (e.g., nutrients, wastes, and respiratory gases) with the interstitial fluid. The transport of solutes across cell membranes is fundamental to the survival of all cells, and the transport mechanisms are therefore present in all cells. Specializations in membrane transport mechanisms often underlie tissue function. For example, excitable tissues express many voltage-sensitive membrane transport systems that account for the ability to generate and propagate electrical signals.

The plasma membranes that separate the cytosol from the ECF are formed from phospholipids and are *effective barriers against the free movement of most water-soluble solutes.* Most biologically important substances require a protein-mediated pathway to cross cell membranes. Solute transport can be categorized based on the **use of cellular energy** (Figure 1-3).

- **Active transport** requires adenosine triphosphate (ATP) hydrolysis.
  - **Primary active transport** occurs via membrane proteins that directly couple ATP hydrolysis to solute movement.

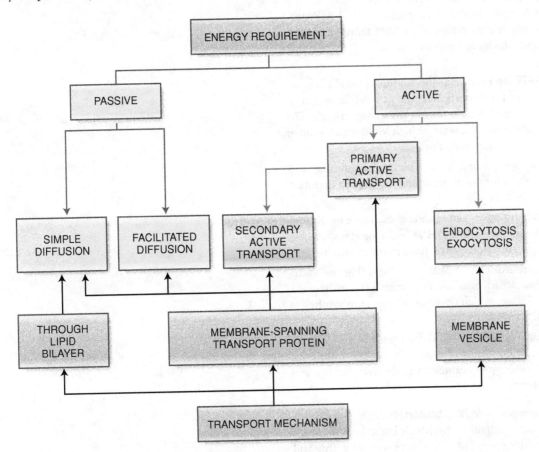

Figure 1-3: Classification of membrane transport systems.

- **Secondary active transport** couples the transport of two or more solutes together. In secondary active transport, energy is used to develop a favorable electrochemical driving force for one solute, which is then used to power the transport of other solutes (e.g., the inwardly directed Na^+ gradient is used to drive glucose uptake from the intestine).

Passive transport does not require ATP hydrolysis or coupling to another solute.

An alternative classification of solute transport is based on the **transport pathway** (Figure 1-3).

Diffusion of lipid-soluble substances (e.g., gases) may occur **directly through the plasma membrane.**

Transport of ions and small molecules more frequently occurs via membrane-spanning proteins, which serve as **pores** or **carriers** through the lipid bilayer.

Movement of macromolecules occurs in **membrane-limited vesicles;** macromolecules enter cells by **endocytosis** and exit cells by **exocytosis.**

▽ Similar to physiologic solutes, drugs also utilize the same fundamental transport processes to reach their target site. For example, **anesthetic gases** are lipid soluble, allowing diffusion through the lipid membranes of the brain. In contrast, most **diuretics** are secreted by membrane transport proteins into the lumen of the nephron to reach their site of action in the kidney. ▼

PRIMARY ACTIVE TRANSPORT Membrane proteins that directly couple ATP hydrolysis to solute transport are called **ATPases.** There are relatively few **examples of primary active transport systems,** some of which are illustrated in Figure 1-4A and discussed below:

The **Na^+/K^+-ATPase** (known as the "sodium pump") is present in all cells and transports $3Na^+$ out of a cell in exchange for $2K^+$, using one ATP molecule in each transport cycle. *The action of sodium pumps accounts for high Na^+ concentration in ECF and high K^+ concentration in ICF.*

Ca^{2+}-ATPases are located in the plasma membrane and endoplasmic reticulum membrane and function to maintain very low intracellular [Ca^{2+}].

H^+/K^+-ATPases pump H^+ out of cells in exchange for K^+ and are present in several epithelia. H^+/K^+-ATPase is responsible for the secretion of acidic gastric juice in the stomach.

H^+-ATPases are expressed inside cells, including the vacuolar H^+-ATPase, which acidifies lysosomes; ATP synthase is a form of H^+-ATPase, which operates in reverse to synthesize ATP in mitochondria.

The **multidrug resistance (MDR) transporters** are ATPases that extrude a wide variety of organic molecules from cells. MDRs are physiologically expressed in the liver, kidney, and blood-brain barrier.

▽ The expression of **MDR transporters** (e.g., P-glycoprotein) is one mechanism by which bacteria and cancer cells can become drug resistant. The effectiveness of a drug will be reduced if it is transported out of the target cell by MDR

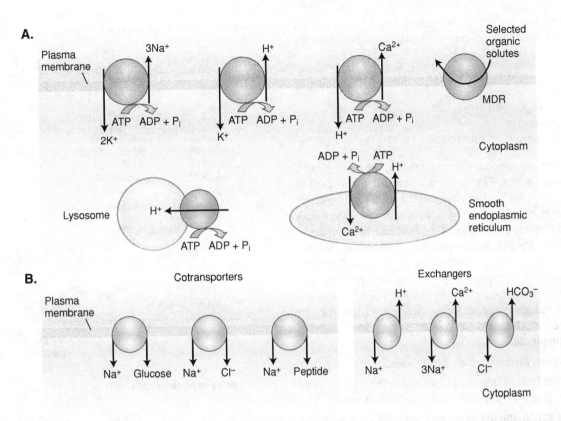

Figure 1-4: Active transport. **A.** Examples of primary active transporters (ATPases) in the plasma membrane and in organelles. **B.** Examples of secondary active transporters; cotransporters transport solutes in the same direction, and exchangers transport solutes in opposite directions. ATP, adenosine triphosphate; ADP, adenosine diphosphate; MDR, multidrug resistance.

transporters. Inhibition of the P-glycoprotein in cancer cells as a potential method of restoring the sensitivity of tumor cells to chemotherapeutic agents has become an intense area of research. ▼

SECONDARY ACTIVE TRANSPORT There are many **examples of secondary active transporters,** some of which are shown in Figure 1-4B and discussed below:

- **Cotransporters (symporters)** couple the movement of two or more solutes in the same direction. Examples of Na^+-driven cotransporters include Na^+/glucose uptake in the intestine and diuretic-sensitive Na^+/K^+/Cl^- and Na^+/Cl^- uptake in the kidney. H^+/peptide cotransport in the intestine is an example of Na^+-independent cotransport.

- **Exchangers (antiporters)** couple the movement of two solutes in the opposite direction. Na^+-driven exchangers include Na^+/Ca^{2+} and Na^+/H^+ exchange, which are important for maintaining low intracellular $[Ca^{2+}]$ and $[H^+]$, respectively. Cl^-/HCO_3^- exchange is an example of an anion exchanger. It is widely expressed, for example, in red blood cells, where it assists in HCO_3^- transport into and out of the cell as part of the blood-CO_2 transport system.

PASSIVE TRANSPORT Passive solute transport can only occur along a favorable electrochemical gradient. **Simple passive transport** is characterized by a linear relationship between the transport rate and the electrochemical driving force. Pathways for simple passive transport include diffusion through the lipid bilayer or via pores or channels in the membrane (Figure 1-5A). **Fick's law of diffusion** describes the simple diffusion of an uncharged solute (s):

$$J_s = -P_s \Delta C_s$$ **Equation 1-2**

J_s = Net flux per unit area
P_s = Permeability
ΔC_s = Concentration difference of s across the membrane

Permeability is a single coefficient relating the driving force for diffusion to net flux. The membrane permeability to a solute is proportional to the lipid solubility of the solute and inversely proportional to its molecular size. *Gases are an example of molecules that are able to move through the lipid bilayer of cell membranes by simple diffusion because they are small and lipid soluble.*

The transport of ions and other small water-soluble molecules across a cell membrane requires transport proteins that span the membrane. There are many examples of passive transport through membrane pores and carriers, the most numerous of which are **ion channels.** Ion channels have the following **general components** (see Figure 1-5B):

1. A **pore region,** through which ions diffuse.

2. A **selectivity filter** within the pore, causing the channel to be highly selective for a particular ion (e.g., Na^+ channels).

3. A **gating mechanism** that opens and closes the channel. In the closed state, no ions flow through a channel but the channel is available for activation. In the open state, ions flow down their electrochemical gradient. Some channels can also enter an inactivated state, where the gating structure is open but other parts of the channel protein block the pore. Recovery from inactivation and passage through the closed state are needed before the inactivated channels can reopen. Channel gates may be controlled by one of the following mechanisms:

  - Membrane voltage (**voltage-gated channels**).
  - Chemicals (**ligand-gated channels**).
  - Mechanical forces in the membrane (e.g., **stretch-activated channels**).

Passive transport can also occur via carrier proteins called **uniporters,** which selectively bind a single solute at one side of the membrane and undergo a conformational change to deliver it to the other side. Solute transport via uniporters is called **facilitated diffusion** because it is faster than simple diffusion. A characteristic feature of facilitated diffusion is the saturation of the transport rate at high solute concentrations (see Figure 1-5C). The GLUT family of related genes encodes uniporters for glucose transport; GLUT transporters are a common example of facilitated diffusion, which mediates glucose uptake in many tissues.

VESICULAR TRANSPORT Macromolecules are transported between the ICF and the ECF using membrane-limited vesicles. **Endocytosis** describes the ingestion of extracellular material to form endocytic vesicles inside a cell. There are three **types of endocytosis:**

1. **Pinocytosis** is the ingestion of small particles and ECF that occurs constitutively in most cells.

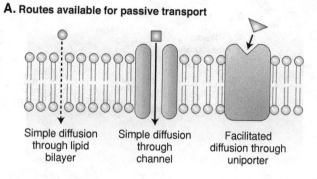

A. Routes available for passive transport

Simple diffusion through lipid bilayer

Simple diffusion through channel

Facilitated diffusion through uniporter

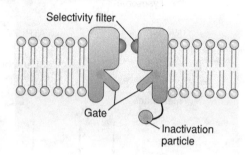

B. Components of ion channels

Selectivity filter

Gate

Inactivation particle

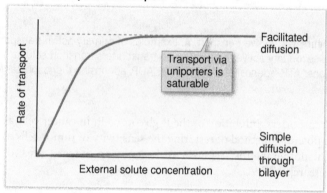

C. Kinetics of passive transport

Rate of transport

Facilitated diffusion

Transport via uniporters is saturable

Simple diffusion through bilayer

External solute concentration

Figure 1-5: A. Passive transport pathways. **B.** General components of ion channels components. **C.** Kinetics of passive transport. Note the linear relationship between simple diffusion and flux; facilitated diffusion via uniporters is faster than simple diffusion but is saturable.

2. **Phagocytosis** is the uptake of large particles (e.g., microorganisms) that occurs in specialized immune cells.

3. **Receptor-mediated endocytosis** allows uptake of specific molecules and occurs at specialized areas of membrane called **clathrin-coated pits** (e.g., uptake of cholesterol bound to low-density lipoproteins).

Exocytosis is the export of soluble proteins into the extracellular space. Such proteins are synthesized in the cell and packaged into intracellular vesicles. When vesicles fuse with the plasma membrane, the soluble proteins are secreted and the vesicle membrane is incorporated in the plasma membrane. There are two **pathways for exocytosis:**

1. The **constitutive pathway** is present in most cells and is used to export extracellular matrix proteins.

2. The **regulated pathway** is present in cells that are specialized for the secretion of proteins such as hormones, neurotransmitters, and digestive enzymes. *An increase in the intracellular Ca²⁺ concentration is a key event that triggers regulated exocytosis.*

▽ **Lambert-Eaton syndrome** is a neurologic condition resulting from autoantibodies that bind to and block Ca²⁺ channels on the presynaptic motor nerve terminals. By blocking the Ca²⁺ channels, the Ca²⁺-dependent exocytosis of vesicles filled with acetylcholine (a neurotransmitter needed for muscle contraction) is inhibited, resulting in muscle weakness. ▼

OSMOSIS

In clinical medicine, the infusion of intravenous fluids requires an understanding of the forces that move water within and between body fluid compartments. *Water transport across a barrier is always passive,* driven either by a diffusion gradient or by a hydrostatic pressure gradient. Osmosis is water movement that is driven by a **water concentration gradient** across a membrane (Figure 1-6A). Water concentration is expressed in terms of total solute concentration; the more dilute a solution, the lower its solute concentration and the higher its water concentration. When two solutions are separated by a **semipermeable membrane** (i.e., one that allows the transport of water but not solutes), *water moves by osmosis away from the more dilute solution.*

OSMOLARITY Osmolarity is an expression of the osmotic strength of a solution and is the **total solute concentration.** The osmolarity contributed by each solute present is the product of the molar solute concentration and the number of particles that the solute dissociates into when dissolved. For example, 1 mol of glucose dissolved in 1 L of water produces a solution of 1 Osm/L; 1 mol of NaCl dissolved in 1 L of water produces a solution of approximately 2 Osm/L. Two solutions of the same osmolarity are termed **isosmotic.** A solution with a greater osmolarity than a reference solution is said to be **hyperosmotic,** and a solution of lower osmolarity is described as **hyposmotic.**

Osmolarity can be converted into units of pressure, which allow osmotic and hydrostatic pressure gradients to be

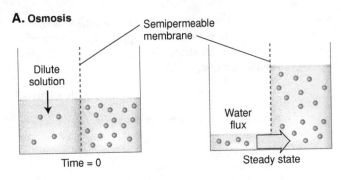

A. Osmosis

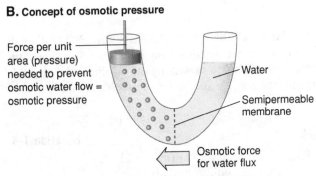

B. Concept of osmotic pressure

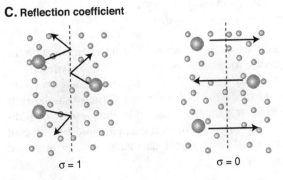

C. Reflection coefficient

Figure 1-6: Osmosis. **A.** Illustration of osmotic water movement across a semipermeable membrane. **B.** The concept of osmotic pressure. **C.** Reflection coefficients: solutes that do not permeate the membrane exert all their osmotic pressure (σ = 1); freely permeable solutes (σ = 0) do not exert any osmotic pressure.

mathematically combined; for example, when considering fluid filtration across capillary walls (see Chapter 4). The concept of osmotic pressure (π) is illustrated in Figure 1-6B and is calculated by the **van't Hoff law:**

$$\pi = g \times C \times RT \qquad \text{Equation 1-3}$$

g = Number of particles produced when the solute dissociates in solution
C = Molar solute concentration
R = Gas constant
T = Temperature

▽ **CLINICAL ESTIMATION OF PLASMA OSMOLARITY** Although blood plasma contains many solutes, a reasonable **clinical estimate of plasma osmolarity** can be obtained by considering only the Na^+, glucose, and urea concentrations:

$$P_{Osm} = 2P_{Na} + \left(P_{glucose}/18\right) + \left(P_{urea}/2.8\right)$$

$$\text{Equation 1-4}$$

P_{Osm} = Plasma osmolarity (mOsm/L)
P_{Na} = Plasma [sodium] (mEq/L)
$P_{glucose}$ = Plasma [glucose] (mg/dL)
P_{urea} = Plasma [urea] (mg/dL)

The measured plasma osmolarity, which is determined in the laboratory, can sometimes be greater than the estimate of plasma osmolarity, calculated using Equation 1-4. This difference between measured and estimated plasma osmolarity is called the **osmolar gap,** and is caused by the presence of additional solutes in plasma. For example, patients with **alcohol intoxication** or **ethylene glycol poisoning** have an increased osmolar gap. ▽

EFFECTIVE OSMOLARITY In many biologic situations, membranes are not completely semipermeable, allowing solutes the ability to permeate the membrane. When the membrane is permeated, the observed osmotic pressure gradient is reduced. The concept of effective osmolarity (or **tonicity**) incorporates the effect of solute permeation. The tendency of a solute to permeate a membrane, and therefore to reduce the effective osmotic gradient, is expressed using the **reflection coefficient** (σ), which is the fraction of the measured osmolarity actually exerted. For solutes that do not permeate a membrane, $\sigma = 1.0$; when the membrane is freely permeable to the solute, $\sigma = 0$ (see Figure 1-6C). The effective osmolarity of a solution is calculated as the product of the osmolarity and the solute reflection coefficient (e.g., if $\sigma = 0.5$, the effective osmolarity exerted is only 50% of the measured osmolarity).

The terms **isotonic, hypotonic, and isotonic** are used to describe the effective osmolarity of a solution relative to a cell.

▪ An **isotonic solution** has the some effective osmolarity as the cells and causes *no net water movement.*

▪ A **hypotonic solution** has a smaller effective osmolarity than the cells and *causes cells to swell.*

▪ A **hypertonic solution** has a larger effective osmolarity than the cells and *causes cells to shrink.*

Because water moves freely across most cell membranes, a steady state condition occurs in which the ECF is isotonic with respect to the ICF. If the steady state is temporarily disrupted, osmotic water movement between ICF and ECF must occur until the tonicity again becomes equal in each compartment. For example, if a patient is intravenously infused with a **hypotonic solution,** the ECF tonicity is initially decreased and water moves into the ICF by osmosis (cells swell). Conversely, if a **hypertonic solution** is infused, the ECF tonicity initially increases and water moves out of the ICF (cells shrink).

MEMBRANE POTENTIALS

The combined action of membrane transport systems in a resting cell results in a steady state condition in which stable ionic concentration gradients exist across the membrane, and the osmolarity remains constant to prevent changes in cellular volume. Ionic gradients are responsible for the generation of a **resting membrane potential difference** across the cell membrane of all cells in which the inside of the cell is electrically negative with respect to the outside (Figure 1-7A). The presence of membrane voltages is fundamental to the function of **excitable tissues** (e.g., nerve and muscle), which are able to generate and propagate electrical signals in the form of **action potentials.** Nonexcitable cells are also affected by their membrane voltage because it contributes to the overall **electrochemical driving force** for ion transport.

IONIC BASIS OF MEMBRANE POTENTIALS

Membrane potentials arise because cell membranes contain ion channels that provide **selective ion permeability** and because there are stable ion diffusion gradients across the membrane. The following steps are involved in the development of a **diffusion potential** (see Figure 1-7B):

1. In the example shown in the figure, two **potassium** chloride (KCl) solutions are separated by a membrane that is permeable to K^+ but *not to Cl^-.*

2. K^+ **diffuses** from the upper to the lower compartment, down its concentration gradient. In this case, *Cl^- cannot follow.*

3. A **voltage difference** develops as the K^+ ions leave the upper compartment, leaving a net negative charge behind. *A very slight separation of KCl ion pairs is enough to generate physiologic voltages.*

4. The negative potential in the upper compartment attracts K^+ ions and opposes the K^+ concentration gradient. An **equilibrium potential** is established when the voltage difference and the concentration gradient are equal but opposite driving forces. *At the equilibrium potential, there is no net movement of K^+.*

This simulated example is analogous to most resting cells, which contain a high $[K^+]$ and have numerous open K^+ channels at rest (*note, however, that the major intracellular anion in cells is protein, not Cl^-*).

A. Resting membrane potential

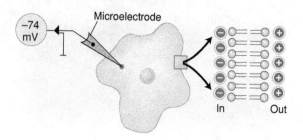

B. Diffusion potentials and Nernst equation

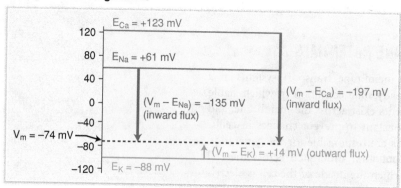

100 mM KCl ("in")

10 mM KCl ("out")

$E_K = (-61.5/z) \log [K^+]_{in} / [K^+]_{out}$
$E_K = -61.5 \log [100] / [10]$
$E_K = -61.5$ mV

C. Electrochemical gradients

$E_{Ca} = +123$ mV

$E_{Na} = +61$ mV

$(V_m - E_{Na}) = -135$ mV (inward flux)

$(V_m - E_{Ca}) = -197$ mV (inward flux)

$V_m = -74$ mV

$(V_m - E_K) = +14$ mV (outward flux)

$E_K = -88$ mV

Figure 1-7: A. The resting membrane potential; all cells have a negative intracellular potential. **B.** Generation of a K⁺ diffusion potential. In this example, K⁺ is the only permeable ion; a small amount of K⁺ diffuses to the lower compartment, creating a negative potential in the upper compartment. The Nernst equation predicts the equilibrium potential (voltage), based on the size of the K⁺ concentration ratio between compartments. **C.** Electrochemical gradients. Membrane potential (V_m) is shown by the dashed line. *Downward arrows* indicate gradients for cation flux into the cell; the *upward arrow* indicates a gradient for cation efflux.

The equilibrium potential is a function of the size of the ion concentration gradient and is calculated using the **Nernst equation:**

$$E_x = \frac{-61.5}{z} \log \frac{[X]_i}{[X]_o} \qquad \textbf{Equation 1-5}$$

E_x = Equilibrium potential for ion x
z = Ion valence (+1 for K⁺, −1 for Cl⁻, +2 for Ca²⁺, and so on)
$[X]_i$ = Intracellular concentration of X
$[X]_o$ = Extracellular concentration of X

Example The only ion channels open in a resting cell are K⁺ channels. If the intracellular [K⁺] = 155 mM/L and the ECF [K⁺] = 4.5 mM/L, predict the resting membrane potential.

The magnitude of the K⁺ diffusion potential that develops is calculated using Equation 1-5:

$$E_x = \frac{-61.5}{z} \log \frac{[K]_i}{[K]_o} \text{ mV}$$

$$E_x = \frac{-61.5}{z} \log \frac{[155]_i}{[4.5]_o} \text{ mV}$$

$$E_x = -94.5 \text{ mV}$$

Table 1-4 lists typical ion concentration gradients and equilibrium potentials for the major ions in excitable and nonexcitable cells.

TABLE 1-4. Ion Concentrations and Equilibrium Potentials

Ion	Intracellular mM	[Extracellular] mM	E_{Nernst} mV
Excitable cells (nerve and muscle)			
Na⁺	12	145	+67
K⁺	155	4.5	−95
Ca²⁺	10⁻⁴	1.0	+123
Cl⁻	4	115	−89
HCO₃⁻	12	24	−19
Nonexcitable cells			
Na⁺	15	145	+61
K⁺	120	4.5	−88
Ca²⁺	10⁻⁴	1.0	+123
Cl⁻	20	115	−47
HCO₃⁻	16	24	−13

RESTING MEMBRANE POTENTIAL The measured membrane potential (V_m) will usually be a composite of several diffusion potentials because the membrane is usually permeable to more than one ion. Ion permeability is best expressed in terms of electrical conductance to reflect ion movement through channels. V_m can then be expressed as the weighted average of ion equilibrium potentials for permeable ions. For example, in the case of a cell with permeability to K^+, Na^+, and Cl^-:

$$V_m = (g_K/g_m)E_K + (g_{Na}/g_m)E_{Na} + (g_{Cl}/g_m)E_{Cl}$$

Equation 1-6

g_x/g_m = Fractional conductance of ion x
E_x = Equilibrium potential for ion x

Example To estimate the membrane potential that will arise, using data in Table 1-4 for a nonexcitable cell and assuming that 80% of total membrane conductance is due to K^+ channels, 5% is due to Na^+ channels, and 15% is due to Cl^- channels:

$$\begin{aligned} V_m &= (0.80)E_K + (0.05)E_{Na} + (0.15)E_{Cl} \\ &= (0.80 \times -88) + (0.05 \times 61) + (0.15 \times -47) \\ &= -74.4 \text{ mV} \end{aligned}$$

In most cells, V_m is primarily a function of ECF $[K^+]$ because *K^+ conductance predominates in most cells at rest.* It should be noted that although the Na^+/K^+-ATPase is electrogenic ($3Na^+$ pumped out of the cell for every $2K^+$ pumped into the cell), its direct contribution to the membrane potential is very small. *The importance of the Na^+/K^+-ATPase in the development of resting membrane potentials is to maintain resting ion concentration gradients.*

Equation 1-6 illustrates the general prediction that changes in V_m will only occur if equilibrium potentials are disturbed (i.e., if ion concentration gradients change), or if the membrane conductance to an ion changes because ion channels open or close. The following terms are used to describe **changes in the membrane potential:**

Depolarization is a change to a less negative membrane potential (membrane potential difference is decreased).

Hyperpolarization occurs when the membrane potential becomes more negative (membrane potential difference is increased).

Repolarization is the return of the membrane potential toward V_m following either depolarization or hyperpolarization.

▽ **Hyperkalemia** is a potentially fatal condition in which the serum $[K^+]$ is increased. An increase in the serum $[K^+]$ depolarizes V_m, which can cause fatal cardiac arrhythmias. Using the following example, consider the effects on the heart when a normal serum $[K^+]$ of 4.5 mM is doubled to 9.0 mM. ▼

Part 1. Calculate the expected resting membrane potential for cardiac cells using the data in Table 1-4 for excitable cells (note $[K^+]_0$ = 4.5 mM) and assuming the following fractional membrane conductances values: g_K/g_m = 0.90, g_{Na}/g_m = 0.05, g_{Cl}/g_m = 0.05.

$$V_m = (0.90)E_K + (0.05)E_{Na} + (0.05)E_{Cl}$$
$$= (0.90 \times -\mathbf{95} \text{ mV}) + (0.05 \times 67 \text{ mV})$$
$$+ (0.05 \times -89 \text{ mV})$$
$$= -\mathbf{87.0} \text{ mV}$$

Part 2. Calculate the expected change in the resting membrane potential when the serum $[K^+]$ is doubled to 9.0 mM. Assume all other variables are unchanged.

The first step is to calculate the new equilibrium potential based on Equation 1-5 (the Nernst equation):

$$E_x = \frac{-61.5}{z} \log \frac{[K]_i}{[K]_o} \text{ mV}$$

$$E_x = \frac{-61.5}{z} \log \frac{[155]_i}{[9]_o} \text{ mV}$$

$$E_x = -76 \text{ mV}$$

Recalculate the resting membrane potential using the new value for E_K:

$$V_m = (0.90)E_K + (0.05)E_{Na} + (0.05)E_{Cl}$$
$$= (0.90 \times -\mathbf{76}) + (0.05 \times 67) + (0.05 \times -89)$$
$$= -\mathbf{69.5} \text{ mV}$$

Depolarizing excitable cardiac myocytes from a membrane potential of −87 mV to −69.5 mV may be enough to trigger extracardiac action potentials, which may lead to a fatal arrhythmia!

ELECTROCHEMICAL GRADIENT The electrochemical gradient for an ion is the *net* driving force for ion flux, which is a combination of the membrane voltage and the ion concentration gradient. An equilibrium potential calculated using the Nernst equation is an expression of the ion concentration gradient in mV. The equilibrium potential can therefore be directly compared to the measured membrane voltage. By convention, the **electrochemical gradient is defined as $(V_m - E_x)$** (see Figure 1-7C).

- For **cations,** a positive value for the calculated electrochemical gradient drives flux *out* of a cell; a negative value represents a net driving force for inward cation flux.

- For **anions,** a positive value for the electrochemical gradient describes a net driving force for *inward* anion flux, whereas a negative value indicates an outwardly directed driving force.

ACTION POTENTIAL

Excitable tissues (i.e., neurons and muscle) are characterized by their ability to respond to a stimulus by rapidly generating and propagating electrical signals. The signal assumes the form of an action potential, which is a constant electrical signal that can be propagated over long distances without decay. An action potential is an **all-or-none impulse** that occurs when an excitable cell membrane is depolarized beyond a **threshold voltage** (Figure 1-8A). Once the threshold has been exceeded, there is a phase of rapid depolarization, which ends abruptly at a peak voltage greater than 0 mV; the **overshoot** is the amount that the peak voltage exceeds 0 mV. A slower repolarizing phase returns membrane potential toward V_m. An **afterhyperpolarization** (undershoot) is observed in nerves (but not in muscle),

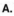

A.

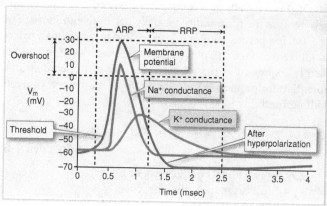

B.

Unmyelinated nerve axon

Continuous conduction

Myelinated nerve axon

Saltatory conduction   Nodes of Ranvier

Myelin sheath

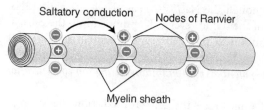

Figure 1-8: A. Nerve action potential. The upstroke of the action potential results from increased Na^+ conductance. Repolarization results from a declining Na^+ conductance combined with an increasing K^+ conductance; afterhyperpolarization is due to sustained high K^+ conductance. **B.** Action potential propagation. Local current flow causes the threshold potential to be exceeded in adjacent areas of the neuron membrane. Because the upstream region is refractory, an action potential is only propagated downstream. In myelinated axons, action potentials propagate faster by "jumping" from one node of Ranvier to the next node by saltatory conduction. ARP, absolute refractory period; RRP, relative refractory period.

in which the membrane potential is transiently more negative than the resting membrane potential.

The characteristic phases of an action potential are explained below by specific **changes in membrane Na⁺ and K⁺ conductance** with time (Figure 1-8A):

1. **Rapid depolarization** after threshold voltage is exceeded is due to the opening of **voltage-gated Na⁺ channels.**

2. The **peak voltage** where rapid depolarization abruptly ends and the membrane enters the repolarizing phase has two components:

   Closure of **inactivation gates** on Na⁺ channels.

   Opening of **voltage-gated K⁺ channels.**

3. **Repolarization** of the membrane potential progresses due to the decreasing Na⁺ conductance and the increasing K⁺ conductance.

4. **Afterhyperpolarization** occurs because K⁺ conductance exceeds that at rest, causing V_m to approach E_K.

REFRACTORY PERIODS In the nervous system, it is necessary to encode the intensity of a stimulus rather than merely indicating whether or not a stimulus is present (e.g., how loud is a sound?). Because individual action potentials all have the same amplitude and *action potentials never summate*, the stimulus intensity must be *encoded by action potential frequency*. The maximum action potential frequency is limited because a **finite period of time** must elapse after one action potential before a second one can be triggered.

   The **absolute refractory period** is the time from the beginning of one action potential when it is *impossible to stimulate another action potential.* The absolute refractory period results from closure of inactivation gates in Na⁺ channels; inactivated channels must close and the gates must be reset before channels can be reopened.

   The **relative refractory period** is the time after the absolute refractory period when another impulse can be evoked, but only *if a stronger stimulus is applied.* A stronger stimulus is needed because a small number of Na⁺ channels have now recovered from inactivation and the membrane is less excitable due to high K⁺ conductance.

Action potential propagation Action potentials are only propagated *in one direction* along a nerve axon or muscle fiber (see Figure 1-8B). The impulse in one area causes **local current flow,** which depolarizes the adjacent area to threshold, generating a new action potential downstream. This process is repeated to propagate the action potential signal; conduction is **unidirectional** because the upstream region is in its refractory period.

   The speed of *action potential conduction is faster in larger diameter fibers* because they have lower electrical resistance than small diameter fibers. *Conduction speed is also increased by the* **myelination** *of nerve axons.* Myelin consists of glial cell plasma membrane, concentrically wrapped around the nerve. In the peripheral nerves, the myelin sheath is interrupted at regular intervals by uncovered **nodes of Ranvier.** Action potentials are propagated from node-to-node rather than conducting along the whole nerve membrane because *voltage-gated Na⁺ channels are only expressed at nodes of Ranvier.* This process, called **saltatory conduction**, is illustrated in Figure 1-8B.

▽ Diseases that result in **demyelination** of either the central nervous system (e.g., multiple sclerosis) or the peripheral nervous system (e.g., Guillain-Barré syndrome) will significantly impede nerve conduction speed, impairing the function of the nervous system. ▼

SYNAPTIC TRANSMISSION

Synapses are specialized cell-to-cell contacts that allow the information encoded by action potentials to pass to another cell. Synapses occur at the junction between the processes of two neurons or between a neuron and an effector cell (e.g., a muscle or gland). There are **two types of synapses:**

1. **Electrical synapses** occur where two cells are joined by **gap junctions,** which conduct current from cell-to-cell via nonselective pores. Cardiac muscle is an example of cells that are electrically coupled via gap junctions.

2. **Chemical synapses** involve the release of a chemical transmitter by one cell that acts upon another cell (Figure 1-9). Action potentials in a presynaptic cell cause the release of the chemical transmitter, which crosses a narrow cleft to interact with specific receptors on a postsynaptic cell. Excitatory neurotransmitters depolarize the postsynaptic membrane, producing an **excitatory postsynaptic potential.** Inhibitory neurotransmitters hyperpolarize the postsynaptic membrane, producing an **inhibitory postsynaptic potential.** Chemical synapses have the following functional characteristics:

   Presynaptic terminals contain neurotransmitter chemicals stored in vesicles. Action potentials in a presynaptic terminal cause Ca²⁺ entry through voltage-gated Ca²⁺ channels, triggering the release of neurotransmitter by **exocytosis.**

   There is always a delay between the arrival of an action potential in the presynaptic terminal and the onset of a response in the **postsynaptic cell.** The delay is short (<1 msec) when the postsynaptic receptor is a ligand-gated ion channel (**ionotropic receptor**), but long (>100 msec) if the receptor is linked to an intracellular second messenger system (**metabotropic receptor**).

   Transmitter action is rapidly terminated. One of three processes can remove transmitter molecules from the synaptic cleft: diffusion, enzymatic degradation by extracellular enzyme (in the case of acetylcholine), or uptake of transmitter into the nerve ending or other cell (usually most important).

SKELETAL MUSCLE

The basic function of all types of muscle is to generate force or movement. Electrical or chemical stimuli are transduced into a mechanical response. The three anatomic types of muscle

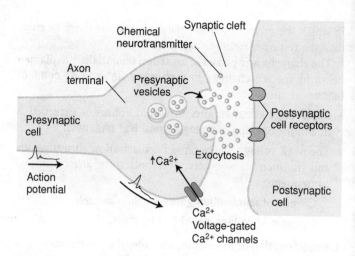

Figure 1-9: Components of a chemical synapse. Action potentials in the presynaptic neuron cause voltage-gated Ca²⁺ channels to open. Ca²⁺ influx triggers exocytosis of neurotransmitter molecules from storage vesicles into the synaptic cleft. Neurotransmitter molecules interact with receptors on the postsynaptic cell membrane to induce either excitatory (depolarizing) or inhibitory (hyperpolarizing) postsynaptic potentials.

are **skeletal, cardiac,** and **smooth.** Both skeletal and cardiac muscle are classified microscopically as **striated muscle.** Skeletal muscle is also referred to as **voluntary** because it *remains relaxed in the absence of nerve stimulation.* Cardiac and smooth muscle can function without nerve input and are referred to as **involuntary.**

NEUROMUSCULAR JUNCTION

Skeletal muscle does not contract until stimulated by action potentials arriving from a motor neuron (Figure 1-10A). The synapse between a motor neuron and a skeletal muscle cell is called a **neuromuscular junction or end plate** (see Figure 1-10B). *Every skeletal muscle cell (fiber) has only one neuromuscular junction,* near its midpoint. An individual neuromuscular junction consists of a small, branched patch of bulb-shaped nerve endings, called **terminal boutons.** Motor neurons branch to activate a group of muscle fibers, known collectively as a **motor unit.** Muscles that are subject to fine control (e.g., muscles of the hand) have many small motor units.

Motor neurons release acetylcholine as their neurotransmitter. Acetylcholine is synthesized in the cytoplasm of presynaptic terminals from acetyl coenzyme A and choline, via the enzyme **choline acetyltransferase,** and is stored in vesicles within the nerve terminal. The amount of acetylcholine within a single presynaptic vesicle is called a **quantum.**

The postsynaptic muscle cell membrane immediately opposite the presynaptic terminals has a high density of **nicotinic acetylcholine receptors.** Nicotinic receptors are ionotropic receptors that function as **nonselective Na⁺ and K⁺ channels.** When opened, nicotinic receptors cause skeletal muscle membrane potential to depolarize because the combined equilibrium potential for Na^+ and K^+ (E_{cation}) is approximately 0 mV. Each quantum of acetylcholine produces a small depolarization of the muscle membrane, called a **miniature end-plate potential** (see Figure 1-10C). Depolarizations from many quanta summate to produce a full end-plate potential in the muscle membrane, which is an example of an **excitatory postsynaptic potential.** *A single motor nerve impulse normally produces an end-plate potential that exceeds the threshold for action potential generation in the muscle cell membrane.*

Acetylcholine within the synaptic cleft is rapidly broken down to choline and acetic acid by the enzyme **acetylcholinesterase,** which is anchored to the muscle cell basement membrane. Choline is taken up by presynaptic nerve terminals and is reused for acetylcholine synthesis. Table 1-5 summarizes the effects of several toxins and drugs that interfere with the neuromuscular junction.

▽ **Myasthenia gravis** is an autoimmune disease in which antibodies are directed against nicotinic acetylcholine receptors, reducing the number at the end plate. Acetylcholine release is normal, but the postsynaptic membrane is less responsive and results in muscle weakness. Treatment of myasthenia gravis is with agents such as neostigmine, which inhibit acetylcholinesterase in the cleft, thereby prolonging the action of acetylcholine at the neuromuscular junction. ▽

A. Motor unit

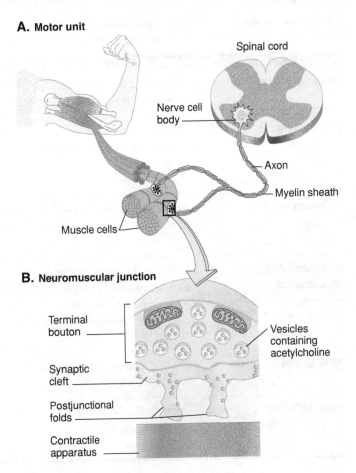

B. Neuromuscular junction

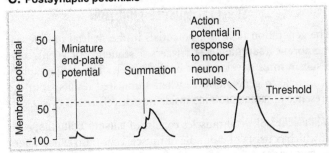

C. Postsynaptic potentials

Figure 1-10: Innervation of skeletal muscle. **A.** Motor units include a motor neuron and the group of muscle fibers that are innervated by its branches. **B.** The neuromuscular junction. Acetylcholine release from motor neuron terminals stimulates nicotinic receptors in the muscle membrane, producing an excitatory postsynaptic potential. **C.** End-plate potentials. Acetylcholine in a single presynaptic vesicle (quantum) evokes a miniature end-plate potential. Action potential in a motor neuron triggers the release of many quanta, and miniature end-plate potentials summate to exceed the threshold for action potential in the muscle fiber.

TABLE 1-5. Drugs and Toxins That Affect Neuromuscular Transmission

Agent(s)	Action	Effect
Botulinum toxin	Enters motor nerve terminal, irreversibly inhibits acetylcholine release	Failure of acetylcholine release; flaccid paralysis of muscle
α-Latrotoxin	Enters motor nerve terminal, promotes massive release of acetylcholine	Initial surge of acetylcholine release followed by irreversible depletion of acetylcholine; contractions followed by flaccid paralysis
ω-Conotoxin	Binds irreversibly to Ca^{2+} channels in motor nerve terminal membrane	Reduced Ca^{2+} entry to nerve terminal, reduced acetylcholine release; flaccid paralysis
_d_-Tubocurarine, pancuronium	Reversible competitive antagonists at nicotinic acetylcholine receptors	Prevents acetylcholine action; flaccid paralysis
α-Bungarotoxin	Irreversible antagonist at nicotinic acetylcholine receptors	Prevents acetylcholine action; flaccid paralysis
Neostigmine	Inhibits acetylcholinesterase in synaptic cleft	Prolongs action of acetylcholine at the end plate
Hemicholinium	Choline reuptake blocker in motor neuron terminal	Depletes acetylcholine in nerve terminals; muscle weakness or flaccid paralysis

SKELETAL MUSCLE FUNCTION

The generation of action potentials in the skeletal muscle cell membrane (**sarcolemma**) triggers a sequence of events that result in force development by the muscle. The unique ability of muscle to generate force when stimulated results from the presence of **motor proteins** inside muscle cells.

SARCOMERES Skeletal muscles consist of **muscle columns,** each of which consists of a bundle of muscle cells (also called **fibers** or **myocytes**) (Figure 1-11A). Muscle cells are multinucleate and are bounded by the sarcolemma. Each myocyte contains several cylindrical **myofibrils,** which display a distinctive pattern of light and dark bands under the light microscope. This striated appearance arises from the orderly arrangement of structural and contractile proteins. Each repeating motif in the striated pattern is called a **sarcomere,** which is the _fundamental contractile unit of skeletal muscle._ Each sarcomere has the following elements (see Figure 1-11B):

A **Z disk** bounds the sarcomere at each end.

Thin filaments, composed of **actin, tropomyosin,** and **troponins,** project from each Z disk toward the center of the sarcomere.

Thick filaments, composed of **myosin,** are present in the center of the sarcomere and are overlapped by thin filaments.

Sarcomeres line up end-to-end within a single myofibril. The darker areas that can be seen microscopically are denoted as **A bands** and correspond to the location of thick filaments. Lighter areas at the ends of sarcomeres are denoted as **I bands** and correspond to thin filaments where no overlap with thick filaments occurs.

MOLECULAR COMPONENTS OF SARCOMERES The orderly array of thin and thick myofilaments produces the characteristic striations of skeletal muscle. **Thin filaments** have three major components (see Figure 1-11C):

1. The backbone of a thin filament is a double-stranded helix of **actin.**

2. The helical groove on the actin filament is occupied by **tropomyosin.** Skeletal muscle contraction is regulated via a protein complex that consists of tropomyosin plus attached troponin subunits.

3. **Troponin** is a heterotrimer consisting of troponins T, C, and I; **troponin T** anchors the trimer to tropomyosin; **troponin C** binds Ca^{2+}, which allows muscle contraction to occur; and **troponin I** inhibits interaction between actin and myosin if the intracellular Ca^{2+} concentration is low.

Thick filaments are composed of **myosin** molecules, which are the molecular motors responsible for the generation of force. Myosin molecules are composed of the following major parts:

- The **myosin head** contains the actin-binding site plus elements necessary for ATP binding and hydrolysis. The heads are cross-bridges that bind to actin during muscle contraction.

- Myosin heads are connected to the tail of the molecule via a **hinge.** The hinge allows the movement of cross-bridges, which is the basis of force generation.

The giant protein **titin** is important for maintaining sarcomere structure and runs from the Z disk to the M line at the center of the sarcomere. In the region of the I band, titin is extensible and is largely responsible for the passive tension that is measured when a relaxed muscle is stretched (see Muscle Mechanics).

SLIDING FILAMENT THEORY The mechanism of active force generation in all muscle types is based on thin filaments being pulled over thick filaments (Figure 1-12). In a relaxed skeletal muscle, contraction is inhibited by the tropomyosin-troponin complexes, which obscure the active site on actin and prevent cross-bridge binding (Figure 1-12, panel 2). When the muscle is stimulated, the intracellular Ca^{2+} concentration increases and **Ca^{2+} binds to troponin C.** The resulting conformational change exposes active sites on actin (Figure 1-12, panel 3). A cycle of events now occurs in which myosin cross-bridges bind to actin,

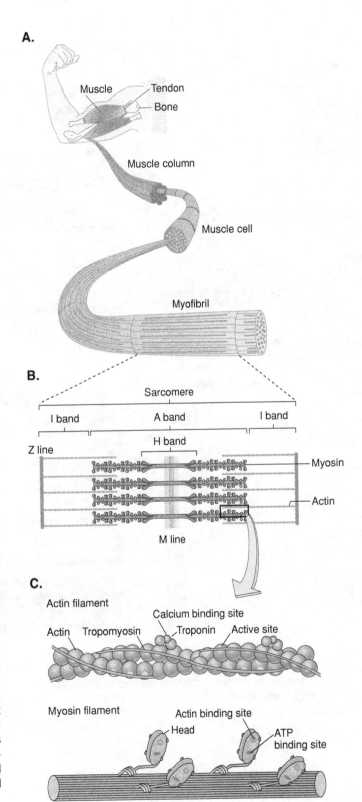

Figure 1-11: A. Structure of skeletal muscle: muscle cells (fibers) contain a group of myofilaments, each composed of sarcomeres aligned end-to-end. **B.** The sarcomere. A regular array of filament proteins between adjacent Z disks comprises a sarcomere. Thin actin filaments extend from Z disks toward a central M line, partially overlapping thick myosin filaments. Under a microscope, the region of thick filaments (A band) appears darker than adjacent areas with only thin filaments (I band), producing the striated appearance of skeletal muscle. Striations in adjacent myofibrils are also aligned. **C.** Molecular components of thin and thick filaments. Thin filaments are composed of actin, with the associated proteins tropomyosin and troponins; thick filaments are composed of myosin. ATP, adenosine triphosphate.

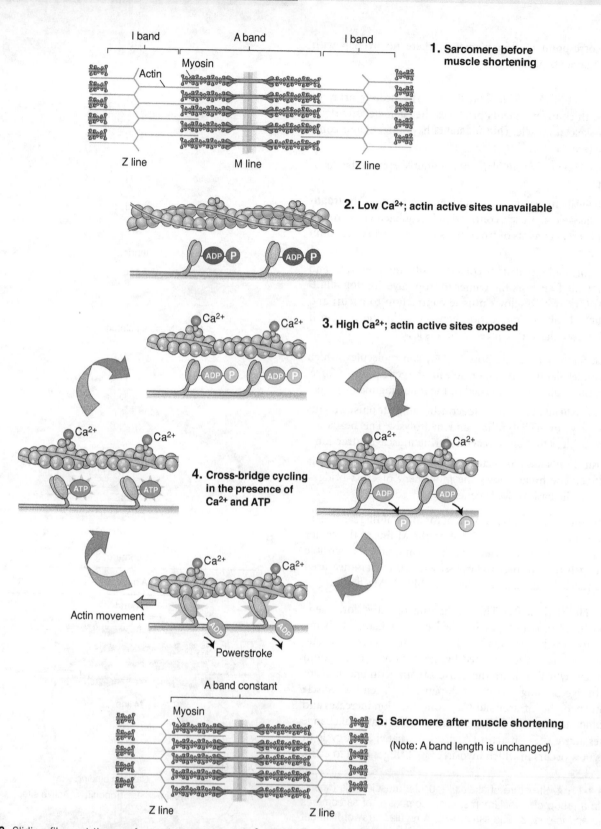

Figure 1-12: Sliding filament theory of muscle contraction. Ca^{2+} binding to troponin C causes actin active sites to be exposed (compare panels 2 and 3). In the presence of adenosine triphosphate (ATP), myosin repeats a cycle of binding to actin, performance of a power stroke, detaching, becoming cocked, and reattaching further along the actin molecule (panel 4). Actin filaments are drawn over myosin. In this example, muscle shortening occurs (compare panels 1 and 5). ADP, adenosine diphosphate.

perform a **powerstroke,** detach, become cocked again, and then reattach (Figure 1-12, panel 4). The cycle repeats in the continued presence of sufficient **Ca²⁺ and ATP.** As a result, thin filaments from each end of the sarcomere move toward the center by sliding over thick filaments, causing neighboring Z disks to approach each other. In the example shown in Figure 1-12, muscle shortening has occurred and the sarcomere length is reduced (compare panels 1 and 5).

▽ When death occurs, ATP production by mitochondria stops and **rigor mortis** (stiffening of the muscles) sets in. ATP is necessary for the myosin heads to detach from the actin filaments after a powerstroke occurs. Once ATP production ceases, the cross-bridges are locked in place, which results in stiff muscles. *Rigor mortis is a sign of death.* ▼

EXCITATION-CONTRACTION COUPLING In all types of muscle, the key event causing contraction is increased intracellular Ca²⁺ concentration. In skeletal muscle, the source of Ca²⁺ for contraction is the **sarcoplasmic reticulum (SR).** Muscle contraction only occurs after an increase in cytosolic Ca²⁺, which follows the generation of a muscle action potential (Figure 1-13). *The only physiologic stimulus for skeletal muscle action potentials is the end-plate potential, developed in response to motor nerve impulses.*

The contractile apparatus of each sarcomere is surrounded by the SR, providing a short diffusion distance for Ca²⁺ to its site of action. The membrane system of the SR is completely enclosed within the cell and is comprised of **longitudinal tubules,** which surround the contractile apparatus and terminate in **lateral sacs** (terminal cisternae). Lateral sacs are closely associated with invaginations of the muscle cell plasma membrane called T tubules. The **T tubules** extend deep into the cell to form blind-ended tubes containing ECF. The lateral sacs from two neighboring sarcomeres converge on a T tubule to form a structure known as a **triad** (Figure 1-14A). Triads are located at the junction of the A band and the I band of every sarcomere.

Action potentials in T tubules induce Ca²⁺ release from the lateral sacs. The Ca²⁺ release mechanism involves **voltage sensors** in the T-tubule membrane (L-type Ca²⁺ channels), which are linked to **Ca²⁺ release channels** (ryanodine receptors) in the SR (see Figure 1-14B). The voltage sensors respond to depolarization in the T tubule with conformational changes that result in the opening of the Ca²⁺ release channels of the SR. The intracellular [Ca²⁺] increases from about 10^{-8} M at rest to about 10^{-5} M during a muscle contraction. To return a muscle to the relaxed state, Ca²⁺ uptake occurs in the longitudinal tubules via **Ca²⁺-ATPases** of the SR. Following Ca²⁺ reuptake, most stored Ca²⁺ is found in the lateral sacs, where it is weakly bound to the protein **calsequestrin.**

FORCE OF CONTRACTION The force of skeletal muscle contraction is controlled by altering the firing pattern of motor nerves to the muscle. The effect of increasing action potential frequency to a muscle is known as **temporal summation** (Figure 1-15). At low stimulation frequency, the muscle briefly generates force and then relaxes. At high stimulation frequency, the muscle does not have time to relax between stimuli. Contractions fuse into a plateau of active force called a **tetanic contraction;** the steady high force level is called the tetanic force. Force does

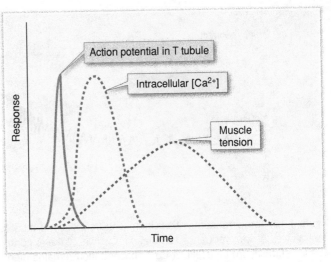

Figure 1-13: E–C coupling sequence in skeletal muscle. Force development depends on increased intracellular Ca²⁺, which is preceded by the muscle action potential.

A. Sarcotubular system of striated muscle cell

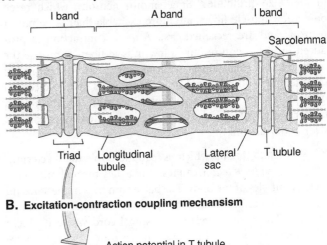

B. Excitation-contraction coupling mechansism

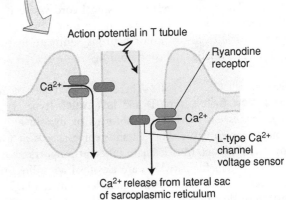

Figure 1-14: A. Muscle triads. Each T tubule is associated with a lateral sac from each of two neighboring sarcomeres to form a triad. **B.** The excitation-contraction coupling mechanism in skeletal muscle. The close association of membranes in the triad allows muscle action potentials to open the sarcoplasmic reticulum Ca²⁺ release channels, through activation of voltage sensors in T tubules.

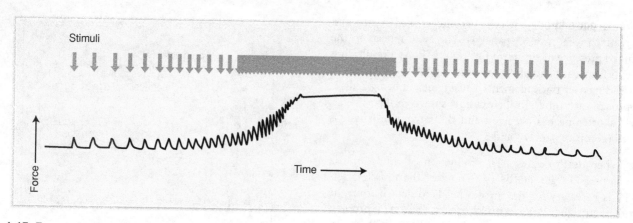

Figure 1-15: Temporal summation. Increased frequency of muscle stimulation (indicated by *downward arrows*) causes increased force of contraction. At low frequency stimulation, Ca^{2+} reuptake is complete and the muscle relaxes completely between stimuli. With high frequency stimulation, intracellular Ca^{2+} concentration remains high; the contraction force reaches a plateau (tetanus) when all the troponin C sites are filled with Ca^{2+}.

not increase if the stimulation frequency is further increased because cross-bridge attachment is already maximal; at this point, the muscle is said to be **tetanized.**

If a greater force of muscle contraction is needed, the number of active motor neurons increases. Recruitment of motor units is called **spatial summation** and is organized according to the "**size principle.**" Small motor neurons, which reach only a few muscle fibers, are more excitable than large motor neurons and are recruited first. A weak contraction is produced initially because only a few muscle fibers comprise the motor unit of small motor neurons. Large motor neurons are less excitable and require a stronger stimulus from the central nervous system. When large motor neurons are recruited, a large number of muscle fibers are stimulated to produce a strong contraction.

▽ **Tetanus toxin,** which is produced by the bacterium *Clostridium tetani,* can result in tetany throughout all the skeletal muscles of the body. The bacterium lives in the soil, and once it contaminates a dirty wound, the tetanus toxin is released. The toxin travels to the spinal cord where it blocks inhibitory nerves, allowing the excitatory motor neurons to fire rapidly. Rapidly firing motor neurons summate to produce tetany, a potentially fatal condition! ▽

SKELETAL MUSCLE DIVERSITY There are two types of muscle fibers: **slow twitch** (type I) and **fast twitch** (type II) (Table 1-6). Expression of different isoforms of myosin and other proteins accounts for different shortening speeds of fast and slow twitch fibers. Muscles have different proportions of slow and fast twitch fibers, which are classified according to their function. For example, postural muscles contain a higher proportion of slow twitch fibers because they must maintain tone and resist fatigue. Extraocular muscles are required to make fast, brief movements of the eye and therefore contain a high proportion of fast twitch fibers. There are genetic differences in the general proportions of muscle fiber types that are expressed among individuals, which accounts in part for the tendency for a person to be either a better sprinter (more fast twitch fibers) or have higher endurance (more slow twitch fibers).

TABLE 1-6. Comparison of Slow Twitch and Fast Twitch Muscle Fibers

Characteristic	Slow Twitch (Type I)	Fast Twitch (Type II)
Color	Red (myoglobin)	White (low myoglobin)
Metabolism	Oxidative	Glycolytic
Mitochondria	Abundant	Few
Glycogen content	Low	High
Fatigability	Low	High

MUSCLE MECHANICS

The sliding filament mechanism provides the potential for a muscle to develop force; the characteristics of the resulting contraction depend on a combination of intrinsic muscle properties and the external constraints placed on the muscle. There are **two general modes of muscle contraction:**

1. An **isometric,** or fixed-length contraction, occurs if both ends of a muscle are fixed. In this case, the muscle is able to develop tension but it cannot shorten.

2. An **isotonic,** or fixed-load contraction, occurs if a muscle is able to shorten to carry a given load.

LENGTH-TENSION RELATIONSHIP Muscle length is an important determinant of the force of contraction. The length-tension (length-force) relation is *studied under isometric conditions.* A resting muscle behaves like a rubber band, requiring force to stretch it to different lengths. The **preload** is the amount of force applied to a resting muscle before stimulation, creating **passive tension** (Figure 1-16A, blue curve). When the muscle is stimulated, **active tension** is added to the passive tension. The amount of active tension produced is the difference between passive tension and **total tension** (Figure 1-16A, red curve).

There is an *optimal range of resting muscle length* (preload) that produces maximal contraction. At very short or very long muscle lengths, active force development declines, producing the characteristic length-tension relationship of striated muscle. The **plateau** of the length-tension relation (Figure 1-16B, point y) reflects optimal overlap of thin and thick filaments within sarcomeres, providing maximum myosin cross-bridge binding. On the **ascending limb** (Figure 1-16B, between points x and y), the muscle is too short, resulting in double overlap of thin filaments and attachment of fewer cross-bridges. On the **descending limb** of the curve (Figure 1-16B, points y and z), the muscle is too long, resulting in inadequate overlap of thin and thick filaments. An additional mechanism contributing to the length-tension relationship in cardiac muscle is the increased Ca^{2+}-sensitivity of troponin C as muscle length increases.

Skeletal muscles operate at the plateau of their length-tension relation because preload is set at the optimal level by bony attachments at each end of the muscle. By contrast, preload is not fixed in cardiac muscle but varies according to the amount of venous return. Preload is a key determinant of the force of cardiac muscle contraction (see Chapter 4).

▽ In a healthy heart, an increased **preload** will stretch the cardiac myocytes, resulting in a more forceful and speedy contraction. However, in a diseased heart (e.g., left ventricular hypertrophy), cardiac muscle can become stiff, impairing its ability to stretch. Increasing preload in this setting will mainly increase the pressures in the heart without the benefit of improving contractile force or speed. ▽

FORCE-VELOCITY RELATIONSHIP Muscle performance can be studied under isotonic conditions to produce a force-velocity relation. The resting muscle length is set by adding a given preload, and the **initial velocity of shortening** is then measured as the muscle is stimulated to lift a range of additional weights. The weight a muscle must lift upon stimulation after resting

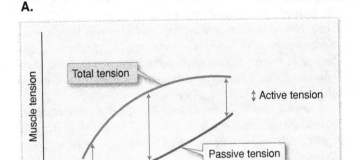

A.

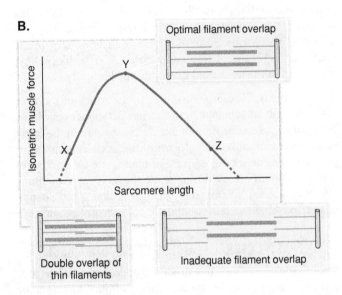

B.

Figure 1-16: The length-tension relationship in skeletal muscle. **A.** Passive tension (preload) is the force required to set the resting length (*blue curve*). Total tension (*red curve*) includes active (developed) tension in addition to passive tension. Maximum active tension is developed from an optimal resting muscle length; short and long resting lengths both reduce developed tension. **B.** Optimal resting muscle length corresponds with optimal overlap of thick and thin filaments in sarcomeres.

length has been established is called **afterload.** *The speed of shortening decreases as the total load increases* (Figure 1-17A). Extrapolating this curve to a theoretical zero load indicates the maximum possible speed of shortening (**V**$_{max}$), which reflects the *rate of myosin ATPase activity.* If preload is increased, there is an increased speed of shortening for any given total load, but without any change in V$_{max}$ (see Figure 1-17B).

In cardiac muscle, increased force and speed of contraction can be produced without changing preload. This is called increased **contractility** *and can be identified by an increase in* V$_{max}$ (see Chapter 4).

SMOOTH MUSCLE

Smooth muscle lines the walls of most hollow organs, including organs of the vascular, gastrointestinal, respiratory, urinary, and reproductive systems. Smooth muscle is an important therapeutic target because it regulates variables such as blood flow, ventilation of the lungs, and gastrointestinal motility.

▽ Homeostasis can be disrupted by too much or too little **smooth muscle tone,** resulting in a pathologic condition. For example, excessive smooth muscle contraction in the respiratory tract can cause difficulty breathing, such as occurs during an asthma attack. An example of inadequate tone occurs in vascular smooth muscle during septic shock; an overwhelming infection releases inflammatory mediators that cause dilation of systemic blood vessels, resulting in severe hypotension. ▼

ULTRASTRUCTURAL FEATURES OF SMOOTH MUSCLE

Smooth muscle cells are not striated in appearance (as are skeletal and cardiac muscle) because *thin and thick filaments are not organized as sarcomeres.* A network of dense bodies in the cytoplasm of smooth muscle cells serves as attachment points for actin filaments; thick filaments overlap thin filaments in an irregular array (Figure 1-18A). The irregular arrangement of actin and myosin allows smooth muscle cells to *generate force over a larger range of preloads* than is possible in striated muscle. There is no T tubule or muscle triad structure in smooth muscle; SR is present but it has an irregular arrangement.

Histologically, there are two general **types of smooth muscle:**

1. **Visceral smooth muscle** is the most common type, in which cells are arranged in large bundles. Cells within a bundle behave as a functional **syncytium** due to the presence of gap junctions between cells.

2. **Multiunit smooth muscle** cells function individually because the cells are not connected by gap junctions. There is a dense nerve supply from autonomic neurons (see Chapter 2). A characteristic of multiunit smooth muscle is fine control over force development in a manner similar to spatial summation in skeletal muscle. For example, multiunit smooth muscle is found in the **iris,** where it provides fine control over the diameter of the pupil.

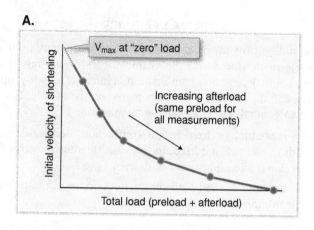

A.

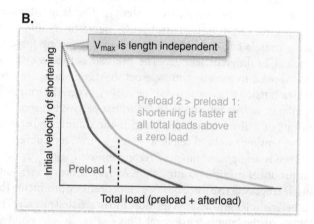

B.

Figure 1-17: The force-velocity relationship in skeletal muscle. **A.** Shortening velocity decreases with increasing total load. The theoretical maximum shortening velocity, V$_{max}$, indicates intrinsic myosin ATPase activity. **B.** Effect of preload on shortening velocity. Increased preload increases the velocity of muscle shortening in a loaded muscle but does not change V$_{max}$.

EXCITATION-CONTRACTION COUPLING

The contraction of smooth muscle begins when the intracellular Ca^{2+} *concentration increases* (see Figure 1-18B). The source of Ca^{2+} is usually from the ECF. Ca^{2+} enters the cell through **voltage-gated Ca^{2+} channels** when the cell membrane becomes depolarized. Depolarization of the membrane potential to threshold for Ca^{2+} channel opening may result from excitatory neurotransmitters or hormones or from spontaneous oscillations in membrane voltage. Contraction can also result from second messenger-stimulated Ca^{2+} release from the SR.

The regulation of smooth muscle contraction involves **myosin phosphorylation** because *smooth muscle myofilaments do not contain troponins.* The relative activity of the antagonistic enzymes **myosin light chain kinase** and **myosin light chain phosphatase** determines whether myosin is activated. When smooth muscle is stimulated and the intracellular $[Ca^{2+}]$ increases, the result is the formation of **Ca^{2+}-calmodulin complexes.** Activated calmodulin stimulates myosin light chain kinase to phosphorylate and thereby activate myosin. When Ca^{2+} levels decrease, the muscle relaxes because the activity of myosin light chain phosphatase predominates, causing myosin to become dephosphorylated.

An important feature of some smooth muscles (e.g., sphincters) is the *ability to maintain force over long periods.* The maintenance of muscle tone without high rates of ATP consumption is possible because cross-bridges can remain attached to actin for extended periods. This is called the **latch bridge state,** and results from slow rates of cross-bridge detachment in smooth muscle.

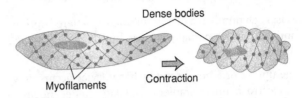

A. Morphology of single smooth muscle cells

Dense bodies

Myofilaments   Contraction

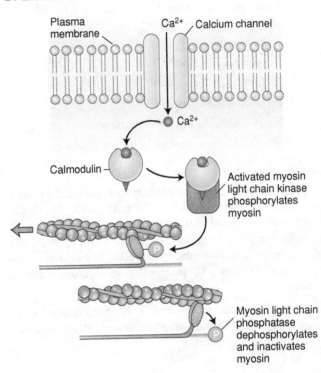

B. Excitation-contraction coupling in smooth muscle

Plasma membrane Ca^{2+} Calcium channel

Ca^{2+}

Calmodulin

Activated myosin light chain kinase phosphorylates myosin

Myosin light chain phosphatase dephosphorylates and inactivates myosin

Figure 1-18: A. Structure of a smooth muscle cell. No sarcomeres are present; actin filaments are anchored to dense bodies and overlap myosin in an irregular array; no muscle triads are present. **B.** Excitation contraction coupling in smooth muscle. In most cases, Ca^{2+} enters the cell from the extracellular fluid (ECF) via voltage-gated Ca^{2+} channels. Ca^{2+} binds to calmodulin, resulting in activation of myosin light chain kinase. Phosphorylation of myosin triggers cross-bridge cycling and force development.

STUDY QUESTIONS

Directions: Each numbered item is followed by lettered options. Some options may be partially correct, but there is only *ONE BEST* answer.

1. The uptake of a novel drug by hepatocytes occurs down an electrochemical gradient. Uptake is independent of other solutes, and the rate of uptake is saturated at high extracellular drug concentrations. Which membrane transport process is most likely to account for all these characteristics of drug uptake?

   A. Antiport with Cl^-

   B. Cotransport with Na^+

   C. Facilitated diffusion

   D. Primary active transport

   E. Simple diffusion through ion channels

   F. Simple diffusion through plasma membrane

Questions 2 and 3

A segment of normal human intestine was perfused in vitro. The lumen was perfused with 150 mM NaCl. The bathing solution contained 300 mM mannitol (an inert sugar). The reflection coefficients of NaCl and mannitol were 0.9 and 1.0, respectively. Assume that NaCl dissociates completely into Na^+ and Cl^-; mannitol does not dissociate in solution.

2. When compared to the osmolarity of the luminal solution, which of the following best describes the osmolarity of the bathing solution?

   A. Isosmotic

   B. Hyperosmotic

   C. Hyposmotic

3. Under the conditions described, what net water movement is expected to occur?

   A. Water moves into the intestine from the bathing solution

   B. Water moves out of the intestine

   C. No net water transport occurs

Questions 4–6

A study of a secretory airway epithelial cell was conducted using methods that allowed the control of ionic composition inside and outside of the cell.

Intracellular concentrations:

   $[K^+] = 135$ mM

   $[Na^+] = 10$ mM

   $[Cl^-] = 20$ mM

Extracellular concentrations:

   $[K^+] = 5$ mM

   $[Na^+] = 140$ mM

   $[Cl^-] = 110$ mM

Nernst equilibrium potentials were calculated: $E_K = -88$ mV, $E_{Na} = +70$ mV, $E_{Cl} = -46$ mV.

4. Under control conditions, membrane conductance was found to be entirely due to open K^+ channels. Under control conditions, resting membrane potential was closest to

   A. −40 mV

   B. −50 mV

   C. −60 mV

   D. −70 mV

   E. −80 mV

   F. −90 mV

   G. −100mV

5. Treatment of the airway epithelial cells with an agonist caused the opening of many Cl^- selective channels in the plasma membrane. Assuming that K^+ channels were unaffected by the agonist, what change in resting membrane potential will occur in response to the agonist?

   A. Depolarization

   B. Hyperpolarization

   C. Repolarization

   D. No change

6. Opening Cl^- channels in the membrane provides a pathway for Cl^- flux across the membrane. In which direction would net Cl^- flux occur?

   A. Cl^- moves out of the cell

   B. Cl^- moves into the cell

   C. There is no net Cl^- flux

7. A 25-year-old man suffered muscle paralysis due to poisoning with ω-conotoxin. This molluscan peptide toxin is known to interfere with voltage-sensitive Ca^{2+} channels at the neuromuscular junction. Which of the following is the most likely explanation for muscle paralysis in this patient?

   A. Failure of action potential conduction in the motor nerve terminal

   B. Failure of acetylcholine synthesis in the motor nerve terminal

   C. Failure of acetylcholine release from the motor nerve terminal

   D. Accelerated breakdown of acetylcholine in the synaptic cleft

   E. Inhibition of postsynaptic nicotinic acetylcholine receptors

8. A 37-year-old woman with worsening muscle weakness was diagnosed with myasthenia gravis. She was treated with the acetylcholinesterase inhibitor neostigmine, and reported improved muscle strength within 1 day of starting treatment. Which of the following is the most likely reason for improved muscle performance in response to neostigmine treatment?

   A. Increased action potential frequency in the motor nerves

   B. Increased acetylcholine synthesis in the motor nerve terminals

   C. Decreased acetylcholine breakdown at the neuromuscular junctions

   D. Decreased reuptake of choline by the presynaptic motor nerves

   E. Direct agonism at the nicotinic acetylcholine receptors

9. A skeletal muscle was stimulated to produce an isotonic contraction. Significant muscle shortening was observed. Which part of the sarcomere would retain a constant length during this type of muscle contraction?

   A. A band

   B. Distance between adjacent Z disks

   C. Distance from Z disk to M line

   D. Distance between adjacent M lines

   E. I band

10. A 49-year-old woman was found to have high blood pressure due to increased vascular smooth muscle tone. Which event occurring inside the vascular smooth muscle cells may contribute to development of high blood pressure in this case?

    A. Decreased opening of voltage-sensitive Ca^{2+} channels in the sarcolemma

    B. Decreased intracellular concentration of calmodulin

    C. Decreased calcium sensitivity of troponin C

    D. Decreased myosin light chain kinase activity

    E. Decreased myosin light chain phosphatase activity

ANSWERS

1—C. Facilitated diffusion only occurs passively down the solute electrochemical gradient; it occurs via uniporters, with no dependence on other solutes and is saturable.

2—A. Lumen osmolarity = $2 \times 150 = 300$ mOsm/L; bathing solution osmolarity = $1 \times 300 = 300$ mOsm/L. The solutions are therefore isosmotic.

3—B. Effective osmolarity (tonicity) = osmolarity × reflection coefficient. Lumen tonicity = $300 \times 0.9 = 270$ mOsm/L; bath tonicity = $300 \times 1.0 = 300$ mOsm/L. The luminal solution is hypotonic with respect to the bathing solution; water therefore moves out of the intestine by osmosis.

4—F. When the cell membrane is selectively permeable for one ion (in this case K^+), an electrochemical equilibrium for that ion is established. Membrane potential is therefore equal to E_K (−88 mV).

5—A. Opening Cl^- channels results in total membrane conductance being shared between K^+ and Cl^-. V_m is the weighted average of E_K and E_{Cl}. No fractional conductances are given, but V_m lies between E_K (−88 mV) and E_{Cl} (−46 mV) and is thus depolarized compared to the control condition.

6—A. The electrochemical gradient ($V_m - E_{Cl}$) is the driving force for Cl^- flux. Under the initial conditions $V_m - E_{Cl} = -88 - (-46) = -42$ mV. By convention, a negative electrochemical gradient directs outward anion flux. Opening Cl channels would shift V_m (−88mV) toward E_{Cl} (−46 mV), such that V_m would become less negative; negatively charged Cl^- ions must move out of the cell to make the cell interior less negative.

7—C. Voltage-operated calcium channels in the presynaptic membrane open in response to action potentials in the motor nerve. Calcium entry triggers the release of acetylcholine by exocytosis. The neurotoxic peptide ω-conotoxin causes this to fail.

8—C. Acetylcholinesterase breaks down acetylcholine to choline and acetic acid within the synaptic cleft. In myasthenia gravis, there is reduced nicotinic acetylcholine receptor availability in the skeletal muscle membrane. Blocking acetylcholinesterase increases the amount and duration of acetylcholine presence in the synaptic cleft, increasing the probability of muscle stimulation.

9—A. The A bands are composed of thick filaments and have a fixed length. Contraction with muscle shortening causes Z disks to approach each other and the I band to shorten, as thin filaments are drawn over thick filaments.

10—E. Excitation contraction coupling in smooth muscle involves activation of thick filaments by phosphorylation. Myosin phosphorylation is determined by a balance between myosin light chain kinase and myosin light chain phosphatase enzymes. A decrease in myosin light chain phosphatase activity favors myosin phosphorylation and greater smooth muscle tone.

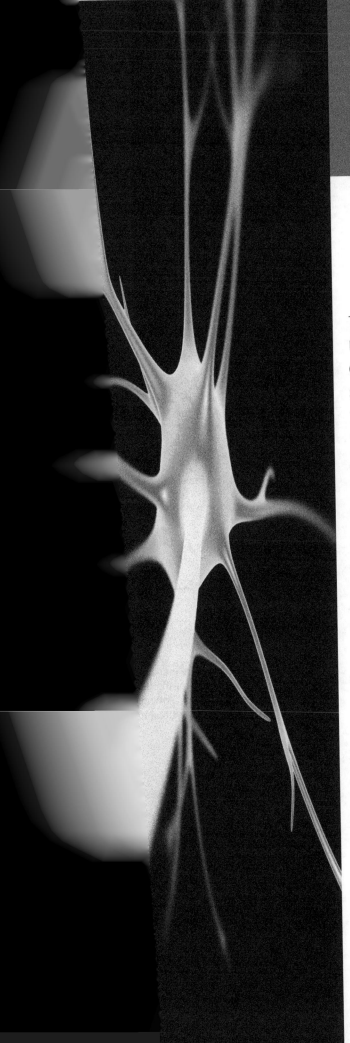

CHAPTER 2

NEUROPHYSIOLOGY

THE NERVOUS SYSTEM

OVERVIEW OF THE NERVOUS SYSTEM

The nervous system mediates a tremendous range of functions, from the unconscious control of visceral functions to sensory perceptions, voluntary movement, behavior, emotions, dreams, and abstract thinking. Nervous tissue is composed of **neurons** and numerous support cells called **glia.** The human brain contains approximately 10^{11} neurons, creating almost limitless potential for neuronal circuits and patterns of connectivity. There is great regional specialization within the nervous system that accounts for its ability to perform diverse functions (e.g., a region for vision, hearing, and movement). As a result, *damage to a specific part of the nervous system usually causes a set of predictable symptoms that aid in the clinical diagnosis of neurologic lesions.*

Neuroscience encompasses the study of the nervous system at many levels, from molecular genetics to behavior and cognition. Neurophysiology is only one part of neuroscience, and is concerned with mechanisms of function. This chapter will mainly discuss the nervous system at the cellular and systems levels. First, an introduction to neuroanatomy will provide the terminology necessary to discuss function. Later in the chapter, more details will be provided about the functions of each of the major anatomic structures.

ANATOMIC TERMINOLOGY The meaning of several **anatomic references** must be understood to describe the location and orientation of structures in the nervous system (Figure 2-1).

- **Rostral** and **caudal** denote toward the "head" and "tail," respectively. These directions are readily visualized below the level of the midbrain; however, above the midbrain, rostral indicates toward the front of the brain and caudal indicates toward the back of the brain.

- **Dorsal** and **ventral** indicate toward the back and front of the body, respectively; below the midbrain level, the terms are used in a similar manner. Above (rostral) the midbrain, dorsal refers to the top of the brain and ventral refers to the bottom of the brain.

- **Anterior** and **posterior** are used consistently to indicate toward the front or back of the body (or brain), respectively.

- **Superior** and **inferior** are used consistently to indicate toward the top of the cerebral cortex or the sacral end of the spinal cord, respectively.

When viewed dorsally, it is apparent that the nervous system can be divided along the midline (**median sagittal plane**) into two equal halves, with one being the mirror image of the other:

- **Medial** and **lateral** indicate toward or away from the midline, respectively.

- **Ipsilateral** indicates two points on the same side of the midline; **contralateral** indicates two points on opposite sides of the midline.

Structures in the nervous system can be viewed from several orientations:

- **Coronal** "slices" are vertically oriented at ninety degrees to the sagittal plane.

- The **horizontal plane** is perpendicular to both the sagittal and coronal planes.

▽ Interpretation of **neuroimaging studies** (e.g., CT or MRI) relies on the ability to visualize neuronal structures in the aforementioned planes (i.e., sagittal, coronal, and horizontal) and to mentally reconstruct them into a three-dimensional structure. ▼

THE PROTOTYPIC NEURON The major parts of a neuron and the terminology used to describe collections of neurons are briefly described below and are shown in Figure 2-2:

- A **soma** is the cell body of a neuron that contains the cell nucleus and the rough endoplasmic reticulum.

- **Neurites** are thin cellular processes extending from the soma.

- The **axon** is the cellular process that carries action potentials away from the soma. Axons are often long and may have multiple branches.

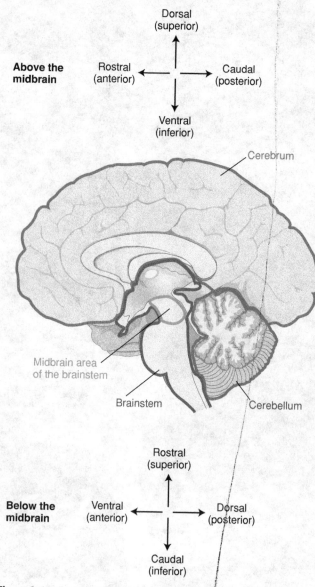

Figure 2-1: Neuroanatomic references. The three major areas of the adult brain are the cerebrum, the cerebellum, and the brainstem. Arrows indicate the different terminology used for anatomic references above and below the midbrain area of the brainstem.

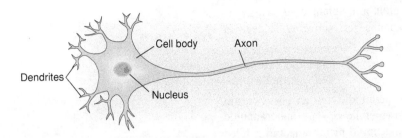

Terms Referring to Collections of Neurons	Description
Gray matter	A general term for neuronal cell bodies in the CNS; the cut surface of the brain appears gray at these sites
Cortex	Thin sheets of neurons, usually at the brain surface and most often used in reference to the cerebral cortex, but there are other examples (e.g., olfactory cortex)
Nucleus (plural: nuclei)	A clearly defined mass of neurons, usually fairly large and deeply placed in the brain (e.g., caudate nucleus of the deep cerebral nuclei)
Locus (plural: loci)	Clearly defined groups of neurons, but smaller than a nucleus (e.g., the locus ceruleus of the brainstem)
Substantia	A less well-defined group of neurons (e.g., the substantia nigra of the midbrain)
Ganglion (plural: ganglia)	Applied to collections of neurons in the PNS (except for the basal ganglia in the CNS)

Terms Referring to Collections of Axons	Description
White matter	A general term for axon groups in the CNS; the cut surface of the brain appears white at these sites
Tract	A collection of axons with a common origin and a common destination (e.g., corticospinal tract)
Capsule	A group of axons connecting the cerebrum and brain stem (e.g., internal capsule)
Commissure	A collection of axons connecting one side of the brain to the other (e.g., anterior commissure connecting the temporal lobes)
Lemniscus	A "ribbon-like" tract (e.g., medial lemniscus that conveys touch sensation through the brain stem)
Nerve	A bundle of axons in the PNS (except the optic nerve)

Figure 2-2: The prototypic neuron. Many processes (neurites) extend from the neuron cell body. A single process, the axon, carries electrical signals away from the cell body; dendrites are processes receiving information from other neurons. The table summarizes terms that apply to collections of neurons where cell bodies are concentrated and terms used to describe collections of axons.

Dendrites have a structure similar to axons but receive impulses from other neurons. Many neurons have an extensive set of dendrites, referred to as the **dendritic tree.**

DIVISIONS OF THE NERVOUS SYSTEM

For descriptive purposes, the nervous system can be divided into the **central nervous system (CNS)** and the **peripheral nervous system (PNS).**

The **CNS** consists of the **brain** and **spinal cord,** which are covered by three membranous layers known collectively as the **meninges.**

1. The **dura mater** is the outermost layer and consists of tough connective tissue.

2. The **arachnoid mater** is the middle layer and lies beneath the dura, which it closely follows. The **subarachnoid space** lies beneath the arachnoid membrane and is filled with **cerebrospinal fluid (CSF).**

3. The **pia mater** is the innermost layer. It is a delicate vascular membrane that closely follows the surface of the brain and spinal cord.

▼   Infection (i.e., viral, bacterial, or fungal) of the meninges results in **meningitis,** whereas infection of the brain parenchyma results in **encephalitis. Meningoencephalitis** results when both the meninges and the brain parenchyma are involved, and commonly occurs as a progression from acute bacterial meningitis, a potentially fatal condition. *The classic clinical triad of meningitis is fever, headache, and nuchal rigidity (stiff neck).* The patient with encephalitis will commonly present with confusion, behavioral abnormalities, an altered level of consciousness, and/or focal neurologic abnormalities. ▼

The **PNS** consists of neurons and glia, which are located outside the meninges. Structures in the PNS include spinal nerves, cranial nerves, and sensory receptors. **Sensory nerves** that convey information from the periphery to the CNS are called **afferent nerves.** Nerves that carry information from the CNS to the periphery are called **efferent nerves;** the efferent nerves that carry information to skeletal muscle are called **motor nerves** and are involved in muscle control.

The **autonomic nervous system (ANS)** is concerned with control of visceral functions such as digestion, blood flow, temperature regulation, and reproduction. The ANS has three divisions:

1. The **sympathetic nervous system** is generally excitatory and is associated with "fight or flight" responses.

2. The **parasympathetic nervous system** is generally antagonist to the sympathetic nervous system and is associated with "rest and digest" functions.

3. The **enteric nervous system** is a large system of neural networks within the walls of the gastrointestinal tract (see Chapter 7).

The functions of the ANS are contrasted with those of the **somatic nervous system,** in which sensory and motor communication occurs between the CNS and the skin, skeletal muscles, and joints. *The autonomic and somatic nervous systems both consist of afferent and efferent nerves, and both have structures located within the CNS and PNS.*

STRUCTURES OF THE CNS

The CNS consists of the brain and spinal cord. The anatomic organization of the CNS is such that predictable deficits result from neural lesions. The pattern of functional deficits observed clinically is therefore helpful in determining the general anatomic site of a neural lesion (e.g., the brain versus the brainstem versus the spinal cord).

The **brain has three major parts** (Figure 2-1):

1. The **cerebrum** is the most obvious part of the brain, and is divided down the middle into the **two cerebral hemispheres** by the **longitudinal fissure.** Each hemisphere receives sensations from and controls the movements of the contralateral side of the body. For example, a cerebral vascular accident (CVA, or stroke) of the right cerebral hemisphere will result in left-sided dysfunction of the affected body part.

2. The **cerebellum** lies behind the cerebrum, and is a key part of the motor system that is required for the maintenance of equilibrium and the coordination of muscle actions.

3. The **brainstem** is a conduit for the flow of information between the cerebrum and the spinal cord. It is a site of regulation of vital body functions, including breathing and consciousness. Although it is described as a "primitive" brain region, the brainstem is the most important area of the brain necessary for basic survival. *The loss of brainstem function is fatal.*

The **spinal cord** is attached to the brainstem and passes downward within the bony vertebral column. *If the spinal cord is transected, there is total loss of sensation and paralysis of muscles below the affected spinal level.* This reflects the function of the spinal cord as the major conduit of sensory and motor information between the brain and the periphery. The spinal cord is connected to the periphery via **spinal nerves,** which are part of the PNS (see Figure 2-3A). Each spinal nerve attaches to the spinal cord by two branches, a **dorsal root** and a **ventral root.** *The dorsal root brings afferent information into the cord, and the ventral root carries efferent information away from the cord.*

A horizontal view through the **spinal cord** reveals a characteristic pattern of **gray matter** and **white matter** (see Figure 2-3B). Gray matter consists of nerve cell bodies; white matter consists of nerve axons covered in **myelin** (an insulating lipid material). The gray matter is shaped like a butterfly, with each "wing" having an upper **dorsal horn** that is separated from a lower **ventral horn** by an **intermediate zone.** *The dorsal horn receives afferent input from the dorsal nerve roots, and the ventral horn sends efferent axons to the ventral nerve roots.* Cells in the intermediate zone integrate sensory information with descending inputs from higher brain centers, which together shape the efferent output via the ventral horn. The white matter consists of several defined nerve tracts arranged in **columns** that carry information either to or from the brain:

  The **dorsal columns** carry only sensory information via ascending tracts.

  The **ventral and lateral columns** convey both sensory and motor information via ascending and descending tracts, respectively.

EMBRYOLOGIC DEVELOPMENT OF THE BRAIN The complex structural relationships of the adult brain are more easily understood in conjunction with a knowledge of basic embryology. The CNS

A.

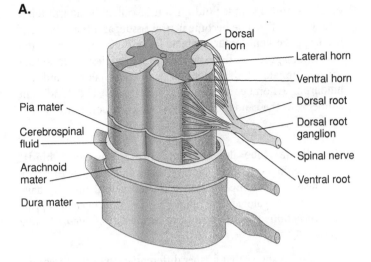

B.

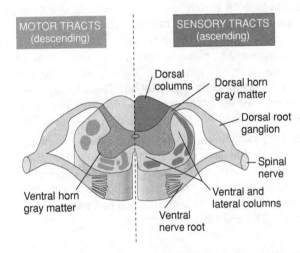

Figure 2-3: The spinal cord. **A.** Spinal nerves connect the spinal cord with the periphery. Each spinal nerve has a ventral root containing axons of efferent neurons and a dorsal root containing axons of afferent neurons. The dorsal root ganglion is a swelling containing the cell bodies of sensory neurons. The spinal cord is covered in three membranes that comprise the meninges: the pia, the arachnoid, and the dura mater. **B.** Cross-section through the spinal cord indicating a butterfly-shaped central area of gray matter. Sensory neurons enter the dorsal horn, and motor neurons leave the ventral horn. The surrounding white matter consists of dorsal, lateral, and anterior columns, each containing nerve tracts running to and from the brain. The ascending and descending tracts shown are present on both the left and right sides.

develops from a simple fluid-filled tube called the **neural tube.** The walls of the tube become neural tissue, and the tube itself becomes the **ventricular system.** Early differentiation of the neural tube produces three primary brain vesicles: the **forebrain** (prosencephalon), the **midbrain** (mesencephalon), and the **hindbrain** (rhombencephalon) (Figure 2-4). The hindbrain connects to the caudal neural tube, which becomes the spinal cord.

▽ **Neural tube defects** (e.g., anencephaly, spina bifida, meningocele, meningomyelocele, and myelocele) occur as a result of incomplete closure of the neural tube by days 26–28 of embryologic development. *Folic acid supplement prior to conception may reduce the incidence of neural tube defects.* ▼

Figure 2-4 shows that further differentiation of the forebrain and hindbrain produces a tube with five vesicles, which are precursors of the major parts of the adult brain:

1. The **telencephalon** greatly enlarges to become the **cerebral hemispheres (cerebral cortex).** The cortex eventually becomes organized with particular regions related to a specific function (e.g., motor cortex). The parts of the body are spatially mapped within each region, illustrating the principle of **somatotopic organization.** The telencephalon includes parts of the **basal ganglia,** which are involved in motor control (see Motor Neurophysiology).

2. The **diencephalon** becomes the most rostral part of the brainstem, the **thalamus** and the **hypothalamus.** *The thalamus is the main integrating center for sensory information coming from the periphery to the cortex,* where it will reach conscious perception. The hypothalamus has many connections to the **ANS** and **endocrine system.**

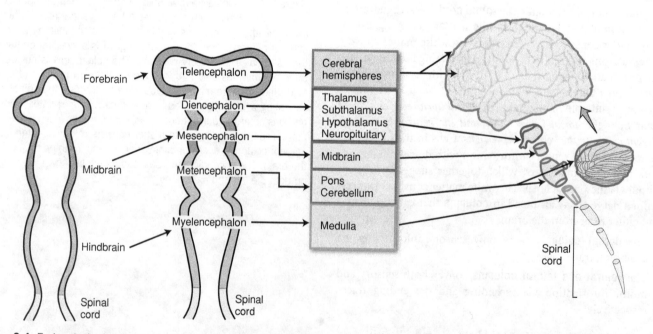

Figure 2-4: Embryologic development of the major anatomic parts of the central nervous system. Early development produces the forebrain, midbrain, and hindbrain vesicles, which subsequently develop into the five vesicles shown in the center of the figure. Differentiation of each of the five vesicles produces the major brain structures indicated in the image on the right side of the figure.

3. The **mesencephalon** develops into the **midbrain,** a small region containing many neuronal tracts.

4. The **metencephalon** becomes the **cerebellum** and the **pons.**

5. The **myelencephalon** becomes the **medulla oblongata,** which is the most caudal part of the brainstem connecting the brain to the spinal cord.

FOREBRAIN STRUCTURES The cerebrum is the largest part of the brain, and is the seat of thoughts, perceptions, and voluntary actions. The term "**cortex**" is often used interchangeably with cerebrum, but it really refers to the surface layer of gray matter. The surface area of the brain is increased by its many folds (**gyri**), which are separated by fissures (**sulci**). The larger sulci are structures that subdivide the cortex into the **frontal, parietal, occipital, and temporal lobes** (Figure 2-5A). The **insular lobe** is not visible from the surface of the brain, but is seen when the margins of the lateral sulcus are pulled open.

Many areas of the cortex can be assigned specific functions (e.g., vision or somatic sensation). In the early twentieth century, Korbinian Brodmann described a map of the brain based on areas with common cytoarchitecture; Brodmann's areas are sometimes used to refer to specific brain areas (see Figure 2-5B). Large areas of cortex *cannot* be assigned specific functions and are called **association cortex;** these areas are involved with interpretation and meaning of sensory information, formation of intentions, and "higher functions" of the mind.

The lower part of the forebrain is the diencephalon, which consists of the thalamus and the hypothalamus. The **thalamus** is an egg-shaped structure that lies deep in the forebrain (Figure 2-6A). It is a relay station through which each of the sensory pathways for somatic sensation, vision, and hearing (audition) synapse as they travel to the cortex. *Sensory pathways in each side of the thalamus continue to the cerebral hemisphere of the same side of the body but convey information from the opposite side of the body.*

Myelinated axons pass from the thalamus to the cortex in a broad band of white matter called the **internal capsule,** which is continuous in the cerebrum with the **cortical white matter.** When viewed in a coronal section, as shown in Figure 2-6B, the cortical white matter is extensive and most of the fibers present are **interneurons** that communicate between cortical neurons. A third band of white matter, the **corpus callosum,** provides a link between the left and right hemispheres and is one important pathway that permits one side of the brain to know what the other side is doing.

There are large collections of gray matter located lateral to the thalamus, called the **deep cerebral nuclei or basal ganglia,** which include the **caudate nucleus, putamen, and globus pallidus.** Many of the descending axons from the motor cortical areas that travel through the internal capsule are destined for the brainstem and spinal cord. Others will influence movements through synapses in the basal ganglia. *Damage to the basal ganglia causes movement disorders (e.g., hemiballismus, which is characterized by involuntary wild flinging movements of one half of the body).*

The **hypothalamus** lies ventral to the thalamus (Figure 2-6B). It is a command center for the ANS, and also for much of the

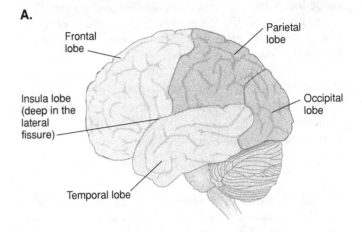

A.

Frontal lobe

Parietal lobe

Insula lobe (deep in the lateral fissure)

Occipital lobe

Temporal lobe

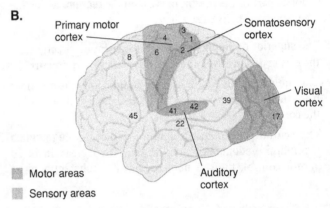

B.

Primary motor cortex

Somatosensory cortex

8   6   4   3   1   2

Visual cortex

45   41   42   39   17

22

Motor areas

Sensory areas

Auditory cortex

Figure 2-5: The cerebrum. **A.** Lobes of the cerebral cortex, named according to the skull bones under which they are located. **B.** Functional classification of regions of the cerebral cortex showing the location of major functional areas. Selected examples of Brodmann's brain areas are indicated (e.g., areas 1, 2, and 3 are in the primary somatosensory cortex, area 4 is the primary motor cortex, area 6 is the premotor cortex, area 8 is the frontal eye field, area 17 is the primary visual cortex, areas 41 and 42 are the auditory cortex, areas 22 and 39 encompass Wernicke's language area, and area 45 is part of Broca's speech area).

endocrine system, through its control of the pituitary gland (see Chapter 8). In addition, the hypothalamus is a source of several basic motivational drives, including the desire to satisfy drives for hunger, thirst, and sex.

There are several other forebrain structures (some of which are discussed in later sections), including:

- The **amygdala and hippocampus** (involved in emotions and memory).
- The **retina** and **optic nerve** of the eye.
- The **olfactory bulb** (involved in the sense of smell).

MIDBRAIN STRUCTURES The midbrain is a narrow region that is part of the brainstem, and is a conduit for all the nerve tracts passing between the forebrain and hindbrain (Figure 2-6A). The dorsal part of the midbrain is called the **tectum,** which has two conspicuous pairs of swellings:

1. The **superior colliculus** receives sensory input directly from the eye, and is involved in the control of eye movements.
2. The **inferior colliculus** is a relay station for sensory input from the ear before it passes to the thalamus and onward to the cortex.

The ventral part of the midbrain is called the **tegmentum** (or **cerebral peduncles**), and contains two areas involved in motor control, the **red nucleus** and the **substantia nigra** (Figure 2-7A).

▼ Degeneration of the **substantia nigra** reduces dopaminergic transmission in the basal ganglia, resulting in parkinsonism. Prominent symptoms of this disorder include lead-pipe rigidity, akinesia, and resting tremor. ▼

HINDBRAIN STRUCTURES The rostral half of the hindbrain (metencephalon) becomes the pons and the cerebellum. The **cerebellum** ("little brain") has two hemispheres, which are connected by a midline region called the **vermis.** The cerebellum is physically connected to the brainstem via the superior, middle, and inferior **peduncles.** The cerebellum receives an enormous number of axons from both the forebrain and spinal cord. *Descending inputs from the forebrain relay information about the intentions for movements, and ascending inputs from the spinal cord relay information about the position of the body in space (known as proprioception).* The cerebellum processes this information to determine the correct sequence of muscle contractions needed to coordinate accurate movement. *Damage to the cerebellum causes jerky movements that are poorly coordinated and inaccurate, referred to as* **ataxia.**

The **pons** bulges out from the ventral surface of the brainstem. The most prominent structural feature of the pons is the massive number of **transverse pontine fibers** that cross from one side to the other (see Figure 2-7B). Most of the descending axons from the cortex synapse in the pons and then cross to the opposite side to enter the cerebellum.

The **medulla** is the most caudal part of the brainstem and connects the pons superiorly to the spinal cord inferiorly. The anterior (ventral) surface has prominent swellings on each

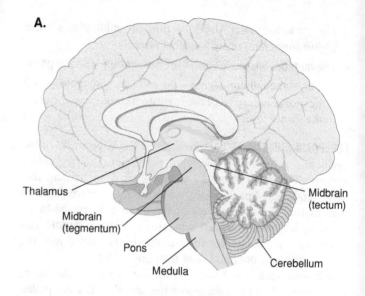

A.

Thalamus

Midbrain (tegmentum)

Pons

Medulla

Midbrain (tectum)

Cerebellum

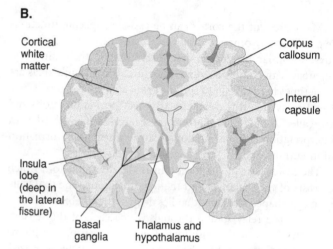

B.

Cortical white matter

Insula lobe (deep in the lateral fissure)

Basal ganglia

Thalamus and hypothalamus

Corpus callosum

Internal capsule

Figure 2-6: Sections through the brain. **A.** Median sagittal section showing the medial surface of the brain and all the structures of the brainstem from the thalamus superiorly to the medulla inferiorly. **B.** Coronal section at the junction of the thalamus and cerebrum. This view shows the position of the insula lobe; the basal ganglia are visible lateral to the thalamus. Major areas of white matter are visible in this plane, including the internal capsule, the cortical white matter, and the corpus callosum.

side, called **medullary pyramids** (see Figure 2-7C). Each of the pyramids contains a **corticospinal (pyramidal) nerve tract.** These tracts carry axons of motor neurons that command movement; as the name suggests, the corticospinal tract travels from the motor cortex to the spinal cord. The medullary pyramids are the site of **decussation** (crossing from one side to the other) of this motor pathway, which explains why *movement of one side of the body is controlled by the opposite cerebral hemisphere.*

▽ **Decussation of motor neurons** in the medullary pyramids is another example of how the anatomic organization of the CNS lends itself to predictable patterns of deficits. For example, motor neurons that originate in the primary motor cortex of the left cerebral hemisphere decussate in the medullary pyramids, resulting in innervation of the right side of the body. Therefore, *a stroke that damages the left primary motor cortex will result in* **right-sided hemiplegia.** ▼

The brainstem must act as a conduit for the many nerve tracts passing between the forebrain and the spinal cord. The midbrain, pons, and medulla also contain several collections of nerve cell bodies (nuclei), many of which are associated with the **cranial nerves** (Table 2-1).

STRUCTURES OF THE PNS

The PNS consists of 31 pairs of spinal nerves and 12 pairs of cranial nerves. The spinal nerves are named according to the segment of the vertebral column they are associated with:

- C1–C8 are the **cervical** spinal nerves.
- T1–T12 are the **thoracic** spinal nerves.
- L1–L5 are the **lumbar** spinal nerves.
- S1–S5 are the **sacral** spinal nerves.
- Coccygeal 1 is the sole **coccygeal** spinal nerve.

The optic nerve (CN II) can be considered part of the CNS because it is located within the meninges. The other 11 pairs of cranial nerves exit the brain and pass, via foramina (holes), in the skull. With the exception of the vagus nerve, all of the cranial nerves serve the head and neck region; the vagus nerve serves visceral structures in the thorax and abdomen. The names and major functions of each cranial nerve are summarized in Table 2-1.

BRAIN EXTRACELLULAR FLUIDS

The total volume of the brain, including cells and extracellular fluids, is limited by the bony skull. If the volume of intracellular or extracellular fluid increases, there is a risk that increased intracranial pressure will result in reduced brain perfusion. Therefore, the volume of brain extracellular fluid is carefully regulated. The composition of brain extracellular fluid is critical because changes in the ionic environment affect the electrical behavior of neurons and will disrupt function. The CNS has **three extracellular fluid compartments** (Figure 2-8).

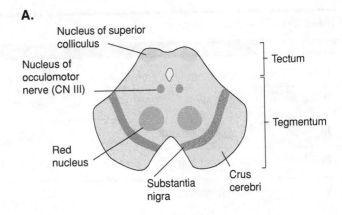

A.

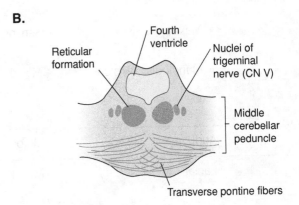

B.

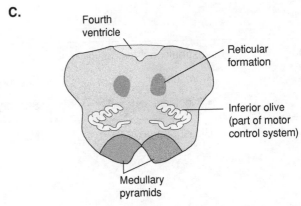

C.

Figure 2-7: Sections through the brainstem at different levels. **A.** The midbrain at the level of the superior colliculus. The midbrain has two major parts, the tectum dorsally and the tegmentum ventrally. The substantia nigra and the red nucleus are part of the motor system. Nuclei of cranial nerves III (oculomotor) and IV (trochlear) are present in the midbrain. **B.** The pons, showing massive crossover of descending fibers in the ventral pons, which are destined for the cerebellum. **C.** The medulla, showing the large medullary pyramids ventrally, which are the site of crossover of the descending corticospinal tracts. Several cranial nerve nuclei, as well as ascending and descending tracts, are present in the medulla but are not shown in the figure.

TABLE 2-1. The Cranial Nerves

Number of Nerve	Name of Nerve	Type	Major Function(s)
I	Olfactory	Sensory	• Smell
II	Optic	Sensory	• Vision
III	Occulomotor	Motor	• Eye movements and constriction of the pupil
IV	Trochlear	Motor	• Eye movements
V	Trigeminal		
	• Ophthalmic division	Sensory	• Cornea and skin of the forehead, scalp, nose, and eyelid
	• Maxillary division	Sensory	• Maxillary facial skin, upper teeth, maxillary sinus, and palate
	• Mandibular division	Mixed	• Sensory to skin over mandible, lower teeth, inside of mouth, and anterior part of the tongue
			• Motor to muscles of mastication
VI	Abducens	Motor	• Eye movements
VII	Facial	Mixed	• Sensory function includes taste from anterior two thirds of the tongue
			• Motor to facial muscles
			• Parasympathetic secretomotor fibers to salivary and lacrimal glands
VIII	Vestibulocochlear		
	• Vestibular	Sensory	• Position and movement of the head
	• Cochlear	Sensory	• Hearing
IX	Glossopharyngeal	Mixed	• Sensory to the pharynx and posterior third of the tongue; carotid sinus baroreceptor and carotid body chemoreceptor
			• Motor to muscles of swallowing
			• Parasympathetic secretomotor to salivary gland
X	Vagus	Mixed	• Major parasympathetic nerve to heart, lungs, and upper gastrointestinal system
XI	Accessory	Motor	• Spinal root: sternomastoid and trapezius muscles
			• Cranial root: muscles of palate, pharynx, and larynx
XII	Hypoglossal	Motor	• Muscles of the tongue

1. **Blood plasma** contained inside the vascular system (approximately 70 mL).

2. **Interstitial fluid** located outside the vascular system in contact with neural cells and glia (approximately 250 mL).

3. CSF located within the **ventricular system** and **subarachnoid space** (approximately 150 mL).

The interstitial fluid surrounding neurons is protected from changes in the plasma composition by a **blood-brain barrier.** However, *there is free exchange of water and solutes between the brain interstitial fluid and the CSF* across the **ependymal cells,** which line the ventricular system. Therefore, it follows that the composition of CSF must be carefully regulated, which is achieved by actively secreting CSF, via the **choroid plexus epithelia.**

THE VENTRICULAR SYSTEM

The ventricular system is a series of interconnected chambers inside the CNS that are filled with **CSF.** The lumens of the embryonic brain vesicles develop into the ventricular system (Figure 2-9A).

- The lumen of the telencephalon becomes the **lateral ventricles** of the **cerebrum.** Each lateral ventricle forms a large C shape as the ventricle curves around from the frontal lobe into the temporal lobe.

- The lumen of the diencephalon becomes the slit-like **third ventricle,** which is located in the midline and is closely associated with the **thalamus.** The lumen of the third ventricle is continuous with each lateral ventricle through an **interventricular foramen (the foramen of Monro).**

- The lumen of the mesencephalon becomes a narrow channel, called the **cerebral aqueduct** (a characteristic feature of the **midbrain**), which connects the third and fourth ventricles.

- The lumen of the whole hindbrain becomes the **fourth ventricle,** which includes the **pons** and **medulla** as its floor and the **cerebellum** as its roof. The fourth ventricle is continuous inferiorly with the **central canal** of the spinal cord.

Each ventricle contains a choroid plexus epithelium, which continuously secretes CSF into the ventricles. CSF exits the ventricular system via holes in the fourth ventricle (the **foramina of Luschka and Magendie**) into the subarachnoid space. CSF flows over the surface of the brain and spinal cord and eventually drains back into the venous system at specialized areas of arachnoid membrane called **arachnoid granulations.** *To maintain a stable CSF volume, the rate of production of CSF by the choroid plexus must be the same as the rate of CSF absorption at arachnoid granulations.* The circulation of CSF replaces the CSF volume approximately four times per day.

▽ **Hydrocephalus** can be defined in general terms as an increase in CSF volume or pressure as a result of an imbalance in CSF production, flow, or absorption. In **communicating hydrocephalus,** there is a free flow of CSF from the ventricles to the subarachnoid space. Communicating hydrocephalus may be caused by oversecretion of CSF (e.g., choroid plexus papilloma) or impaired return of CSF to the venous system (e.g., meningitis can impair the flow of CSF through the

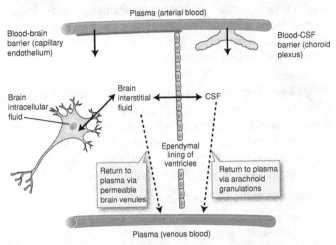

Figure 2-8: Relationships between fluid compartments in the brain. Movement of solutes from arterial plasma into the brain is restricted by the blood-brain barrier and the blood-cerebrospinal fluid (CSF) barrier. There is regulated exchange between the brain interstitial fluid and the brain intracellular fluid compartment across the cell membranes of neurons and glia. There is free exchange between CSF and brain interstitial fluid across ependymal cells lining the ventricles. Brain interstitial fluid can return to the systemic circulation via permeable venules, and CSF returns to systemic venous blood via arachnoid granulations (specialized projections of the arachnoid membrane).

arachnoid granulations) In **noncommunicating hydrocephalus,** an obstructed path occurs, preventing the free flow of CSF through the ventricular system (e.g., a pineal tumor that occludes the cerebral aqueduct). ▼

▽ **Normal pressure hydrocephalus** is a special type of communicating hydrocephaly that primarily affects the elderly. The indolent nature of this condition results in enlarged lateral ventricles and relatively normal CSF pressures. *The classic clinical triad for normal pressure hydrocephalus consists of dementia, gait ataxia, and urinary incontinence.* ▼

Functions of the CSF include:

▢ To act as a shock absorber to **protect the brain** from contact with the skull during movement.

▢ To assist in the maintenance of a **constant internal environment** in the CNS.

▢ To provide a route for **removal of metabolites** from the brain.

CSF SECRETION CSF is secreted by the choroid plexuses, which consist of a highly vascular core surrounded by fronds of epithelial tissue that project into the ventricular lumen. The **choroid plexus epithelial cells** actively secrete CSF via a transcellular mechanism (see Figure 2-9B).

▢ The **Na⁺/K⁺-ATPase** is utilized at the luminal membrane to drive Na⁺ secretion.

▢ **K⁺-Cl⁻ cotransport** is utilized to secrete Cl⁻ into the CSF; much of the K⁺ that is cosecreted with K⁺ is recycled via the Na⁺/K⁺-ATPase.

▢ Water is readily secreted by osmosis through **aquaporin water channels** in the cell membranes.

The **blood-CSF barrier** is maintained by tight junctions between the choroid plexus epithelial cells, which do not allow free diffusion of molecules from the plasma into the CSF. CSF is an isotonic fluid with a composition similar to plasma, with the notable exception that there is little protein in CSF. As a result, CSF has a low buffering capacity, which allows the **central chemoreceptors** to sense changes in blood-carbon dioxide levels through small changes in CSF pH (see Chapter 5).

▽ Breakdown of the blood-CSF barrier occurs in **bacterial meningitis.** Bacterial invasion of the choroid plexus epithelial cells allows the bacteria to gain access to the CSF, a medium that facilitates bacterial replication due to its paucity of host immune cells. *The critical event in bacterial meningitis is the triggering of the host immune system by the invading bacteria.* Once the host immune system is activated, inflammatory cytokines and immune cells induce meningeal inflammation, causing the barriers between the brain extracellular fluids to become leaky and dysfunctional. As a result, serum proteins and inflammatory cells enter the subarachnoid space, producing a purulent exudate and diffuse cerebral edema. This sequence of events explains the **classic CSF abnormalities in bacterial meningitis:**

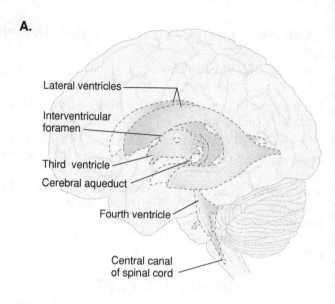

A.

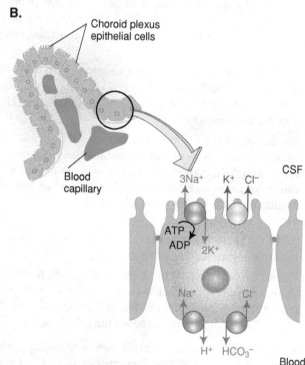

B.

Figure 2-9: The ventricular system. **A.** Location of the ventricles of the brain. **B.** The choroid plexus epithelium and the cellular mechanism of cerebrospinal fluid secretion.

1. **Elevated white blood cell count** (typically polymorpho-nuclear leukocytes).

2. **Decreased glucose concentration,** thought to be due to inflammation resulting in reduced glucose transport into the CSF.

3. **Increased protein concentration.**

4. **Increased pressure,** apparent as an increased "opening pressure" of a lumbar puncture. ▼

THE BLOOD-BRAIN BARRIER

The interstitial fluid of the brain surrounds neurons and glia. The volume of the brain interstitial fluid is small due to the very high density of cells in neural tissue. The small volume of brain interstitial fluid causes it to be vulnerable to changes in composition. The **capillary endothelial cells** that enclose brain capillaries form the selective blood-brain barrier between the brain interstitium and plasma. Neighboring endothelial cells are connected by **tight junctions** that prevent the free diffusion of plasma constituents into the brain (Figure 2-10A). *Solutes that enter the brain from the blood must pass across the capillary endothelial cells.*

A few highly lipid-soluble substances are able to diffuse through capillary endothelial cell membranes (e.g., oxygen, carbon dioxide, urea, nicotine, and ethanol). Most solutes that are not lipid soluble (e.g., electrolytes) are unable to diffuse into the brain; **glucose** is an important exception and is a crucial substrate for neuronal tissue. Glucose enters the brain by **facilitated diffusion via GLUT1** carriers present in capillary endothelial cell membranes. Other transport systems are expressed by brain capillary endothelial cells, which allow, for example, Na$^+$ flux into the brain and the removal of K$^+$ from the brain (see Figure 2-10B).

A few small areas of the brain, known as **circumventricular organs,** lack a blood-brain barrier; that is, the *area postrema, posterior pituitary, subfornical organ, median eminence, pineal gland, and organum vasculosum laminae terminalis* (OVLT). This arrangement allows certain neurons to be directly exposed to solutes in the blood, which facilitates some neuroendocrine control processes. For example, in the median eminence of the **hypothalamus,** capillaries must be leaky to take up hypothalamic hormones (see Chapter 8); leakiness at the OVLT allows circulating **cytokines** to signal to the body temperature control system to generate a **fever** response.

▼ **Brain (cerebral) edema** is an increase in the volume of fluid within the CNS, and may result in reduced brain perfusion and serious brain damage. There are two broad types of brain edema:

1. **Cytotoxic edema** occurs when cells are starved of oxygen, causing cellular swelling (e.g., ischemia).

2. **Vasogenic edema** occurs when brain capillaries are damaged and become more permeable than normal (e.g., brain tumor, trauma), resulting in increased brain interstitial fluid volume.

Regardless of the cause, increased intracranial pressure can be fatal because it may result in brain herniation. Clinical signs and symptoms of increased intracranial pressure include

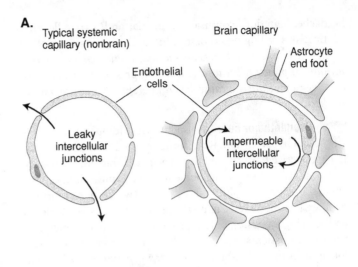

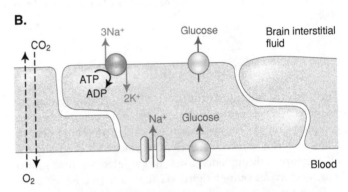

Figure 2-10: The blood-brain barrier. **A.** Comparison between a typical nonbrain systemic capillary, which has spaces between endothelial lining cells that allow free exchange between the plasma and interstitial fluid, and a brain capillary, which has continuous tight junctions that seal the junctions between endothelial cells. Brain capillaries are also surrounded by glia (astrocytes). **B.** Transcellular transport across the blood-brain barrier; oxygen and carbon dioxide can diffuse freely through endothelial cells; glucose enters the brain by facilitated diffusion.

headache, agitation, confusion, diplopia, and/or papilledema (optic disk swelling noted on funduscopic examination). *Note: an elevated intracranial pressure is a contraindication to performing lumbar puncture because releasing the pressure from below the opening in the skull can cause the brain to shift downward, inducing herniation.* ▼

▽ **Pseudotumor cerebri,** also known as idiopathic intracranial hypertension, is a disorder of unknown etiology and is characterized by chronically elevated intracranial pressure that primarily affects young obese women. Typical clinical presentation includes chronic daily headache (worse in the morning or after bending over), nausea, and vision changes (diplopia and graying of vision). The prolonged elevated intracranial pressure in patients induces papilledema, putting them at risk for optic atrophy and blindness. *Note: hypervitaminosis A and ingestion of outdated tetracycline antibiotics can cause pseudotumor cerebri.* ▼

CELLULAR NEUROSCIENCE

The sophisticated higher functions of the nervous system are possible because neurons are able to communicate through complex circuits. The basic features of the prototype neuron allow a neuron to receive signals from potentially thousands of other neurons through dendrites, and to integrate these inputs and produce an output signal via the axon (see Figure 2-3). Because the size, shape, and functional properties of neurons vary tremendously, several **overlapping systems of classification** are employed.

1. The **number of neurites** (processes) is used to classify three basic types of neuron (Figure 2-11A):

   Unipolar neurons have a single neurite (e.g., primary sensory neurons with the cell body located in the dorsal root ganglia of spinal nerves).

   Bipolar neurons have two neurites (e.g., a retinal bipolar cell).

   Multipolar neurons have three or more neurites. This is the most common type of neuron (e.g., spinal motor neuron).

   Multipolar neurons usually have a large dendritic tree that provides a large range of possible inputs for that neuron. In contrast, unipolar and bipolar neurons have a highly specific input and are associated with specialized functions (e.g., sensing touch at a specific body location).

2. The **organization of dendrites** varies widely. In the cerebral cortex, two general patterns describe the overall shape of the neuron:

   Pyramidal neurons

   Stellate (star-shaped) neurons

   Dendrites function as antennae, receiving signals from other neurons and, as a result, the cell membrane is a rich site of postsynaptic receptor expression. In most cases, there are tiny dendritic spines at the sites where axons synapse with the dendrite. The presence or absence of spines is also used to describe neurons as **spiny** or **aspiny.**

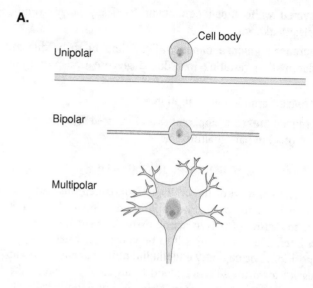

A.

Unipolar — Cell body

Bipolar

Multipolar

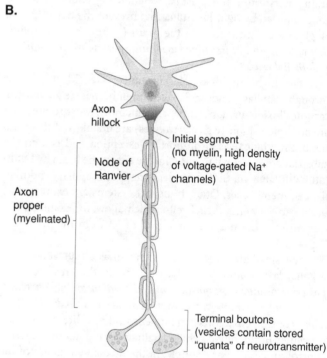

B.

Axon hillock

Initial segment (no myelin, high density of voltage-gated Na+ channels)

Node of Ranvier

Axon proper (myelinated)

Terminal boutons (vesicles contain stored "quanta" of neurotransmitter)

Figure 2-11: Neuronal structures. **A.** Classification of neurons based on the number of neurites extending from the cell body. Unipolar neurons have a single neurite; bipolar neurons have two neurites; and multipolar neurons are the most common type and have three or more neurites. **B.** Regions of the axon. The axon originates from the soma at a tapering region called the axon hillock. The initial segment lacks myelin and is the site of action potential stimulation. The axon proper may be myelinated or nonmyelinated and may vary greatly in length from one neuron to another; axons may have collateral branches (not shown). The axon terminal is a swollen area called the terminal bouton, which has many vesicles containing neurotransmitter.

3. **Axon length** is used to classify neurons:

  - **Golgi type I neurons** have long axons and project from one region of the nervous system to another.
  - **Golgi type II neurons** have short axons that contribute to local circuits in the region of the cell body.

4. A broad **functional classification** is used to describe neurons:

  - **Primary sensory neurons** have neurites at the body surface, which convey sensory information to the CNS.
  - **Motor neurons** end on muscles and initiate muscle contraction.
  - **Interneurons** only form connections with other neurons. *Most neurons are interneurons.*

5. The **type of neurotransmitter** released by the axon of a neuron is used to classify neurons (e.g., neurons that release acetylcholine as the neurotransmitter are "cholinergic").

AXONS AND PRESYNAPTIC TERMINALS

The axon carries the output signal from a neuron after integration of incoming signals by the dendrites and soma. There are **three major functional axon regions** that have been described (see Figure 2-11B):

1. The axon originates at a tapering region of the soma called the **axon hillock.** The **initial segment,** or *spike initiation zone,* is just beyond the axon hillock. If a depolarizing stimulus is applied, *action potentials are readily triggered at the initial segment due to the extremely high level of voltage-gated Na^+ channels expressed in the cell membrane at this site.*

2. The **axon proper** has a constant diameter and may extend over a very long distance. The axon diameter varies between different types of neurons and is an important determinant of the conduction velocity of action potentials; *large diameter axons have lower electrical resistance and faster conduction velocities.*

3. The end of an axon is called the **axon terminal,** or **terminal bouton,** which is the point of **synapse** formation with the target neuron or effector cell. The axon terminal contains numerous **synaptic vesicles** containing neurotransmitter molecules.

AXOPLASMIC TRANSPORT If an axon is cut at a proximal site, the distal part of the axon degenerates through a process known as Wallerian degeneration. Degeneration occurs because the soma contains the synthetic machinery of the neuron, and the axon depends upon transport up and down the axon to ferry materials to and from the parent cell body. Axoplasmic transport is mediated by the cytoskeleton, which has three components:

1. **Microtubules** run longitudinally along neurites and are formed from polymers of **tubulin** molecules. **Microtubule-associated proteins** (e.g., tau) are required to correctly organize microtubules in the axon.

2. **Microfilaments** are polymers of actin molecules.

3. **Neurofilaments** are long protein molecules (rather than polymers of subunit proteins).

The microtubules function like train tracks and transport material up and down the axon. The movement of materials is driven by **motor proteins** along the microtubule tracks.

- **Anterograde transport** is movement from the soma toward the axon terminal. An example of anterograde transport is the movement of vesicles containing neurotransmitters from the cell body to the axon terminal.

- **Retrograde transport** is movement from the axon terminal toward the neuron cell body. The uptake of nerve growth factor at the axon terminal by endocytosis and its transport to the soma (where is stimulates protein synthesis) is an example of retrograde transport.

- **Motor proteins** function as "legs" that walk along microtubules carrying a payload such as a vesicle or mitochondrion. The motor protein **kinesin** *powers anterograde transport, and* **dynein** *powers retrograde transport.*

▼ Many infectious agents (e.g., herpesvirus, polio virus, rabies virus, and tetanus toxin) utilize axonal transport to reach their site of action. For example, the oral **herpesvirus** that causes **cold sores** is an example of a virus that uses the axonal transport mechanism to infect neurons. In this case, the virus enters nerve endings at the mouth and is transported back to the cell body, where it is dormant for a period of time. When reactivated, the virus replicates and returns to the axon terminals, causing a cold sore to form. ▼

NEUROGLIA

Glia are close partners of neurons and support neuronal function in many ways. There are about 10 times more glial cells than neurons in the brain, and they occupy about half of the brain volume. **Three major types of glia** are found in the brain: astrocytes, microglia, and oligodendrocytes.

1. **Astrocytes** are highly branched cells that envelope neurons and brain capillaries (Figure 2-12A). Several functions have been ascribed to astrocytes, including:

- To provide a structural **scaffold** for neurons.

- To provide neurons with **lactate** as an energy source. Astrocytes take up glucose from the blood and release lactate into the brain extracellular fluid. Astrocytes store most of the glycogen in the brain, which is converted to lactate for neuronal use.

- To **maintain a stable [K⁺]** in the brain extracellular fluid by uptake of K^+ that is released from active neurons. Without rapid K^+ reuptake, [K⁺] increases and depolarizes neuronal resting membrane potentials (see Chapter 1).

- To **remove neurotransmitters** from brain extracellular fluid in the region of synapses (e.g., uptake of the excitatory transmitter glutamate).

- To **synthesize neurotransmitter precursors** for neurons (e.g., glutamine synthesis for glutaminergic neurons).

▼ **Gliosis** is a term used to describe astrocyte proliferation in response to an injury (e.g., stroke) that results in scar formation in the CNS. Gliosis, along with neuronal loss, is a

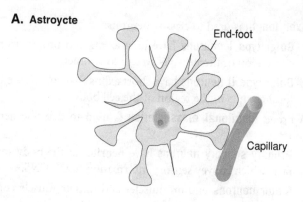

A. Astroycte

End-foot

Capillary

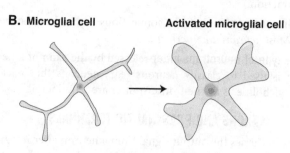

B. Microglial cell   **Activated microglial cell**

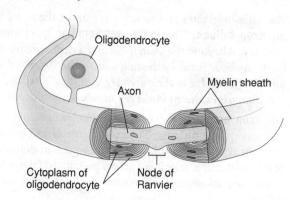

C. Oligodendrocyte

Oligodendrocyte

Axon

Myelin sheath

Cytoplasm of oligodendrocyte

Node of Ranvier

Figure 2-12: Neuroglia. **A.** Astrocytes are the most common glial cell type. **B.** Microglia are activated by infection and coordinate the brain's immune response. **C.** Oligodendrocytes form the myelin sheath around neurons in the central nervous system.

prominent feature in many diseases that affect the CNS, including Alzheimer's disease, multiple sclerosis, and stroke. ▼

2. **Microglia** are highly reactive cells that are activated by injury or infection, which causes them to proliferate and become phagocytic (see Figure 2-12B). *Microglia are the main antigen-presenting cells* in the CNS and function like peripheral **macrophages.**

3. **Oligodendrocytes** produce and maintain the **myelin sheaths** around neurons in the CNS by wrapping around the axons many times (see Figure 2-12C). The cytoplasm of the oligodendrocyte is squeezed out of the concentric wrappings to produce multiple layers of compressed cell membrane that comprise myelin. A single oligodendrocyte myelinates multiple neurons. **Schwann cells** are the equivalent of oligodendrocytes in the PNS; each Schwann cell myelinates a single axon.

▽ Although the successes and failures of **neuronal regeneration** are still a mystery today, it is recognized that axonal regeneration occurs in the PNS but has very limited success in the CNS. Many factors are likely to contribute to this difference. However, one key factor thought to be critical for axonal regeneration is the makeup of the extracellular environment. In the PNS, Schwann cells actively regenerate and produce neuron growth factors (e.g., laminin and fibronectin) that stimulate the formation and growth of the axon. In addition to the absence of these critical growth factors in the mature CNS, the glial cells also produce growth inhibitory proteins. The loss of growth-stimulating proteins and the presence of growth-inhibitory proteins in the extracellular environment of the mature CNS may, at least partially, explain the loss of regenerative capacity of the CNS. ▼

SYNAPTIC TRANSMISSION

Chemical synapses mediate most communication between neurons. The basic elements of communication via chemical synapses were introduced in Chapter 1 in the discussion about neuromuscular transmission. Similar features are present at synapses within the nervous system:

  Presynaptic axon terminals store neurotransmitter molecules in vesicles.

  Action potentials in the axon depolarize the axon terminals.

  Depolarization causes Ca^{2+} entry into the axon terminal.

  Exocytosis of vesicles occurs, causing release of neurotransmitter into the narrow synaptic cleft.

  Neurotransmitter interacts with a specific receptor on the postsynaptic membrane, causing a postsynaptic event. Activation of ionotropic receptors causes direct changes in ion permeability of the postsynaptic membrane; activation of metabotropic receptors usually triggers a G-protein–coupled second messenger signal in the postsynaptic cell.

  Neurotransmitter signaling is terminated by removal from the synaptic cleft through diffusion, enzymatic degradation, or, most commonly, active reuptake of neurotransmitter molecules.

There are several configurations of synaptic inputs that can occur, with the most common being synapses between axon terminals and the dendritic spines of another neuron (Figure 2-13).

INTEGRATION OF POSTSYNAPTIC POTENTIALS The flow of information between neurons is mediated by changes in the membrane potential of the postsynaptic cell (see Figure 2-13A).

▪ **Excitatory postsynaptic potentials (EPSPs)** result if a neurotransmitter depolarizes the postsynaptic membrane potential.

▪ **Inhibitory postsynaptic potentials (IPSPs)** result if a neurotransmitter hyperpolarizes the postsynaptic membrane potential.

The postsynaptic neuron will generate action potentials when the sum of EPSPs and IPSPs in the region of the initial axon segment is depolarized beyond a threshold potential. If an IPSP occurs at about the same time and the same place as an

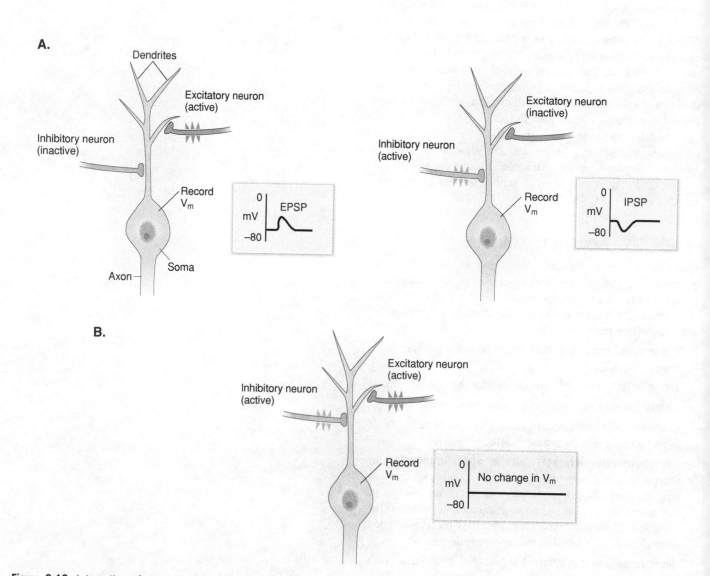

Figure 2-13: Integration of postsynaptic potentials. **A.** Excitatory neurons cause depolarization; inhibitory neurons cause hyperpolarization. **B.** Summation of synaptic inputs occurs to produce a net postsynaptic potential. In this example, a single excitatory input is cancelled out by a single inhibitory input. EPSP, excitatory postsynaptic potential; IPSP, inhibitory postsynaptic potential.

EPSP, it tends to cancel out the excitation and prevents stimulation of the postsynaptic neuron (see Figure 2-13B).

Even in the absence of IPSPs, the ability of EPSPs to reach the initial segment and to evoke action potentials depends on the properties of dendrites. Postsynaptic potentials are **graded potentials,** which decay with time and distance from the point of synaptic contact (Figure 2-14A).

- The **time constant (τ)** is the time that it takes for a membrane potential to decay to 37% of its peak value. If a dendrite has a long time constant, there is more time for individual EPSPs to summate. **Temporal summation** occurs when a series of axon potentials arrive via the same excitatory afferent nerve and the EPSPs summate (see Figure 2-14B).

- The **space constant (λ)** is the distance along the dendrite that a postsynaptic potential has traveled when it has decayed to 37% of its maximum value. If the space constant is large, then EPSPs from widely spaced synaptic inputs are able to summate, which is known as **spatial summation** (see Figure 2-14C).

The time and space constants both vary significantly between dendrites due to differences in their size and shape and to differences in ion channel expression in the dendritic cell membrane.

NEUROCHEMISTRY The enormous diversity of function in the nervous system is mainly the result of the complexity of neuronal circuits rather than the diversity of neurotransmitters and their postsynaptic receptors. Although there are over 100 different neurotransmitters present in the nervous system, many fewer transmitters mediate the majority of synaptic events. There are **two major classes of neurotransmitters** (Table 2-2):

1. The **small molecule transmitters** include **acetylcholine,** certain **amino acids,** and the **monoamine neurotransmitters.**

2. The **large molecule transmitters** are **neuropeptides** of various sizes.

In some cases, there is a pattern to the distribution of neurons that use a particular neurotransmitter and, as a result, the neurotransmitter assumes a prominent role in a given function (e.g., dopaminergic neurons are important in the control of movement).

▽ The primary inhibitory neurotransmitters of the CNS are γ-aminobutyric acid (GABA) and glycine, examples of small molecule transmitters. **Sedative-hypnotic drugs** (e.g., benzodiazepines, barbiturates, and alcohols) target the GABA$_A$ receptor, which, through the action of increased Cl$^-$ influx, results in membrane hyperpolarization. Caution must be used with these drugs because there is a dose-dependent depression of the CNS: sedation → anxiolysis → hypnosis → anesthesia → medullary depression (respiratory depression) → coma. Synergism with other CNS depressants occurs, increasing the risk for potentially lethal overdoses. *Note: the dose-response relationship for benzodiazepines flattens out at medullary depression, giving it a better safety profile than other sedative drugs.* ▽

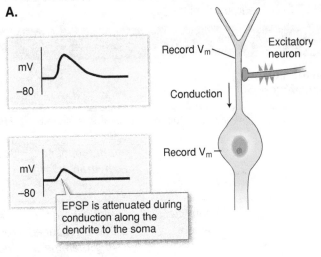

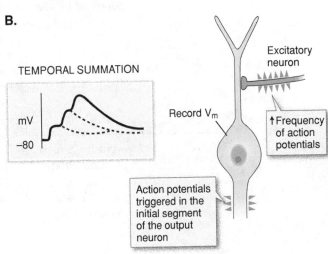

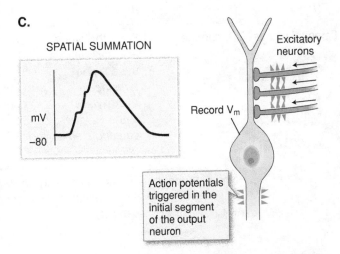

Figure 2-14: Temporal and spatial summation of synaptic inputs. **A.** Attenuation of an excitatory postsynaptic potential (EPSP) during conduction along a dendrite. **B.** Temporal summation of EPSPs produced by a sequence of action potentials in the afferent neuron. **C.** Spatial summation of EPSPs produced by several different afferent neurons.

TABLE 2-2. Neurotransmitter Systems

Class	Chemical	Synthesis	Postsynaptic Receptors	Signal Termination	General Function(s) in the Nervous System
Small molecule transmitters					
	Acetylcholine	Choline + acetyl CoA, via the enzyme *choline acetyltransferase*	*Nicotinic* (cation channel) *Muscarinic* (G-protein–coupled)	Extracellular hydrolysis by *acetylcholinesterase*	• Movement control • Cognition
	Glutamate & aspartate	Available from the diet and produced from *glutamine supplied by glia*	*Metabotropic receptors* *Inotropic receptors* • NMDA (Ca^{2+} permeable channels) • AMPA (Na^+/K^+ channel) • Kainate (Na^+/K^+ channel)	*Reuptake*	• General excitation (most rapid synaptic events in the brain are mediated by *glutaminergic signaling*, which evokes EPSPs through the opening of cation channels)
	GABA	From the amino acid *glutamate* via the enzyme *glutamic acid decarboxylase*	$GABA_A$ (Cl^- channel) $GABA_B$ (G-protein–coupled)	*Reuptake*	• General inhibition (most rapid inhibitory synapses in the brain use *GABA* to evoke an IPSP)
	Glycine	Available from the diet	Glycine receptor (Cl^- channel)	*Reuptake*	• General inhibition
Catecholamines	Dopamine	From the amino acid *tyrosine* via the enzyme *tyrosine hydroxylase* in the *catecholamine pathway*	D_1 (stimulatory G-protein–coupled) D_2 (inhibitory G-protein–coupled)	*Reuptake*	• Movement control • General affect
	Norepinephrine	From dopamine in the *catecholamine pathway*	α & β *Adrenergic receptors*	*Reuptake* or breakdown via the enzymes *monoamine oxidase* and *catechol-O-methyltransferase*	• Alertness • General affect
	Epinephrine*				
	Serotonin (5-HT)	From the amino acid tryptophan via the enzyme *tryptophan hydroxylase*	Several subtypes, both ion channels, and G-protein–coupled	*Reuptake*	• Mood (*5-HT reuptake blockers are commonly prescribed antidepressants*) • General arousal

Class	Chemical	Synthesis	Postsynaptic Receptors	Signal Termination	General Function(s) in the Nervous System
Large molecule transmitters**					
Opioids	β-Endorphin Dynorphin Metenkephalin Leuenkephalin	Protein synthesis in the neuron cell body	μ-Receptors (β-endorphin) κ-Receptors (dynorphin) δ-Receptors (enkephalins)	Metabolism by extra-cellular *neuropeptidase* enzymes	• Control of pain
	Substance P		Neurokinin receptor		• Transmission of pain signals

* Epinephrine is produced in the adrenal medulla (see Autonomic Nervous System).

**Only selected neuropeptides are included.

NMDA, *N*-methyl-D-aspartate; AMPA, α-amino-3-hydroxy-5-methylisoxazole-4-propionic acid; EPSP, excitatory postsynaptic potential; IPSP, inhibitory postsynaptic potential; GABA, γ-aminobutyric acid.

SENSORY NEUROPHYSIOLOGY

The sensory systems provide information about the external environment that is crucial to human survival (e.g., location of food; sources of danger). The state of the internal body environment is also constantly monitored as part of the homeostatic feedback control systems of the body. Sensory systems are each specialized to measure a different type of energy but are organized according to a set of common principles (Figure 2-15):

- The **stimulus** is a distinct type of energy (e.g., **light, sound, and heat; mechanical and chemical**).

- Specialized **receptors** are available to detect each type of stimulus (i.e., **photoreceptors** for light; **mechanoreceptors** for mechanical stimuli; **thermoreceptors** for heat; and **chemoreceptors** for chemical composition). *Receptors are transducers that convert the stimulus energy into electrical signals in neurons.*

- Specific **pathways** organize and convey the sensory information to the CNS.

- **Interpretation** of sensory input occurs in specific areas of the CNS. Integration of inputs produces the **perception** of a stimulus. The nature of the CNS pathway is important for perception; for example, stimulation of the optic nerve is always perceived as light, even if the stimulation is pressure applied to the eye (a concept referred to as the **labeled line**). Subjective factors are important in perception (e.g., physical detection of a stimulus could be disturbing or pleasurable, depending on previously learned information).

Any sensory system must be able to encode **four attributes of a stimulus:**

1. The **modality** is the type of stimulus. The five traditional sensory modalities are touch, vision, hearing, taste, and smell. In reality, many sensations require a combination of basic modalities (e.g., detecting that something is wet

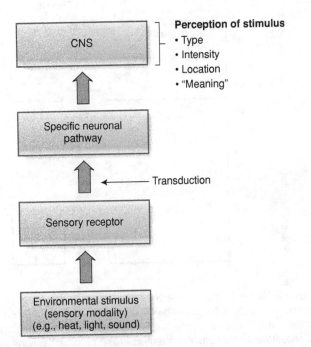

Figure 2-15: General model of sensory perception.

without seeing the object combines the sensations of touch and temperature).

2. The **intensity** of stimulus refers to the amount of stimulation (e.g., the loudness of a sound or the pressure applied to the skin).

3. The **duration** of a stimulus.

4. The **location** of a stimulus, which might be a position in a three-dimensional space (e.g., source of a sound) or a location could be a site on the body surface. The location of a stimulus is determined by the neuronal pathway and final destination of the signal in the CNS.

SENSORY TRANSDUCTION

Most sensory receptors are highly specialized structures that preferentially respond to a single type of stimulus. The **adequate stimulus** is the stimulus for which a receptor has the lowest threshold for detection. Receptors transduce the stimulus energy into a graded electrical potential called a **generator potential,** which will trigger action potentials in the sensory neuron if the threshold potential is exceeded (Figure 2-16).

Receptors encode stimulus duration by producing generator potentials that correspond with the duration of the stimulus. *Receptors transduce stimulus intensity by producing larger generator potentials in response to increased stimulus intensity.* In the case of the first generator potential shown in Figure 2-16, the stimulus intensity was small and the resulting generator potential failed to reach the threshold potential to trigger action potentials in the sensory nerve. More intense stimulation produces a larger generator potential, which is *encoded*

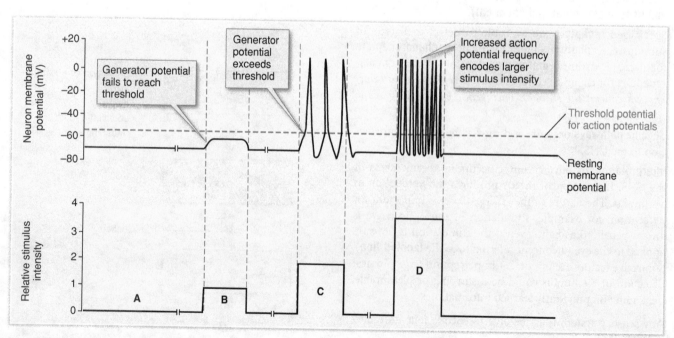

Figure 2-16: Frequency coding of stimulus intensity. The lower part of the figure shows four stimuli (A–D) of increasing intensity (e.g., pressure applied to the skin); the upper part of the figure shows responses in the sensory neuron to this stimulation. **A.** No stimulus; the sensory neuron is at the resting membrane potential. **B.** Weak stimulus; the resulting generator potential does not depolarize the sensory neuron beyond threshold. **C.** Moderate stimulus; action potentials are recorded in the sensory nerve because the generator potential exceeds threshold. **D.** Large (intense) stimulus; the generator potential amplitude and the action potential frequency are increased.

as a higher frequency of action potentials in the sensory neuron. When there is a large depolarization at the spike initiation zone, new action potentials are generated immediately after the refractory period of the previous action potential has ended. The higher frequency of action potentials is interpreted by the CNS as larger stimulus intensity, referred to as **frequency coding.** Information about the stimulus intensity is supplemented by **population coding,** which refers to the number of receptors that respond to the same stimulus. A receptor can only transduce a stimulus that is applied to a restricted area (the concept is referred to as the **receptive field**). Locations that have a high density of receptors with overlapping receptive fields will yield action potentials from a larger number of sensory neurons when stimulus intensity increases (e.g., pressing harder on an area of skin stimulates more receptors).

ADAPTATION OF SENSORY RECEPTORS The neuron depicted in Figure 2-16 shows a constant train of action potentials produced in response to a sustained stimulus, referred to as a **tonic** response. In most cases, however, the action potential response declines when a constant stimulus is applied (a **phasic** response), due to a phenomenon called **adaptation.** The mechanism of adaptation in most cases occurs at the level of the receptor. The generator potential declines over time with a constant stimulus, causing the frequency of action potentials in the sensory nerve to decrease. Receptors can be **slowly adapting** or **rapidly adapting,** depending on the rate of decay of the generator potential (Figure 2-17). Receptor adaptation is necessary so that constant environmental stimuli can be partially ignored, preventing a flood of sensory information into the CNS. Rapidly adapting receptors are useful in situations where the rate of change of a stimulus is important (e.g., the tension of a working muscle).

THE SOMATOSENSORY SYSTEM

The somatic sensory system conveys sensations from the skin and muscle. There are four **cutaneous sensory modalities:** touch, vibration, pain, and temperature. The somatosensory system includes **proprioception,** which relates to sensory information from the musculoskeletal system (see Motor Neurophysiology). Primary sensory neurons travel to the CNS in the peripheral spinal and the cranial nerves. The area of skin supplied with afferent nerve fibers by a single dorsal root is referred to as a **dermatome** (Figure 2-18).

▽ In the clinical setting, it is useful to have a **knowledge of the dermatomes** to better determine the localization of lesions in the sensory pathways. For example, "**sciatica**" is a general term that refers to back pain that radiates down the leg. The most common cause of "sciatica" is spinal disk herniation that impinges upon a spinal nerve, resulting in a dermatomal pattern to the pain. Compare and contrast the pain pattern of an L5 versus an S1 nerve root injury:

L5: pain radiates from the back to the buttock, posterolateral thigh, and anterolateral lower leg to the large toe.

S1: pain radiates from the back to the buttock, posterolateral thigh, and calf to the lateral border of the foot. ▽

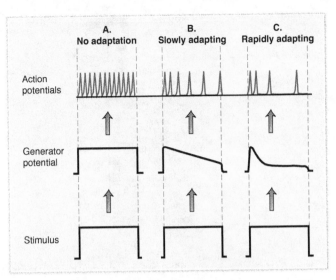

Figure 2-17: Receptor adaptation. An equivalent stimulus is applied to three different sensory receptors. **A.** If there is no receptor adaptation, a constant generator potential and action potential frequency are recorded. **B.** Slowly adapting receptors respond to a constant stimulus with a gradual decline in the generator potential and the action potential frequency. **C.** Rapidly adapting receptors have a generator potential and an action potential frequency that declines rapidly in response to a constant stimulus.

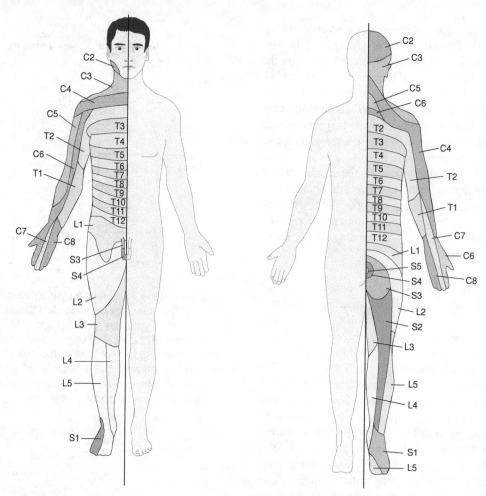

Figure 2-18: Skin dermatomes.

TOUCH SENSATION Discriminative touch allows the precise sense of the location of contacts with the skin and detailed information about the texture of objects to be gained. This kind of fine touch sensation is transduced by specialized receptors, including those listed below and shown in Figure 2-19:

- **Merkel's disks** and **Meissner's corpuscles** are both located near the skin surface and have small receptive fields that are suited to fine discrimination. Merkel's disks are slowly adapting and are suited to sensing steady pressure. Meissner's corpuscles are more rapidly adapting and are better suited to sensing rapid changes in skin contacts.

- **Ruffini's endings** contribute to the sensation of touch but have large receptive fields and are slowly adapting, making them useful for sensing local stretching of the skin rather than fine discriminative touch.

- **Pacinian corpuscles** are very rapidly adapting receptors that respond to rapidly changing stimuli, and therefore can sense **vibration.**

- **Hair follicles** have a nerve plexus that transduces displacement of the hair.

The spatial resolution of touch sensation varies widely in different areas of the body. **A two-point discrimination test** measures the minimum distance between two points of contact that can be perceived as two distinct stimuli. *The greatest spatial resolution is found on the fingertips and lips, and the lowest spatial resolution is found on the skin of the calf and lower back.* The high two-point discrimination of the fingertips is due to a high density of Merkel's disks and Meissner's corpuscles, which have small receptive fields. The associated sensory pathway for somatic sensation in the fingertips also contains a large number of neurons, including a large area of the somatosensory cortex.

The **main pathway for touch, vibration, and proprioception** involves a three-neuron chain (Figure 2-20):

1. The **first-order neuron** is the somatosensory receptor neuron. The afferent fiber is in the peripheral spinal nerve, the cell body is in the dorsal root ganglion, and the axon ascends the **dorsal column** white matter of the spinal cord to the brainstem.

2. The **second-order neuron** is located in the **dorsal column nuclei** of the caudal medulla. *The axon crosses to the opposite side and ascends through the brainstem to the thalamus in a tract called the **medial lemniscus.***

3. The **third-order neuron** is located in the **thalamus** and ascends to the primary somatosensory cortex via the white matter of the internal capsule.

▽ The **dorsal column-medial lemniscus (DCML)** sensory pathway conveys fine touch and vibratory and proprioceptive sensory input. *Note: the site of decussation for the DCML tract is at the level of the medulla.* Thus, any unilateral damage to this tract below the level of the medulla will result in an ipsilateral loss of sensation, whereas any damage to this tract above the medulla will result in a contralateral loss of sensation. ▼

▽ **Tabes dorsalis** is a late manifestation of syphilis and presents as signs and symptoms associated with impaired sensations as a result of demyelination of the dorsal columns. Signs include an ataxic wide-based gait as a result of loss of touch and proprioception, paresthesias (altered sensations), bladder dysfunction (e.g., urinary retention), and a positive **Romberg sign** (unable to maintain a steady posture while standing with feet together and eyes closed; the inability to maintain a steady posture while standing with feet together and eyes open indicates cerebellar dysfunction, not a DCML impairment). ▼

THE SOMATOSENSORY CORTEX The basic perception of touch and the ability to perform the kind of elaborate processing that allows us to recognize an object from its touch alone occurs in the cortex. The **primary somatosensory cortex** is located in the **postcentral gyrus** of the parietal lobe. Lesions in this area impair somatic sensations, and electrical stimulation evokes somatic sensations in specific parts of the body. The body surface is represented as a **somatotopic map** (often called the **homunculus**) in the primary somatosensory cortex. The homunculus has two striking features (Figure 2-21):

1. *The somatotopic map is discontinuous*, with the genitals represented below the feet and the hand represented between the head and the face.

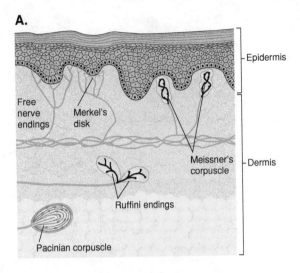

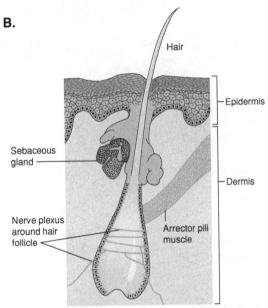

Figure 2-19: Touch receptors in the skin. **A.** Merkel's disks and Meissner's corpuscles just beneath the epidermis mediate discriminative touch. Ruffini's endings sense stretch and Pacinian corpuscles sense vibration. **B.** In hairy skin, the displacement of hairs contributes to touch sensation via a plexus of nerve endings wrapped around the hair root.

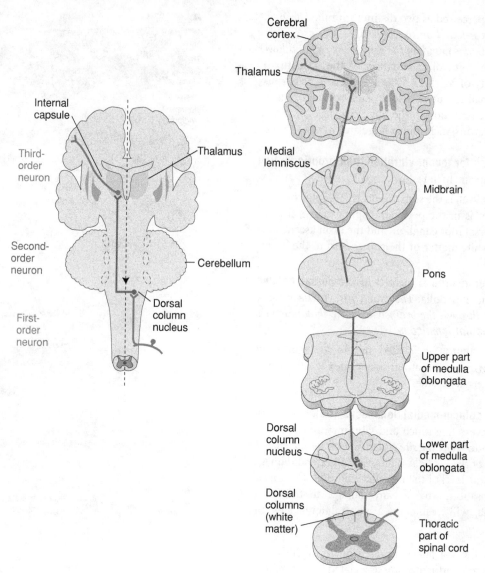

Figure 2-20: Neural pathway for discriminative touch and vibration. The pathway is a three-neuron chain. The first-order neuron ascends in the dorsal column of the spinal cord; the second-order neuron crosses over the midline in the medulla, and the third-order neuron ascends from the thalamus to the somatosensory cortex.

2. *The amount of cortex representing a given area reflects the importance of the sensory input.* For example, the fingers and mouth occupy a disproportionately large amount of cortex compared to the surface area of skin involved.

There are several secondary somatosensory areas, including the **posterior parietal cortex,** which integrates the sense of touch with other sensations such as vision. Lesions in this area may cause **agnosia,** which is the inability to recognize objects despite the presence of normal sensations. **Astereognosia** refers to the specific inability to recognize objects through touch.

▽ To test for **astereognosia,** a simple object such as a pen-
cil is placed in a bag; with eyes closed, the patient reaches into the bag. A patient with astereognosia will be able to describe the shape and feel of the object but will be unable to identify it. ▼

TEMPERATURE SENSATION The subjective sensations of "warm" and "cold" reflect two populations of thermoreceptors in the skin. Thermoreceptors are free nerve endings that only respond to temperature.

Cold fibers are the most numerous type of thermoreceptor and fire action potentials across a broad range of temperatures, with a peak response of about 30°C (86°F). Temperatures lower than approximately 16°C (60°F) are sensed as painful.

Warm fibers respond to a narrower range of temperatures, with a peak response at about 43°C (109°F).

Both types of thermoreceptors are rapidly adapting, which explains why a sudden change in temperature (e.g., entering a cold ocean) transmits an initial shock that quickly subsides. The superficial thermoreceptors play an important role in providing protection against exposure to objects or environments that are too hot or too cold, and contribute significantly to the ability to recognize complex modalities like wetness or slipperiness. However, these peripheral thermoreceptors play a minor role in the homeostatic control of core body temperature (see Integrative Functions of the Nervous System).

PAIN SENSATION In the somatosensory system, pain can be described as **superficial pain** (arising from the body surface) or **deep pain** (arising from muscles and joints). The term **nociceptor** is used to describe pain receptors, which are free nerve endings in the skin. Nociceptors have a high threshold of activation and should be silent unless a noxious stimulus is applied. Nociceptors can respond to excessive mechanical, thermal, or chemical stimuli. **Superficial pain** has two components:

1. **Initial pain** is a sharp, highly localized pain. The onset of pain sensation is fast because the nociceptors use larger myelinated nerve fibers with rapid conduction velocities.

2. **Delayed pain** is a diffuse burning sensation that lasts longer than initial pain. The onset is delayed because the nociceptors involved are unmyelinated neurons with a slow conduction velocity.

It is unfortunate, but biologically necessary, that nociceptors are slowly adapting so that a constantly applied noxious stimulus continues to be perceived as a painful stimulus. When tissue injury occurs, chemosensitive nociceptors are stimulated by K^+ released from damaged cells and by local inflammatory mediators (e.g., histamine released from mast cells). The inflammation response causes sustained hyperalgesia around the injured area (e.g., even a minor burn is very sensitive for a prolonged period), which is caused by inflammatory mediators such as prostaglandins and leukotrienes.

▼ The **analgesic effect of nonsteroidal anti-inflammatory drugs (NSAIDs)** (e.g., ibuprofen) is related to inhibiting the production of inflammatory pain sensitizers (e.g., prostaglandins and leukotrienes). By inhibiting the production of prostaglandins and leukotrienes, NSAIDs can limit the sustained hyperalgesic state induced by these pain sensitizers. ▼

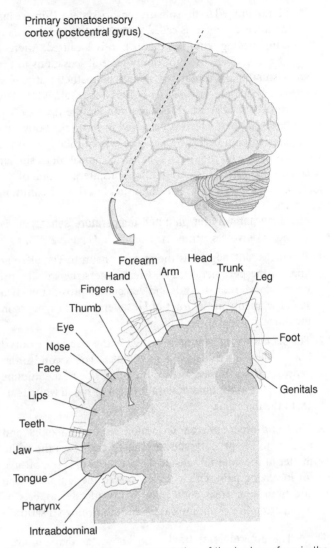

Figure 2-21: Somatotopic representation of the body surface in the primary somatosensory cortex.

Pain is not limited to the somatic sensory system. Pain arising from the internal organs is called **visceral pain,** which is usually a dull, burning sensation that is poorly localized. Afferent fibers of the ANS are used to convey visceral sensations to the CNS: visceral pain sensations follow sympathetic afferents, whereas physiologic visceral sensations (e.g., satiety) follow parasympathetic afferents. Noxious stimuli in the viscera often cause **referred pain,** which is perceived to be on the body surface. Referred pain occurs because the afferent fibers from the viscera converge on the spinal cord via the dorsal roots, similar to somatic pain afferents, and results in misinterpretation of the location source. Table 2-3 lists the usual location of common examples of referred pain.

The **main pathway for pain and temperature sensation** via spinal nerves involves a three-neuron chain (Figure 2-22):

1. The **first-order neuron** is the receptor neuron. The afferent fiber in the peripheral nerve, which enters the spinal cord via the dorsal root, ascends and descends approximately two spinal segments in the **tract of Lissauer** prior to synapse in the dorsal horn gray matter.

2. The **second-order neuron** is located in the area of the dorsal horn, called the **substantia gelatinosa.** The second-order neuron crosses immediately to the other side of the midline and ascends in the **anterolateral system** of spinal white matter to the thalamus.

3. The **third-order neuron** is located in the **thalamus** and ascends to the **primary somatosensory cortex** via the white matter of the internal capsule. This projection is responsible for localizing pain. Other projections to the temporal lobe and brainstem areas contribute to the affective aspects of pain perception as an unpleasant and disturbing sensation.

▽ The **anterolateral tract** (also known as the spinothalamic tract) conveys pain and temperature sensory input. Because of the ascending and descending tracts of Lissauer, the site of decussation for the anterolateral tract is within 1–2 spinal cord segments above and below the level where the peripheral afferent neuron enters the spinal cord. *Thus, any unilateral damage to the ALS tract will result in a contralateral loss of sensation beginning 1–2 spinal cord segments below the level of the lesion.* ▽

▽ **Syringomyelia** is characterized by progressive cavitation of the central spinal canal, most commonly occurring in the cervical spinal cord. Anatomically, the decussating second-order neurons associated with the ALS tract are in close proximity to the spinal canal, rendering them susceptible to damage early in this disease as the central canal expands. As a result, *patients present with bilateral loss of pain and temperature in a "cape-like" distribution of the shoulders and upper extremities.* As the cavitation progresses, *motor neurons that reside in the ventral horn of the spinal cord become compressed, resulting in bilateral flaccid paralysis of the upper extremities.* ▽

The pain pathway is modulated by a mechanism known as **pain gating,** which occurs at the site where the first-order neuron synapses with the second-order neuron. Many people are familiar with the notion that pain can be relieved by gently

TABLE 2-3. Typical Sites of Referred Pain

Pathologic Conditiont	Site(s) of Referred Pain (Variation in Site Does Occur)
Myocardial infarction	Left chest wall, left neck or jaw, left shoulder, left arm
Diaphragm irritation from cholecystitis or hepatitis	Right shoulder
Diaphragm irritation from ruptured spleen	Left shoulder
Stomach ulcer or cancer	Epigastrium, midback between the scapula
Lower lobe pneumonia	Upper quadrant abdominal pain on the same side as the pneumonia
Appendicitis	Periumbilical area (Note: right lower quadrant pain associated with appendicitis is not referred pain, it indicates somatic pain caused from the inflamed appendix irritating the parietal peritoneum)
Kidney stone	Flank radiating to groin, including testicle or labia majora

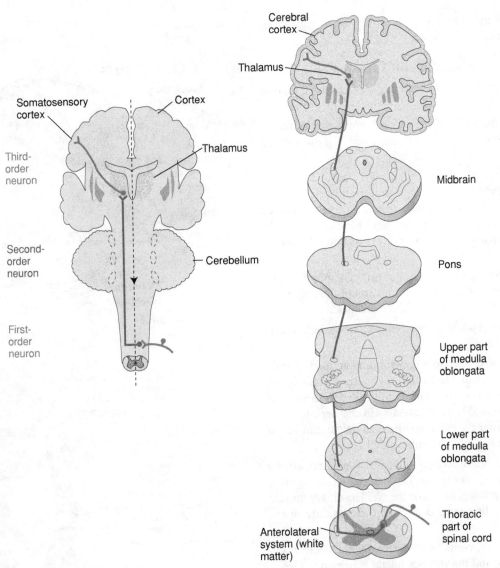

Figure 2-22: Neural pathway for pain and temperature. The pathway is a three-neuron chain. The first-order neuron synapses in the dorsal horn of the spinal cord; the second-order neuron immediately crosses the midline and ascends to the brainstem in the anterolateral white matter of the spinal cord; and the third-order neuron ascends from the thalamus to the somatosensory cortex

rubbing the injured area. The mechanism behind this response involves a circuit within the dorsal horn of the spinal cord. Touch fibers entering the same dorsal root as the pain fiber send a collateral branch that synapses on inhibitory interneurons within the spinal gray matter. The inhibitory interneurons release **opioids** both pre- and postsynaptically to inhibit transmission in the pain pathway between the first- and second-order neurons.

THE VISUAL SYSTEM

The optics of the eye focus light on specialized retinal **photoreceptor cells,** which transduce light into a neuronal signal. The visual field has a highly ordered representation on the retina and throughout the visual pathway from the retina to the cerebral cortex. Central processing occurs in the primary visual cortex and surrounding visual association cortex and allows interpretation of the complex qualities of vision (e.g., form, color, depth, motion, and distance).

ANATOMY OF THE EYE

The **major structures of the eye** are described as follows (Figure 2-23A):

The **sclera** is the white of the eye. It is composed of tough connective tissue, which is continuous with the dura mater around the optic nerve.

The **retina** forms the inner cellular layer around most of the eye. The **fovea** is a small depression in the center of the retina, which is surrounded by a region called the **macula.** Light is focused on this part of the retina, which has *the highest level of visual acuity (i.e., the ability to distinguish between two-point light sources).*

The **optic nerve** exits the eye posteriorly. The point of exit of the optic nerve causes a discontinuation of the retina and produces a small "blind spot" in the visual field.

The **cornea** is the curved transparent area where light enters the front of the eye.

The **iris** is the colored diaphragm running across the anterior part of the eyeball. The **pupil** is the aperture at the center of the iris, the diameter of which is controlled by muscles of the iris. The pupil dilates (**mydriasis**) in the dark to allow more light to enter the eye and constricts (**miosis**) in bright light to prevent the excessive entry of light.

The **lens** lies behind the cornea and consists of a transparent viscous gel encased in a capsule. The lens and cornea together constitute the **optic apparatus** of the eye. The **ciliary muscle** and **suspensory ligaments** determine the curvature of the lens.

The cavity of the eye contains fluids; the **aqueous humor** is in front of the lens, and the **vitreous humor** is behind the lens.

Table 2-4 highlights examples of conditions that involve different structures of the eye.

FLUID COMPARTMENTS OF THE EYE The intraocular fluids of the eye keep the eyeball distended. Vitreous humor is a stable gelatinous mass, but aqueous humor is continually secreted. **Intraocular pressure** is maintained within a normal range of approximately 15 mm Hg (±3 mm Hg) by a balance between the secretion and absorption of aqueous humor. The aqueous humor is secreted by the ciliary body and is absorbed via the canal of Schlemm.

Epithelial cells projecting from the **ciliary body** actively secrete aqueous humor into the space between the iris and the lens (the posterior compartment) (see Figure 2-23B).

Aqueous humor flows through the pupil into the space between the iris and the cornea (the anterior compartment).

The **canal of Schlemm** leaves the anterior chamber, at the angle between the iris and cornea, and drains into the extraocular veins.

▽ **Glaucoma** is associated with a pathologic increase in intraocular pressure, which occurs as a result of an

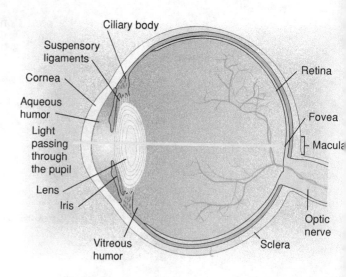

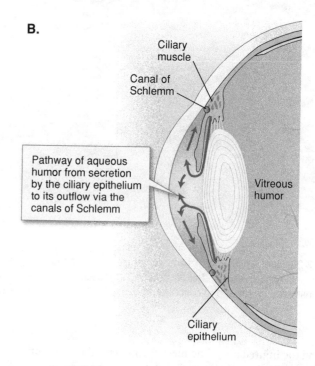

Figure 2-23: A. Anatomy of the eye. **B.** Secretion and reabsorption of aqueous humor. The ciliary epithelium secretes aqueous humor, which enters the anterior compartment of eye via the pupil and drains into the venous system via the canal of Schlemm.

imbalance between aqueous humor production and drainage. Glaucoma may result in damage to the optic nerve and progressive loss of vision. Patients with **acute closed-angle glaucoma,** which results from rapid increases in intraocular pressure, present with a painful, red eye and are at risk of rapid permanent vision loss. *Acute closed-angle glaucoma is considered a medical emergency!* **Open-angle glaucoma,** on the other hand, is much more common and presents as an insidious onset of painless progressive loss of vision; typically, the peripheral vision is affected first, and the central vision is affected later. ▼

OPTICAL PRINCIPLES

Light rays bend as they enter the eye and become focused at the retina. The bending of light at a curved surface is called **refraction.** The degree of refraction depends on how curved the surface is and on the **refractory index** of the material. Materials with a high refractory index cause the light to slow more as it enters the eye, resulting in more refraction.

The cornea and lens are both convex surfaces that cause light to be focused toward a **focal point;** the distance beyond the lens where light focuses is the **focal distance** (Figure 2-24A). When an image is viewed through a convex lens, *the projected image is turned upside down, with the two sides reversed* (see Figure 2-24B). This occurs at the eye, but the brain is able to perceive images in their correct orientation.

The *refractive power* of a lens is measured using **diopter** ("D") units. A spherical lens that focuses light 1 m beyond the lens has a power of +1 D; a lens with 10 times this refractory power (+10 D) focuses light 10 cm beyond the lens. *A concave lens disperses light* and has refractory powers described in negative dioptric units.

MECHANISM OF ACCOMMODATION The total refractory power of the eye is approximately +60 D, with two thirds of refraction occurring at the cornea and most of the remaining refraction occurring at the lens. The lens has a variable curvature that provides **refractive plasticity** by contributing between +13 D (in its most flattened state) to +26 D (in its most curved state). The ability to voluntarily change the refractive power of the lens allows objects at different distances to be focused on the retina. For example, if a distant object moves toward the eye, the lens becomes more curved to keep the object in focus. Changing the shape of the lens to focus an object is called **accommodation.**

The mechanism of accommodation depends on the elastic properties of the lens and the tension placed on it by the suspensory ligaments. If a lens is isolated from the eye, it becomes almost spherical. However, inside the eye, the lens is placed under tension by the suspensory ligaments, and in the resting condition, the lens remains fairly flat. The ciliary muscle is located at the attachment of the suspensory ligaments to the eyeball; contraction of the ciliary muscles reduces tension in the ligaments and allows the lens to assume a more rounded shape. Contraction of the ciliary muscles is controlled by the parasympathetic nerves (see Autonomic Innervation of the Eye).

ERRORS OF REFRACTION People with normal vision (**emmetropia**) focus distant objects clearly, with the

TABLE 2-4. Conditions Involving the Major Structures of the Eye

Major Eye Structure	Disease/Condition
Sclera	**Osteogenesis imperfecta:** The sclera appear blue because the genetic defect in the type I procollagen allows the underlying (blue) choroid layers to be seen.
Retina	**Hypertensive retinopathy:** Severity and duration of hypertension are the key determinants of retinopathy. One classification system is based on funduscopic examination findings: grade 1, arterial narrowing, "copper/silver wiring"; grade 2, arteriovenous nicking; grade 3, flame-shaped hemorrhages, cotton-wool spots (infarcted zones), hard exudates (extravasated lipid); grade 4, papilledema.
Macula	**Tay-Sachs disease:** A neurodegenerative disease caused by hexosaminidase A deficiency. Patients have a characteristic macular "cherry-red" spot.
Optic nerve	**Multiple sclerosis:** Optic neuritis is a common initial presenting symptom of multiple sclerosis characterized by decreased visual acuity, ocular pain (especially with movement), and color desaturation.
Cornea	**Herpes:** Dendritic ulcers of the cornea are characteristic of herpetic eye infections.
Iris	**Neurofibromatosis type I:** A genetic condition that results in characteristic neurofibromas (benign Schwann cell tumors), café au lait spots (freckling of non-sun-exposed skin), and Lisch nodules (iris hamartomas).
Lens	**Marfan's syndrome:** A genetic defect in fibrillin production that results in the classic clinical triad: ocular lens dislocation, aortic dilation, and long thin extremities.

ciliary muscle completely relaxed (Figure 2-25A). To focus objects at close range, the ciliary muscle is contracted to provide the appropriate amount of accommodation. There are **four basic refraction errors:** ▼

1. **Myopia** (nearsightedness) occurs when light from distant objects is focused in front of the retina with the ciliary muscle relaxed. There is no way for the maximally flattened lens to refract the light any less, resulting in a limiting "far point" for clear vision. However, accommodation still occurs to allow clear focus on closer objects. *Myopia is usually caused by an eyeball that is too long; the refraction error can be corrected using eyeglasses with a concave lens* (see Figure 2-25B).

2. **Hyperopia** (farsightedness) occurs when the resting position of the lens does not adequately refract the light from distant objects, causing the focal point to lie behind the retina. The hyperopic patient is able to voluntarily use the accommodation mechanism to increase the refractive power of the lens and bring distant objects into focus. The remaining range of ciliary muscle contraction available to accommodate near objects may be reduced, causing the "near point" to recede. *Hyperopia is most commonly the result of a short eyeball; the refraction error is corrected using eyeglasses with a convex lens* (see Figure 2-25C).

3. **Presbyopia** is the reduced ability to accommodate near or distant objects due to a dramatic decrease in the elasticity of the lens, which occurs with increasing age. In most people older than the age of 70, the curvature of the lens becomes fixed, resulting in the inability to focus on near objects (e.g., reading); distance vision is also limited because the lens flattens less than it does in younger people. Bifocal lenses, which have an upper half of the lens focused for distance vision and a lower part focused for near vision, are often prescribed.

4. **Astigmatism** is caused by incorrect curvature of the eye in one plane. Two different focal distances are produced, depending on the plane on which light enters the eye. *Eyeglasses with a cylindrical lens are needed to correct the refraction error of astigmatism.*

THE RETINA

The retina is the site of phototransduction and is composed of the following **cellular layers** (Figure 2-26A):

- The **retinal pigment epithelium** is the outermost layer of cells. It assists the photoreceptor cells by recycling the visual pigment molecules that are degraded during phototransduction. The pigment epithelium also absorbs stray light, preventing reflection of light back into the eye, which would otherwise disturb phototransduction.

- There are two types of photoreceptor resting on the pigment epithelium: the **rods** and the **cones.**

- Retinal **bipolar cells** form synapses with photoreceptor cells at one pole and with ganglion cells at the other pole.

- **Ganglion cells** are the innermost layer of cells, and they are the output cells of the retina. *The axons of ganglion cells become the optic nerve.*

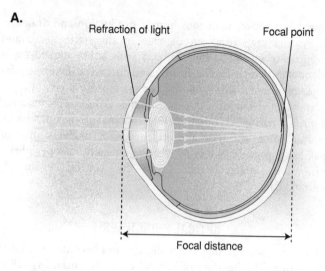

A.
Refraction of light   Focal point

Focal distance

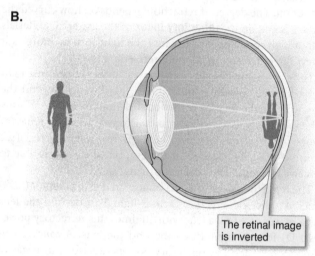

B.

The retinal image is inverted

Figure 2-24: Optical properties of the eye. **A.** The convex cornea and lens cause refraction of light and convergence of light rays to bring objects into focus on the retina. The focal distance is the distance from the front of the eye to the focal point. **B.** Image inversion by the optical apparatus of the eye.

A. Normal vision (emmetropia)

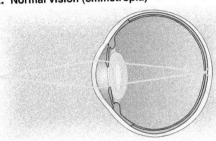

B. Myopia

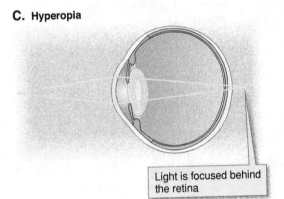

Light is focused in front of the retina

Myopia correction

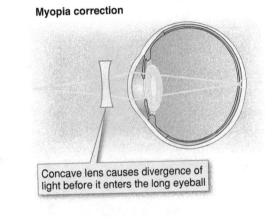

Concave lens causes divergence of light before it enters the long eyeball

C. Hyperopia

Light is focused behind the retina

Hyperopia correction

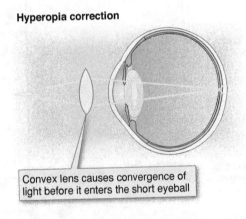

Convex lens causes convergence of light before it enters the short eyeball

Figure 2-25: Myopia (nearsightedness) and hyperopia (farsightedness). **A.** The normal eye focuses light from a distant point on the retina with the ciliary muscles relaxed. **B.** Myopia results when the eyeballs are longer than normal, causing light to be focused on a point in front of the retina. Myopia can be corrected using eyeglasses with a concave lens. **C.** Hyperopia results when the eyeballs are shorter than normal, causing light to be focused behind the retina. Hyperopia can be corrected using eyeglasses with a convex lens.

Horizontal cells have a radial orientation and form synapses in the outer layer of the retina with the photoreceptors and the bipolar cells.

Amacrine cells have a similar orientation to horizontal cells but are located in the inner layer of the retina, where they synapse with bipolar cells and ganglion cells.

PROPERTIES OF RODS AND CONES Rods and cones both have an outer segment and an inner segment (see Figure 2-26B). The outer segment faces the retinal pigment epithelium and is composed of characteristic membrane folds, referred to as **disks.** The disk membrane contains a high concentration of the visual pigment molecule **rhodopsin.** The inner segment synapses with bipolar and horizontal cells. There are key

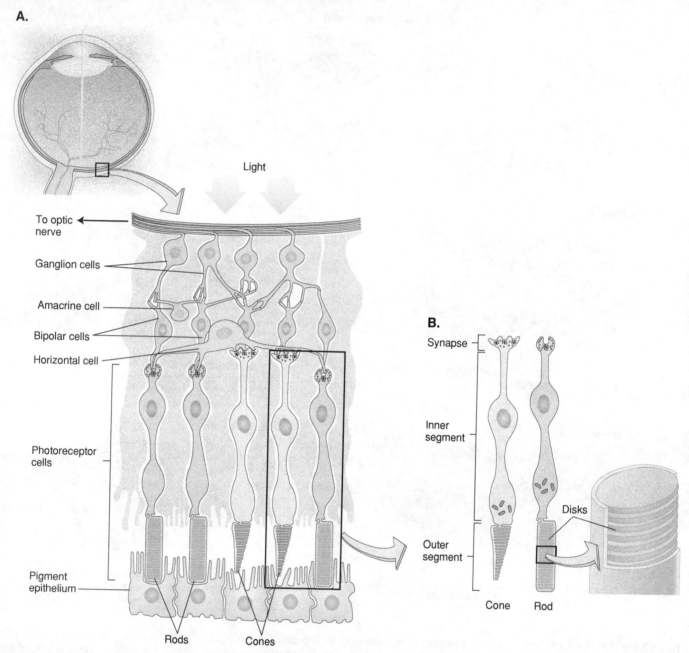

Figure 2-26: The retina. **A.** Incoming light passes through several neuronal layers to reach the photoreceptor cells. The retinal output consists of action potentials in ganglion cells; the axons of ganglion cells are conveyed to the central nervous system via the optic nerve. **B.** Rods and cones. Photoreceptor cells have two major regions, an outer segment resting on the retinal pigment epithelium, and an inner segment that synapses with bipolar and horizontal cells. The outer segment contains stacks of membranous disks containing the visual pigment molecule rhodopsin.

differences in the **properties of rods and cones** that underlie different functional properties of the visual system:

- **Rods** are monochromatic (single color) receptors, which are highly sensitive to light and allow objects to be seen in low intensity light. **Dark adaptation** (increased light sensitivity in response to prolonged darkness) occurs to a much greater extent in rods than in cones.

- **Cones** are less sensitive to light and function best under high light intensity conditions, such as bright sunlight. There are **three types of cone photoreceptors,** with overlapping sensitivity to light of different wavelength (see Mechanism of Color Vision):

1. Blue (or S) cones absorb light of short wavelength.

2. Green (or M) cones absorb light of medium wavelengths most optimally.

3. Red (or L) cones absorb light at the long wavelength end of the visible spectrum.

In most cases, colored light excites each type of cone but to a different degree; *it is therefore the pattern of stimulation from the three types of cones that encodes* **color.**

The fovea only contains cone cells. Most cone cells in the fovea synapse with a single bipolar cell, which in turn synapses with a single ganglion cell. This creates very small receptive fields for the foveal bipolar and ganglion cells, thereby accounting for the high visual acuity of the fovea. Visual acuity decreases dramatically toward the periphery of the eye; a high proportion of rod cells are located in the periphery, and many rods converge on each ganglion cell. Therefore, *central vision has a high resolution but is poor in dim light, whereas peripheral vision has low resolution but allows vision in low light.*

MECHANISM OF PHOTOTRANSDUCTION Phototransduction is the cascade of chemical and electrical events through which light energy is converted into a receptor potential (Figure 2-27). Rods and cones are unusual sensory receptors in that the receptor potential is a **hyperpolarization.** The **phototransduction mechanism** involves the following steps:

1. The photoreceptor membrane potential is depolarized in the dark because **cyclic guanosine monophosphate (cGMP)-activated nonselective cation channels** are open. Continual Na^+ influx is measured as the "**dark current**" of photoreceptors. Depolarization of the photoreceptor causes tonic release of the neurotransmitter **glutamate.**

2. Light is absorbed by the light receptor molecule **rhodopsin.** The rhodopsin molecule is formed from the transmembrane

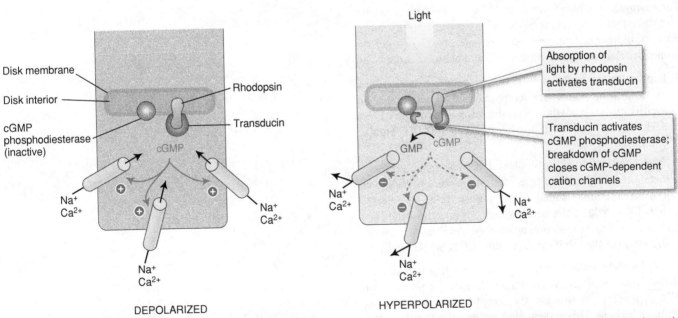

Figure 2-27: Mechanism of phototransduction. The membrane potential of photoreceptors is depolarized in the dark due to sustained opening of cyclic guanosine monophosphate (cGMP)-dependent cation channels. The absorption of light by the visual pigment rhodopsin stimulates the G protein transducin to increase cGMP phosphodiesterase activity. cGMP is broken down to guanosine monophosphate (GMP), which causes cation channels to close and results in a hyperpolarizing receptor potential.

protein **opsin** and an attached **retinal** molecule (retinal is a vitamin A derivative).

3. Photons of light are absorbed by retinal, causing **isomerization** from 11-*cis* retinal to all-*trans* retinal. A resulting conformation change in opsin activates the rhodopsin pigment; activated rhodopsin is called **metarhodopsin II.**

4. Opsin is associated with the guanosine triphosphate (GTP)-binding protein **transducin,** which triggers a second-messenger response inside the photoreceptor.

5. When rhodopsin absorbs light, transducin is activated, resulting in the stimulation of a **cGMP phosphodiesterase.** cGMP is the diffusible second messenger that is responsible for maintaining the dark current. Activation of the phosphodiesterase increases the rate of cGMP breakdown and causes cGMP-activated cation channels to close.

6. Inhibition of the dark current causes the photoreceptor membrane to hyperpolarize, which reduces the tonic release of glutamate on bipolar cells.

7. Termination of phototransduction involves the inactivation of metarhodopsin II by the ever-present enzyme **rhodopsin kinase.** All-*trans* retinal and opsin separate soon after light is absorbed, and are recycled over a period of several minutes to regenerate rhodopsin.

Signal amplification is a key feature of the phototransduction mechanism, whereby a few photons of light produce a large change in intracellular cGMP concentration and closure of many nonselective cation channels.

RETINAL PROCESSING The output from the retina occurs in the form of action potentials from retinal ganglion cells. Each ganglion cell may receive input from a single bipolar cell (e.g., at the fovea) or from the convergence of many bipolar cells (e.g., at the periphery of the eye). There is significant refinement of the visual signal by the retina before central pathways are involved. For example, our highly developed ability to detect contrasts and the edges of objects is based on the presence of different types of bipolar cell. Some bipolar cells respond to glutamate with a depolarization and others with a hyperpolarization.

Depolarization of the bipolar cell occurs when it expresses the ionotropic glutamate receptor. These bipolar cells are excited in the dark when photoreceptors produce the tonic dark current, and are therefore referred to as **OFF bipolar cells.**

Hyperpolarization of the bipolar cell occurs when it expresses metabotropic glutamate receptors, which convert glutamate into an inhibitory signal. These bipolar cells are referred to as **ON bipolar cells** because they are excited in the light (Figure 2-28A). Stimulation by light reduces glutamate release and weakens the inhibitory stimulus in ON bipolar cells.

A point light source moving across the retina will cause a variable pattern of action potential frequencies from ganglion cells, depending on whether the receptive field is excited or inhibited by light. This pattern of signaling helps the visual system to perceive contrasts such as edges and borders. The ability to perceive contrasts is greatly increased by the property of **antagonistic center-surrounds** in the receptive fields of bipolar

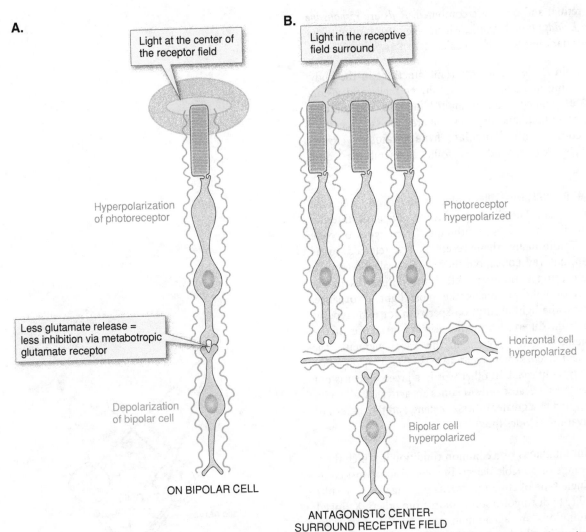

A.

Light at the center of
the receptor field

Hyperpolarization
of photoreceptor

Less glutamate release =
less inhibition via metabotropic
glutamate receptor

Depolarization
of bipolar cell

ON BIPOLAR CELL

B.

Light in the receptive
field surround

Photoreceptor
hyperpolarized

Horizontal cell
hyperpolarized

Bipolar cell
hyperpolarized

ANTAGONISTIC CENTER-
SURROUND RECEPTIVE FIELD

Figure 2-28: Center-surround organization of bipolar cell receptive fields. **A.** Stimulation of an ON bipolar cell when light is shone in the center of its receptive field through a direct pathway between the photoreceptor and bipolar cell. **B.** Inhibition of an ON bipolar cell when light is shone in the area of the retina surrounding the receptive field center. Hyperpolarization of the photoreceptor results in hyperpolarization of the bipolar cell through an indirect pathway that includes horizontal cells.

cells. Whatever the electrical response of a bipolar cell is to light in the center of the receptive field, the opposite response occurs if light is applied to the immediate surrounding area (see Figure 2-28B). When a point light source moves across the retina, an ON bipolar cell is inhibited as the light moves across one edge of its receptive field surround. When the light moves to the center of the receptive field, the bipolar cell is strongly stimulated. However, when the light moves to the other side of the receptive field surround, the output signal is again decreased.

DARK AND LIGHT ADAPTATION Retinal sensitivity must be altered in response to changing levels of light or images appear washed out and uniform in bright light or, conversely, images are invisible in dim light conditions. In sustained bright light, a large proportion of rhodopsin will dissociate to retinal and opsin. Therefore, *the retina becomes adapted to light by having less visual pigment available for phototransduction.* Conversely, the retina becomes more sensitive to light with increasing time spent in darkness. Rhodopsin stores are built up as all the available retinal and opsin are combined. *Rods are responsible for the dark adaptation response*, which takes 30–40 minutes of continuous darkness to reach a peak.

▽ Vitamin A has many important functions in the body, including maintenance of healthy epithelia and vision. **Vitamin A deficiency** results in **night blindness** (rod cell dysfunction), **xerophthalmia** (dry eyes that are prone to ulceration and infection), and **follicular hyperkeratosis** (rough elevations of skin around hair follicles resembling goose bumps). ▽

MECHANISM OF COLOR VISION Color is determined by the wavelength of light. The phototransduction of light of differing wavelengths is achieved by the three different types of cone receptors. Traditionally, these receptors are referred to as **blue, green, and red cones,** but they are also called S (short), M (medium), and L (long) to reflect the differences in the wavelengths of light producing the most light absorbance. Differences in the light absorption spectrum for each type of cone arise from differences in the primary structure of the opsin protein, which is present in the visual pigment. *The nervous system decodes color according to the relative stimulation of the three types of cones.* In other words, a green object is not perceived as green because only M cones are activated; all cones may be activated to a greater or lesser extent, and the pattern of overall activation decodes the color.

▽ "**Color blindness**" is a common condition in which there is a range of possible defects in color vision. Most commonly, a single type of cone receptor is missing, which results in the inability to distinguish some colors from others. X-linked recessive mutations are a common cause of defective color vision, resulting in a higher proportion of males than females with this condition.

▪ **Monochromacy** (true color blindness) is the lack of two out of three of the cone receptor types and is rare.

▪ **Dichromacy** is the lack of one type of cone receptor. The selective loss of the blue cone (**tritanopia**) is rare. Most commonly, either the red cone (**protanopia**) or the green cone (**deuteranopia**) is missing. There is extensive overlap in the spectral sensitivity of red and green cones for wavelengths of light between 500 and 600 nm. The loss of either red or green cones results in difficulty distinguishing between green, yellow, orange, or red colors. *Patients have particular difficulty distinguishing between red and green and are therefore said to have* **red-green color blindness.**

▪ **Anomalous trichromy** is caused by defective (not missing) L cones with absorbance spectra between the normal L and M ranges. ▽

THE VISUAL PATHWAY

The **main visual pathway** conveys signals from the retina to the primary visual cortex as follows (Figure 2-29):

▪ Axons from retinal ganglion cells enter the **optic nerve** in each eye.

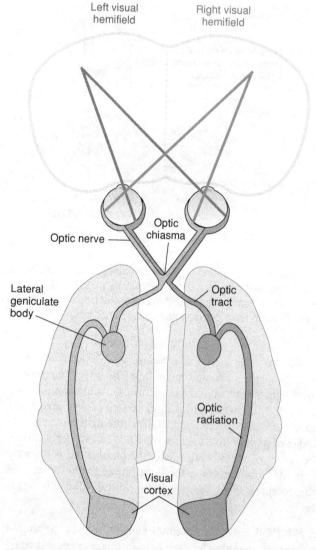

Figure 2-29: The main visual pathway. The binocular visual field is shown, divided into equal left and right halves. Light from the left visual hemifield stimulates the right half of each retina; light from the right visual hemifield stimulates the left half of each retina. Nerve impulses originating from stimuli in the left hemifield are transmitted to the right visual cortex, whereas those from the right hemifield are transmitted to the left visual cortex.

The optic nerves meet at the **optic chiasm,** where some axons cross the midline.

An **optic tract** leads from each side of the optic chiasm to the **lateral geniculate body** of the thalamus, where retinal ganglion cells synapse.

Second-order sensory neurons follow a course to the primary visual cortex via the **optic radiation.**

The visual fields of each eye overlap extensively to produce binocular vision. Images from each half of the visual field are processed by the contralateral side of the visual cortex (e.g., the left visual cortex is concerned with information from the right half of the visual field). As a result, *axons from the nasal half of each retina must cross the midline at the optic chiasm, whereas axons from the temporal half of each retina remain on the ipsilateral side.* For example, light from the right half of the visual field projects onto the nasal half of the right retina and will cross at the optic chiasm before continuing on to the left visual cortex, whereas the light that projects on the temporal half of the left retina will not cross at the optic chiasm and will continue on to the left visual cortex (Figure 2-29).

▽ The visual pathway between the retina and the visual cortex can be interrupted at several locations, resulting in characteristic **visual field defects.** Table 2-5 summarizes the defects caused by different lesions in the visual pathway. ▼

TABLE 2-5. Visual Field Defects Caused by Lesions in the Visual Pathway

Site of Lesion	Description of Visual Field Defect	Defect	Possible Cause
Optic nerve	Blindness in the affected eye	Monocular blindness	Optic neuritis, retinal artery occlusion
Optic chiasm	Loss of fibers crossing the midline from the nasal half of each retina causes loss of temporal visual field on both sides	Bitemporal heteronymous hemianopia	Pituitary tumor (e.g., craniopharyngioma) pressing on the optic chiasm from below
Optic tract	Loss of fibers for the visual field on the opposite side to the lesion	Homonymous hemianopia	Brain tumor
Optic radiation	Loss of fibers for the visual field on the opposite side to the lesion	Homonymous hemianopia	Brain tumor; occlusion of a branch of the posterior cerebral artery
Visual cortex (one side)	Loss of visual processing for the visual field on the opposite side to the lesion	Homonymous hemianopia with macular sparing	Posterior cerebral artery thrombosis; however, the central (macula) vision is maintained due to collateral circulation between the posterior and middle cerebral arteries

Visual fibers are not restricted to the main visual pathway. Information about light levels and the visual scene project to the following brain areas:

- The **suprachiasmatic nuclei,** for control of circadian rhythms.
- The **superior colliculi** of the midbrain, for the control of eye movements.
- The **pretectal nuclei** of the midbrain, for the reflex control of eye movement associated with changing the focus of vision and for the **pupillary light reflex.**

EYE MOVEMENTS

Movements of the eyes must be extremely fast and accurate to serve the demands of the visual system. For example, the control of eye movement must be able to fix the gaze on objects at different distances, to maintain focus on objects as the head moves, and to follow moving objects in the visual field. The movement of both eyes must also be exactly integrated to maintain binocular vision. Movements of the eye are mediated by three pairs of muscles, which receive motor innervation from cranial nerves III (oculomotor), IV (trochlear), and VI (abducens) (Figure 2-30):

1. The **medial and lateral rectus** muscles, which move the eyes side to side.

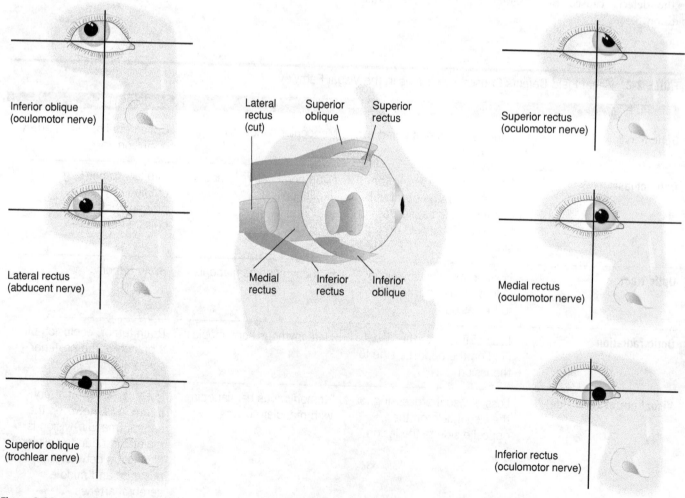

Figure 2-30: Extraocular muscles. The individual action of each muscle is shown for the right eye. The nerve supply of each muscle is shown in parentheses.

2. The **superior and inferior rectus** muscles, which move the eyes upward and downward.

3. The **superior and inferior oblique** muscles, which prevent rotation of the eyeball and move the eyes upward and downward.

Fixation movements of the eye lock the gaze on a specific object, allowing it to be focused on the central part of the retina. Once a particular object is selected, *the gaze is locked by the involuntary fixation pathway,* which begins in the visual association areas surrounding the primary visual cortex. Involuntary fixation on the object is maintained by reflexes that are coordinated by the **superior colliculus.** The eyes continuously make small movements, which cause the image on the fovea to move slightly. If the image moves close to the edge of the fovea, there is a rapid reflex flicking movement of the eyes to restore the position of the image to the center of the fovea. *The gaze is unlocked by the* **voluntary fixation pathway.** The voluntary selection of a new object originates from an area in the frontal lobe, close to the premotor cortex. Cortical fibers descend to the brainstem nuclei that control cranial nerves III, IV, and VI.

Saccadic movements of the eyes are rapid movements in the position of the eyes (saccades). Saccadic movement is necessary when objects in the visual field are moving or when the head is moving. A succession of fixation points is selected to survey the "highlights" of the moving visual scene. Reading is an example of saccadic movement, where the brain becomes trained to use saccades to survey a static visual field for highlights. If an object is moving in a regular cycle, saccadic movements quickly become smooth "pursuit" movements as the central visual processing mechanisms adapt and produce programmed eye movements.

▽ **Nystagmus** is defined as rhythmic oscillations of the eyes characterized by a slow drifting component and a fast saccadic component in the opposite direction. Although nystagmus can be physiologic, it can also indicate underlying serious pathologic conditions, including demyelinating diseases (e.g., multiple sclerosis), cerebellar or brainstem lesions, drug intoxication (anticonvulsants or alcohol), or vestibular dysfunction (e.g., Ménière's disease). *A complete neurologic examination should be performed on all patients presenting with nystagmus.* ▽

DEPTH PERCEPTION

To achieve binocular vision, the visual image of interest must be projected onto the fovea of both eyes simultaneously. This is achieved even during rapid saccadic eye movements, and the brain fuses the images from each eye into the perception of a single image. One major advantage of binocular vision is improved **depth perception (stereopsis).** Because the eyes are placed about 5 cm apart, the images projected onto the two retinae are not precisely the same, particularly for objects that are close to the eyes. This slight difference is computed by the brain to provide depth perception in the visual scene.

▽ **Strabismus** refers to misalignment of the eyes, which results in two images being projected to the brain, causing **diplopia** (double vision) in adults. In children, however, uncorrected strabismus can result in **amblyopia** (reduced vision) of the misaligned eye. Amblyopia occurs because the developing brain has the ability to suppress the images from the deviated eye, thereby preventing diplopia at the expense of reduced vision in the affected eye. ▼

AUTONOMIC INNERVATION OF THE EYE

When the gaze changes to fix on a new object at a different distance from the eye, the lens must rapidly accommodate to focus the object on the retina. The brain cortical areas that control fixation movements of the eye also control accommodation of the lens. Cortical signals descend to the oculomotor nucleus in the midbrain (see Figure 2-7A). **The oculomotor nucleus has two efferent parts:**

1. A **motor nucleus,** giving rise to motor fibers to the extraocular muscles.

2. A visceral part (the **Edinger-Westphal nucleus**), giving origin to parasympathetic preganglionic fibers, which pass in cranial nerve III to the **ciliary ganglion.** Postganglionic neurons pass to the eye and innervate the ciliary muscles for accommodation of the lens.

The same pathway from the Edinger-Westphal nucleus is used by parasympathetic neurons that innervate the iris to bring about constriction of the pupil. The **pupillary light reflex** assists the eye in adapting to variable light levels; reflex constriction of the pupils occurs when light is shone into the eyes. Afferent signals from some retinal ganglion cells pass (via the optic nerve) to the **pretectal nucleus** of the midbrain; interneurons connect the pretectal area to the Edinger-Westphal nucleus on both sides. Efferent parasympathetic neurons innervate muscles of the iris, resulting in constriction of the pupil. The pupillary light reflex is consensual (i.e., light shone in one eye constricts both pupils). *Brainstem damage can result in an absent pupillary light reflex and/or the presence of different sized pupils.*

▼ A detailed understanding of the **pupillary light reflex pathway** is essential to diagnosing the location of an associated lesion. Consider afferent versus efferent lesions in the pathway:

■ **Afferent (optic nerve, CN II) lesion.** When light is shone in the affected eye, the direct and consensual reflex is absent; when light is shone in the unaffected eye, the direct and consensual reflex is intact.

  • **Explanation.** The afferent nerve must be intact to trigger an efferent (pupillary constriction) response. *Because neurons project from the pretectal area to the Edinger-Westphal nucleus on both sides, any afferent stimulus that reaches the pretectal nucleus will trigger an efferent response in both eyes (assuming an intact efferent pathway).*

■ **Efferent (CN III or Edinger-Westphal nucleus) lesion.** Light shone in the eye of the affected side will trigger a consensual reflex but not a direct reflex; light shone in the eye of the unaffected side will trigger a direct reflex but not a consensual reflex.

  • **Explanation.** The afferent nerves on both sides are intact and will transmit a stimulus to the pretectal nucleus, which will trigger an efferent response in an intact efferent pathway.

Note: a lesion of CN III will result in weakness of the extraocular muscles, innervated by CN III, in addition to defects in the pupillary light reflex. ▼

Sympathetic innervation to the eye is relayed from the first thoracic segment of the spinal cord and reaches the eye via the **superior cervical ganglion.** Postganglionic fibers travel along the outer surface of blood vessels to the eye. Sympathetic neurons innervate the iris to cause dilation of the pupil.

▽ **Horner's syndrome** is caused by the interruption of the sympathetic nerves to the face and head and therefore has the following consequences:

- **Persistent constriction of the pupil** on the affected side, due to loss of the sympathetic dilator response.

- **Persistent vasodilatation** of blood vessels on the affected side, due to loss of sympathetic vasoconstriction.

- **Loss of sweating** in the affected area, due to sweat glands being stimulated by sympathetic innervation.

- **Droop of the upper eyelid,** due to loss of contraction of smooth muscle fibers in the eyelid, which receive sympathetic innervation. ▼

THE AUDITORY AND VESTIBULAR SYSTEMS

The auditory and vestibular systems are concerned with the sense of hearing (**audition**) and the sense of **balance,** respectively. A sense of hearing goes beyond simple encoding of stimulus intensity and location, and includes complex higher processing that allows verbal communication with all of its nuances and emotions. In contrast, the vestibular system informs the nervous system about the position of the head and how it is moving; most of the input from the vestibular system is processed subconsciously. The auditory and vestibular systems both use **hair cells** to transduce mechanical forces into action potentials. Hair cells are located in a fluid-filled sensory organ called the **membranous labyrinth.** There is a labyrinth inside a hollowed out part of the temporal skull bone on each side of the head. Each labyrinth has two parts (Figure 2-31):

1. The **cochlea** is the auditory part of the labyrinth. Afferent neurons exiting the cochlea form the auditory (cochlea) nerve, which is part of the vestibulocochlear nerve (CN VIII).

2. The **otolith organs** and the **semicircular canals** form the vestibular part of the labyrinth. Afferent neurons from these organs form the vestibular nerve, which joins with the auditory nerve to form CN VIII.

THE PHYSICAL NATURE OF SOUND

Most sounds that are heard are caused by variations in air pressure. As an object moves, it compresses the air in front of it (increasing the pressure), whereas the air behind it becomes less dense (decreasing the pressure). For example, the vibrations of a guitar string set up periodic variations in air pressure that travel as a **sound wave** (Figure 2-32). All sound waves travel at the same speed through air (343 m/s, or 768 m/h), but they

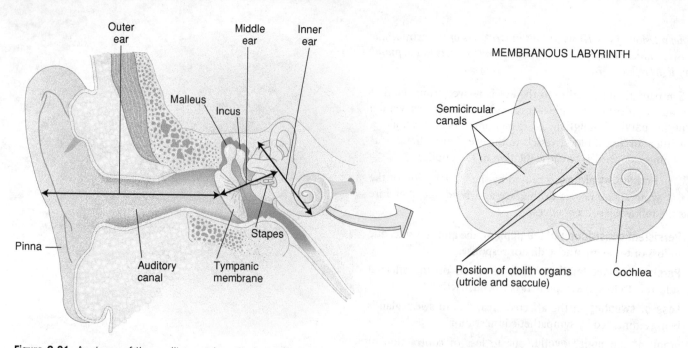

Figure 2-31: Anatomy of the auditory and vestibular apparatus. The outer ear is comprised of the pinna and auditory canal; the middle ear consists of the tympanic membrane and the three ossicles, the malleus, incus, and stapes. The inner ear is comprised of the membranous labyrinth; the cochlea is the auditory part of the labyrinth; and the semicircular canals and the otolith organs form the vestibular part of the inner ear.

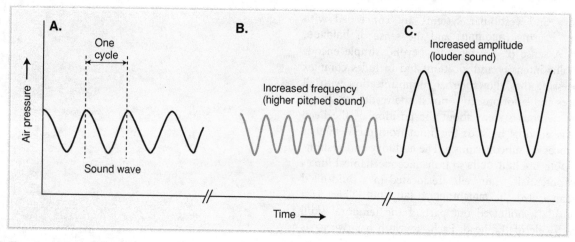

Figure 2-32: The physical nature of sound. **A.** Sound waves produced by cyclic variation in air pressure. **B.** Increased frequency of sound waves is perceived as a higher pitch sound. **C.** Increased amplitude of sound waves is perceived as a louder sound.

have the variable properties of **frequency** and **amplitude.** The frequency is the number of cycles of peaks and troughs in air pressure per second, measured in **hertz (Hz).** *The sound frequency determines the pitch (high or low tone) that we perceive. The amplitude of pressure cycles in a sound wave reflect the **intensity** of the sound and are perceived as its loudness.*

THE OUTER AND MIDDLE EAR

The visible outer ear (**pinna**) funnels sound down the **auditory canal** to the **tympanic membrane** (eardrum). The middle ear is an air-filled space beyond the tympanic membrane, containing a chain of three small bones (**ossicles**) called the **malleus,** the **incus,** and the **stapes.** Sound waves cause movements of the tympanic membrane, which are transferred across the middle ear by the ossicles to a second membrane, the **oval window.** The stapes bone moves like a piston in response to sound waves and passes sound vibrations into the fluid of the cochlea through the oval window. *The structures of the middle ear amplify the force of sound waves* in two ways, resulting in pressure forces at the oval window that are approximately 20 times greater than at the tympanic membrane:

1. The ossicles act as **levers** that transform the large movements of the tympanic membrane into smaller, more forceful vibrations of the oval window.

2. The **oval window** has a much smaller surface area than that of the tympanic membrane.

Other accessory structures of the middle ear include the eustachian tube and two small muscles, the **tensor tympani** and the **stapedius,** which are attached to the ossicles. The **eustachian tube** links the cavity of the middle ear to the nasal cavity and provides a route to equalize air pressure between the middle ear and the atmosphere (e.g., during ascent and descent of an airplane). The muscles of the middle ear mediate the **attenuation reflex** in response to excessively loud sounds. Contraction of the muscles stiffens the ossicles and reduces transmission of vibrations to the inner ear. The attenuation reflex has several functions:

- **Protection of hair cells** from damage due to excessive vibrations. However, the reflex has a long latency, approximately 0.1 s, so that sudden loud sounds are still damaging.

- **Prevention of saturation** of the hair cell transduction mechanism by a prolonged loud noise.

- **Discernment of speech** against ambient noise. Compared to higher frequency sounds (e.g., speech), the attenuation reflex suppresses low-frequency sounds more effectively and helps to dampen ambient noise.

▽ Vibration of the stapes is regulated by the stapedius muscle (the smallest muscle in the human body), which is innervated by the facial nerve (CN VII). A lesion of CN VII can result in paralysis of the stapedius, allowing excessive vibration of the stapes, which the patient will sense as **hyperacusia** (excessive sensitivity to sounds). ▽

THE INNER EAR

The inner ear includes all of the structures of the membranous labyrinth, although only the cochlea is concerned with the transduction of sound. The cochlea consists of three coiled tubes, located side by side: the **scala vestibuli,** the **scala media,** and the **scala tympani** (Figure 2-33A). The spiral coils of the cochlea are encased in a bony shell and are wrapped around a central bony pillar (the **modiolus**). The scala vestibuli is separated from the scala media by **Reissner's membrane,** and the scala media is separated from the scala tympani by the **basilar membrane.**

At the base of the cochlea, the oval window meets the scala vestibuli, and the **round window** meets the scala tympani. When the oval window bulges inward and compresses fluid in the cochlea, the round window can bulge outward to prevent excessive pressure changes within the cochlea. Movement of the oval

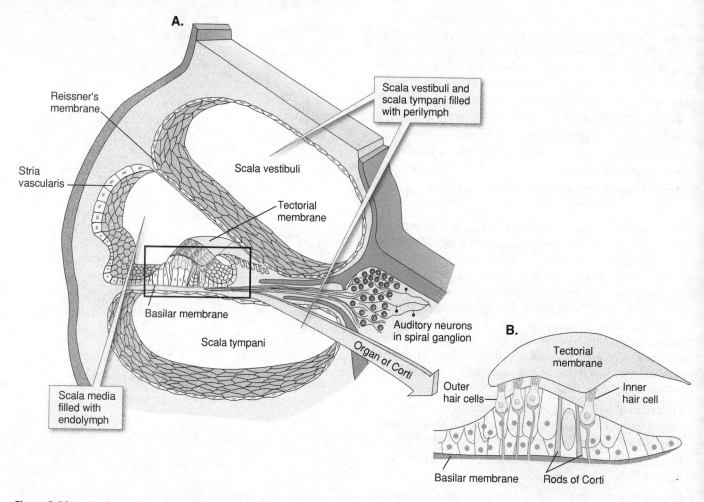

Figure 2-33: A. Cross-section through the cochlea. **B.** The organ of Corti.

window sets up a "traveling wave" that flexes the basilar membrane. *Movement of the basilar membrane is the key mechanical event that excites hair cells and results in action potentials in auditory neurons.*

The auditory receptors are located in the **organ of Corti,** which sits on top of the basilar membrane (see Figure 2-33B). The sensory hair cells rest on the basilar membrane and extend upward to a supporting membrane, the **reticular lamina,** which is anchored to the basilar membrane by **the rods of Corti.** The roof of the organ of Corti is formed by the gelatinous **tectorial membrane.** When a traveling wave passes along the basilar membrane, the hair cells, reticular lamina, and rods of Corti move as one unit toward the tectorial membrane. Traveling waves in the basilar membrane bend the stereocilia, which project from the surface of hair cells; *the deformation of stereocilia is the crucial event in the transduction of sound waves into a receptor potential.*

FLUIDS OF THE INNER EAR The inner ear is filled with fluid that facilitates the generation of traveling waves in the basilar membrane in response to movements of the oval window. Differences in the composition of the cochlea fluids are important for generation of receptor potentials in response to the traveling wave. The scala vestibuli and scala tympani are both filled with **perilymph,** which has a similar composition to other extracellular fluids; that is, low $[K^+]$ and high $[Na^+]$.

The scala vestibuli and the scala tympani are continuous with each other at the apex of the cochlea via a hole called the **helicotrema.** The scala media is a blind-ended structure that contains **endolymph,** *an unusual extracellular fluid because it has a high [K+] of 150 mM and a low [Na+] of 1 mM.* Endolymph is actively secreted by a layer of endothelial lining cells along one wall of the scala media, called the **stria vascularis.** The difference in [K+] between perilymph and endolymph creates an **endocochlear potential** difference across Reissner's membrane of about +80 mV in the endolymph.

▽ **Jervell and Lange-Nielsen syndrome** is a rare condition characterized by congenital deafness and cardiac arrhythmia. A genetic mutation occurs, which affects a K+ channel in the heart and in the inner ear. In the inner ear, this results in a decreased [K+] in the endolymph and therefore disruption of the endocochlear potential difference. Patients also have a prolonged cardiac action potential, which results in a long Q-T segment on the electrocardiogram. These K+ channel mutations result both in congenital deafness and the risk of sudden cardiac death! ▼

TRANSDUCTION OF SOUND

When vibration of the oval window causes a traveling wave in the basilar membrane, hair cells are pushed against the tectorial membrane. Hair cells have a tall **kinocilium** at one edge of the cell, which is surrounded by approximately 100 stereocilia. When stereocilia are in the upright position, the resting membrane potential of hair cells is approximately -70 mV. Displacement of the stereocilia toward the kinocilium opens mechanically gated, nonselective cation channels in the tips of stereocilia, resulting in membrane depolarization. Figure 2-34 shows that the hair cell body is bathed in perilymph, whereas the tips of stereocilia pierce the reticular lamina and are bathed in K+-rich endolymph. If displacement of the stereocilia opens cation channels, there is an influx of K+ and depolarization. This is contrary to the effect of opening K+ channels in other cells, but the presence of very high [K+] in endolymph and the positive endocochlear potential drive K+ influx into hair cells. A depolarizing receptor potential causes influx of Ca2+ and exocytosis of neurotransmitter (probably glutamate) from storage granules at the base of the cell. Conversely, displacement of stereocilia away from the kinocilium closes cation channels, thereby hyperpolarizing the hair cell membrane potential and decreasing neurotransmitter release.

FUNCTIONS OF INNER AND OUTER HAIR CELLS The hair cells located between the rods of Corti and the modiolus are referred to as inner hair cells, and those lateral to the rods of Corti are referred to as outer hair cells (Figure 2-33B). *Inner hair cells are responsible for the transduction of sound* because almost all the neurites from auditory nerves are associated with inner hair cells. The neurites that contact inner hair cells extend from neurons located in a swelling on the auditory nerve, called the **spiral ganglion** (Figure 2-33A). Axons from spiral ganglion neurons form the auditory nerve and enter the auditory pathway.

Outer hair cells are collectively referred to as the **cochlear amplifier** because they amplify the traveling wave that passes along the basilar membrane. Outer hair cells respond to sound

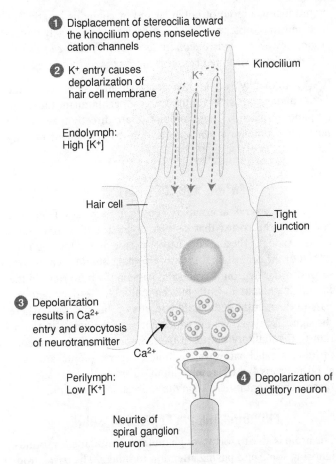

① Displacement of stereocilia toward the kinocilium opens nonselective cation channels

② K+ entry causes depolarization of hair cell membrane

Kinocilium

K+

Endolymph: High [K+]

Hair cell

Tight junction

③ Depolarization results in Ca2+ entry and exocytosis of neurotransmitter

Ca2+

Perilymph: Low [K+]

④ Depolarization of auditory neuron

Neurite of spiral ganglion neuron

Figure 2-34: Mechanotransduction of sound by a hair cell. Deformation of the stereocilia toward the large kinocilium results in the opening of mechanically gated cation channels. The resulting entry of K+ from the K+-rich endolymph causes depolarization of the hair cell and Ca2+ entry. Release of neurotransmitter by exocytosis from the base of the cell excites the neurites of auditory neurons.

by producing a receptor potential and by changing length. The mechanism of outer hair cell function is not completely understood; however, *selective damage to outer hair cells can lead to deafness, demonstrating the importance of the cochlear amplifier.*

▽ **Ototoxicity** is a known potential adverse effect of the **aminoglycoside antibiotics** (e.g., gentamicin, tobramycin, and amikacin). These antibiotics are directly toxic to the hair cells of the inner ear and can lead to permanent hearing loss. ▽

CENTRAL AUDITORY PATHWAYS

There are several alternative neuronal pathways from the cochlea to the cortex that synapse at intermediate brainstem nuclei. Axons of the auditory nerve synapse first in the **cochlear nuclei** of the brainstem. In one of the **main auditory pathways,** second-order neurons branch and pass up the brainstem in the **lateral lemniscus** to both **inferior colliculi.** Tertiary neurons pass to the **medial geniculate nucleus** of the thalamus, where the signal is relayed via the white matter of the **acoustic radiation** to the **auditory cortex** in the temporal lobe. The presence of other parallel pathways, multiple crossover points, and binaural neurons (which receive inputs from both ears) suggests that *no single brainstem lesion can cause unilateral deafness.*

ENCODING THE PROPERTIES OF SOUND

The brain is able to sort through multiple simultaneous sounds, ignoring some and paying attention to others. The basic properties of sounds that must be encoded to allow higher level processing are **intensity, frequency,** and **location.**

ENCODING SOUND INTENSITY The perception of the loudness of a sound correlates with the number of active auditory neurons and their rate of firing. More intense sounds cause larger vibrations that are spread across a larger area of the basilar membrane, thereby involving more hair cells and activation of more auditory neurons. Loudness is also correlated with the rate of action potential generation because larger distortions of hair cells produce larger receptor potentials, which increase action potential frequency in auditory neurons.

ENCODING SOUND FREQUENCY The frequency of sound waves determines the perception of pitch. Frequency encoding depends on the mechanical properties of the basilar membrane. At the base of the cochlea, the basilar membrane is narrow and stiff, whereas at the apex it is wider and more compliant (Figure 2-35A). High-frequency sounds produce traveling waves that peak near the base, and low-frequency sounds produce traveling waves that propagate all the way to the apex. As a result, each section of the basilar membrane has a **characteristic frequency** that produces a maximal deflection and a large hair cell response (known as the "**place code**") (see Figure 2-35B). The systematic organization of auditory nerves produces a map of the basilar membrane in the cochlear nuclei that represents the characteristic frequencies. This **tonotopic map** is preserved throughout the auditory pathway, so that the location of an active neuron reflects the frequency of the sound that excited it.

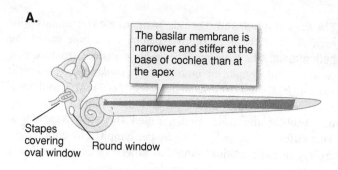

A.

The basilar membrane is narrower and stiffer at the base of cochlea than at the apex

Stapes covering oval window   Round window

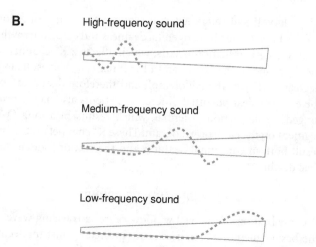

B.

High-frequency sound

Medium-frequency sound

Low-frequency sound

Figure 2-35: Place code for sound frequency. **A.** An uncoiled cochlea showing the nonuniform geometry of the basilar membrane. **B.** Representations of traveling waves produced in the basilar membrane by sounds of different frequencies. High-frequency sounds produce a traveling wave toward the base of the cochlea, whereas low-frequency sounds are represented by traveling waves reaching the apex of the cochlea.

LOCALIZATION OF SOUND The ability to localize the origin of a sound is important for survival (e.g., locating a moving vehicle). A major location cue is the **interaural time delay** between sounds arriving at both ears. Whenever a sound does not occur directly ahead or behind a person, it takes slightly longer for the sound to reach one ear compared to the other. A similar mechanism operates for a continuous tone because the phases of sound waves received by each ear are not exactly synchronized.

The second cue to location is the **interaural intensity difference,** which occurs because the head obstructs the passage of sound waves and casts a "sound shadow." For example, the head casts a sound shadow to the right if the sound comes directly from the left. In this case, the left ear receives a more intense stimulus than the right ear. The difference in neuronal responses between the ears, for the same sound, is used to encode location.

The outer ear is important in locating sounds moving in the vertical plane for which there are no differences in interaural timing or intensity. Sounds are reflected off the folds of the pinna, creating delays between sound waves that enter the auditory canal directly and those that are reflected off the pinna.

▽ **Deafness** can be characterized as either conductive or sensorineural hearing loss. **Conductive hearing loss** can be caused by a defect in any of the sound-conducting structures (e.g., auricle, external auditory canal, tympanic membrane, or the middle ear, including the ossicles). On the other hand, **sensorineural hearing loss** can be a result of a lesion of the inner ear or CN VIII (vestibulocochlear nerve).

The **Weber and Rinne tuning fork tests** are used to differentiate conductive hearing loss from sensorineural hearing loss. The Weber test is performed by placing the stem of a vibrating tuning fork on top of the patient's skull, an equal distance from each ear. The patient is asked to indicate in which ear the sound is heard louder. The normal response is to hear the sound with both ears equally. The Rinne test is performed by initially placing the vibrating tuning fork against the mastoid process behind the ear until the sound is no longer heard; the fork is then immediately placed in the air just outside the ear. The normal response is to detect sound by air conduction better than bone conduction.

- In *unilateral conductive hearing loss,* the Weber test will result in lateralization of the vibrations toward the affected side because the ambient room noise is absent on this side; the Rinne test will indicate bone conduction greater than air conduction.

- In *unilateral sensorineural hearing loss,* the Weber test will result in lateralization of the vibrations to the unaffected side; the Rinne test will indicate air conduction greater than bone conduction. ▽

THE VESTIBULAR LABYRINTH

The function of the vestibular system is to provide a **sense of balance and equilibrium.** Input from the vestibular system is also important in the control of **eye movement and body posture.** *Vestibular dysfunction is manifested by uncontrolled* *eye movements and feelings of nausea and vertigo.* There are two types of structures in the inner ear that provide vestibular sensation, the otolith organs and the semicircular canals, both of which are hollow organs containing endolymph.

1. The **otolith organs** (the utricle and saccule) detect tilting of the head and linear acceleration.

2. The **semicircular canals** detect angular acceleration produced by rotation of the head.

THE OTOLITH ORGANS The otolith organs include two chambers within the labyrinth, the **utricle** and the **saccule** (Figure 2-36A). Hair cells are located in a sensory epithelium called the macula. The tips of hair cell stereocilia project into a gelatinous cap, which is covered in small calcium carbonate crystals called **otoliths** (see Figure 2-36B). Movement of the head displaces otoliths and bends the stereocilia, resulting in development of a receptor potential in the same way as that described for auditory hair cells. The otolith organs transduce two types of information, the static angle (tilting) of the head and the presence of linear acceleration.

1. **Tilting of the head** changes the angle between the otolith organs and the direction of the force of gravity. Different degrees of tension are placed on hair cell stereocilia, depending on their orientation. All possible angles are represented because the *macula of each utricle is oriented horizontally and the macula of each saccule is oriented vertically.*

2. **Linear acceleration** (e.g., starting and stopping when riding in a vehicle) also displaces the otoliths and excites hair cells in the maculae. *(Note: when traveling at a **constant velocity**, there is no acceleration, resulting in the sensation of being perfectly still.)*

THE SEMICIRCULAR CANALS There are three semicircular canals arranged at right angles to each other. The hair cells of each canal are located in a swelling called the **ampulla;** the cilia of the hair cells project into a gelatinous mass called the **cupula** (Figure 2-37). Movements of the cupula cause generation of receptor potentials in the hair cells. The presence of three semicircular canals provides information about all possible orientations.

Rotation of the head produces **angular acceleration forces.** When the head begins to rotate, there is a lag in the movement of the endolymph, causing the cupula to be deflected like a sail being hit by the wind. The semicircular canals respond to rotation in different planes as follows:

The **superior canal** senses rotation front to back (e.g., nodding the head for "yes").

The **horizontal canal** senses rotation left to right (e.g., shaking the head for "no").

The **posterior canal** senses rotation in the plane from the left to the right shoulder.

The position of the semicircular canals on one side of the head is the mirror image of those on the other side. In this arrangement, any rotation will cause stimulation on one side and inhibition on the other side, thereby augmenting the vestibular stimulus to the brain.

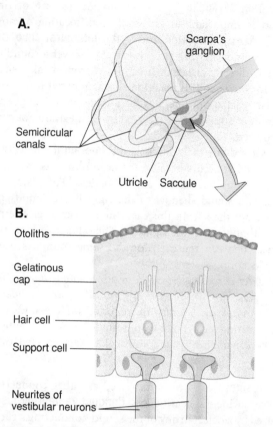

Figure 2-36: The otolith organs. **A.** Location of the utricle and saccule (cochlea removed). **B.** Cross-section through an otolith organ showing the sensory epithelium (macula). Stereocilia of vestibular hair cells are embedded in a gelatinous cap, which is covered in otolith crystals. Tilting of the head, or linear acceleration forces, displace the stereocilia, resulting in the generation of a hair cell receptor potential.

If constant rotation occurs for approximately 30 seconds, the movement of endolymph "catches up" so that the canal and endolymph move together at the same speed. The angular acceleration is now zero, and the cupula is no longer deflected. If rotation is suddenly stopped, inertia causes the endolymph to bend the cupula in the opposite direction, which is accompanied by the sensation of spinning in the opposite direction.

THE CENTRAL VESTIBULAR PATHWAYS The primary afferent vestibular neurons are located in a swelling on the vestibular nerve called **Scarpa's ganglion.** Neurites extend to the vestibular hair cells, and action potential firing is modulated by the depolarizing or hyperpolarizing receptor potentials produced by hair cells. Axons of primary afferent neurons travel in the vestibular part of CN VIII to the **vestibular nucleus** of the brainstem. The vestibular nucleus has several parts, and sends **neuronal projections** to the following targets above and below the brainstem:

- **Projections to the cortex** occur via the thalamus as with other sensory pathways, although there is no equivalent "vestibular cortex" to the auditory and visual areas.

- There is a rich supply of second-order vestibular neurons to the **cerebellum** to coordinate movements, using information about body position.

- More direct vestibular input to motor neurons of the **lower limb** occurs via the **vestibulospinal tract,** which assists in the automatic maintenance of balance.

- Vestibular input to motor neurons of the **neck** facilitates independent maintenance of head position.

- Projections to the motor neurons for **extraocular muscles** are particularly important in keeping the eyes focused on an object as the body moves. The **vestibuloocular reflex** causes the eyes to turn in the direction opposite that of the rotation of the head. For example, if the gaze is fixed on a particular object, turning to the right causes both eyes to move toward the left, thereby keeping the object precisely in view. The vestibuloocular reflex relies on projections from the vestibular nucleus to nuclei of cranial nerves III, IV, and VI, which control eye movements.

▽ **Vertigo,** often imprecisely referred to as dizziness, is the sensation that either the body or the environment is moving when actually both are stationary, and is classically described as a spinning sensation. Spatial orientation and posture are controlled by three sensory systems: vestibular, visual, and somatosensory. A mismatch between any of these three systems can result in vertigo; *vestibular dysfunction is the most common cause of pathologic vertigo.* Vertigo is commonly accompanied by nausea, nystagmus, postural unsteadiness, and gait ataxia. Several clues obtained during the physical examination can help to differentiate peripheral causes of vertigo (e.g., Ménière's disease, benign positional vertigo, or labyrinthitis) from central causes of vertigo (e.g., cerebellar infarct or mass).

A finding in **peripheral vertigo** is nystagmus that is unidirectional and has fast saccadic eye movements in the opposite

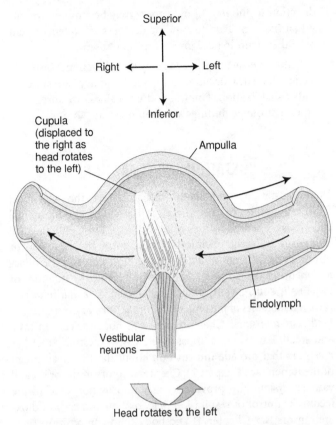

Figure 2-37: Cross-section through the ampulla of a semicircular canal. The movement of the cupula in the horizontal canal is shown as the head rotates to the left.

direction to the lesion; nystagmus may be suppressed with visual fixation. Tinnitus and/or deafness are often present, but other neurologic signs are typically absent.

In **central vertigo**, nystagmus may be bidirectional or unidirectional, vertical or purely horizontal, and does not suppress with visual fixation. Tinnitus and/or deafness are absent, but other neurologic findings are often present. ▼

GUSTATION AND OLFACTION

Taste (gustation) and **smell** (olfaction) are the two most familiar examples of chemoreception in which environmental chemicals are sensed by the nervous system. The ability to smell numerous different chemicals results from the existence of hundreds of different **olfactory receptor proteins** in the olfactory neurons. In contrast, there are only five basic qualities of taste: **salt, sour, sweet, bitter,** and **umami.** *The ability to perceive the subtleties of flavor depends on the normal functioning of both taste and smell.* Chemoreception is not restricted to taste and smell. For example, most of the gastrointestinal tract has receptors that provide information about the chemical milieu of the lumen (see Chapter 7). Chemoreceptors in the brain and vascular system also provide sensory information used in the feedback control of respiration (e.g., oxygen and carbon dioxide sensors; see Chapter 4) and body fluid composition (e.g., osmoreceptors; see Chapter 6).

GUSTATORY RECEPTORS

Taste receptors are located on projections from the surface of the tongue called **papillae.** Each papilla has numerous **taste buds,** which open onto the surface of the tongue at a small depression called the **taste pore.** Each taste bud contains approximately 100 **taste receptor cells,** which bear microvilli that project into the taste pore (Figure 2-38A). The microvilli are the chemically sensitive region of the cell. Sensory neurons form synapses at the base of taste receptor cells.

There are different transduction mechanisms underlying the five primary qualities of taste, which are summarized below (see Figure 2-38B). Most taste receptor cells have more than one of the transduction mechanisms and can therefore respond to two or more of the basic tastes. *Every taste transduction mechanism causes depolarization of the receptor cell,* which causes Ca^{2+} entry into the cell and exocytosis of neurotransmitters (as yet unknown) to stimulate gustatory neurons.

1. **Salt** receptors use a Na^+ channel to sense the $[Na^+]$ in the mouth. Na^+ enters the receptor cell, causing a graded receptor potential; an increase in $[Na^+]$ in the mouth drives more Na^+ entry, resulting in a larger depolarization.

2. **Sourness** receptors respond to *acidity.* H^+ binds to and inhibits a type of K^+ channel in the cell membrane, resulting in reduced K^+ conductance and membrane depolarization.

3. **Sweetness** receptors use intracellular second messengers (see Chapter 8 for a discussion of intracellular second messenger systems). For example, binding of a sugar may stimulate formation of cyclic adenosine monophosphate (cAMP),

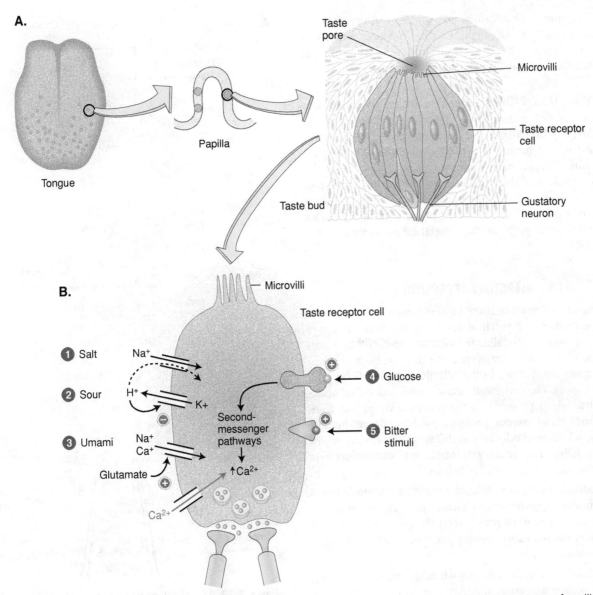

Figure 2-38: Taste receptors. **A.** Location of taste receptors within taste buds on the tongue, which are located on various types of papillae. Taste buds consist of a collection of taste receptor cells, each of which communicates with a sensory neuron. **B.** Sensory transduction mechanisms for the primary qualities of taste (*note: some taste receptors do not express every transduction mechanism*).

which inhibits a K⁺ channel and depolarizes the receptor cell membrane.

4. **Bitterness** receptors use more than one transduction mechanism, depending on the tastant. Mechanisms include direct binding to K⁺ channels and changes in second messengers.

5. **Umami** (Japanese word meaning "delicious") receptors respond to amino acids, particularly glutamate. An ionotropic glutamate receptor mediates depolarization. The umami receptor accounts for the desirable flavor of amino acids, such as the culinary additive **monosodium glutamate (MSG).**

▽   **MSG** consumption has been implicated in a collection of symptoms, known as the **Chinese restaurant syndrome,** which some people experience after eating Chinese food. The symptom complex includes headache, flushing, sweating, perioral numbness and tingling, chest pains, and occasionally more severe symptoms such as cardiac arrhythmias and airway swelling and obstruction. Although MSG has not been proven to cause this syndrome, the Food and Drug Administration has mandated that food labels include MSG warnings. ▼

THE CENTRAL TASTE PATHWAY Afferent information about taste from the anterior two thirds of the tongue is carried in the **facial nerve (CN VII);** taste sensation from the posterior one third of the tongue is carried in the **glossopharyngeal nerve (CN IX).** Primary sensory neurons synapse in the gustatory nucleus of the medulla. Second-order neurons cross the midline and ascend to the thalamus; third-order neurons are relayed from the thalamus to the primary **gustatory cortex** in the postcentral gyrus of the parietal lobe and then to the insular lobe.

OLFACTORY RECEPTORS

The olfactory receptor cells are bipolar neurons. A peripheral neurite extends into a patch of nasal membrane in the upper part of the nasal cavity called the **olfactory epithelium.** A central axon joins an olfactory nerve and enters the brain through one of many small holes in the **cribriform plate** of the skull (Figure 2-39A). The peripheral neurite bears cilia, called **olfactory hairs,** which project into the mucus covering the nasal membrane. Nasal mucus contains soluble **odorant-binding proteins,** which help odorants to diffuse to the surface of the olfactory hairs. The **sensory transduction mechanism** that detects the odorant functions as follows:

▪ The odorant binds to an **olfactory receptor protein** (a transmembrane receptor) in an olfactory hair. There are several hundred different olfactory receptor proteins, and each olfactory neuron expresses only one type of olfactory receptor protein.

▪ All olfactory receptor proteins stimulate the G protein G_{olf} when occupied by an odorant.

▪ Adenylyl cyclase is stimulated, which increases the concentration of the intracellular second messenger **cAMP.**

▪ cAMP opens **nonselective cation channels,** causing membrane depolarization.

▪ **Voltage-gated Ca^{2+} channels** open in response to depolarization.

▪ Depolarization is augmented by the opening of **Ca^{2+}-activated Cl^- channels.**

▪ When the receptor potential reaches threshold, action potentials are generated in the cell body and axon of the olfactory neuron.

The olfactory response is terminated when odorants diffuse away and when enzymes within the mucus break down the odorants.

THE CENTRAL OLFACTORY PATHWAY In contrast to the three-neuron chain of the gustatory pathway, *the main olfactory pathway includes only two neurons and does not synapse in the thalamus.* Axons of the olfactory receptor neurons enter the **olfactory bulb,** an ovoid structure on the inferior surface of the frontal

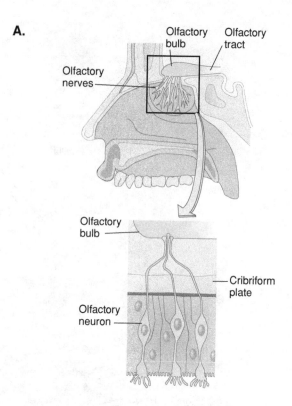

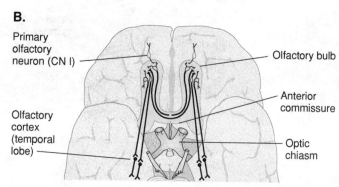

Figure 2-39: The olfactory system. **A.** The olfactory epithelium is located in a patch of nasal membrane. Primary sensory neurons pass via small holes in the cribriform plate of the skull to enter the olfactory bulb. **B.** The main central olfactory pathway conveys second-order neurons from the olfactory bulb directly to the olfactory cortex in the temporal lobe. Some fibers pass between olfactory bulbs by crossing the midline via the anterior commissure.

lobe, where they synapse with second-order neurons. The second neuron in the chain sends axons via the **olfactory tract** to the **olfactory cortex** in the temporal lobe (see Figure 2-39B). Some second-order neurons cross the midline via a band of white matter, called the anterior commissure, to synapse in the opposite olfactory bulb.

▽ **Kallmann syndrome** is an X-linked disorder characterized by congenital anosmia (lack of smell) and gonadotropin-releasing hormone (GnRH) deficiency. During embryologic development, anosmin, the mutated protein associated with this syndrome, is needed to mediate migration of the olfactory bulb and GnRH-producing neural progenitor cells. The lack of neural migration results in this syndrome. ▼

MOTOR NEUROPHYSIOLOGY

OVERVIEW OF THE SOMATIC MOTOR SYSTEM

The human skeleton is a system of levers that are moved by contraction of skeletal muscles. The motor system is comprised of skeletal muscles and the neurons that control them. Muscle contraction only occurs in response to action potentials in **alpha motor neurons,** which originate in the ventral gray matter of the spinal cord (and brainstem nuclei) and constitute the **final common path** for motor control (see Chapter 1). The **hierarchy of motor control** within the CNS is as follows:

- The highest level of control resides in areas of **association cortex** and the **basal ganglia,** which determine the goal of movements.
- The **primary motor cortex** and **cerebellum** determine the correct sequence of commands that will allow the goal to be achieved.
- Neuronal circuits in the **spinal cord** are the lowest level of control and function to implement descending commands.

SPINAL CONTROL OF MOVEMENT

There are **three inputs to alpha motor neurons** that determine which muscle fibers will contract: upper motor neurons, spinal interneurons, and sensory neurons.

1. **Upper motor neurons** from the cortex or brainstem are important mediators of voluntary movements and are mainly inhibitory in nature.
2. **Spinal interneurons** may be excitatory or inhibitory and form an extensive circuitry within the spinal cord. Basic motor programs (e.g., walking) are encoded in spinal circuits known as **central pattern generators,** which include many spinal interneurons. Spinal circuits are accessed and modulated by higher centers as appropriate.
3. **Sensory neurons from muscle proprioceptors** provide feedback about muscle length and tension.

PROPRIOCEPTORS Sensory information and feedback is needed at every stage of motor control to ensure smooth, coordinated, and accurate movements. Sensory information about body position and its relationship to the environment is relayed from the vestibular, visual, and auditory systems. A large amount of somatosensory information comes from receptors (e.g., Pacinian corpuscles) in the skin and joint capsules. In addition, **muscles contain two types of proprioceptors** that provide feedback about muscle length and tension:

1. **Muscle spindles** consist of several specialized muscle fibers called **intrafusal fibers,** which are contained in a fibrous capsule (Figure 2-40A). Intrafusal fibers are connected at both ends to the force-generating extrafusal muscle fibers. The middle portion of a muscle spindle is expanded because sensory axons are wrapped around the intrafusal fibers at this location. The sensory fibers are large myelinated axons, known as type Ia, and have very fast conduction speeds. *Muscle spindles provide information to the CNS about muscle stretch (length) and the speed with which muscle length is changing.*

2. **Golgi tendon organs** are sensory nerve terminals that are encapsulated within tendons (see Figure 2-40B). They are arranged *in series* with extrafusal muscles fibers, with one end attached to the extrafusal muscle fibers and the other end attached to the collagen fibers of the tendon. The sensory axons are smaller than type Ia fibers and are designated type Ib. *Golgi tendon organs provide information about muscle force.*

GAMMA MOTOR NEURONS Although the central region of a muscle spindle is not contractile, there are contractile filaments at each end. The motor supply to contractile filaments within muscle spindles is from gamma motor neurons and is referred to as the **fusimotor system.** The cell bodies of gamma motor neurons are located in the ventral gray matter of the spinal cord. *Contraction of intrafusal fibers alters the sensitivity of muscle spindles.* For example, intrafusal fibers and extrafusal fibers must shorten at the same time to prevent the muscle spindles from becoming slack, which would inappropriately decrease their rate of action potential generation. Modulating the tone of intrafusal fibers through the activity of the fusimotor system allows the activity of muscle spindles to be maintained as muscle length and tension vary.

THE MYOTACTIC REFLEX The myotactic (**muscle stretch**) reflex is demonstrated by tapping a tendon with a reflex hammer; for example, when testing the **knee jerk reflex** (Figure 2-41).

- Tapping the patellar tendon causes a small degree of **stretch in the quadriceps muscle,** which results in the generation of action potentials in Ia afferents from muscle spindles.

- A **monosynaptic reflex arc** is formed when sensory afferents enter the spinal cord, via the dorsal root, and synapse directly on the alpha motor neurons; reflex contraction of the quadriceps causes the knee jerk response.

The physiologic function of the monosynaptic myotactic reflex is to resist gravity. When a load is placed on a muscle, it is stretched, which results in reflex contraction of the muscle to take up the load.

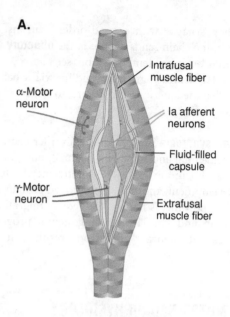

A.

- Intrafusal muscle fiber
- α-Motor neuron
- Ia afferent neurons
- Fluid-filled capsule
- γ-Motor neuron
- Extrafusal muscle fiber

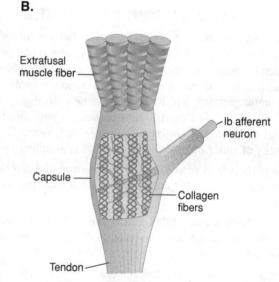

B.

- Extrafusal muscle fiber
- Ib afferent neuron
- Capsule
- Collagen fibers
- Tendon

Figure 2-40: Muscle proprioceptors. **A.** Muscle spindle. Intrafusal muscles fibers are arranged in parallel with the extrafusal muscle fibers. Muscle length is monitored by myelinated Ia afferent neurons coiled around the midsection of intrafusal fibers. Gamma motor neurons contract intrafusal fibers to maintain spindle tension when surrounding extrafusal fibers contract. **B.** A Golgi tendon organ arranged in series with muscle fibers at the junction between the muscle and tendon. Sensory endings of Ib afferent neurons are intertwined with collagen filaments and detect the force of muscle contraction.

A lesion in any part of the myotactic reflex circuit will result in **areflexia.** The following deep tendon reflexes (and their associated spinal segments) are important to know when performing a neurologic examination:

- Brachioradialis (C5–C6)
- Biceps (C5–C6)
- Triceps (C6–C7)
- Knee (L2–L4)
- Ankle (S1)

RECIPROCAL INHIBITION In many cases, muscles work in antagonistic pairs (e.g., the biceps and triceps muscles of the arm, or the quadriceps and hamstring muscles of the thigh). When a muscle produces movement by shortening, it is referred to as an **agonist;** muscles that oppose the action of the agonist are **antagonists.** To execute a simple movement (e.g., flexion of the elbow), the contraction of biceps is accompanied by relaxation of its antagonist, the triceps muscle; this phenomenon is known as **reciprocal inhibition** and is mediated by spinal interneurons. Reciprocal inhibition also occurs in the myotactic reflex because collateral branches of the Ia afferents synapse on inhibitory interneurons that supply alpha motor neurons of the antagonist muscle (Figure 2-41).

THE REVERSE MYOTACTIC REFLEX The reverse (inverse) myotactic reflex is the reflex inhibition of muscle contraction stimulated by active contraction of the muscle itself. The reverse myotactic response protects a muscle from a potentially damaging overload during extreme contraction. However, its more important function in muscles under normal loading conditions is to provide a *tension feedback system* that regulates muscle tension during a sustained contraction. For example, when picking up a fragile object such as an egg, a steady force that is not too powerful must be applied. As muscle tension increases, the reverse myotactic reflex slows muscle contraction. As muscle tension then decreases, the activity of the reflex declines and allows tension to increase; this balance allows the maintenance of a steady controlled force. *The reverse myotactic reflex is mediated by Golgi tendon organs;* sensory afferents enter the dorsal root and synapse on inhibitory interneurons, which suppress alpha motor neurons of the agonist muscle.

THE FLEXOR WITHDRAWAL REFLEX Spinal interneurons are not always inhibitory, as demonstrated by the flexor withdrawal response, which protects the affected limb by rapidly removing it from an injurious stimulus. The **steps of the flexor withdrawal reflex response** can be illustrated, for example, when a painful stimulus is applied to one leg (Figure 2-42):

- **Pain receptors** are activated at the site of stimulation.
- **Afferent pain fibers** enter the dorsal root and send collaterals to several spinal segments.
- **Excitatory interneurons** that synapse with alpha motor neurons serving flexors are stimulated. Contraction of flexors removes the limb from the aversive stimulus.

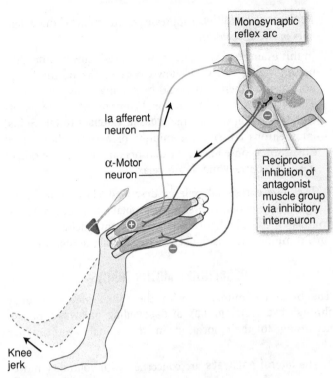

Figure 2-41: The knee jerk reflex, an example of the myotactic (stretch) reflex. Muscle contraction is stimulated by a monosynaptic pathway following activation of muscle spindle afferents. Reciprocal inhibition of antagonist muscles occurs simultaneously, via inhibitory spinal interneurons.

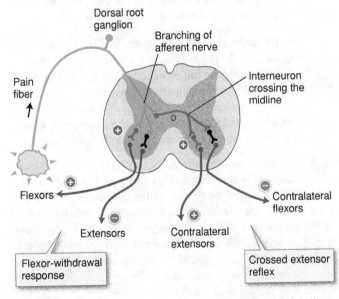

Figure 2-42: The flexor withdrawal reflex pathway. If a painful stimulus is applied to one side of the body, flexors contract and extensors relax on that side to rapidly remove the body part from the stimulus. The opposite response occurs on the contralateral side of the body to maintain posture; this crossed extensor reflex is mediated by spinal interneurons.

■ **Reciprocal inhibition** suppresses contraction of the extensors of the affected limb.

■ In this example, where one leg would suddenly be lifted, the person would rarely fall down because the postural support of the other limb would be simultaneously increased. This occurs due to an additional component of the flexor-withdrawal reflex, called the **crossed extensor reflex.** Spinal interneurons crossing the midline orchestrate the crossed extensor response in which extensors on the opposite side of the body contract and flexors relax.

The different spinal reflexes described above provide an insight into the extensive network of spinal interneurons. Motor commands from higher centers are frequently delivered to the final common path via the network of spinal interneurons.

DESCENDING MOTOR TRACTS

The brain communicates with the spinal motor circuitry through **two major groups of descending pathways,** named according to their location in the spinal white matter (Figure 2-43A):

1. The **lateral pathways** are concerned with voluntary movement of the distal muscles (e.g., muscles of the arm and hand). There are **two major pathways** in this group, the corticospinal tract and the rubrospinal tract.

   ■ The **corticospinal (pyramidal) tract** contains fibers that mostly originate from the motor cortex; the fibers descend through the internal capsule and upper brainstem to the medullary pyramids, where the tract crosses the midline.

   ▽ Similar to the sensory pathways, the site of decussation of the **lateral corticospinal tract** has significant clinical implications. *Lesions above the medullary pyramids will result in contralateral muscle weakness; lesions below the pyramidal decussation will produce an ipsilateral muscle weakness.* ▽

   ■ The **rubrospinal tract** is a much smaller pathway that originates in the red nucleus of the midbrain. Neurons are active in simpler voluntary actions such as walking. Many functions of the rubrospinal tract are redundant in humans due to the presence of a highly developed corticospinal tract. However, *if the corticospinal tract is damaged, some of its functions may be recovered via the rubrospinal tract.*

   ▽ For the comatose patient, "posturing" can clue the physician to the site of neurologic damage. **Decorticate posturing,** characterized by flexion of the elbows and wrists and supination of the arms, indicates damage immediately rostral to the red nucleus of the midbrain. An intact red nucleus allows the upper extremities to undergo flexion. In contrast, **decerebrate posturing,** characterized by extension of the elbows and wrists with pronation, indicates a midbrain lesion that involves the level of the red nucleus. ▽

2. The **ventromedial pathways** originate in the brainstem and innervate the proximal and axial muscles to help maintain head position and posture. Sensory information about the body position and balance is derived from the visual and vestibular systems and is conveyed via **three major tracts:**

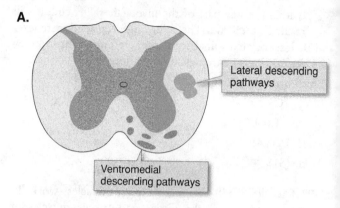

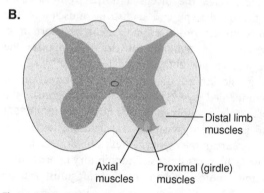

Figure 2-43: A. Descending motor pathways in the spinal white matter. **B.** Organization of alpha motor neurons in the ventral gray matter of the spinal cord. Note that a major function of the lateral pathways is to mediate voluntary control of the (laterally placed) alpha motor neurons to the distal limb muscles.

The **vestibulospinal tract** originates in the vestibular nuclei and provides one of the links between the sensors for balance and the extensor muscles, which are important for maintaining posture.

The **tectospinal tract** originates in the superior colliculus of the midbrain, which receives input from the retina and visual cortex and has reciprocal connections with the vestibular nuclei. The main function of the tectospinal tract is to direct the head and eyes to move toward a selected object in the visual field.

The **reticulospinal tract** originates in the reticular formation and consists of two antagonistic pathways: one from the pontine reticular area and the other from the medullary reticular area. A balance between the activities of these pathways facilitates fine control of posture through actions on the extensor muscles of the lower limb.

The **lower motor neurons** in the spinal cord are organized in a predictable manner that is consistent with the function and location of the descending motor tracts (see Figure 2-43B). The group of alpha motor neurons that serves a single muscle is known as the **motor neuron pool.** Motor neuron pools that control a particular action (e.g., flexion of the wrist) are located close to each other in the ventral horn of the spinal cord. Thus, there is a **medial to lateral organization,** with the distal muscles of the limbs represented most laterally, the axial muscles of the trunk represented medially, and the motor neurons for the proximal limb (girdle) muscles located in an intermediate position.

▽ Interpreting the cause of motor weakness necessitates distinguishing an upper motor neuron lesion from a lower motor neuron lesion. Each has characteristic physical findings:

Upper motor neuron lesions are characterized by spastic paresis (an incomplete paralysis), hyperreflexia, hypertonia, and a positive Babinski sign (upturned toes when the lateral edge of the sole is stroked with a blunt object; the normal response is downturned toes and is referred to as the plantar response). *Note: the key to understanding the signs of an upper motor neuron lesion is remembering that upper motor neurons are typically inhibitory in nature.* Thus, *a lesion that disrupts upper motor neurons will remove the inhibition, resulting in* **spasticity.**

Lower motor neuron lesions are characterized by flaccid paralysis, areflexia, hypotonia, absent Babinski sign, fasciculations (visible muscle twitches), and atrophy. ▼

▽ **Poliomyelitis** is an example of a pure lower motor neuron lesion. The poliovirus infects and selectively destroys the motor neuron cell bodies located in the ventral horn of the spinal cord, typically in the lumbar region. ▼

▽ **Amyotrophic lateral sclerosis** (also known as ALS or Lou Gehrig's disease) is a progressive motor neuron disease that affects both upper and lower motor neurons. Although cranial nerve involvement does occur, this disease typically begins in the cervical spine. Patients with both an upper and a lower motor neuron lesion at the level of the cervical spine will present with *flaccid paresis of the upper extremities* and *spastic paresis of the lower extremities.* ▼

CORTICAL CONTROL OF MOTOR FUNCTIONS

The creation of instructions for movement engages many areas of the cerebral cortex, allowing perceptions about the spatial relations of the body to be combined with abstract thought and decision making. Axons found in the corticospinal tracts may therefore originate from one of several areas of the cerebral cortex; there are numerous connections between the cortical areas related to motor function. Much of the outflow to the corticospinal tract is relayed from the **primary motor cortex,** which is located in the precentral gyrus (Figure 2-5B) and has several characteristic features:

▨ Movements can be **stimulated by applying very weak electrical currents** to this area of the cortex.

▨ There is a detailed **somatotopic map** (similar to that of the primary sensory cortex); destruction of cortex in this area produces specific movement deficits.

▨ Neuronal output can be traced directly to spinal motor neurons and, in the case of the limbs, **produces movements in the contralateral side of the body.**

▼ The **middle cerebral artery** supplies the majority of the lateral surface of the cortex, including the section of primary motor cortex (and primary sensory cortex) responsible for movement (and sensation) of the face and upper extremities. The area responsible for the lower extremities is supplied by the **anterior cerebral artery.** An occlusion of the middle cerebral artery will cause contralateral spastic paresis (and impaired sensation) of the face and upper extremities, whereas occlusion of the anterior cerebral artery will have similar effects of the lower extremities. ▼

The area of cortex immediately rostral to the primary motor cortex is an extension of the motor cortex and has two defined areas:

1. The **supplementary motor cortex** is located medially and directs many axons to distal limb muscles via the corticospinal tract.

2. The **premotor cortex** is located laterally and communicates with the reticulospinal neurons controlling the proximal muscles.

Larger electrical currents must be applied to the supplemental and premotor areas to stimulate movements; the movements elicited by stimulating these areas are less discrete and may involve both sides of the body.

THE BASAL GANGLIA The basal ganglia are forebrain structures that consist of several interconnected **deep cerebral nuclei** (Figure 2-44A):

▨ The **striatum** (divided into the **caudate nucleus** and **putamen**).

▨ The **globus pallidus.**

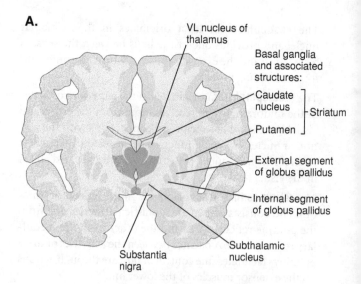

A.

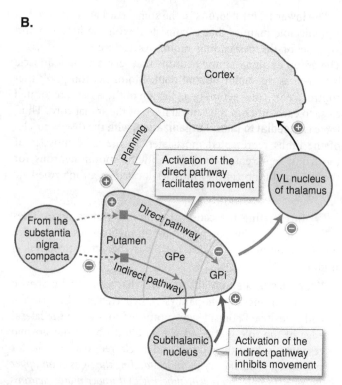

B.

Figure 2-44: The basal ganglia. A. Coronal section through the forebrain at the midthalamic level, showing the position of the basal ganglia. **B.** The major motor loop mediates a cycle of positive feedback from the cortex, through the basal ganglia, and back to the cortex via the ventrolateral (VL) nucleus of the thalamus. Excitatory cortical input to the basal ganglia is via the putamen; output from the basal ganglia is inhibitory via the internal segment of the globus pallidus and the pars reticulata of the substantia nigra (not shown). The direct pathway through the basal ganglia inhibits the output nuclei, resulting in disinhibition of the VL nucleus and facilitation of movement. The indirect pathway through the basal ganglia passes, via the external segment of the globus pallidus and subthalamic nucleus, and augments the inhibitory output nuclei. Dopaminergic inputs from the pars compacta of the substantia nigra promote motor behaviors by stimulating the direct pathway and inhibiting the indirect pathway.

- The **subthalamic nucleus.**
- The **substantia nigra** of the midbrain (although not part of the forebrain, it is a functional part of the basal ganglia).

The basal ganglia are a key part of a **motor loop,** which begins and ends in the cortex and is important in the initiation of voluntary movements. Therefore, a **cycle of positive feedback** occurs in which the basal ganglia provide the boost that initiates a movement from intentions into actions.

- Excitatory input from large areas of cortex involved in developing the strategy for a voluntary movement are funneled into the basal ganglia via the **striatum** (the putamen in particular).
- The final excitatory output from the basal ganglia back to the cortex arrives at the supplemental motor area, via the **ventral lateral nucleus (VLN)** of the thalamus.
- The output from the basal ganglia to the VLN is a tonic inhibitory stimulus, which is conveyed via the **internal segment of the globus pallidus** and the **pars reticulata of the substantial nigra.** Stimulation of the VLN occurs when the tonic inhibitory signal from the output nuclei is suppressed.

There are two distinct **pathways connecting the input and output nuclei of the basal ganglia** (see Figure 2-44B):

1. The **direct pathway** from the putamen to the internal segment of the globus pallidus is an inhibitory connection that suppresses the tonic inhibitory output nuclei. *Activation of the direct pathway therefore facilitates movement* by allowing positive feedback through the thalamocortical pathways.

2. The **indirect pathway** is conveyed to the output nuclei of the basal ganglia via the external segment of the globus pallidus and the subthalamic nucleus. Excitatory neurons from the subthalamic nucleus boost the activity of the output nuclei. *Stimulation of the indirect pathway therefore inhibits movement* by suppressing the VLN.

Disorders of the basal ganglia A fine balance between the activity of the direct and indirect pathways is necessary to ensure normal motor behaviors. The relative overactivity of the indirect pathway will result in paucity of movement (**hypokinesia**), whereas underactivity will lead to uncontrollable movements that lack purpose (**hyperkinesia**).

▽ In **Parkinson's disease,** there is degeneration of the dopaminergic neurons that project from the substantia nigra to the striatum. Dopaminergic input to the striatum has two main effects: (1) to stimulate the direct pathway, via activation of D_1 receptors, which facilitates movement; and (2) to inhibit the indirect pathway, via activation of D_2 receptors, which facilitates movement circuitously by inhibiting an inhibitory pathway. Thus, when dopaminergic input to the striatum decreases (as occurs in Parkinson's disease), the resulting imbalance favors paucity of movement (bradykinesia). The cardinal signs of **parkinsonism** are bradykinesia, rigidity, and a resting "pill-rolling" tremor. *The goal of therapy in Parkinson's disease is to rebalance the direct and indirect basal ganglia pathways to favor movement*, achieved by stimulating the direct path and/or inhibiting the indirect path. Administering **levodopa,** the metabolic precursor to dopamine, in combination with carbidopa (a decarboxylase inhibitor that blocks peripheral conversion of levodopa to dopamine, thereby increasing CNS bioavailability), accomplishes this goal. Utilization of direct dopamine-receptor agonists (e.g., bromocriptine) also improves symptoms. Another approach in therapy is to alter the cholinergic influence on the striatum. Acetylcholine drives the indirect pathway, decreasing movement. Use of anticholinergics (e.g., benztropine) will reduce indirect pathway stimulation, shifting the balance toward direct pathway output and movement. ▼

▽ **Huntington's disease** is a fatal autosomal dominant disorder in which patients present with an insidious onset of **chorea** (quick random involuntary movements, often of the extremities), progressive **dementia,** and **behavioral disorders.** The key pathologic lesion that characterizes this condition is severe idiopathic degeneration of GABA neurons in the striatum, resulting in atrophy of the caudate nucleus. ▼

▽ **Hemiballismus** most commonly results from a hypertensive lacunar infarct of the subthalamic nucleus and is clinically characterized by wild, violent flinging movements, typically of the upper extremities. *Note: the affected limb is contralateral to the involved subthalamic nucleus.* ▼

THE CEREBELLUM

The cerebellum ("little brain") is caudal to the occipital lobe and is attached to the posterior aspect of the brainstem by the paired inferior, middle, and superior **cerebellar peduncles.** The cerebellum receives a very large amount of input from the motor cortical areas as well as from the somatosensory, vestibular, visual, and auditory systems. The role of the cerebellum is to compare the intended movement with what is actually happening and to instruct the motor cortex to make the necessary adjustments to achieve smooth coordinated movements. *Cerebellar lesions produce a characteristic movement disorder called* **ataxia,** *in which movements become inaccurate and are poorly coordinated.*

▽ **Chronic alcohol abuse** can lead to cerebellar degeneration, most profoundly seen in the vermis, causing patients to have gait ataxia. ▼

Different structural and functional classifications can be used to describe the cerebellum. The gross anatomy of the cerebellum reveals two lateral hemispheres that are separated by a midline ridge called the vermis. These structures correlate with important **functional divisions** as follows:

▪ Output from the **vermis** is directed mainly to the ventromedial descending pathways controlling the axial musculature.

▪ Output from the **lateral hemispheres** is directed to the cerebral cortical areas, which then control limb movements via the lateral descending pathways.

Anatomic descriptions of the cerebellum utilize surface fissures to further define cerebellar lobes and lobules. The major lobes are the **anterior, posterior, and flocculonodular lobes**

(Figure 2-45). Most of the output from the cerebellum is relayed via three pairs of **deep cerebellar nuclei:** the **fastigial, interposed,** and **dentate** nuclei.

An alternative functional classification is often used, based on the **evolution of cerebellar functions:**

The **vestibulocerebellum** correlates with the flocculonodular lobe. *It is the most primitive system and contributes to the control of balance and eye movements.* Input arrives from the vestibular and visual systems and output is relayed to the vestibular nuclei of the brainstem.

The **spinocerebellum** correlates with the vermis and medial areas of the lateral hemispheres (referred to as the intermediate zone). Output from the vermis projects to the fastigial nucleus, and output from the intermediate zones projects via the interposed nucleus. *The spinocerebellum contributes to the control of posture and walking and modulates spinal reflex activity.*

▽ **Friedreich's ataxia** is the most common inherited form of ataxia. Degeneration of the spinocerebellar tracts, lateral corticospinal tracts, and dorsal columns are the predominant lesions associated with this condition, of which gait ataxia is the most common initial symptom. ▽

The **cerebrocerebellum** represents the highest level of evolution and occupies most of the lateral cerebral hemispheres. The motor cortical areas provide a massive neuronal projection via the pons to the lateral cerebellum. A **motor loop** is completed by output from the lateral cerebellum back to the motor cortex and premotor cortex via the dentate nucleus and VLN of the thalamus. *The cerebrocerebellum is crucial in the decisions regarding the detailed sequence and timing of muscle contractions needed to effect a coordinated movement.*

▽ In addition to ataxia, **cerebellar dysfunction** commonly presents with an intention tremor, dysmetria, and dysdiadochokinesia. An **intention tremor** is absent at rest and most prominent during voluntary movement toward a target. **Dysmetria** (past-pointing) is the inability to estimate distance as it relates to a voluntary movement and is assessed during the finger to nose test. Patients with dysmetria will often overshoot or undershoot their intended target. **Dysdiadochokinesia** is the impaired ability to perform rhythmic, rapid alternating movements, such as rapidly alternating supination and pronation of the hands; the movements become slow, poorly timed, and uncoordinated. *Note: physical findings are ipsilateral to the cerebellar lesion (i.e., a patient will fall toward the side of the cerebellar lesion).* ▽

In summary, the somatic motor system represents interactions between multiple areas of the nervous system. Imagine standing still, waiting to cross a busy street—the spinal circuits and the ventromedial descending pathways are stimulating antigravity muscles to maintain posture and are helping to coordinate head and eye movements to survey the traffic. The motor cortical areas are active in planning a movement strategy to cross the street, based on visual and auditory predictions of how fast automobiles are moving. As the moment to cross

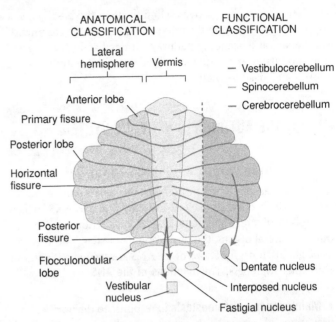

Figure 2-45: The cerebellum. The cerebellum is divided into anterior, posterior, and flocculonodular lobes by surface fissures (shown on the left). The functional regions of the cerebellum are the vestibulocerebellum, spinocerebellum, and cerebrocerebellum (shown on the right); the output pathways of the functional cerebellar areas via the cerebellar nuclei are shown (*note: the nuclei are bilateral but are only shown on the right*).

the street approaches, active cycling through the basal ganglia triggers movement, and the motor cortex sends the commands via the lateral descending pathways. Immediately, the cerebellum modulates and sequences the descending outputs into a coordinated dash to safety!

THE AUTONOMIC NERVOUS SYSTEM

OVERVIEW OF AUTONOMIC FUNCTION

The CNS has only two output systems: the somatic motor system, which controls skeletal muscles, and the ANS, which controls **involuntary functions.** The ANS is distributed throughout the visceral organs, the cardiovascular system, and the exocrine glands; most functions of the ANS are carried out without conscious awareness. The **functions of the ANS** can be broadly categorized in three areas:

1. **Maintenance of homeostasis** in response to the normal fluctuations of controlled variables (e.g., the negative feedback regulation of blood pressure).

2. **Integration of the stress response,** including the response to exercise and the classic "fight or flight" response.

3. **Integration of visceral function** (e.g., coordination of organs in the digestive system after the ingestion of food).

The divisions of the ANS are the **sympathetic, parasympathetic,** and **enteric nervous systems** (see Chapter 7, the Enteric Nervous System). The functions of the ANS are closely integrated with the endocrine system, largely because the **hypothalamus** controls both efferent ANS activity and the secretion of hormones by the **pituitary gland** (see Chapter 8).

In general, the actions of the sympathetic and parasympathetic divisions oppose each other (Table 2-6). *The activation of the sympathetic division is characterized by a widespread pattern of activation and occurs in* **response to stress.**

- In the cardiovascular system, **heart rate and contractility increase** and blood is redistributed to the muscles, heart, and brain by constriction of arterioles in the skin and viscera.

- Tissue metabolism is directed toward **energy utilization** by glycogenolysis in the liver and lipolysis in adipose tissue.

- Actions of the sympathetic division on **smooth muscle** include contraction of sphincters in the gastrointestinal and urinary tracts and the dilation of the bronchioles and pupils.

The functions of the parasympathetic division generally act to conserve and restore energy reserves. Heart rate is decreased, and the digestive functions of the gastrointestinal system are stimulated (see Chapter 7). In some cases, the sympathetic and parasympathetic divisions act cooperatively; for example, during the male sexual response, penile erection is mediated by parasympathetic neurons, whereas ejaculation is coordinated by the sympathetic division (see Chapter 9).

CIRCUITS OF THE ANS The general organization of the ANS includes correlates of the upper and lower motor neurons of the

TABLE 2-6. Effects of the Autonomic Nervous System on Effector Organs

Organ	Sympathetic Response	Sympathetic Receptor Type	Parasympathetic Response (All Mediated via Muscarinic Receptors)
Heart			
Sinoatrial node	Increased heart rate	β_1	Decreased heart rate
Atrioventricular node	Increased conduction speed	β_1	Decreased conduction speed
Myocardium	Increased contractility	β_1	–
Vascular smooth muscle	Constriction in skin, abdominal viscera, and kidney	α_1	–
	Dilation in skeletal muscle	β_2	–
Bronchiolar smooth muscle	Relaxation	β_2	Constriction
Gastrointestinal tract			
Circular smooth muscle	Reduced motility	α_2, β_2	Increased motility
Sphincters	Constriction	α_1	Relaxation
Secretion	Inhibition	α_2	Stimulation
Liver	Glycogenolysis and gluconeogenesis	β_2	–
Adipose tissue	Lipolysis	β_1, β_3	–
Kidney	Renin secretion	β_1	–
Urinary bladder			
Detrusor	Relaxation of bladder wall	β_2	Contraction of bladder wall
Sphincter	Constriction	α_1	Relaxation
Genitalia	Ejaculation; vaginal contraction	α_1	Erection
Eye			
Pupil	Dilation	α_1	Constriction
Ciliary muscle	–		Contraction (accommodation)

somatic motor system. The **hierarchy of ANS control** represents all levels of the nervous system:

1. The highest level of control incorporates motivational behaviors and responses to emotions, which are driven by the hypothalamus and the **limbic system** (see Integrative and Behavioral Functions of the Nervous System).

2. The **brainstem** is an important ANS control center, which contains nuclei that coordinate many basic homeostatic functions; for example, the **nucleus of the solitary tract** in the medulla is a site of cardiovascular, respiratory, and gastrointestinal control.

3. Reflexes at the level of the **spinal cord** also contribute to autonomic control (e.g., micturition, defecation, and ejaculation).

4. The lowest level of the ANS hierarchy is the **lower motor neurons,** which innervate target structures in the periphery. The cell bodies of lower motor neurons in the ANS are located outside the CNS, in **autonomic ganglia.** These neurons are referred to as **postganglionic neurons,** and are controlled by **preganglionic** neurons located either in the spinal cord or the brainstem.

THE SYMPATHETIC NERVOUS SYSTEM

Preganglionic sympathetic neurons originate in the **lateral horn** of the spinal cord and may synapse either in the **paravertebral ganglia,** which are arranged in a chain called the **sympathetic trunk,** or in the **collateral ganglia.** A preganglionic fiber can follow one of three pathways to its synapse with a postganglionic neuron (Figure 2-46):

1. Most sympathetic preganglionic axons are short; the myelinated axons exit the spinal cord, via ventral nerve roots, to join a spinal nerve and pass, via **white rami communicantes,** to synapse in a paravertebral ganglion.

2. Some fibers ascend or descend within the sympathetic trunk because *preganglionic sympathetic neurons only arise from spinal segments T1 to L2.* Therefore, some preganglionic axons from the upper thoracic spinal segments must ascend to the **cervical ganglia.** Some fibers from the lower lumbar spine descend to serve pelvic organs (e.g., bladder and reproductive organs) via the **sacral ganglia.**

3. Some preganglionic neurons in the thoracic region pass through the sympathetic trunk without synapsing. These neurons form the **splanchnic nerves,** which pass to the collateral ganglia associated with major abdominal blood vessels (i.e., the **celiac, superior mesenteric, inferior mesenteric, and renal arteries**).

The neurotransmitter released by preganglionic neurons is **acetylcholine,** which binds to **nicotinic (ionotropic) acetylcholine receptors** on the postganglionic neuron (*note: this is a different receptor than that expressed at the neuromuscular junction*). The binding of acetylcholine results in depolarization of the postganglionic neuron. There are **three possible routes taken by postganglionic sympathetic neurons** (Figure 2-47):

1. Postganglionic fibers destined for somatic structures in the body wall (e.g., skin, blood vessels, and sweat glands) are distributed in **spinal nerves.** Postganglionic fibers are unmyelinated and exit the paravertebral ganglia, via **gray rami communicantes,** to rejoin the spinal nerve.

2. Fibers from paravertebral ganglia, which are destined for internal organs, may form anatomically distinct nerves (e.g., **cardiac nerves**).

3. Postganglionic fibers may also be distributed in nerves that pass along the outside of the **arteries.** For example, fibers passing to the head via cervical ganglia and fibers originating in the collateral ganglia utilize this pathway.

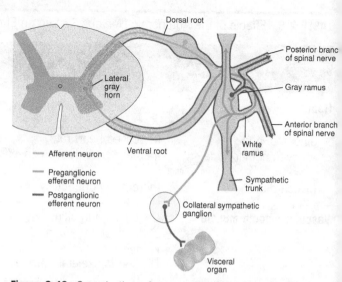

Figure 2-46: Organization of neurons in the sympathetic nervous system. Preganglionic neurons arise from the lateral horn of the spinal cord; myelinated fibers enter the sympathetic trunk via the white ramus. Preganglionic fibers may synapse in the sympathetic trunk at the same spinal level; they may ascend or descend within the sympathetic trunk or pass to collateral ganglia. Postganglionic fibers are unmyelinated and leave the sympathetic trunk via the gray ramus.

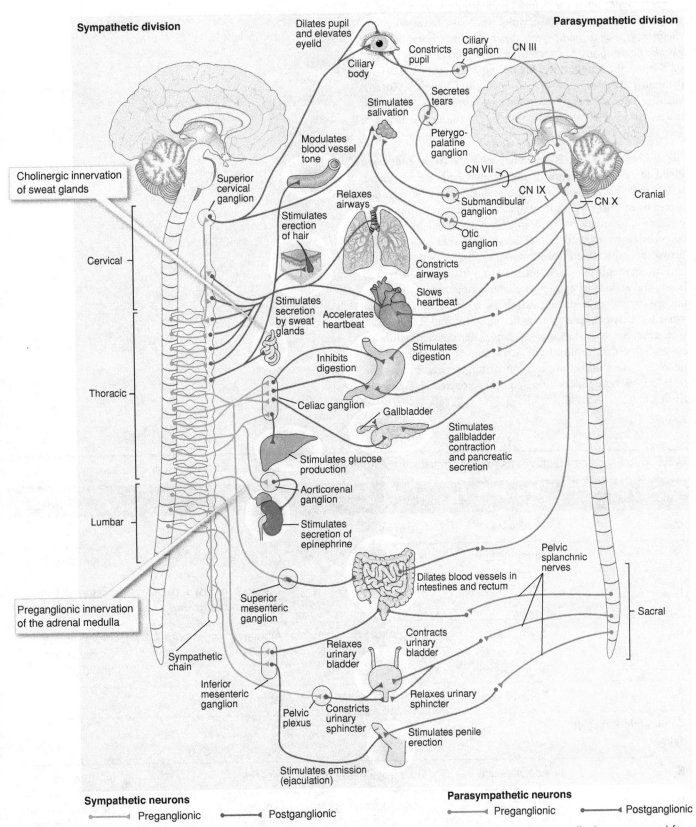

Figure 2-47: Organ-specific autonomic innervation. Acetylcholine is the neurotransmitter released from all preganglionic neurons and from parasympathetic postganglionic fibers. Sympathetic postganglionic fibers release norepinephrine (with the exception of cholinergic neurons to sweat glands). (*Note: the names of the parasympathetic ganglia serving the head and those of the collateral sympathetic ganglia are shown in the figure*).

Norepinephrine is the primary neurotransmitter released by postganglionic sympathetic neurons, with the exception of the cholinergic postganglionic sympathetic neurons serving the sweat glands. The responses of target cells to norepinephrine depend on the specific **adrenergic receptor type** (i.e., α_1, α_2, β_1, β_2, or β_3) that is expressed (see Table 2-6; see also Chapter 8, Adrenal Gland). The adrenergic receptors are important targets for drugs; some selective agonists and antagonists are listed in Table 2-7.

THE ADRENAL MEDULLA The adrenal medulla is an **endocrine gland** located at the core of the adrenal (suprarenal) gland, which is comprised of endocrine cells that may be regarded as modified postganglionic sympathetic neurons. Sympathetic preganglionic neurons pass to the adrenal gland, via the splanchnic nerves, and release acetylcholine as an excitatory neurotransmitter. Medullary endocrine cells secrete **epinephrine** and norepinephrine in a ratio of approximately 4:1. The hormonal actions of epinephrine are complementary to those elicited by norepinephrine acting as a neurotransmitter at synapses between postganglionic neurons and target cells (see Chapter 8). The increased plasma concentration of epinephrine that results from activation of the sympathetic nervous system allows stimulation of target cells that receive little sympathetic innervation (e.g., hepatocytes and adipose tissue).

TABLE 2-7. Signaling Mechanisms and Pharmacology of Autonomic Receptor Subtypes

Adrenergic-Receptor Type	Physiologic Agonist	Signaling Mechanism	Pharmacologic Agonist	Pharmacologic Antagonist
α_1	Norepi $\geq$ Epi	IP_3/DAG/Ca^{2+}	Phenylephrine	Prazosin
α_2	Norepi $\geq$ Epi	$\downarrow$ [cAMP]	Clonidine, methyldopa	Yohimbine
β_1	Epi > Norepi	$\uparrow$ [cAMP]	Dobutamine ($\beta_1 > \beta_2$), isoproterenol ($\beta_1 = \beta_2$)	Metoprolol
β_2	Epi > Norepi	$\uparrow$ [cAMP]	Albuterol, isoproterenol ($\beta_1 = \beta_2$)	Propranolol (nonselective β_1 and β_2)
β_3	Epi > Norepi	$\uparrow$ [cAMP]	Isoproterenol	
Cholinergic-Receptor Type				
N_1	Acetylcholine	Ionotropic receptor	Nicotine	D-Tubocurarine
N_2	Acetylcholine	Ionotropic receptor	Nicotine	Hexamethonium, mecamylamine
M_{1-5}	Acetylcholine	Various	Bethanechol, methacholine, pilocarpine	Atropine, benztropine, ipratropium

cAMP, cyclic adenosine monophosphate; DAG, diacylglycerol; Epi, epinephrine; IP_3, inositol 1,4,5-triphosphate; M_{1-5}, muscarinic receptors (five subtypes); N_1, nicotinic receptor at the neuromuscular junction; N_2, nicotinic receptor at autonomic ganglia; Norepi, norepinephrine.

THE PARASYMPATHETIC NERVOUS SYSTEM

In general, the parasympathetic preganglionic fibers are long and synapse with postganglionic neurons that are either in ganglia close to the target organ or are within the target organ itself. Most preganglionic fibers originate in the brainstem in nuclei that coordinate the autonomic responses of their target organs. Axons are contained in **four cranial nerves** (Figure 2-47):

1. The **occulomotor nerve** (CN III) conveys axons from the **Edinger-Westphal nucleus** in the midbrain to the ciliary ganglion; most postganglionic neurons supply the **ciliary muscles of the eye.**

2. The **facial nerve** (CN VII) relays preganglionic fibers from the **superior salivary nucleus** of the medulla; postganglionic neurons are relayed to the submandibular and sublingual salivary glands via the submandibular ganglion. Other preganglionic fibers pass via the pterygopalatine ganglion, which gives origin to postganglionic neurons serving the **lacrimal and nasal glands.**

3. The **glossopharyngeal nerve** (CN IX) contains preganglionic fibers from the **inferior salivary nucleus** of the medulla. A complex pathway relays fibers via the otic ganglion to the **parotid salivary gland.** The *glossopharyngeal nerve also carries afferent neurons from the sensory organs that monitor blood pressure (the* **carotid sinus***) and blood gas composition (the* **carotid body***).*

4. *The* **vagus nerve** *(CN X) carries the largest collection of preganglionic parasympathetic fibers.* The neurons originate in the **nucleus ambiguus** and **dorsal motor nucleus** of the medulla. Vagal fibers terminate in the heart and lungs and the gastrointestinal system.

Parasympathetic innervation of the pelvic organs originates in the gray matter of the sacral spinal cord, from segments **S2 to S4**. Preganglionic axons initially exit the spinal cord via the ventral nerve roots and exit the spinal nerves to form the **pelvic splanchnic nerves.** Preganglionic fibers terminate in the **hypogastric nerve plexuses** of the pelvis; unmyelinated postganglionic fibers pass to the **distal large intestine**, the **bladder,** and the **reproductive organs.**

INTEGRATIVE AND BEHAVIORAL FUNCTIONS

Many neuronal circuits in the cortex are integrated to produce complex phenomena such as emotions, motivated behavior, consciousness, language, memory, and cognition. Three areas of the brain are particularly important for the **implementation of integrative functions:**

1. The **hypothalamus** is the major controller of the endocrine and ANS. It is a key site for the control of homeostatic functions and motivated behaviors, including eating, circadian rhythms, and the sex drive.

2. The **reticular formation** consists of several well-defined nuclei that give origin to monoaminergic neurons; the widespread connections of these neurons form the **diffuse modulatory systems** of the brain. The functional concept is one of an **ascending reticular activating system** for the forebrain,

which is essential for determining the level of consciousness and general arousal.

3. The **limbic system** is the seat of emotions, and is formed from a series of cortical and subcortical structures that have reciprocal connections with the reticular formation and hypothalamus. *Dysfunction of the limbic system and diffuse modulatory systems underlie psychiatric diseases such as major depression, bipolar disorder, and schizophrenia.*

THE HYPOTHALAMUS

The hypothalamus orchestrates many homeostatic functions via the autonomic and endocrine systems. It is also a key output pathway for the limbic system, playing a role in the expression of emotions. The hypothalamus occupies the small area below the thalamus and extends from the optic chiasm anteriorly to the mamillary bodies posteriorly; the lower part of the third ventricle lies in the center of the hypothalamus. The hypothalamus consists of **groups of nuclei,** the names and functions of which are summarized in Figure 2-48.

The hypothalamus receives many **afferent inputs:**

Collaterals from the **visceral and somatic sensory pathways** (e.g., via the medial lemniscus and the reticular formation) serve the hypothalamus in its role as an integrator of homeostatic and visceral function. The hypothalamus can directly monitor changes in plasma composition through the circumventricular organs, where the blood-brain barrier is permeable (see Brain Extracellular Fluids).

Afferent fibers from the **frontal lobe** and parts of the **limbic system** link the hypothalamus with the higher centers for mood and emotion.

The **major efferent connections** of the hypothalamus are:

Descending pathways via the reticular formation (e.g., **reticulospinal tract**) control the **peripheral ANS.** The hypothalamus sends efferents to the brainstem nuclei for parasympathetic outflow and to the lateral horn of the spinal cord for sympathetic outflow.

Output to the **endocrine system** is via connections with the pituitary gland, via the **hypothalamohypophyseal tract,** to the posterior pituitary and **hypophyseal portal blood supply** to the anterior pituitary (see Chapter 8).

Output is conveyed to the **limbic system** through several pathways (e.g., the **mammillothalamic tract**).

REGULATION OF FOOD INTAKE Body weight is determined by the balance between food intake and energy expenditure. The hypothalamus is the main site where food intake is regulated. There are **two areas of the hypothalamus that are important in the regulation of eating:**

1. The **ventromedial nucleus** is the **satiety center;** damage to this area causes unrelenting hunger.

2. The **lateral hypothalamic area** is the **feeding center;** damage to this area causes profound loss of the desire to eat.

The neurochemistry of circuits within the feeding control centers is complex, although several **orexigenic (stimulate**

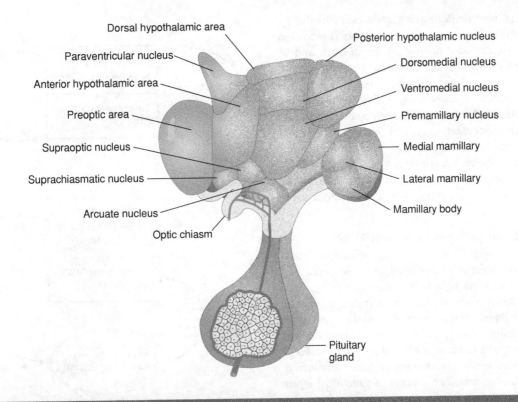

Figure 2-48: Anatomy of the hypothalamic nuclei and the homeostatic functions of the hypothalamus.

Function of the Hypothalamus	Area of the Hypothalamus
Secretion of hormonal release factors controlling the pituitary gland	Arcuate and paraventricular nuclei; periventricular area
Activation of sympathetic nervous system	Dorsal and posterior areas
Eating behavior	Ventromedial and arcuate nuclei; lateral area
Drinking behavior and thirst	Lateral area
Water and electrolyte balance	Supraoptic and paraventricular nuclei
Body temperature regulation	Preoptic area
Sexual behavior	Preoptic and anterior area
Circadiam rhythms	Suprachiasmatic nucleus

feeding) and **anorexigenic (inhibit feeding) factors** are known, including:

- **Corticotropin-releasing hormone (CRH)** and the **cocaine and amphetamine-regulated transcript (CART),** which are among the neurotransmitters in the ventromedial nucleus that suppress the desire to eat.

- **Neuropeptide Y** (NPY) and the **orexins,** which are neurotransmitters in the lateral hypothalamic area that stimulate eating.

The drive to eat is influenced by both short-term factors related to the daily pattern of meals and by long-term factors related to the energy stores in adipose tissue (Figure 2-49). In the short term, hunger is induced by **hypoglycemia** and by the gastrointestinal peptide hormone **ghrelin** (see Chapter 7). After a meal is consumed, the sensation of satiety is mediated via the vagus nerve, due to distention of the stomach and by the release of the gastrointestinal hormone **cholecystokinin.** The major long-term regulator of eating is **leptin,** a polypeptide hormone released by adipocytes, which **stimulates the expression of CART and inhibits NPY** thereby inhibiting eating. Plasma leptin concentration reflects the size of the total body fat store; there is a feedback loop in which high levels of body fat should increase leptin levels and decrease feeding. Patients who are obese are poorly responsive to leptin, which may contribute to the development and maintenance of overeating.

▽ In general, the pathogenesis of **obesity** relates to an imbalance of energy intake versus expenditure, such that a net positive caloric balance occurs, resulting in increased adiposity. Researchers are working to unlock the molecular-genetic mystery behind the etiology of individuals prone to obesity. Dysregulation of **leptin** has been implicated as a potential explanation. It is known that loss of function mutations in leptin or in leptin receptors result in obesity. However, most obese people have increased leptin levels but do not have mutations in either leptin or its receptors. The concept of functional leptin resistance has been used to describe this situation and is a current topic of research. ▽

REGULATION OF BODY TEMPERATURE Body temperature is one of the key physiologically controlled variables and is regulated by negative feedback via the hypothalamus. *Body temperature is stable when the rate of heat generation from cellular metabolism equals the rate of heat loss to the environment.* **Heat exchange occurs via four processes:**

1. **Radiation** transfers heat as electromagnetic energy between objects that are not in contact. Heat transfer may be bidirectional and occurs from warm objects to cooler objects.

2. **Conduction** of heat occurs down a temperature gradient between objects that are in direct contact.

3. **Convection** is the transfer of heat in fluids and occurs in the direction of a temperature gradient. For example, when immersed in cold water, the body heats the surrounding water, setting up convection currents that carry warm water away from the body. Another example of convection is the transfer of heat from the body core to the body surface via circulating blood.

4. **Evaporation** is an example of unidirectional heat transfer in which body heat is used to evaporate water on the skin. The rate of evaporation depends on the gradient of water vapor pressure (i.e., evaporation cannot occur when the humidity of air is 100%).

The active regulation of heat transfer is controlled by the hypothalamus. **Afferent input regarding body temperature** is derived from two sources:

1. **Peripheral thermoreceptors** in the skin provide information about body surface temperature that is used to anticipate threats to core body temperature.

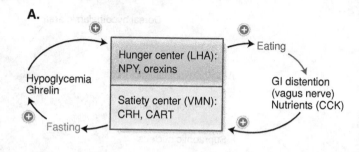

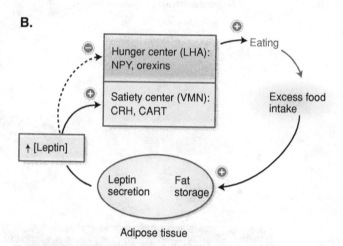

Figure 2-49: Hypothalamic control of feeding behavior. The lateral hypothalamic area (LHA) stimulates feeding, whereas the ventromedial nucleus (VMN) inhibits feeding. **A.** Short-term control of eating involves stimulation of hunger through the LHA by hypoglycemia and the gastrointestinal peptide ghrelin. Acute satiety signals acting through the VMN include distention of the stomach and the release of gastrointestinal peptides, particularly cholecystokinin (CCK). **B.** Long-term control of eating in relation to body energy stores occurs by leptin signaling to the hypothalamus. Excess energy is stored as fat in adipose tissue, which increases leptin secretion; leptin stimulates the VMN and inhibits the LHA, thereby reducing food intake.

2. **Central thermoreceptors** mostly consist of temperature-sensitive neurons in the hypothalamus that monitor the core body temperature. Warm receptors are most abundant and are localized in the preoptic area of the hypothalamus. *Physiologic responses are dominated by changes in core temperature rather than by changes in skin temperature.*

The normal set-point value for core body temperature of about 37°C (98.6°F) is determined by the hypothalamus; a negative feedback response occurs if body temperature deviates from the set point. There are several **effectors for body temperature regulation:**

Skin circulation is regulated by the adrenergic sympathetic tone; active vasoconstriction minimizes heat loss in response to cold. A reduction in sympathetic tone occurs when the body is hot, which vasodilates blood vessels in the skin and results in increased heat loss. Further vasodilation occurs as part of the sweating response.

Metabolic rate may vary acutely in response to body temperature changes. A low body temperature increases cellular metabolism via activation of the sympathetic nervous system and through increased thyroid hormone secretion. **Shivering** occurs when the core body temperature falls below approximately 35°C (95°F); it is coordinated by the hypothalamus and occurs first in the proximal muscles. *Shivering generates a large amount of heat from muscle but is a short-term response.*

Sweating is the most important response to increased body temperature due to the large amount of heat needed to evaporate water. Sweat is a hypotonic saline solution secreted by the eccrine sweat glands in the skin in response to **cholinergic** postganglionic sympathetic innervation. The corelease of other peptide transmitters along with acetylcholine, or possibly the local generation of bradykinin by the sweat glands, also causes vasodilation.

▽ **Sweating** can be viewed as a symptom of many underlying pathologic conditions. Because the sympathetic nervous system innervates sweat glands (albeit through cholinergic receptors), sweating can be a byproduct of any condition that drives sympathetic output. For example, excessive sweating (**diaphoresis**) is a prominent feature during a myocardial infarction, amphetamine intoxication, or hypoperfusion states (e.g., hypovolemic shock) in which sympathetic discharge is needed to maintain cardiac output. ▽

Behavioral changes that minimize both heat and cold stress occur in response to thermal discomfort; for example, wearing more clothing, eating more, and increasing physical activity in cold weather, or seeking shade, eating less, and reducing activity in hot weather.

▽ **Fever** is a regulated increase in body temperature in response to infection or disease. The mechanism of fever generation involves several phases (Figure 2-50A):

Secretion of **cytokines** by immune cells in response to an infection; cytokines function as **circulating pyrogens (e.g., interleukin 6).**

■ Access of cytokines to the brain across the leaky blood-brain barrier at the **OVLT**, one of the circumventricular organs.

■ Generation of **prostaglandin E2** (PGE$_2$) by the capillary endothelial cells of the OVLT stimulates the hypothalamus to raise the set point for body temperature. *This accounts for the efficacy of cyclooxygenase inhibitors (e.g., NSAIDs) at reducing fever because PGE$_2$ formation is reduced.*

As fever is generated, the body temperature is below the new higher set-point value, resulting in sensations of cold discomfort ("**the chills**"), which is associated with vasoconstriction and even shivering. When a fever "breaks," the set point suddenly decreases to normal, resulting in the elevated body temperature being higher than the normalized set-point value. In this stage of fever, a sensation of heat discomfort occurs, which is associated with sweating and vasodilation (see Figure 2-50B). ▼

▽ **Hypothermia** is defined as core body temperature below 35°C (95°F), the point at which compensatory heat conserving mechanisms begin to fail. To prevent significant morbidity and mortality, patients should be removed from the cold environment and rewarmed. ▼

GENERATION OF CIRCADIAN RHYTHMS Most of the body's major controlled variables exhibit regular cyclical variation throughout a 24-hour period. For example, body temperature varies by about 1°C, and is lowest in the early morning and highest in the evening. The plasma concentrations of several hormones also exhibit striking circadian rhythms (e.g., cortisol levels peak about 8 AM, whereas growth hormone levels are highest during sleep). Circadian rhythms are generated by an **endogenous body clock** because they persist in people who are isolated from all time and light and dark cues. The body clock is created by neurons of the **suprachiasmatic nucleus** of the hypothalamus, the activity of which oscillates spontaneously in a daily cycle. The endogenous clock has a free running period of about 25 hours, and is entrained to a 24-hour period by the normal light and dark cycle and other social cues. The suprachiasmatic nucleus receives afferent fibers directly from the retina via the **retinohypothalamic tract,** which provides information about daylight.

▽ Air travel across time zones produces the unpleasant sensations of "**jet lag**" (e.g., fatigue and being unable to eat and sleep properly when in the new time zone). Jet lag is caused by the mismatch between the endogenous circadian rhythms and the new time zone, and several days are required to entrain the body clock to the new time. A similar problem is faced by shift workers who are expected to suddenly switch their routines from nights to days or vice versa. ▼

THE RETICULAR FORMATION AND DIFFUSE MODULATORY SYSTEMS

The reticular formation is an anatomic concept that describes networks of neurons that extend throughout the core of the brainstem. It can be roughly categorized as three columns: **median, medial,** and **lateral.** An important characteristic of

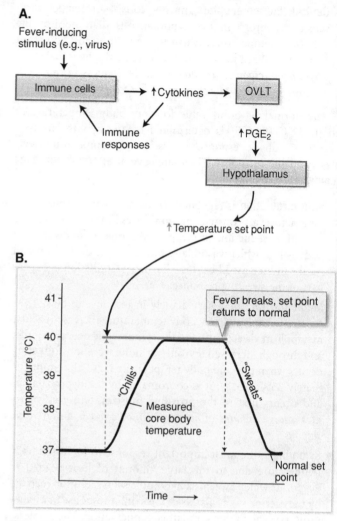

Figure 2-50: A. The mechanism of fever generation. Infections cause cells of the immune system to secrete cytokines, which cross the blood-brain barrier at the organum vasculosum laminae terminalis (OVLT). Endothelial cells of the OVLT produce prostaglandin E$_2$ (PGE$_2$) in response to cytokines, resulting in an increase in the hypothalamic set point for body temperature. **B.** The phases of fever. Changes in the hypothalamic set point during episodes of fever induce effector responses that cause the measured body temperature to change. At the beginning of a fever, the body temperature is initially below the set point; the patient feels cold and experiences "chills" (vasoconstriction and possible shivering) until the fever is established. When a fever "breaks," the body temperature is suddenly above the set point temperature; the patient feels hot and experiences vasodilation and sweating until the body cools.

neurons in the reticular formation is their widespread connectivity throughout the CNS. The concept of a **reticular activating system** recognizes that the activity of neurons in the reticular formation has an important influence on the degree of wakefulness because lesions may result in loss of consciousness and even coma.

▽ Consciousness requires proper functioning of the reticular activating system and both cerebral hemispheres. Therefore, the **principal causes of unconsciousness or coma** are:

1. Lesions that damage the reticular activating system.

2. Diffuse damage to both cerebral hemispheres.

3. Global suppression of the cerebrum and/or reticular activating system by drugs (e.g., sedative-hypnotics or alcohol) or metabolic derangements (e.g., anoxia, hypercapnia, hypoglycemia, or hepatic encephalopathy). ▽

Many of the structures and functions of the reticular formation are correlated with the functional concept of diffuse modulatory systems, which are categorized according to the principal neurotransmitter that is used. There are **four major diffuse modulatory systems:**

1. The **serotonergic system** originates in the **raphe nuclei,** which form a seam on either side of the midline throughout much of the brainstem and release the neurotransmitter serotonin (5-hydroxytryptamine, known as 5-HT). *Serotonergic neurons of the raphe nucleus are central to the control of wakefulness and sleep-wake cycles and to the control of mood and emotions.*

2. The **noradrenergic system** originates in the **locus coeruleus** of the pons, which functions as an "alarm center" that becomes most active when new environmental stimuli appear. Noradrenergic neurons are widely distributed throughout the CNS and mediate an increase in the general state of arousal. *The noradrenergic system, taken together with the serotonergic system, correlates with the concept of a reticular activating system.*

3. **Dopaminergic neurons** are widespread in the CNS. Several dopaminergic systems have been identified, including:

   The **nigrostriatal system**, which is a functional part of the basal ganglia and connects the substantia nigra of the midbrain to the striatum. Dopaminergic neurons are important in the initiation of **voluntary movement** (see Disorders of the Basal Ganglia).

   The **mesocorticolimbic system,** which originates in the tegmentum of the midbrain and ramifies throughout the limbic system. Dopaminergic neurons play an important role in the brain's **reward system,** which includes the **nucleus accumbens** at the base of the forebrain and the **prefrontal cortex.** For example, cocaine and amphetamines both increase dopaminergic transmission in the mesocorticolimbic system by inhibiting dopamine reuptake. *The reward system is short circuited by **addictive drugs,** including cocaine, amphetamines, alcohol, nicotine, and opiates, which all increase dopaminergic transmission in the nucleus accumbens.*

4. **Cholinergic neurons** are widespread in the CNS and include diffuse modulatory systems originating in the basal forebrain and brainstem. *Cholinergic neurons are involved in the ability to direct selective attention to a particular task and are important for learning and memory.*

▽ **Cholinergic neurons** in the **nucleus basalis of Meynert,** a forebrain structure, are involved in the pathogenesis of **Alzheimer's disease.** ▽

▽ **MOOD DISORDERS** The two major **affective (mood) disorders** are **major depression** and **bipolar disorder.** Bipolar disorder is expressed by periods of depression alternating with bouts of mania (sustained emotional highs). *Drugs that enhance the diffuse serotonergic and noradrenergic modulatory systems are among the most effective treatments available for mood disorders.* For example, the **monoamine oxidase inhibitors (MAOIs)** reduce the rate of norepinephrine and serotonin breakdown, which elevates the levels of these transmitters in the brain. More recently, **serotonin-selective reuptake inhibitors (SSRIs)** such as fluoxetine (e.g., Prozac) have been developed. The effectiveness of these drugs supports the monoamine hypothesis that low activity of serotonin and norepinephrine is the basis of mood disorders. However, the SSRIs and MAOIs require weeks to become fully effective, suggesting that long-term regulation of downstream pathways is involved. ▽

▽ **SCHIZOPHRENIA** Schizophrenia is a group of **psychotic disorders** characterized by a loss of the normal perceptions of reality evidenced by delusions, hallucinations, and disordered speech and behavior. **Dopamine antagonists** are effective when used as **antipsychotic (neuroleptic) drugs** due to the inhibition of dopamine signaling in the mesocorticolimbic system. *The antipsychotic actions of dopamine antagonists are mediated by blocking D_2-receptors.* The use of nonselective dopamine antagonists inhibits the nigrostriatal dopaminergic system, resulting in adverse effects that resemble Parkinson's disease. ▽

THE ELECTROENCEPHALOGRAM

The general degree of neuronal activity and synchronization of activity throughout the brain is strongly influenced by the diffuse modulatory systems. The electroencephalogram (EEG) is a method that measures cortical activity, and is an extracellular voltage recording produced by placing electrodes at several locations on the patient's scalp. The voltage differences measured between selected pairs of electrodes reflect the summation of electrical activity in the cortical neurons. Because a large number of neurons must be active to record a voltage signal on the surface of the skull, the size of EEG waves frequently reflects the synchronicity of the neuronal activity. **EEG rhythms** are highly variable but can be categorized based on their frequency, and they can be correlated to general states of alertness (Figure 2-51A). The EEG is particularly useful in diagnosing **seizures,** in which neurons in a given area fire synchronously to produce large spikes or waves.

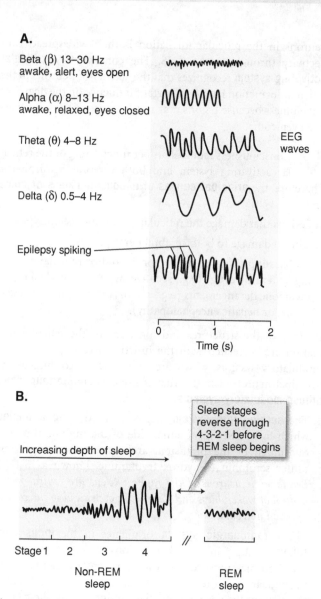

Figure 2-51: The electroencephalogram (EEG). **A.** Basic EEG wave patterns and a spiking pattern associated with epileptic brain activity. **B.** EEG patterns observed during the five stages of sleep. REM, random eye movement.

Patients who regularly suffer seizures are described as having
epilepsy.

▽ Many treatment modalities exist for the **management of epilepsy.** The goals of therapy follow three main mechanisms:

1. **Reduce seizure initiation** by inducing hyperpolarization via stimulating GABA-mediated inhibitory tone (e.g., using barbiturates or benzodiazepines).

2. **Decrease axonal conduction** via blockade of Na^+ channels, thereby inhibiting seizure propagation (e.g., using phenytoin or carbamazepine).

3. **Inhibit depolarization** by blocking presynaptic T-type Ca^{2+} channels in the thalamus (e.g., using valproic acid or ethosuximide). ▼

SLEEP

Sleep is largely controlled by the diffuse modulatory systems. The serotonergic and noradrenergic systems are most active during an awake cycle; activity in these neurons decreases at the onset of sleep. Waking involves a general increase in activity in these neurons as well as in cholinergic pathways in the basal forebrain and histaminergic neurons in the midbrain. The **sleep cycle** has several defined phases, each of which has its own distinct EEG rhythm (see Figure 2-51B):

■ **Non-rapid eye movement (non-REM) sleep** is characterized by a decreasing level of consciousness and an increasing level of rest. The parasympathetic nervous system is active and the heart rate and respiration are reduced; muscles are relaxed and movement is minimal. Non-REM sleep progresses through **four stages;** stages 3 and 4 are the most restful and correlate with **slow-wave sleep,** which can be recorded on an EEG.

■ **REM sleep** is dreaming sleep, which occurs after non-REM sleep has progressed in a cycle through stages 1–4, then back in reverse to stage 1. Paradoxically, REM sleep produces EEG rhythms that resemble the waking state. With the exception of the muscles of ventilation, the extraocular muscles, and the muscles of the middle ear, other skeletal muscles are inactive during REM sleep.

▽ **REM sleep** features an awake brain and a paralyzed body. In addition to these classic features, vivid visual imagery and sexual arousal also occur during this time of the sleep cycle. In fact, evaluation of nocturnal penile tumescence can help to determine whether the cause of **erectile dysfunction** is psychogenic (nocturnal penile tumescence does occur) or organic (nocturnal penile tumescence is limited or does not occur). ▼

The normal adult generally sleeps 7–8 hours per night; each sleep cycle typically is about 90–120 minutes, with approximately 25% of the time spent in REM sleep. Young children sleep for longer periods and have a higher proportion of REM sleep, whereas elderly persons have reduced sleep time and an absent stage 4, often leaving them with the complaint that they do not feel as rested as they used to feel.

THE LIMBIC SYSTEM

The **limbic lobe** is an anatomic concept that describes the cortical areas surrounding the brainstem, including the **cingulate and parahippocampal gyri.** The **limbic system** is a functional concept, which includes a series of structures that are intimately associated with the experience and control of emotions and with learning and memory. It consists of **several cortical structures** with extensive connections to the hypothalamus and reticular formation (Figure 2-52A):

- The **cingulate cortex** is connected to the highest centers of cognition in the prefrontal and association areas of cortex, and is a site where the "sensations" of emotions are perceived.

- The **hippocampus** is a curved elevation of gray matter on the medial surface of the temporal lobe and interacts with the cingulate cortex and the higher association cortex. *The hippocampus is important in the conversion of short-term memory to long-term memory.*

- The **amygdaloid nucleus (amygdala)** is located lateral to the hippocampus and just below the basal ganglia. *The amygdala is involved in strong emotions, including fear and aggression, and linking emotions with memories.*

The **circuits of the limbic system** include fiber tracts passing between cortical and subcortical areas (see Figure 2-52B):

- The **hypothalamus** is an important output route of the limbic system for the expression of emotions because its efferent connections coordinate autonomic and visceral functions. The hypothalamus is connected to higher parts of the limbic system, via the hippocampus, by tracts passing in the **fornix.**

- The activity of the hypothalamus is relayed back to the cortex, via the **mammillothalamic tract,** from the mamillary bodies to the **anterior thalamic nuclei,** thereby providing a pathway linking the expression with the sensation of emotions.

FEAR AND ANXIETY When a situation is perceived as threatening, the sensation of fear together with activation of the **stress response** is experienced in which the sympathetic nervous system and the hypothalamic-pituitary-adrenal hormone axis are stimulated. The *amygdala is a central structure in mediating the fear response;* lesions in this area can prevent fear. Higher cortical areas integrate sensory information with learned experience and produce descending input to the amygdala, which results in the sensation of fear. Output from the amygdala to the hypothalamus results in activation of the "fight or flight" response by the sympathetic nervous system. The hippocampus has a calming effect on activation of the stress response, and provides a **negative feedback pathway to limit the stress response.**

- Increased plasma concentration of **cortisol** is part of the stress response.

- Cortisol stimulates areas of the **hippocampus.**

- The hippocampus inhibits activation of the stress response by the **hypothalamus.**

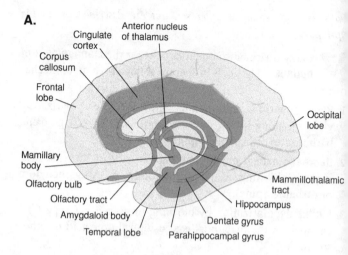

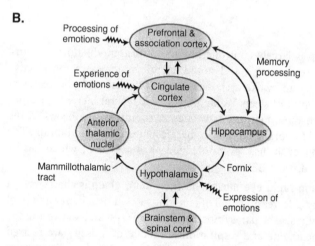

Figure 2-52: The limbic system. **A.** Major anatomic structures forming the limbic system. **B.** The main circuit of the limbic system.

When a person experiences chronic stress, the negative feed-back mechanism appears to be less effective due to persistently high levels of cortisol and resulting damage or downregulation of the hippocampus.

Aggression is an emotion related to fear, and is also mediated by the amygdala and hypothalamus. Surgical or laboratory-induced lesions in the amygdala can result in both a flattening of emotions and loss of fear and also produce a placid state. Aggression is normally suppressed by higher parts of the limbic system in the frontal cortex, which, if severed, may result in uncontrolled rage.

▽ **Klüver-Bucy syndrome** is a rare neurologic disorder that occurs as a result of bilateral lesions of the amygdala (e.g., herpes encephalitis). Patients exhibit **hypersexuality** (lack of social sexual restraint), **hyperorality** (strong compulsion to place objects in the mouth), **visual agnosia** (able to see objects, but unable to identify them), **flat affect,** and **placidity** (able to approach danger without anger or fear). ▽

LEARNING AND MEMORY

The learning process requires that information is stored and can be retrieved (remembered). There are **two general types of memory:**

1. **Declarative memory** relates to facts and events that can be consciously recalled and critically involves structures in the medial temporal lobe.

2. **Nondeclarative memory** uses different mechanisms to store information that is generally not consciously recalled. There are **three types of nondeclarative memory:**

   ▪ The ability to learn a skill or procedure (e.g., riding a bicycle) is called **procedural memory.**

   ▪ The ability to form emotional associations in the memory is called **learned emotion.**

   ▪ **Conditioned reflexes** are a simple form of memory; for example, the habit of hearing a lunchtime alarm at school may be sufficient to induce reflex gastrointestinal activity after a period of regular conditioning that relates the sound of the alarm to eating.

THE MEMORY ENGRAM The engram is the location of a memory in the brain, and is presumed to be the large areas of the association cortex. A memory is thought to be encoded through a distributed network of neurons, which have altered function and connectivity when a memory is created. The **prefrontal cortex** is envisioned as the **working memory** in which new sensory inputs are integrated with previous learning. Declarative memory may only be **short term,** where a fact or event is only recalled for a few seconds or minutes within the working memory (e.g., remembering a telephone number). The conversion of short-term memory into a **long-term memory** is called **memory consolidation,** and is enhanced by repetition and by adding several sensory modalities (e.g., writing out lecture notes) or adding emotional context. *Memory consolidation requires the hippocampus;* damage in this area causes **anterograde amnesia** (the inability to form new declarative memories). The hippocampus can access widespread areas of the cortex for memory storage via the nearby parahippocampal cortex and other parts of the temporal lobe. *The ability to recall long-term memories that are already stored does not require the hippocampus.* The inability to recall previous memories is called **retrograde amnesia.**

▽ **Alzheimer's disease** is the most common cause of dementia in the United States, and manifests as an insidious onset of progressive memory loss followed by a slowly progressive course of dementia, aphasia (loss of language skills), and apraxia (loss of learned motor skills). Late in the disease, there is a loss of judgement, reason, and cognitive ability. **Key pathologic findings** include:

▪ **Diffuse cerebral cortical atrophy** resulting in enlarged ventricles.

▪ **Markedly atrophic hippocampi.**

▪ **Microscopic findings** include senile plaques (Aβ **amyloid**) and neurofibrillary tangles (intraneuronal aggregates of abnormally phosphorylated tau proteins, a microtubule-associated protein). ▽

Additionally, Alzheimer's disease is associated with decreased levels of acetylcholine, thought to be the result of degeneration of cholinergic neurons in the nucleus basalis of Meynert. This disease typically is fatal within 10 years of onset, with death occurring due to secondary causes (e.g., pneumonia).

CELLULAR BASIS OF LEARNING Learning and memory is associated with changes in the structure and function of synapses and is known as **synaptic plasticity.** Repeated synaptic stimulation can result in a persistent change in the sensitivity of a neuron, which usually involves an increased excitability called **long-term potentiation.** At the molecular level, many examples of ion channel phosphorylation, altered intracellular second-messenger activity, and gene expression are thought to be associated with long-term potentiation. In addition to lasting functional changes in neuronal firing patterns, structural changes also occur in which the organization of synaptic contacts may be completely remodeled. Synaptic changes correlate with evidence of learning in the whole organism.

LANGUAGE AND SPEECH

The ability to comprehend language and to speak is among the most sophisticated functions of the human nervous system. It is also one of the most **lateralized brain functions** and is *dominated by centers in the left hemisphere.* There are **two cortical areas specialized for language** (Figure 2-53):

1. **Broca's area** is in the frontal lobe, just anterior to the motor cortical areas that control the mouth.

2. **Wernicke's area** is in the upper part of the temporal lobe, near the auditory cortex.

The following (**Wernicke-Geschwind**) **model** accounts for the basic features of Broca's and Wernicke's aphasias (Figure 2-53):

▪ Inputs of spoken or written words arrive from the **auditory and visual cortex,** respectively, and are relayed to Wernicke's area.

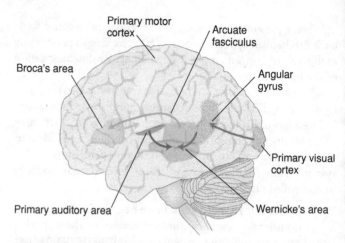

Figure 2-53: Broca's and Wernicke's areas for language and speech. Arrows indicate the Wernicke-Geschwind model for speech production; information about spoken or written words is conveyed from the auditory and visual cortices respectively to Wernicke's area where language comprehension occurs. Output from Wernicke's area, via the arcuate fasciculus, directs Broca's area to develop a motor program for the generation of speech, which is conveyed to the neighboring motor cortex.

Understanding the meaning of words is achieved by processing in **Wernicke's area.**

Output from Wernicke's area to Broca's area occurs via a tract called the **arcuate fasciculus.**

Broca's area generates the commands needed to instruct the neighboring motor cortex to produce the movements of the mouth and tongue needed to speak.

▽ Models such as the **Wernicke-Geschwind** model, which illustrates how language and speech are created, are based on clinical findings in patients with defects in understanding or producing words (i.e., **aphasia**).

Broca's aphasia is characterized by an *inability to produce speech or "find a word,"* whereas comprehension is generally preserved.

Wernicke's aphasia is characterized by fluent production of speech, but the sentences lack meaning and *comprehension of language is poor.* ▼

STUDY QUESTIONS

Directions: Each numbered item is followed by lettered options. Some options may be partially correct, but there is only ONE BEST answer.

1. A novel drug produced by screening snake venoms was found to kill glial cell tumors in culture. However, initial in vivo studies showed that the drug did not enter the brain of experimental animals and therefore could not access glial cells in the intact brain. Which structure is most responsible for preventing the entry of this drug into the brain?

   A. Arachnoid mater

   B. Brain capillary endothelium

   C. Choroid plexus epithelium

   D. Dura mater

   E. Pia mater

2. A 28-year-old woman was prevented from traveling by air to a family wedding due to an acute episode of vertigo. Over the next few months, she experienced several transient, neurologic problems, including blurred vision, sudden muscle weakness in her legs, loss of perineal sensations, and urinary incontinence. What cellular defect is most likely to account for these clinical findings?

   A. Atrophy of skeletal muscles

   B. Demyelination of central nervous system (CNS) neurons

   C. Destruction of preganglionic sympathetic neurons

   D. Loss of CNS dopaminergic neurons

   E. Proliferation of Schwann cells

3. In a laboratory experiment, a cortical neuron was electrically stimulated to produce action potentials. The stimulated neuron made synaptic contact with another neuron in which a recording electrode was located. The recording electrode detected a small depolarization following the electrical stimulation of the first neuron. Which neurotransmitter was most likely to be released at the synapse between these neurons?

   A. GABA

   B. Glutamate

   C. Glycine

   D. Met-enkephalin

   E. Somatostatin

4. A 53-year-old man suffered a vascular lesion to a small area of the lower lumbar spinal cord, which resulted in the loss of touch sensation from his left leg. Sensations of pain and temperature were not affected. Damage to which part of the spinal cord accounts for this pattern of sensory loss?

   A. Right anterolateral tract

   B. Right dorsal column

   C. Right dorsal horn

   D. Right ventral horn

   E. Left anterolateral tract

   F. Left dorsal column

   G. Left dorsal horn

   H. Left ventral horn

5. A 13-year-old boy was referred to a pediatrician due to his unusual height of 196 cm (6 ft 5 in). The boy recently reported visual disturbances. A pituitary tumor was discovered using MRI scans, and was found to be pressing on the center of the optic chiasm from below. What visual field defects are expected in this patient?

   A. Binasal hemianopia

   B. Bitemporal hemianopia

   C. Left homonymous hemianopia

   D. Right homonymous hemianopia

6. A 41-year-old woman was taken to the emergency department after being involved in a motor vehicle accident. Neurologic examination showed that the pupillary light reflex was absent in both eyes when light was shone in the left eye, but was normal in both eyes when light was shone in the right eye. At which location could a lesion account for this pattern of deficit in the pupillary light response?

   A. Left occulomotor nerve (CN III)

   B. Left optic nerve

   C. Right Edinger-Westphal nucleus

   D. Right visual cortex

   E. Superior colliculi

7. A 19-year-old girl visited her family doctor, concerned about poor hearing in her right ear. She had no family history of deafness and could not remember having any ear infections as a child. She admitted listening to loud music through a personal music player, and while at her work in a launderette, she usually listened in her right ear only so that she could still hear the customers. What are the most likely results of the Weber and Rinne tuning fork tests performed by her doctor?

   A. Weber test lateralizes to the left; Rinne test shows air conduction > bone conduction

   B. Weber test lateralizes to the left; Rinne test shows bone conduction > air conduction

   C. Weber test lateralizes to the right; Rinne test shows air conduction > bone conduction

   D. Weber test lateralizes to the right; Rinne test shows bone conduction > air conduction

8. A functional magnetic resonance imaging (fMRI) study of the thalamus showed changes in neuronal activity in the thalamus in response to various sensory stimuli. Which of the following sensory modalities would be associated with the lowest level of thalamic neuronal activity?

   A. Audition

   B. Conscious proprioception

   C. Gustation

   D. Olfaction

   E. Vision

9. A 68-year-old man visits his doctor complaining about a tremor in his hands, which is particularly bad when he tries to perform a task. He demonstrates past-pointing when asked to perform a finger to nose test, and has difficulty producing rapidly alternating supination and pronation movements of the hands. The doctor also notes a wide, awkward gait. Based on these clinical findings alone, in which part of the motor system is a dysfunction expected?

   A. Basal ganglia

   B. Cerebellum

   C. Lateral spinal pathways

   D. Primary motor cortex

   E. Ventromedial spinal pathways

10. A 17-year-old girl was taken to the emergency department because of a drug overdose. She was unconscious and remained comatose for 2 weeks. Her friend reported that she had started taking an unknown recreational drug 1 month earlier. In the days after regaining consciousness, the girl was profoundly depressed and developed unrelenting insomnia. Which of the following nuclei is most likely to have been damaged by her drug abuse?

   A. Amygdaloid   F. Fastigial

   B. Arcuate   G. Paraventricular

   C. Caudate   H. Raphe

   D. Dentate   I. Suprachiasmatic

   E. Edinger-Westphal   J. Supraoptic

ANSWERS

1—B. The blood-brain barrier prevents the free access of most solutes from plasma to the brain extracellular fluid. The blood-brain barrier is formed by the capillary endothelial cells and supporting glial cells. The choroid plexus also contributes, to a lesser extent, by actively regulating cerebrospinal fluid composition.

2—B. The involvement of somatic sensory and motor functions, as well as autonomic functions such as urinary continence, indicates the involvement of many parts of the nervous system. This presentation in a young woman is consistent with a diagnosis of multiple sclerosis, which is caused by the autoimmune destruction of myelin sheaths around neurons in the brain and spinal cord.

3—B. The neurotransmitter produces an excitatory postsynaptic potential in this case. Glutamate is the most common excitatory neurotransmitter in the central nervous system; the others are all inhibitory transmitters. Enkephalin and somatostatin are large molecule transmitters present in lower abundance than the other examples given.

4—F. Touch (as well as vibration and proprioception) sensations are conveyed via the dorsal column white matter to the brain. This pathway crosses over at the level of the caudal medulla, so that touch sensation from the left leg is represented in left side of the spinal cord.

5—B. A tumor pressing on the optic chiasm disrupts optic fibers crossing from one side to the other, from the nasal half of each retina. These neurons are excited by light from the temporal parts of the visual field.

6—B. The absence of both the direct and consensual light reflex response when light is shone in the left eye indicates a problem with the afferent part of the pupillary light reflex pathway on the left. A normal response on both sides when light is shone in the right eye demonstrates that the efferent parts of the reflex pathway, including the Edinger Westphal nucleus and cranial nerve III, are unaffected. The superior colliculus and visual cortex are not involved in the pupillary light reflex.

7—A. The patient is most likely to have damaged hair cells in her right ear by listening to loud music selectively in this ear for a prolonged period of time. This produces a sensorineural hearing loss due to failure of the hair cell transduction mechanism (rather than a failure of sound conduction through the middle ear). In unilateral sensorineural hearing loss, the Weber test lateralizes to the unaffected side and air conduction of sound is better than bone conduction.

8—D. The sensory pathway for olfaction does not involve the thalamus and would therefore result in the least thalamic neuronal activity. The olfactory pathway involves the nasal mucosa, olfactory bulb, and olfactory tract, leading to the olfactory cortex in the temporal lobe. The pathways of all the other sensory modalities listed involve the thalamus.

9—B. The presence of an intention tremor, and the lack of coordination during complex movements, indicates dysfunction in the cerebellar hemispheres. The gait abnormality described is consistent with dysfunction in the circuits of the spinocerebellum.

10—H. The loss of serotonergic neurons in the raphe nucleus is the most consistent with development of mood and sleep problems. Loss of the amygdaloid nuclei reduces aggressiveness. The arcuate, paraventricular, suprachiasmatic, and supraoptic nuclei are all hypothalamic nuclei; the caudate, dentate, and fastigial nuclei are associated with the motor system; and the Edinger-Westphal nucleus is a parasympathetic nucleus.

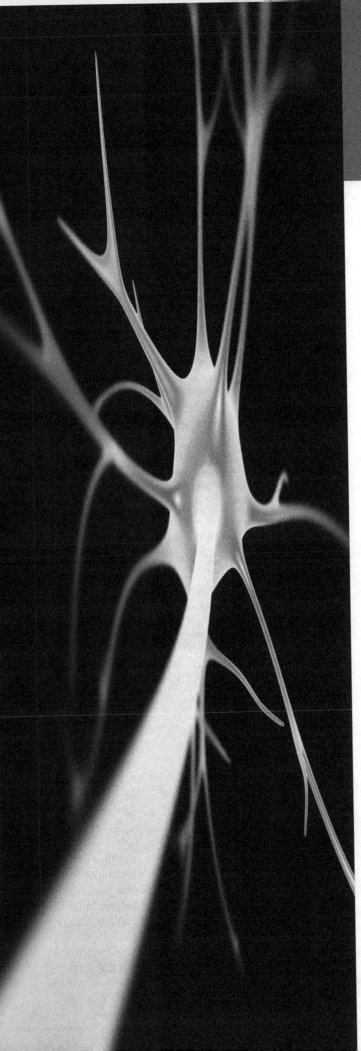

CHAPTER 3

BLOOD

THE COMPOSITION OF BLOOD

Blood circulates within the cardiovascular system to provide a vehicle for the distribution of respiratory gases, nutrients, water, electrolytes, hormones, antibodies, drugs, metabolic waste, and heat throughout the body. Most of the major negative feedback control systems of the body defend normal blood composition (e.g., blood glucose concentration, blood volume, and arterial O_2 partial pressure). Blood is composed of **cellular elements** (i.e., red blood cells, white blood cells, and platelets), which are suspended in blood **plasma.** A person who weighs 70 kg has approximately 5 L of blood, of which about 2 L is occupied by the formed cellular elements and 3 L is plasma.

This chapter will discuss mainly the physiologic regulation of the red blood cell mass and the mechanisms that prevent bleeding.

PLASMA COMPOSITION

Plasma is the part of the extracellular fluid that is contained within the cardiovascular system. It is a dilute solution, which by weight is approximately 92% water, 7% protein, and 1% small dissolved solutes (e.g., ions, urea, glucose, amino acids, and lipids). The normal plasma concentrations of selected ions and small molecules are almost the same as those in the interstitial fluid because of the free exchange of water and small solutes across most blood capillaries (Table 3-1). In contrast, *most capillaries are impermeable to plasma proteins.* The resulting difference in protein concentration between the plasma and the interstitial fluids creates a colloid osmotic (oncotic) pressure gradient that opposes the filtration of plasma out of the capillaries (Chapter 4). **Albumin** is the most abundant type of plasma protein and, therefore, is the greatest contributor to the plasma oncotic pressure. The major types of plasma protein and their functions are listed in Table 3-2.

▽ **Hypoalbuminemia** has many causes, including nephrotic syndrome, liver failure, and severe malnutrition. Regardless of the cause, hypoalbuminemia can result in **anasarca** (generalized massive edema). ▽

THE CELLULAR ELEMENTS OF BLOOD

There are three main **cell types in circulating blood** (Figure 3-1):

1. **Red blood cells (erythrocytes)** are essential for the transport of O_2 and CO_2 in blood (Chapter 5). *There are approximately 5×10^{12} red blood cells per L of blood.*

2. **Platelets (thrombocytes)** are small cellular fragments that play a key role in **hemostasis** by adhering to sites of damage and through participation in the blood clotting system. *There are approximately 300×10^9 platelets per L of blood.*

3. **White blood cells (leukocytes)** are the only fully functional nucleated cells in circulating blood. White cells play a defensive role in destroying infecting organisms and in the removal of damaged tissue. *The total white cell count is approximately 5×10^9 cells per L of blood.* The characteristic features and functions of the **five major types of white blood cells** are described in Table 3-3.

HEMATOPOIESIS

The formation of blood cells (hematopoiesis) occurs in the **bone marrow.** In neonates, most of the skeleton contains active bone marrow, but in adults it is usually found only in the vertebrae, ribs, skull, pelvis, and the proximal femurs. Blood cells are derived from **stem cells** in the bone marrow and are produced after several stages of cell division and differentiation. Blood-forming cells may be divided into four groups, depending on their capacity for self-renewal, cell division, and the ability to form different cell types (see Figure 3-1):

1. **Pluripotent hematopoietic stem cells,** of which there are very few, are capable of forming any type of blood cell.

2. **Multipotential progenitor cells** can form a specific but wide range of blood cells. There are two types of multiprogenitor cells. One differentiates into lymphoid cells, and another differentiates into other types of blood cells; the latter is sometimes referred to as the GEMM (granulocyte erythroid monocyte megakaryocyte) progenitor cell.

3. **Committed progenitor cells** are capable of self-renewal but are able to form only one or two cell types. There is a different type of committed progenitor for each of the mature blood cell types found in circulating blood, with the exception of neutrophils and monocytes, which are both derived from a single type of committed progenitor cell.

4. **Maturing cells** do not divide again and are undergoing structural differentiation to form a specific type of blood cell.

The process of blood cell formation therefore involves sequences of cell division and differentiation. **Erythropoiesis** is the process of red blood cell formation; **thrombopoiesis** is the process of platelet production; and **leukopoiesis** is a general term describing white blood cell production.

TABLE 3-1. Normal Plasma Composition

Substance	Normal Value	Normal Range
Sodium	140 mM	136–146 mM
Potassium	4.5 mM	3.5–5.5 mM
Chloride	100 mM	96–106 mM
Bicarbonate	24 mM	22–28 mM
Calcium*	2.5 mM	2.2–2.8 mM
pH (arterial)	7.40	7.35–7.45
P_{CO_2} (arterial)	40 mm Hg	38–42 mm Hg
P_{O_2} (arterial)	90 mm Hg	80–100 mm Hg
Glucose (fasting)	80 mg/dL	70–99 mg/dL
Urea (BUN)	12 mg/dL	9–18 mg/dL
Protein	7 g/dL	6–8 g/dL

*Approximately 50% is protein bound.
BUN, blood urea nitrogen.

TABLE 3-2. The Major Types of Plasma Proteins

Plasma Protein	Major Source	Examples and Functions
Albumin	Liver	Main component of plasma oncotic pressure; binding of various substances
α-Globulins & β-Globulins	Liver	Examples (there are many) include hormone-binding proteins and the iron carrier protein transferrin
Coagulation proteins	Liver	Examples include plasminogen, prothrombin, antithrombin III, and fibrinogen
Immunoglobulins	Lymphoid tissue	Host defense reactions
Complement proteins	Liver	Host defense reactions

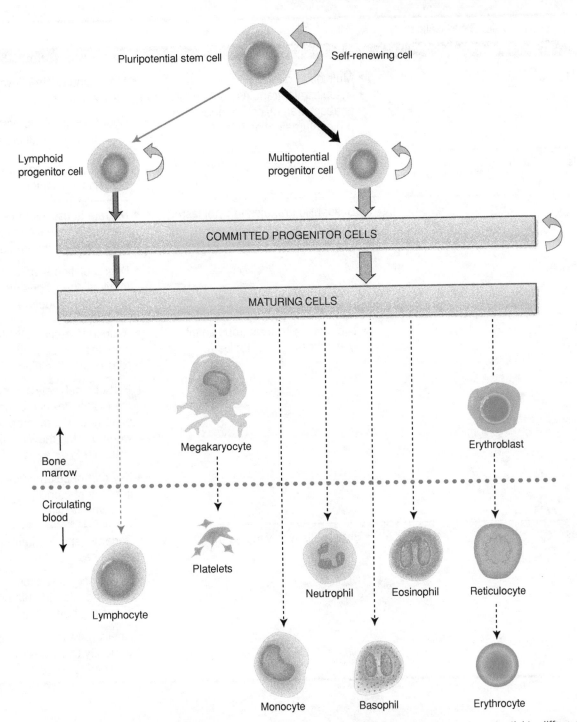

Figure 3-1: Hematopoiesis. Pluripotential stem cells in the bone marrow are self-renewing cells that have the potential to differentiate into any type of blood cell. Cell division and differentiation produces stem cells that are committed to produce particular types of blood cell. Most bone marrow cells are in a phase of maturation, on the way to becoming one of the cell types in circulating blood.

 Bone marrow (hematopoietic cell) transplant may be used in the treatment of many different hematologic and immunologic diseases, including acquired conditions such as leukemia, lymphoma, and aplastic anemia, and inherited conditions such as sickle cell anemia and severe combined immunodeficiency. **Hematopoietic stem cells** have several features that make transplantation clinically feasible:

▦ A remarkable *regenerative capacity.*

▦ An innate *ability to "home"* to the bone marrow of the recipient.

▦ An ability to *survive cryopreservation.* ▼

TABLE 3-3. Types of White Blood Cells

Cell Type	Relative Abundance (%)	Characteristic Feature(s)	Major Function(s)
Neutrophils	50–70	• Multilobed nucleus • Cytoplasmic granules containing antibacterial, digestive, and proinflammatory agents	• Ingest and destroy invading microorganisms • Coordination of the early phase of acute inflammation
Eosinophils	5	• Acidophilic granules in cytoplasm	• Phagocytic, especially against parasitic infestation
Basophils	0.5	• Basophilic granules in cytoplasm; contents include histamine	• Migrate to tissues to become mast cells; release of histamine contributes to inflammation • Degranulation is a key feature in allergic reactions mediated by immunoglobulin E
Monocytes	1–5	• Large cell with numerous small lysosomes in the cytoplasm	• Respond chemotactically to invading microorganisms and sites of inflammation • Part of a cell network, called the monocyte-macrophage system; called macrophages when outside the vascular system • Key part of cell-mediated immune response, in concert with lymphocytes
Lymphocytes	20–40	• Small cells with variable morphology	• Generate specific immune responses • B lymphocytes become plasma cells and secrete antibodies, mediating humoral immunity • T cells provide cell-mediated immunity (e.g., destruction of virally infected cells)

Because of the tremendous regenerative capacity of a stem cell, only a small percentage of the donor's bone marrow is needed for complete replacement of the recipient's entire lymphohematopoietic system. Mouse models have shown that transplantation of a single stem cell can completely replace the entire lymphohematopoietic system of the adult mouse.

ERYTHROPOIESIS

The **erythron** is a dispersed organ that consists of the whole mass of mature red blood cells and their progenitors in the bone marrow. The production of red blood cells is regulated to provide an adequate O_2-carrying capacity in blood. The hormone **erythropoietin (EPO)** is the primary regulator of erythropoiesis, and is released from the kidney when O_2 tension in the renal parenchyma is reduced (see Chapter 6). Committed erythroid stem cells in the bone marrow are responsive to EPO, which increases the rate of cell division and the differentiation into mature red cells.

The maturation of red cells in the bone marrow requires several factors; most notably **iron,** for the synthesis of the O_2-carrying pigment hemoglobin, and the essential nutrients **folic acid** and **vitamin B$_{12}$.** There are several **general features of the process of stem cell differentiation** into mature red cells:

- Cells **decrease in size.**
- **Hemoglobin** is produced, which fills the cytoplasm and causes the characteristic red coloration.
- The number of cell **organelles** decreases; *all organelles eventually disappear from red cells.*
- The **nucleus** gradually condenses and disappears.

In the final stage of differentiation, immature red cells are called **reticulocytes,** which are characterized by the presence of organelle remnants. *There is normally less than 1% of circulating red blood cells in the immature reticulocyte stage.* However, the appearance of larger numbers of reticulocytes reflects a rapid increase in the demand for red blood cells (e.g., after acute hemorrhage). *The reticulocyte count is therefore a useful index of the rate of red blood cell production.*

THROMBOPOIESIS

Platelets are small disk-shaped cell fragments without a nucleus. The cytoplasm contains an extensive cytoskeleton, which allows the shape of a platelet to change upon activation. There are also many secretory granules containing factors that regulate hemostasis. Platelet production (thrombopoiesis) occurs in the bone marrow by the cytoplasmic **fragmentation of megakaryocytes** (Figure 3-1). Megakaryocytes are the largest cells in the bone marrow and are formed when committed progenitor cells undergo repeated nuclear division without cell division. The rate of platelet formation is regulated by the cytokine **thrombopoietin (TPO)** (note: the term "cytokine" is used to describe peptide hormones that regulate cell differentiation or immune functions). TPO is constitutively secreted by the liver and kidneys, although *the plasma concentration of TPO is mostly determined by the number of platelets in circulation.* Platelets remove TPO from the circulation and so high levels of TPO result when there is a low platelet count **(thrombocytopenia).** Increased TPO concentrations stimulate megakaryocytes to produce more platelets and thereby restore a normal platelet count.

LEUKOPOIESIS

The **characteristics of white blood cell production** vary depending on the cell type. The development of **lymphoid progenitor cells** in bone marrow yields only primitive precursor cells. *The final differentiation of lymphocytes occurs in peripheral lymphoid tissues as part of a specific immune response;* **T lymphocytes** differentiate in the thymus gland, and **B lymphocytes** mainly differentiate in the lymph nodes. **Myelopoiesis** is the formation of the other (nonlymphoid) white blood cells through immature **myeloid cell** stages in the bone marrow into fully differentiated cells.

The **granular white blood cells** (i.e., neutrophils, eosinophils, and basophils) all have morphologically similar stages of cell differentiation in the bone marrow. Granulocytes are released from the bone marrow as mature cells. *In the case of neutrophils, a large pool of cells is maintained in the bone marrow* and can be rapidly mobilized in response to an infection.

Monocytes leave the bone marrow soon after their formation. In contrast to neutrophils, there is no pool of mature monocytes in the bone marrow. Monocytes typically spend 2–3 days in the circulation before entering the tissues to become macrophages.

▽ **Differential white blood cell counts** include both the total number of white cells and the proportion of each type of white cell present (Table 3-3). The production of white blood cells (leukopoiesis) is under the control of several cytokines, which are collectively known as **colony-stimulating factors.** An important element in the regulation of leukopoiesis is the secretion of colony-stimulating factors by active white blood cells. For example, *bacterial infections are usually associated with an increased proportion of neutrophils and monocytes, whereas viral infections increase the proportion of lymphocytes.* ▽

▽ If a malignant transformation occurs in a white blood cell lineage, a person can develop **leukemia** or **lymphoma.** *Leukemia is a general term used to describe a malignancy that is primarily based in the bone marrow and blood, whereas lymphomas are solid tumors that are primarily based in the lymph nodes.* In acute leukemia, the bone marrow becomes infiltrated with malignant blast cells (immature white blood cells). When these blast cells are of myeloid lineage, the condition is called **acute myeloid leukemia;** when the blast cells are of lymphoid lineage, **acute lymphoblastic leukemia** occurs. Regardless of cell lineage, *the symptoms associated with acute leukemia are typically due to bone marrow failure, which includes suppressed red blood cells (presenting as anemia), suppressed white blood cells (presenting as infection), and suppressed platelet formation (presenting as bleeding tendency).* Chronic leukemia, on the other hand, has a much more gradual onset, typified by very high leukocyte counts and by cells that have a mature appearance (e.g., chronic myeloid leukemia and chronic lymphocytic leukemia). ▽

RED BLOOD CELLS

Mature erythrocytes are disk-shaped anucleate cells, approximately 7–8 μm in diameter. The extensive cytoskeleton of red cells causes them to be extremely pliable and allows them to pass through the microcirculation. Red cells can also withstand large osmotic pressure differences, which are encountered when they pass through the renal medullary circulation (see Chapter 6). When red cells leave the bone marrow, they contain several **key cytoplasmic proteins:**

Hemoglobin is the major protein present in red blood cells, and is responsible for the large O_2-carrying capacity of blood (see Chapter 5).

Glycolytic enzymes are needed because red cells have no mitochondria and must synthesize adenosine triphosphate (ATP) via glycolysis.

Carbonic anhydrase is used to catalyze the following equilibrium reaction, which is essential for CO_2 carriage in blood (see Chapter 5):

$$H_2O + CO_2 \leftrightarrow H_2CO_3 \leftrightarrow HCO_3^- + H^+$$

The normal lifespan of a red blood cell in the circulation is approximately 100–120 days. *Erythropoiesis must therefore replace approximately 0.8% to 1.0% of the circulating red cells daily to maintain a stable red cell mass.* Aging red blood cells become progressively more fragile and are ultimately removed from the circulation by scavenging macrophages, particularly in the spleen. The end product of hemoglobin breakdown in macrophages is **bilirubin,** which is conjugated in the liver and excreted in the bile (see Chapter 7).

A critical balance must be maintained between the rate of red cell production and the rate of red cell loss from the circulation. The concept of a balance between the rate of erythropoiesis and red cell loss provides a physiologic basis for understanding disorders when the red cell mass is either decreased **(anemia)** or increased **(polycythemia).**

RED BLOOD CELL INDICES

Several indices are routinely reported in a **complete blood count (CBC)** to characterize the red cell mass (Table 3-4).

The **size of the total red cell mass** is described by three variables:

1. **Hemoglobin concentration (Hb)** is the amount of hemoglobin in a volume of blood.

2. **Hematocrit (Hct) or packed cell volume (PCV)** is the ratio of the volume of red cells to the volume of whole blood. It may be determined by centrifuging a sample of blood and comparing the height of the column of packed red cells at the bottom of the tube to the total height of the column.

3. **Red blood cell count (RBC)** is the number of red cells per liter of blood.

The **average size of a red blood cell** is described using the **mean cell volume (MCV),** which is the average volume of a single red cell expressed in femtoliters ($fL = 10^{-15}$ L). MCV is calculated by dividing the Hct by the red blood cell count. *MCV < 80 fL indicates that red cells are small* (**microcytosis**); *MCV > 100 fL indicates that red cells are large* (**macrocytosis**).

Two other variables are derived to describe the **adequacy of hemoglobin synthesis:**

1. **Mean cell hemoglobin (MCH)** is the average amount of hemoglobin in the average red cell, expressed in picograms ($pg = 10^{-12}$ g). MCH is calculated by dividing the hemoglobin concentration by the red blood cell count.

TABLE 3-4. Red Blood Cell Indices

Index	Units/Calculation	Normal Range
Hemoglobin concentration (Hb)	g/dL	• Adult man, 14–18 g/dL • Adult woman, 11–15 g/dL
Hematocrit (Hct)	%	• Adult man, 40–54% • Adult woman, 34–46%
Red blood cell count (RBC)	10^{12}/L	• Adult man, 4.5–6.5 • Adult woman, 3.9–5.6
Mean cell volume (MCV)	(% Hct ÷ 100)/RBC (fL)	82–98 fL
Mean cell hemoglobin (MCH)	(Hb × 10)/RBC (pg)	27–33 pg
Mean cell hemoglobin concentration (MCHC)	(100 X MCH)/MCV (g/dL)	30–35 g/dL (g %)

2. **Mean cell hemoglobin concentration (MCHC)** is the average concentration of hemoglobin in red cells, calculated by dividing MCH by MCV.

Example A 42-year-old woman visits her family doctor complaining of recent heavy menses and a constant feeling of fatigue. A CBC reveals Hb of 8 g/dL, Hct of 24%, and RBC of 2.6×10^{12}/L. Calculate the MCV, MCH, and MCHC.

$$MCV = (\%Hct \div 100)/RBC \text{ L}$$
$$= 24 \div 100/2.6 \times 10^{12} \text{ L}$$
$$= 92 \times 10^{-15} \text{ L} = 92 \text{ fL (normal range} = 82\text{--}98)$$

$$MCH = (Hb \times 10)/RBC \text{ g}$$
$$= (8 \times 10)/2.6 \times 10^{12} \text{ g}$$
$$= 30.8 \times 10^{-12} \text{ g} = 30.8 \text{ pg (normal range} = 27\text{--}33)$$

$$MCHC = (100 \times MCH)/MCV \text{ g/dL}$$
$$= (100 \times 30.8)/92 \text{ g/dL}$$
$$= 33.5 \text{ g/dL (g\%) (normal range} = 30\text{--}35)$$

This patient has anemia, as defined by her low hemoglobin concentration and low Hct; her red blood cell count is decreased in proportion to the decreased Hct. Therefore, the reduced red cell mass consists of normally sized cells (rather than abnormally sized cells), which contain a normal concentration of hemoglobin.

As a complement to the red cell indices, a **blood smear** is viewed under the microscope to investigate variations in cell size and in cell shape, which can indicate errors in red cell maturation. A **reticulocyte count** is determined in patients with anemia to assess the rate of red cell production. Establishing the cause of anemia requires other studies, including measurements of the nutrients required for hemoglobin synthesis (particularly iron, vitamin B_{12}, and folic acid). When defects in red cell production are indicated, an aspirate of the bone marrow may also be studied.

▽ **ANEMIA AND POLYCYTHEMIA Anemia** is defined as a reduced red cell mass and is most often recognized when laboratory test results are abnormal. Anemia is more easily diagnosed if historic data for a patient are available because there is considerable physiologic variation in the Hct (Table 3-4). The *symptoms of advanced anemia* include fatigue, dizziness, and shortness of breath. A physical examination may indicate signs of compensatory increases in cardiac output, such as strong peripheral pulses and tachycardia. Upon auscultation, flow murmurs may be heard over the branch points of large arteries due to the low viscosity of the blood. ▼

There are many specific causes of anemia, but the physiology of red cell production provides a basis for diagnosis (Figure 3-2). When a reduced hemoglobin concentration and Hct indicate the presence of anemia, *a reticulocyte count can be used to determine if the rate of red cell production is normal.* A high reticulocyte count suggests an increased rate of erythropoiesis, which reflects physiologic compensation for an increased rate of red cell loss. There are **two general causes of decreased red cell survival:**

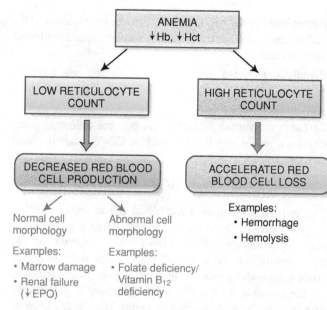

Figure 3-2: General causes of anemia. Accelerated loss of red blood cells stimulates red blood cell production, increasing the proportion of reticulocytes in circulating blood. Anemia caused by inadequate red blood cell production is characterized by a reduced reticulocyte count. EPO, erythropoietin; Hb, hemoglobin concentration; Hct, hematocrit.

1. **Hemorrhage** causes immediate loss of red cells. When plasma volume is restored, the reduced red cell mass is revealed by a low Hct.

2. In **hemolytic anemia,** the rate of red cell breakdown is increased. Hemolytic anemia can be caused by a wide range of conditions, but is uncommon. For example, in **hereditary spherocytosis,** the cell cytoskeleton is defective, resulting in increased red cell fragility. **Hemoglobinopathies** (e.g., **sickle cell disease**) are inherited defects in hemoglobin structure that can result in the deformation and increased destruction of red cells.

In cases of anemia where the reticulocyte count is normal or reduced, a defect in red cell production or maturation is indicated. There are **three requirements for normal red cell production:**

1. **Functional bone marrow.** Hypoproliferation of red cells may result if the bone marrow is damaged (e.g., aplastic anemia).

2. **Erythropoietin.** Secretion of EPO is needed to stimulate the bone marrow. *Low EPO levels are found in patients with renal insufficiency.*

3. **Adequate nutrient supply for hemoglobin synthesis.** *The most common cause of anemia worldwide is iron deficiency.* Other examples in which there is a failure of the normal maturation of red cells include dietary deficiency of vitamin B_{12} or folic acid.

▽ **Iron deficiency** is the most common cause of a **microcytic anemia,** whereas the major causes of a **macrocytic (or megaloblastic) anemia** are **vitamin B_{12}** and/or **folate deficiency.** ▼

▽ **Polycythemia** is an abnormally high level of circulating red blood cells, and is less commonly encountered than anemia. *A high red cell mass increases the viscosity of blood and increases the risk of thrombosis (formation of an intravascular blood clot).* The most common causes of polycythemia are associated with increased levels of EPO. For example, conditions that result in reduced arterial O_2 content, such as lung disease, carbon monoxide poisoning, or living at a high altitude, all stimulate EPO secretion. ▼

BLOOD CLOTTING

An essential property of the blood is the ability to clot, which aids in preventing blood loss. Precisely regulated interactions between blood vessel walls, circulating platelets, and clotting proteins in the plasma account for the ability to quickly stop blood loss (i.e., **hemostasis**). The formation of a stable blood clot is followed by the orderly breakdown of the clot (**fibrinolysis**) as wound healing proceeds. *A fine balance must be achieved between the activation of hemostatic mechanisms to prevent* **bleeding** *and excessive activation, which can cause* **intravascular thrombosis and embolism** *(blood vessel occlusion).*

OVERVIEW OF HEMOSTASIS

Three physiologic mechanisms interact to **prevent hemorrhage:**

1. **Vasoconstriction** of small vessels reduces blood flow and increases the likelihood of vessel closure. At a site of injury, platelet activation and clot formation result in the release of the vasoconstrictors. Platelets release the vasoconstrictors **serotonin and thromboxane A₂;** the clotting protein thrombin stimulates endothelial cells to secrete the highly potent vasoconstrictor **endothelin-1.**

2. **Platelet plug formation** occurs at the site of damage in capillaries, arterioles, and venules. Plug formation is called **primary hemostasis.**

3. **Clot formation** occurs in which a fibrin mesh forms together with platelets and other trapped blood cells. Clot formation is called **secondary hemostasis,** and is closely coordinated with primary hemostasis.

▽ **Increased tissue pressure** is an effective means to prevent bleeding; for example, this can be achieved by applying a surgical clamp, a tourniquet, or by applying direct pressure to a wound. Increasing the tissue pressure reduces blood vessel radius and decreases local blood flow; hemostatic mechanisms are facilitated by preventing the washout of procoagulant factors. ▽

▽ *Key elements in a patient's history can help to differentiate bleeding due to a **platelet disorder** versus bleeding due to a plasma coagulation defect (**coagulopathy**).* Bleeding that results from defective platelet function typically occurs superficially in sites such as the skin (e.g., petechiae and ecchymosis) and mucous membranes. In contrast, patients who bleed secondary to clotting factor dysfunction will suffer "deep" bleeds, such as in the deep subcutaneous tissues or muscles causing a hematoma, or in the joints causing hemarthrosis.

PLATELET FUNCTION

There are **three phases of primary hemostasis:**

1. **Platelet adhesion** to the exposed subendothelial extracellular matrix occurs at a site of injury (Figure 3-3). Adhesion is mediated by a variety of different platelet receptors, including:

   ▫ Receptors of the **integrin family** are important for binding to extracellular matrix proteins (e.g., collagen).

   ▫ The **von Willebrand factor** (vWF) is a ligand present in plasma and is released by endothelial cells and by activated platelets. The binding of vWF to a type of platelet receptor promotes platelet adhesion; vWF forms crosslinks between platelets and with collagen.

   ▫ Other receptor types bind ligands associated with platelet activation (e.g., **thromboxane A₂**) and blood clotting (e.g., **thrombin**), which further promote platelet adhesion and activation.

▽ **von Willebrand's disease (vWD)** is the most common inherited bleeding disorder and is characterized by either a deficiency or a functional defect in vWF. Because vWF is also a cofactor for the procoagulant factor VIII, *a defect in vWF*

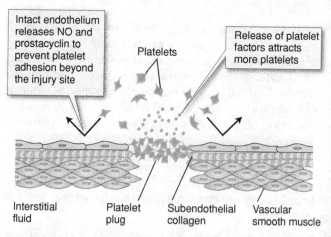

Blood vessel lumen

Intact endothelium releases NO and prostacyclin to prevent platelet adhesion beyond the injury site

Platelets

Release of platelet factors attracts more platelets

Interstitial fluid   Platelet plug   Subendothelial collagen   Vascular smooth muscle

Figure 3-3: Primary hemostasis. A platelet plug is rapidly formed to stop blood loss from an injured vessel. Adhesion of platelets to subendothelial collagen is accompanied by the release of platelet factors, resulting in recruitment and aggregation of more platelets. Intact endothelial cells release factors such as nitric oxide (NO) and prostacyclin, which prevent platelet adhesion beyond the site of injury.

will result in both platelet dysfunction and coagulopathy, a characteristic feature of this disease that is shared with very few other conditions (e.g., disseminated intravascular coagulopathy [DIC]). ▼

2. **Platelet activation.** Several intracellular signaling pathways are activated when ligands bind to platelet receptors. The result is *exocytosis of the contents of platelet granules* and a morphologic change from a smooth membrane surface to one with finger-like cytoplasmic projections. Adherent platelets therefore release many locally acting agents and undergo physical changes that increase adhesion and aggregation with other platelets. Activated platelets release many factors that promote hemostasis, including:

   - **Adenosine diphosphate (ADP)** is a potent activator of other platelets, amplifying the platelet activation response.
   - **Serotonin** and **thromboxane A$_2$** assist hemostasis as vasoconstrictors.
   - **vWF** augments platelet adhesion and aggregation.
   - **Ca^{2+}** and the clotting factors **fibrinogen** and **factor V** facilitate coagulation.
   - **Platelet-derived growth factor** promotes wound healing by stimulating growth and migration of fibroblasts and smooth muscle cells at the site of injury.

3. **Platelet aggregation** completes the formation of a platelet plug (Figure 3-3). The signaling molecules released during platelet activation amplify the platelet adhesion and activation responses and recruit more platelets to the site of injury. The platelet plug is prevented from extending beyond the site of injury by **prostacyclin** and **nitric oxide,** which are secreted from intact endothelial cells and inhibit platelet activation.

   ▽ **Antiplatelet drugs** are used to prevent thrombosis (e.g., cardiovascular disease) and target many of the steps of platelet activation and adhesion. A few examples include:

   - **Aspirin** and NSAIDs, which inhibit the production of thromboxane A$_2$ by blocking the key enzyme cyclooxygenase (COX). These agents therefore inhibit platelet activation and secretion.
   - **Clopidogrel** (Plavix) and **ticlopidine** (Ticlid), which antagonize the actions of adenosine diphosphate and therefore inhibit platelet activation.
   - **Eptifibatide** (Integrilin) is a competitive inhibitor of glycoprotein IIb/IIIa, a platelet specific adhesion molecule in the integrin family. Blockade of this important adhesion receptor prevents the binding of fibrinogen, vWF, and other adhesion molecules to activated platelets. ▼

   ▽ **Thrombocytopenia** (low platelet count) has many causes, which can be broadly classified into three categories:

1. **Decreased platelet production** by the bone marrow (e.g., leukemia or tumor infiltration of the marrow).

2. **Splenic sequestration of platelets** (e.g., splenomegaly secondary to portal hypertension).

3. **Increased destruction of platelets** (e.g., antibody-mediated platelet destruction in idiopathic thrombocytopenic purpura [ITP]).

Regardless of the cause, thrombocytopenia results in an increased **bleeding tendency.** ▼

THE BLOOD COAGULATION MECHANISM

A blood clot is formed when the plasma protein **fibrinogen** is proteolytically cleaved to produce **fibrin,** which subsequently becomes cross-linked into a stable mesh. Clotting can occur in the absence of platelet activation, but there is usually parallel activation of primary and secondary hemostasis and cross talk between the pathways to ensure coordinated activation. In the classic description of coagulation, clotting may be initiated by one of two pathways: the **intrinsic pathway** or the **extrinsic pathway** (Figure 3-4). Each pathway consists of a cascade of reactions, in which inactive circulating precursor proteins ("**clotting factors**") become activated, in most cases by proteolytic cleavage. These chain reactions normally are not activated in the circulation because clotting factors are present

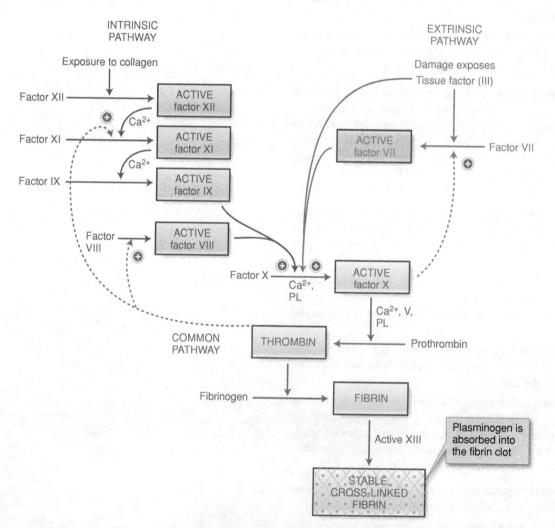

Figure 3-4: Secondary hemostasis. A cascade of coagulation reactions results in the formation of a stable fibrin mesh to prevent bleeding from a site of injury. The intrinsic pathway for coagulation is triggered by the exposure of subendothelial collagen; the extrinsic pathway is activated when tissue factor (a cell membrane lipoprotein) is exposed in injured tissue. The intrinsic and extrinsic pathways converge at the activation of factor X, resulting in the generation of thrombin, which converts fibrinogen to fibrin. PL, phospholipid

at low concentration in plasma. The *intrinsic pathway is triggered when blood contacts a negatively charged surface* (e.g., exposed subendothelial collagen; aggregations of platelets). The *extrinsic pathway is activated when blood contacts cells outside the vascular endothelium*; nonvascular cells express a ubiquitous membrane protein called **tissue factor,** which initiates the extrinsic pathway.

The intrinsic and extrinsic pathways converge at the **common pathway** for coagulation, which begins with the activation of factor X. The plasma protein **prothrombin** is cleaved by activated factor X to produce the protease **thrombin** (Figure 3-4). Thrombin is responsible for the cleavage of fibrinogen and for the activation of factor XIII, which cross-links fibrin into a stable mesh. *The extrinsic pathway is thought to be the most important pathway for initiating thrombin activation, whereas the intrinsic pathway is thought to be more important for maintaining thrombin generation.*

The current understanding of the clotting pathways shows that rather than the intrinsic, extrinsic, and common pathways being independent, they form a network with reciprocal connections. For example, activated factor IX of the intrinsic pathway activates factor VII of the extrinsic pathway. In the reverse direction, a complex formed from tissue factor, activated factor VII, and Ca^{2+} in the extrinsic pathway can activate factors IX and XI of the intrinsic pathway. *Thrombin plays a central role in the coordination of the clotting cascades* because it stimulates the downstream events in the common pathway, resulting in the formation of a fibrin clot, and it mediates positive feedback stimulation at upstream points in the intrinsic and extrinsic pathways (Figure 3-4).

CLOTTING INDICES Several tests are used to assess the function of primary and secondary hemostatic mechanisms, including:

- The **bleeding time** is a sensitive test of platelet function. A small standardized incision is made in the underside of the forearm, and the amount of time it takes for bleeding to stop is recorded. *Drugs such as aspirin, which inhibits platelet function, increase the bleeding time.*

- The **prothrombin time (PT)** evaluates the extrinsic coagulation pathway. A sample of blood plasma is incubated with tissue factor in the presence of an excess of Ca^{2+}. Because there are variations between assays, corrections may be applied that normalize the prothrombin time of a sample to that of a normal sample (e.g., the **prothrombin ratio** and **international normalized ratio [INR]**). *The anticoagulant drug warfarin increases the prothrombin time.*

- The **partial thromboplastin time (PTT)** indicates the performance of the intrinsic pathway. The intrinsic pathway is triggered by adding an activator surface (e.g., silica) plus phospholipid and Ca^{2+} to a plasma sample. *The anticoagulant drug heparin increases the partial thromboplastin time.*

▽ **Clotting factors II, VII, IX, and X** (and the anticoagulant proteins C and S) are produced in the liver and rely upon a **vitamin K-dependent** enzymatic reaction, γ-carboxylation of a glutamyl residue, which has significant clinical implications. In select patients (e.g., those at risk of developing a blood clot secondary to atrial fibrillation), it can be advantageous to block the function of γ-glutamyl carboxylase to induce a coagulopathy. The anticoagulant medication **warfarin** (Coumadin) inhibits the enzyme vitamin K epoxide reductase, making vitamin K unavailable for the γ-carboxylation reaction, which will halt the production of the vitamin K-dependent coagulation factors. *Careful monitoring of the prothrombin time or the INR is required to ensure that excessive anticoagulation does not occur.* ▽

▽ The bleeding disorders **hemophilia A** (classic hemophilia) and **hemophilia B** (Christmas disease) are X-linked recessive disorders that result in the deficiency of clotting factors VIII and IX, respectively. *An increase in PTT is expected in both conditions because both factor VIII and factor IX are part of the intrinsic pathway.* ▽

ANTICOAGULANTS

The blood clotting cascades have the effect of amplifying a stimulus for coagulation, so it is essential that blood clotting is restricted to the site where it is needed. Random blood clotting in the circulation is normally prevented by the presence of anticoagulant factors. *The capillary endothelium is the main source of anticoagulant factors.*

▪ **Tissue factor pathway inhibitor (TFPI)** is anchored to the endothelial cell membrane and blocks the action of activated factor VII in the extrinsic pathway.

▪ **Antithrombin III** inhibits coagulation by binding to activated factor X and thrombin; the binding of antithrombin III is augmented by heparan sulfate molecules on the surface of endothelial cells.

▪ **Thrombomodulin** inhibits coagulation by binding to thrombin.

▪ **Proteins C and S** act together to inactivate activated factors V and VIII, which are cofactors in the clotting cascades.

▽ **Heparin** is a glycosaminoglycan molecule that is released endogenously from mast cells and basophils, and is widely used as an anticoagulant drug. *Heparin functions by augmenting the anticoagulant effects of antithrombin III.* ▽

▽ **Hypercoagulable states** occur when there is a defect in the anticoagulant pathway. For example, a *deficiency of antithrombin III, protein C, or protein S* will increase a patient's risk for thrombosis. The most common inherited cause of hypercoagulability is the **factor V Leiden** mutation. In this condition, factor V undergoes a mutation that renders it *resistant to the anticoagulant actions of protein C*, which allows factor V to remain activated, prolonging its thrombogenic effect. ▽

FIBRINOLYSIS

When a blood clot is initially formed, it is a semisolid mass consisting of platelets and a fibrin mesh, which also traps red and white blood cells and contains plasma. The clot solidifies as platelets contract and squeeze out plasma water. The protein **plasminogen** is among the serum proteins that are adsorbed into the clot at the time of its formation. The cleavage of plasminogen produces the protease **plasmin,** which breaks down fibrin and fibrinogen. The breakdown products of the fibrin mesh are released from the blood clot and are scavenged by macrophages.

Fibrinolysis begins soon after a clot is formed. The activation of plasminogen is mainly regulated by two factors, which are released from capillary endothelial cells: **tissue plasminogen activator** and **urokinase-type plasminogen activator** (Figure 3-5). It is important that plasmin is not active in the circulation because it can also break down fibrinogen. If plasmin escapes from the clot, it is rapidly bound and inactivated by the circulating plasma protein α_2-**antiplasmin.**

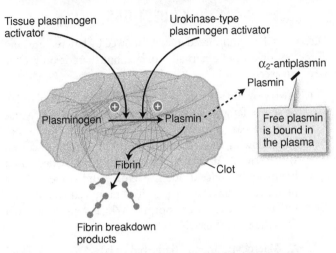

Figure 3-5: Fibrinolysis. The plasma protein plasminogen is incorporated into the fibrin mesh when a clot forms. The cleavage of plasminogen produces the protease plasmin, which breaks down fibrin. Tissue plasminogen activator and the urokinase-type plasminogen activator are factors secreted from endothelial cells, which catalyze the conversion of plasminogen to plasmin.

STUDY QUESTIONS

Directions: Each numbered item is followed by lettered options. Some options may be partially correct, but there is only *ONE BEST* answer.

1. A 61-year-old woman visits her family doctor complaining of severe fatigue, which has become progressively worse over the past 6 months. She is referred to a hematologist following the results of a complete blood cell count, which shows decreased hematocrit (24%), decreased hemoglobin concentration (8 g/dL), and decreased red blood cell count 2.6 x 10^{12}/L. The mean cell volume and reticulocyte counts are normal. Which type of anemia does the patient have?

   A. Macrocytic anemia (large red cells)

   B. Microcytic anemia (small red cells)

   C. Normocytic, hypoproliferative anemia

   D. Normocytic, hyperproliferative anemia

   E. No anemia is present

2. A 21-year-old woman returns to the United States from a student exchange visit to Australia. The morning after her flight, she is awakened because she is experiencing a pain throughout her right leg, which is of pale blue color. She is taken to the emergency department, where a clinical diagnosis determines that she has deep vein thrombosis. Which of the following laboratory findings would be consistent with this history?

   A. Antithrombin III defect

   B. Decreased hematocrit

   C. Decreased fibrinogen

   D. Decreased platelet count

   E. Factor VIII defect

3. The addition of sodium citrate to banked blood inhibits coagulation. By what mechanism do citrate ions inhibit coagulation?

   A. Antagonist to adenosine diphosphate

   B. Antagonist to thromboxane A_2

   C. Binds to factor VII

   D. Binds to factor X

   E. Chelates Ca^{2+} ions

4. A 42-year-old man with a family history of stroke and heart attack decides to take a daily aspirin tablet, having seen a television commercial. What is the main mechanism by which aspirin reduces the likelihood of intravascular blood clot formation?

   A. Inhibition of the extrinsic clotting pathway

   B. Inhibition of the intrinsic clotting pathway

   C. Inhibition of platelet function

   D. Stimulation of anticoagulant synthesis

   E. Stimulation of fibrinolysis

   F. Vasodilation

5. A 29-year-old woman with Crohn's disease develops mild vitamin K deficiency despite trying to eat a healthy diet. How will this vitamin deficiency manifest when blood clotting indices are measured?

   A. Decreased platelet count

   B. Decreased international normalized ratio (INR)

   C. Prolonged bleeding time

   D. Prolonged prothrombin time (PT)

   E. Prolonged partial thromboplastin time (PTT)

ANSWERS

1—C. Low hemoglobin concentration and hematocrit demonstrate the presence of anemia. Mean cell volume is normal because the red blood cell count is reduced in proportion to the reduced hematocrit; therefore a normocytic anemia is present. The reticulocyte count is not increased, as would occur, for example, in hemorrhage or hemolytic disease, indicating that the anemia is hypoproliferative (low red cell production).

2—A. The patient is likely to be in a hypercoagulable state, predisposing her to deep vein thrombosis. Defects in anticoagulants, such as antithrombin III, produce a hypercoagulable state. Decreased platelets, fibrinogen, or factor VIII all oppose coagulation; hematocrit is not directly relevant.

3—E. Citrate ions chelate Ca^{2+}, which is required as a cofactor for several steps in the coagulation cascades.

4—C. Aspirin and other NSAIDs inhibit the production of *thromboxane A_2* by blocking the key enzyme cyclooxygenase (COX). These agents therefore inhibit platelet activation.

5—D. Vitamin K deficiency reduces the production of prothrombin (and other clotting factors) in the liver. In mild vitamin K deficiency, the prothrombin time is therefore prolonged. Platelet production is not dependent on vitamin K; bleeding time is an indicator of platelet function and is not affected. The INR provides a normalized value of the prothrombin time and would therefore also be increased. Prolonged partial prothromboplastin time reflects function of the intrinsic clotting pathway and does not become affected until vitamin K deficiency is severe.

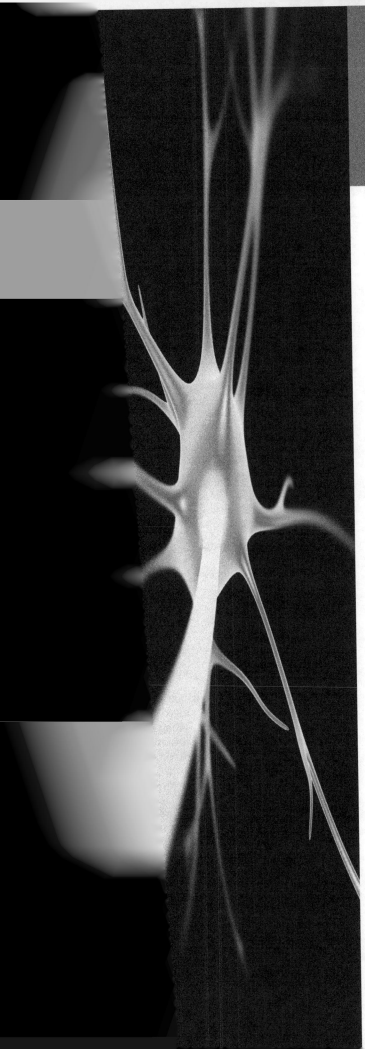

CHAPTER 4

CARDIOVASCULAR PHYSIOLOGY

THE CARDIOVASCULAR SYSTEM

OVERVIEW

The cardiovascular system consists of the heart, blood vessels, and blood. Its primary function is to transport materials to and from all parts of the body. The heart pressurizes blood and provides the driving force for its circulation through the blood vessels. Blood is propelled away from the heart in the arteries and returns to the heart in the veins. Substances transported throughout the cardiovascular system can be categorized as (1) materials entering the body from the external environment (e.g., O_2 and nutrients); (2) materials moving between cells within the body (e.g., hormones and antibodies); and (3) waste products, from cells, requiring elimination (e.g., heat and CO_2). The exchange of materials between blood and interstitial fluid occurs across capillaries in the microcirculation.

ANATOMIC ORGANIZATION OF THE CARDIOVASCULAR SYSTEM

The heart has four chambers. The two **atria** serve as reservoirs for blood returning to the heart. The two **ventricles** are pumps that propel blood through the circulation (Figure 4-1). A **septum** divides the heart into right and left sides. The right atrium is the reservoir serving the right ventricle, which pumps blood to the **pulmonary circulation** via the pulmonary artery. Blood returns from the lungs to the left atrium via the pulmonary veins. The left ventricle propels blood, via the aorta, to all other organs in the body through the **systemic circulation.**

Circulation of blood is completed as the blood from the systemic circulation drains into the right atrium via the superior and inferior venae cavae. The term "**right side**" of the circulation refers to the pulmonary circulation, which is served by the right ventricle. The term "**left side**" of the circulation refers to the systemic circulation, which is served by the left ventricle. The right side of the heart propels deoxygenated blood to the lungs, and the left side of the heart propels oxygenated blood to the tissues.

▽ **Heart failure** results from conditions that impair the ability of the heart to fill with, or to pump out, sufficient blood. Either side of the heart may be affected, or both sides may be affected in some patients. In right-sided heart failure, there is a buildup of pressure that begins with the failing right ventricle and then moves to the right atrium and back to the systemic veins. Clinical signs include jugular venous distention and peripheral edema. *The most common cause of right-sided heart failure is preexisting left-sided heart failure.* In **left-sided heart failure,** pressure begins to build in the left ventricle, then back to the left atrium and into the lungs. Clinical signs include pulmonary edema and shortness of breath. *The most common cause of left-sided heart failure is myocardial infarction.* ▽

The pulmonary and systemic circulations are in series with each other, and *all blood passing through one system must flow through the other system.* In the pulmonary circulation, blood normally flows at low pressure and receives the entire output of the right ventricle. In **pulmonary hypertension,** which can cause right-sided heart failure, pressure in the pulmonary artery is elevated, resulting in strain on the right ventricle.

Blood flow from the left ventricle is the same as that from the right ventricle because the two sides operate in series. Output from the left ventricle is distributed at higher pressure through organ systems arranged in parallel. One-way valves between the atria and the ventricles, between the ventricles and their receiving arteries, and within the systemic veins ensure that blood flows in one direction around the circulation.

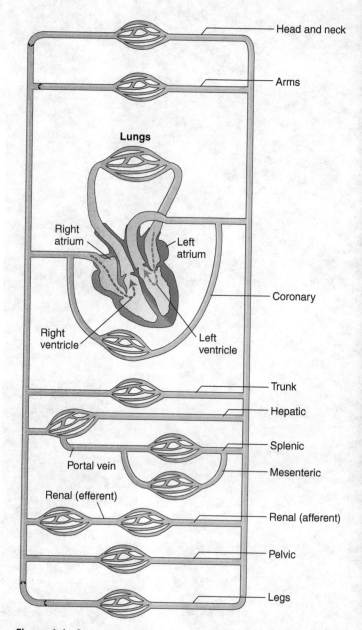

Figure 4-1: Overview of the cardiovascular system. Systemic and pulmonary circulations are arranged in series. Organ blood supply in the systemic circulation is arranged in parallel. Blue indicates deoxygenated blood; red indicates oxygenated blood.

HEMODYNAMICS

Blood flow around the circulation is driven by a difference in pressure between the arteries and the veins. The amount of blood flow produced for a given pressure gradient depends on how much resistance to flow is offered by the vascular system.

PRESSURE

Pressure is defined as a force exerted per unit area. Units of mm Hg are used clinically—1 mm Hg is equivalent to a pressure exerted by a 1 mm Hg column of mercury acting on an area of 1 cm². **Flow** of fluid occurs as the result of a difference in pressure between two points. In a closed system of fluid-filled tubes, such as the cardiovascular system, *the difference in pressure between the aorta and the large central veins drives blood flow through the systemic circulation.* Blood is an incompressible fluid, and its volume cannot decrease when the ventricles contract. Instead, blood is pressurized, creating the potential energy for blood flow. Blood pressure decreases over distance as potential energy is lost through friction between blood and blood vessel walls and between blood cells. For a given pressure difference between two points, the amount of flow that occurs depends on **resistance.**

According to **Ohm's law,** flow is proportional to the driving pressure gradient (ΔP) and inversely proportional to resistance (R):

$$Q = \Delta P / R \qquad \text{Equation 4-1}$$

Q = Flow
ΔP = Difference in pressure $P_1 - P_2$
R = Resistance

▽ Ohm's law may be applied in many situations. For example, **stenosis (severe narrowing) of the aortic valve** increases resistance to ejection of blood from the left ventricle. According to Ohm's law, left ventricular pressure must increase significantly to maintain sufficient cardiac output. Chronically high left ventricular pressures can result in left ventricular hypertrophy and heart failure. ▼

RESISTANCE

A tube will offer greater resistance (R) to fluid flow if its length (L) increases or if the radius (r) is decreased. Resistance is also greater if the fluid moved has a higher viscosity (η).

Poiseuille's law describes the determinants of resistance:

$$R = 8L\eta \, / \, \pi r^4 \qquad \text{Equation 4-2}$$

R = Resistance
L = Length of tube
η = Viscosity of fluid
r = Radius of tube

Radius is the dominant variable that determines resistance because radius is raised to the fourth power, as indicated in Equation 4-2. Figure 4-2 applies the principles of Equations 4-1 and 4-2 and shows that doubling the vessel radius increases flow by a factor of 16. Physiologic control of vascular resistance is achieved by altering the blood vessel diameter through **vasoconstriction** and **vasodilatation.**

▽ Poiseuille's law is also applied when selecting an appropriate sized intravenous catheter to achieve **rapid fluid infusion.** For example, when attempting resuscitation of a hemodynamically unstable patient, a catheter is selected that maximizes radius and minimizes length to reduce its resistance.

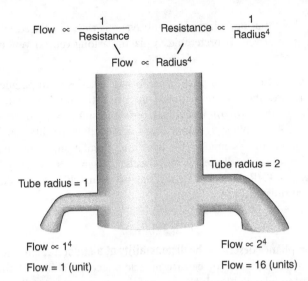

$$\text{Flow} \propto \frac{1}{\text{Resistance}} \qquad \text{Resistance} \propto \frac{1}{\text{Radius}^4}$$

$$\text{Flow} \propto \text{Radius}^4$$

Tube radius = 1

Tube radius = 2

Flow $\propto 1^4$
Flow = 1 (unit)

Flow $\propto 2^4$
Flow = 16 (units)

Figure 4-2: Vessel radius is the main determinant of resistance and flow. If radius is doubled, resistance decreases by a factor of $2^4 = 16$. Flow increases 16-fold, assuming the driving pressure stays the same.

In this situation, a large bore intravenous catheter placed in a peripheral vein is preferable to placing a long central venous line. ▼

Resistance in the circulation can occur in series or in parallel. When resistances are arranged in series, the total resistance (R_T) is the sum of individual resistances: $R_T = R_1 + R_2 + R_3 \cdots + R_n$. When resistances are arranged in parallel, such as in organ systems in the systemic circulation, individual resistances contribute as reciprocals: $1/R_T = 1/R_1 + 1/R_2 + 1/R_3 \cdots + 1/R_n$, and the total resistance is much less than for serial resistances.

COMPLIANCE

Compliance describes the **distensibility of a structure.** Changes in the compliance of cardiac muscle affect the ability of the heart to fill with blood. Altered compliance of blood vessel walls changes the volume and pressure of blood.

Compliance is defined as the volume change produced by a given pressure change:

$$C = \Delta V / \Delta P \qquad \textbf{Equation 4-3}$$

C = Compliance
ΔV = Volume change
ΔP = Pressure change

If a structure has low compliance (i.e., it is stiff), applying a normal pressure change (ΔP) will produce a small volume change (ΔV). Alternatively, delivering a normal volume will be associated with a large pressure change.

▽ Low compliance is the central pathology in **diastolic heart failure.** Chronic hypertension renders the left ventricle thickened and noncompliant, impairing relaxation and diastolic filling. Ventricular compliance may be improved by treatment with calcium channel blockers to aid relaxation of the cardiac myocytes during diastole. ▼

STRUCTURE AND FUNCTION OF CARDIAC MUSCLE

Atria and ventricles are composed of cardiac muscle cells, together with supporting connective tissue. A fibrous ring perforated by **four valve openings** electrically isolates the atria from the ventricles.

1. The **tricuspid valve** permits blood flow from the right atrium to the right ventricle.

2. The **pulmonic valve** conveys blood from the right ventricle to the pulmonary artery.

3. The **mitral valve** allows blood to flow from the left atrium into the left ventricle.

4. The **aortic valve** conducts blood from the left ventricle into the aorta.

The mitral and tricuspid valves are termed **atrioventricular** (AV) valves; the pulmonic and aortic valves are referred to as **semilunar** valves. The relationships between heart valves, heart chambers, and blood vessels are shown in Figure 4-3.

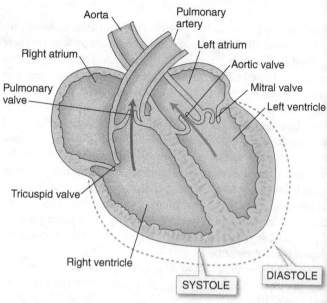

Figure 4-3: Anatomy of heart chambers and valves. The right ventricle pumps deoxygenated blood (*blue arrow*) to the lungs via the pulmonary arteries. The left ventricle pumps oxygenated blood (*red arrow*) to the systemic circulation via the aorta. Systole, in which the semilunar valves are open and the atrioventricular valves are closed, is shown.

▽ To understand the clinical implications of **congenital heart diseases,** it is necessary to have a knowledge of the structure and function of a normal (healthy) heart. Congenital heart diseases can be divided into cyanotic versus noncyanotic. Cyanosis is a bluish coloration of the skin due to the presence of deoxyhemoglobin. In cyanotic heart disease, a right-to-left shunt occurs, whereby deoxygenated blood returning to the right side of the heart bypasses the lungs and reenters the systemic circulation. Structural anomalies responsible for noncyanotic heart disease allow deoxygenated blood to reach the lungs and become oxygenated. ▽

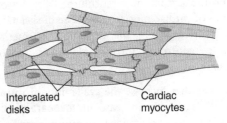

Figure 4-4: Electrical coupling of cardiac myocytes. Gap junctions in the intercalated disks provide a low-resistance pathway for the spread of electrical excitation.

CELLULAR ANATOMY OF VENTRICULAR MUSCLE

▨ Cardiac muscle is striated and has an intracellular sarcomere structure that is very similar to that of skeletal muscle (see Chapter 1). Figure 4-4 shows that cardiac muscle cells (myocytes) form a highly branched network.

▨ Myocytes are surrounded by a sarcolemma (plasma membrane), with transverse tubules (T tubules) that extend into the cell interior.

▨ Sarcoplasmic reticulum is associated with every T tubule.

▨ Myocyte connections occur at structures called intercalated disks. The presence of gap junctions in intercalated disks accounts for high electrical conductance (low resistance) between myocytes.

▨ A single adequate stimulus for action potential in one myocyte results in the rapid spread of excitation to all myocytes via gap junctions. This is known as the **all-or-none electrical response of the heart.**

▽ In the patient with **coronary ischemia,** areas of heart muscle can begin to randomly depolarize. These myocytes are referred to as "irritable." Depolarization of one irritable myocyte rapidly propagates via the all-or-none principle, which can lead to a fatal arrhythmia (ventricular fibrillation or ventricular tachycardia). *Fatal arrhythmias are the most common cause of sudden death during a myocardial infarction.* ▽

EXCITATION-CONTRACTION COUPLING

Cardiac muscle cells contract without nervous stimulation. Pacemaker cells spontaneously generate action potentials, which spread through gap junctions. Action potentials conducted along T tubules are associated with opening of the voltage-gated Ca^{2+} channels and entry of extracellular Ca^{2+} into the cells. Ca^{2+}-induced Ca^{2+} release is triggered from internal sarcoplasmic reticulum stores. Almost all Ca^{2+} that interacts with troponin C to initiate contraction is derived from internal stores. Contraction occurs via the same sliding filament mechanism as described in Chapter 1. Relaxation of cardiac muscle depends on the removal of free cytosolic Ca^{2+}. In cardiac muscle, Ca^{2+} is moved back into the extracellular fluid via the Na^+/Ca^{2+} exchangers in the sarcolemma, which couple the inward transport of $3Na^+$ from the extracellular fluid to the outward transport of one intracellular Ca^{2+}. In addition, Ca^{2+}-ATPase is used by all types of muscle and pumps Ca^{2+}

back into the sarcoplasmic reticulum. Table 4-1 compares the properties of cardiac muscle with those of skeletal and smooth muscle. Differences in the excitation-contraction coupling process, the control of force development, and other factors are highlighted.

▽ Drugs that increase the availability of intracellular free Ca^{2+} cause an increase in **myocardial contractility.** Digitalis is a cardiac glycoside with multiple cardiac effects, one of which is to increase myocardial contraction via greater loading of intracellular Ca^{2+} stores. This is accomplished via the following steps:

▨ Digitalis blocks the Na^+/K^+-ATPase on the myocyte of the cardiac cell membrane, yielding an increase in intracellular $[Na^+]$.

▨ Increased intracellular $[Na^+]$ alters the electrochemical driving force for Na^+/Ca^{2+} exchange and results in the reversal of the normal transport direction, bringing Ca^{2+} into the cell.

▨ Increased intracellular $[Ca^{2+}]$ causes more Ca^{2+} to be stored in the sarcoplasmic reticulum.

▨ Subsequent excitation releases more Ca^{2+}, resulting in increased myocardial contraction (a positive inotropic effect). ▽

TABLE 4-1. Comparison of Muscle Types

Characteristic	Cardiac Muscle	Skeletal Muscle	Smooth Muscle
Histologic appearance	Striated	Striated	Not striated
Stimulus for excitation	Pacemaker potentials and electrical coupling via gap junctions	Transmission at the neuromuscular junction	Variable: • Synaptic • Hormonal • Pacemakers • Coupling via gap junctions
Electrical activity	Long action potential plateau	No action potential plateau	Variable
Excitation-contraction coupling	Ca^{2+}-induced Ca^{2+} release from sarcoplasmic reticulum	Voltage sensor triggers Ca^{2+} release from sarcoplasmic reticulum	Variable: • Ca^{2+} entry via L-type channels • IP_3-mediated Ca^{2+} release from stores
Molecular basis of contraction	Ca^{2+}-troponin C	Ca^{2+}-troponin C	Ca^{2+}-calmodulin
Ending contraction	Repolarization of action potential	Breakdown of acetylcholine in neuromuscular junction	Myosin light chain phosphatase activity
Control of force developed	Regulation of Ca^{2+} entry	Spatial and temporal summation	Latch bridge state
Metabolism	Oxidative	Oxidative and glycolytic fiber types	Oxidative

CARDIAC ELECTROPHYSIOLOGY

THE CONDUCTING SYSTEM

The **sinoatrial (SA) node** is the normal **pacemaker of the heart** and the origin of each normal heartbeat. The SA node is a collection of specialized myocytes near the site where the superior vena cava enters in the wall of the right atrium. Spontaneous depolarization of the SA node occurs, resulting in the generation of action potentials. Figure 4-5 illustrates the pathway by which excitation (**depolarization**) spreads through the heart. Action potentials from the SA node spread rapidly throughout the atria via gap junctions between adjacent myocytes.

The **atrioventricular (AV) node** is the only electrical communication between the atria and the ventricles. It is characterized by very slow electrical conduction, ensuring that atrial contraction is completed before the ventricles are activated. The AV node is continuous with the ventricular conducting system, which consists of the atrioventricular bundle (bundle of His), the left and right bundle branches, and the Purkinje fiber system.

The **ventricular conducting system** is composed of columns of specialized myocytes containing a small amount of contractile protein. The large diameter of cells reduces electrical resistance and promotes rapid conduction. A thick connective tissue sheath insulates the ventricular conducting system, ensuring that the first electrical connection with working ventricular muscle occurs through Purkinje fibers. Action potentials spread rapidly through the ventricular muscle via gap junctions between the adjacent myocytes. The typical sequence of ventricular activation is from the left side of the ventricular septum near the apex of the heart, and then to the inner surface of the myocardium in both ventricles in the region of the apex. The general spread of excitation is from the inner (endo-) myocardium to the outer (epi-) myocardium and from the apex toward the base.

▽ In **Wolff-Parkinson-White syndrome**, there is an accessory conduction pathway that creates a bidirectional link between the atria and the ventricles. A normal impulse that conducts from the atria down the AV node to the ventricles can travel up the accessory pathway to reexcite the atria. Alternatively, an atrial impulse can first conduct down the accessory pathway, depolarizing the ventricles, and then travel up the AV node (retrograde) and reactivate the atria. Either possibility can lead to paroxysmal supraventricular tachycardia, which manifests as palpitations, syncope, hypotension, and sometimes heart failure. ▼

VENTRICULAR MUSCLE ACTION POTENTIAL

Action potentials arriving at the ventricular muscle from the ventricular conducting system trigger the rapid spread of action potentials in all ventricular myocytes. The ventricular muscle action potential has a very long duration (250 ms). Figure 4-6 illustrates the following **five phases of the ventricular muscle action potential,** 0 through 4:

▪ **Phase 4** is the interval between action potentials when the ventricular muscles are at their stable **resting membrane potential.**

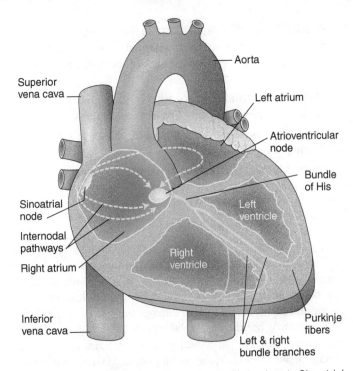

Figure 4-5: Electrical conducting system of the heart. Sinoatrial node → atrial muscle → atrioventricular node → bundle of His → bundle branches → Purkinje fibers → ventricular muscle.

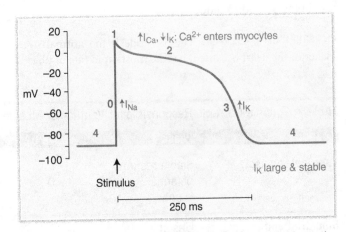

Figure 4-6: Ventricular action potential. Phase 4 = stable resting membrane potential; phase 0 = rapid depolarization upon stimulation; phase 1 = partial repolarization; phase 2 = plateau phase; and phase 3 = repolarization. I_{Na}, Na$^+$ current; I_{Ca}, Ca^{2+} current; I_K, K$^+$ current.

- **Phase 0** is the **initial rapid upstroke** that occurs immediately after stimulation. Membrane potential moves from its resting value of about −90 mV to a peak of about +30 mV during phase 0.

- **Phase 1** is a **partial repolarization** of the membrane potential from its peak value of +30 mV to about 0 mV.

- **Phase 2,** also known as the **plateau phase,** is a dramatic slowing of repolarization.

- **Phase 3** is the **repolarization** of membrane potential back to the resting value.

SA NODE ACTION POTENTIAL

Figure 4-7 illustrates the SA node action potential. SA nodal cells are pacemakers because their membrane potential difference depolarizes spontaneously during phase 4, which is called the **pacemaker potential** or **diastolic depolarization.** The maximum membrane potential difference in pacemaker cells is about −60 mV, but *there is no stable period of resting membrane potential.* When the pacemaker potential reaches a threshold voltage of about −40 mV, the action potential is triggered in the cells of the SA node. When compared with ventricular muscle, phase 0 in the SA node is slow and the action potential duration is shorter. Action potential generation in the AV node is qualitatively the same as in the SA node but has a significantly slower phase 4 depolarization. Table 4-2 contrasts the ionic basis of nodal and ventricular muscle action potentials.

▽ A knowledge of the ventricular action potential helps in the understanding of the mechanism of antiarrhythmic agents. There are **four classes of antiarrhythmics,** based on their site of action: class I, sodium channel blockers; class II, beta blockers; class III, potassium channel blockers; and class IV, calcium channel blockers. The SA node and AV node action potential upstroke (phase 4) is Ca^{2+} dependent, whereas the ventricular upstroke (phase 0) is Na^+ dependent. As such, class I antiarrhythmics are effective in the treatment of ventricular ectopy (additional heart beats of ventricular origin), and class II and class IV antiarrhythmics are effective in slowing conduction in the SA and AV nodes. ▽

HIERARCHY OF PACEMAKERS The SA node is the normal pacemaker of the heart because it has the most rapid rate of phase 4

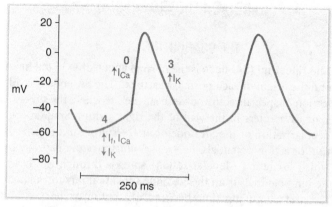

Figure 4-7: Nodal action potential. Phase 4 = unstable pacemaker potential; phase 0 = slow depolarization upon stimulation; and phase 3 = repolarization. I_f, nonselective cation current; I_{Ca}, Ca^{2+} current; I_K, K^+ current.

TABLE 4-2. Ionic Currents Responsible for Ventricular Muscle and Nodal Action Potentials

Location	Phase 4	Phase 0	Phase 1	Phase 2	Phase 3
Ventricular muscle	Stable resting potential: I_K only	I_{Na} ↑ (fast)	I_{Na} ↓ I_{Cl} & I_K ↑	Plateau phase: I_{Ca} ↑ I_K ↓	Repolarization: I_{Ca} ↓ I_K ↑
Sinoatrial and atrioventricular nodes	Unstable pacemaker potential: I_f & I_{Ca} ↑ I_K ↓	I_{Ca} ↑ (slow)			Repolarization: I_{Ca} ↓ I_K ↑

(diastolic) depolarization. A person is in **normal sinus rhythm** when cardiac excitation progresses from the SA node through the entire conduction pathway. The intrinsic rate of SA node firing is about 100 beats/min. Normal parasympathetic tone reduces the SA node firing rate to about 70 beats/min at rest. Endurance athletes have enhanced parasympathetic tone, which results in the classic finding of a slow resting heart rate in trained individuals. The AV node becomes the pacemaker if the SA node fails or transmission to the AV node fails. These patients are in nodal rhythm and typically have resting heart rates of 45–55 beats/min.

In patients with **complete heart block** (see normal and abnormal heart rhythm), there is no transmission through the AV node; the His-Purkinje fibers pace the heart between 20 and 40 beats/min. Slower pacemaker activity in distal parts of the conducting system allows the heart to continue beating if the SA node fails. However, these patients are likely to have **bradycardia** (slow heart rate) and reduced cardiac output. For example, **sick sinus syndrome** occurs when the SA node becomes fibrotic and loses its ability to spontaneously depolarize. Patients have bradycardia and symptoms of hypoperfusion such as dizziness, syncope, weakness, and fatigue. Abnormal heart rhythms can be diagnosed by observing an electrocardiogram (ECG). ▼

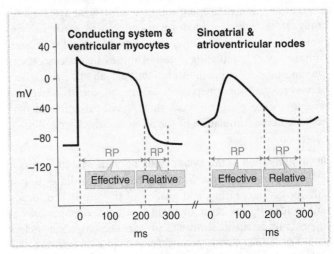

Figure 4-8: Cardiac action potentials. Cardiac action potentials have long refractory periods (RP). No stimulus can produce another action potential during the effective refractory period.

REFRACTORY PERIODS

The normal mechanical pumping cycle of the heart requires a single excitation event. Any additional action potentials spread rapidly through coupled myocardial cells and produce additional **arrhythmias** (inappropriate heart beats). If the ventricular rate is excessive, there is insufficient time between beats for the ventricles to fill.

Figure 4-8 shows that ventricular muscle cells have a long, **effective (absolute) refractory period** from the onset of phase 0 to midway through phase 3. This protects against circular (reentry) conduction, in which control by the pacemaker fails and each spread of excitation through the ventricles triggers the next. Treatment with drugs such as beta blockers and calcium channel blockers, which extend the refractory period, can be effective at preventing reentry arrhythmias. The long refractory period of the AV nodal cells also protects against conduction of rapid atrial arrhythmias to the ventricles. For example, in **atrial fibrillation,** the atrial rate is between 350 and 500 impulses per minute. Without the refractory properties of the AV node, the ventricular rate would correspond with the atrial rate, which would be incompatible with life.

AUTONOMIC REGULATION OF HEART RATE

If the autonomic nerves to the heart are cut (such as may occur during a heart transplant), the spontaneous heart rate at rest is approximately 100 beats/min. Parasympathetic tone reduces the typical resting heart rate to approximately 70 beats/min, and parasympathetic stimulation reduces the heart rate further and produces a **negative chronotropic effect.** Parasympathetic nerves release acetylcholine, which acts via the muscarinic receptors on the nodal cells. The muscarinic receptor antagonist **atropine** can be used to treat **symptomatic bradycardia.** Atropine blocks parasympathetic tone, allowing sympathetic tone to continue unchecked. Sympathetic nerve stimulation or circulating catecholamines increase the heart rate and produce a **positive chronotropic effect.** Sympathetic nerves release norepinephrine, acting on the β_1-adrenergic receptors. Figure 4-9 contrasts the parasympathetic and sympathetic nerve stimulation of the SA node, which underlies the effects on heart rate.

▽   **Activation of the sympathetic nervous system** occurs in response to stress. Signs include tachycardia as well as pale cool skin, sweating, and dilation of the pupils. It is important to identify the cause of sympathetic drive, which may be intrinsic or extrinsic. Examples of intrinsic activation include pain, fear, anxiety, or hypotension; examples of extrinsic activation include the use of drugs such as caffeine, cocaine, methamphetamines, or ephedrine. ▽

THE ECG

The collective spread of action potentials through the myocytes produces small voltages that can be measured on the surface of the body with an ECG. A standard ECG is obtained by placing an electrode on each limb and at six specific locations on the anterior chest wall. In a lead, one electrode is regarded as the positive side of a voltmeter and another is the negative side. A lead reports changes in voltage difference between the positive and negative electrodes. By varying which electrode is regarded as positive or which is negative, a standard set of 12 leads provides a range of views of electrical events in the heart. Figure 4-10 illustrates the major waves on an ECG, together with standard intervals and segments and standard calibrations of time and voltage. Electrical activity in nodal and conducting tissue is not seen on an ECG because the amount of tissue is too small to produce measurable voltage differences at the body surface.

ECG waveforms are produced by momentary changes in voltage differences during the spread of cardiac excitation.

▨ The **P wave** represents atrial depolarization.

▨ The **QRS complex** is produced by ventricular depolarization.

▨ The **T wave** results from ventricular repolarization.

▨ Atrial repolarization is obscured by the QRS complex.

▽   The QT interval is mostly determined by the duration of phase 2 of the ventricular action potential (Figure 4-6). A longer phase 2 is represented on the ECG as a prolonged QT interval, which may set up a dangerous form of ventricular tachycardia called **torsade de pointes.** Class III antiarrhythmic drugs cause a prolonged phase 2 of the action potential because repolarization is delayed when the K⁺ channels are blocked. Careful monitoring of the QT interval is a must when initiating therapy with a class III drug (e.g., amiodarone). ▽

▽   **Heart muscle mass is depicted as amplitude on the ECG.** For example, the P wave is smaller than the QRS

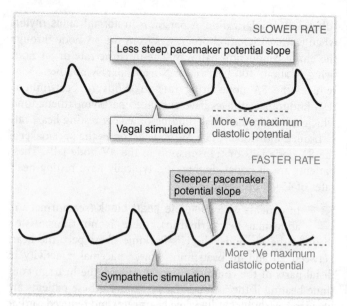

Figure 4-9: Effects of autonomic nerve stimulation on nodal action potentials. Parasympathetic (vagal) stimulation reduces the heart rate by hyperpolarizing the nodal cells and reducing the slope of pacemaker potentials. Sympathetic stimulation increases the heart rate by depolarizing the nodal cells and increasing the slope of pacemaker potentials.

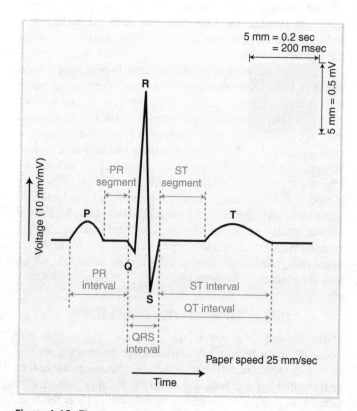

Figure 4-10: Electrocardiogram (ECG). Typical recording from lead II, showing ECG waves, segments, and intervals, and standard calibrations for time and voltage.

complex because atria have less mass than ventricles. Left ventricular hypertrophy is identified if the sum of voltage deflections for the S wave in lead V_1 and the R wave in leads V_5 or $V_6 \geq 35$ mm. Similarly, right ventricular hypertrophy is characterized by an R wave that is larger than the S wave in V_1. ▼

LEAD SYSTEMS ECG signals are vector quantities, since charge movement through the heart has both direction and magnitude. **Two lead systems** have been devised as follows (Table 4-3):

1. The **frontal (vertical) plane** is defined by **six limb leads.**
2. The **transverse plane** is perpendicular to the frontal plane and is defined by six **precordial chest leads.**

Table 4-3 lists the placement of standard ECG electrodes. Every lead has a unique axis within its plane. **Frontal plane leads** are composed of three bipolar limb leads (I, II, and III), in which the positive electrode placed on one limb is compared to a negative electrode placed on another limb. These electrode connections to the left arm, the right arm, and the left leg form an equilateral triangle with the heart at its center, called **Einthoven's triangle** (Figure 4-11A). Three augmented unipolar limb leads (aV_R, aV_L, and aV_F) are defined by using

TABLE 4-3. Placement and Polarity of Electrocardiogram Electrodes

Lead System	Lead Name	+Ve Electrode	−Ve (reference) Electrode
Frontal plane leads	I	LA	RA
	II	LL	RA
	III	LL	LA
	aV_R	RA	LA & LL combined
	aV_L	LA	RA & LL combined
	aV_F	LL	RA & LA combined
Transverse plane precordial leads	V_1	Fourth intercostal space to the right of the sternum	
	V_2	Fourth intercostal space to the left of the sternum	
	V_4	Fifth intercostal space in the midclavicular line	Virtual reference to center of heart
	V_3	Midway between V_2 and V_4	
	V_6	Fifth intercostal space in the midaxillary line	
	V_5	Midway between V_4 and V_6	

LA, left arm; RA, right arm; LL, left leg.

each limb electrode as a positive electrode referenced to a null point obtained by adding the potential from the other two limb leads.

The frontal plane is a circle in which each lead occupies one axis. The **hexaxial reference system** produced by the six frontal plane leads is shown in Figure 4-11B. This system provides a means of describing the direction of an electrical vector produced by the spread of electrical activity in the heart. The direction of the mean QRS vector is used most often because it is affected by common pathology (e.g., ventricular hypertrophy; bundle branch block). Each precordial chest electrode is a positive electrode terminal and can be compared to the virtual center of the heart, estimated electronically from the average of the limb leads.

ELECTRICAL VECTORS Figure 4-12 illustrates the concept of an electrical vector and how one may appear on different ECG leads. The ECG is an extracellular recording that views cells from the outside. Resting myocytes have a negative voltage on the inside of the cell membrane or, stated differently, they have a positive voltage on the outside of the cell membrane. A region of myocytes that has depolarized is negative on the outside when compared to neighboring cells at rest. This creates a voltage difference between adjacent regions, which is a vector quantity.

Vectors are represented using an arrow to illustrate their size and direction. By convention, the head of the vector (arrow) points toward the positive voltage (toward tissue not yet depolarized). The average vector changes momentarily in size and direction, producing the waves seen on an ECG. All 12 leads simultaneously report the spread of excitation through the heart when viewed from different angles. The waveform is different on each lead because each lead has a different orientation to the heart.

A major event is recorded by a lead when the vector direction is parallel to the axis of the lead. No net deflection is recorded by a lead if the vector is perpendicular to the axis of the lead. This concept is used to estimate the direction of vectors by assessing the ECG. The largest net deflection occurs in the lead that is roughly parallel to the electrical event. If a lead shows no net deflection (i.e., the event is **isoelectric**), then the electrical vector is perpendicular to the axis of that lead. Knowledge of the orientation of leads in the frontal plane is necessary to estimate vector direction in this way.

MEAN ELECTRICAL AXIS OF VENTRICULAR DEPOLARIZATION In principle, the axis (vector direction) of any part of the ECG can be determined. The mean axis of ventricular depolarization is most commonly evaluated by analyzing the QRS complex. The mean QRS axis has a normal range of −30° to +90° on the hexaxial reference system. Axes in the range of −30° to −90° are termed left axis deviation; axes in the range of +90° to +150° are termed right axis deviation.

▽ **Ventricular hypertrophy** is the thickening (or enlargement) of the myocardium and is a common cause of axis deviation. An increased left ventricular mass biases the direction of the net QRS vector toward the left. Similarly, patients with **right ventricular hypertrophy** usually have a **right axis deviation. Left axis deviation** can also occur when the abdominal contents physically push the heart up and to the left, such as occurs in patients who are **obese or pregnant.** ▽

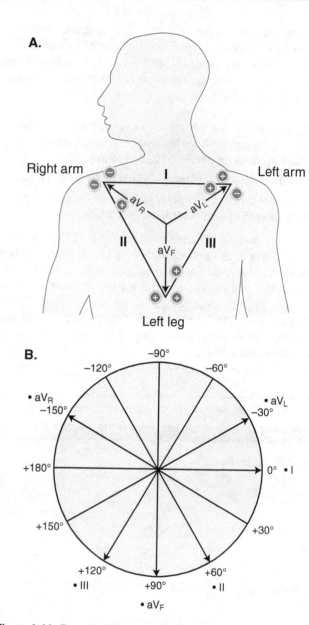

Figure 4-11: Frontal plane electrocardiogram leads. **A.** Einthoven's triangle, formed by bipolar limb leads I, II, and III. Directions of the unipolar limb leads aV$_R$, aV$_L$, and aV$_F$ are also shown. **B.** Hexaxial reference circle, showing the axis of each frontal plane lead.

Mean electrical axis usually can be estimated from an ECG by inspection alone. Figure 4-13 shows an example of left axis deviation. The sum of all deflections (net deflection) in the QRS complex of lead aV_R is near zero. The mean axis is, therefore, approximately perpendicular to this lead, corresponding to the axis of lead III. As expected, there is a large net QRS deflection recorded in lead III, confirming that the electrical vector in this case is roughly parallel to lead III (and perpendicular to aV_R). Because the net deflection is negative in lead III, the QRS vector is directed at the negative end of lead III at an angle of approximately −60° on the hexaxial reference system.

NORMAL AND ABNORMAL HEART RHYTHM

An ECG is routinely used to record heart rate and rhythm. Figure 4-14 compares a normal lead II record with several common arrhythmias. In normal sinus rhythm, a P wave is followed at normal intervals by a QRS complex and a T wave (see Figure 4-14A). Heart rate, in beats/min, is calculated by dividing the R-R interval (expressed in seconds) into 60. Heart rate above 100 beats/min is described as **tachycardia;** a heart rate below 60 beats/min is described as **bradycardia.**

▽ A premature atrial beat is revealed when a P wave occurs earlier than expected and is followed by the usual QRS complex and T wave (see Figure 4-14B). **Paroxysmal atrial tachycardia** is a rapid run of heart beats that begins suddenly and ends abruptly; P waves precede each QRS complex, showing that beats originate in the atria (see Figure 4-14C). In **atrial fibrillation** (see Figure 4-14D), there is chaotic electrical activity; no P waves can be defined, and QRS complexes occur at irregular intervals, reflecting random depolarization of the AV node. The resulting pulse is classically described as "irregularly irregular." In atrial fibrillation, stasis of blood often occurs in the atrial appendages due to the loss of atrial contraction. Anticoagulation therapy may be needed to counter the risk of thromboembolism.

Heart block is a **group of abnormalities** characterized by varying degrees of impaired conduction through the AV node.

▪ In **first-degree heart block,** the PR interval is abnormally long at a normal heart rate, indicating delayed conduction through the AV node (see Figure 4-14E).

▪ **Second-degree heart** block is characterized by intermittent failure of the AV node so that not every P wave is followed by a QRS complex. There are two types of second-degree heart block: **Mobitz type I (Wenckebach)** block is a benign rhythm whose origin is the AV node (see Figure 4-14F). It is characterized by progressive lengthening of the PR interval on consecutive beats, followed by a dropped QRS complex. **Mobitz type II** second-degree heart block is a more ominous rhythm and has its origin in the distal His-Purkinje system. It is characterized by dropped ventricular beats that are not preceded by PR interval lengthening (see Figure 4-14G). The block may persist for two or more beats, yielding an atrial to ventricular ratio of 2:1, 3:1, and so on. *Type II heart block may progress quickly to complete heart block.*

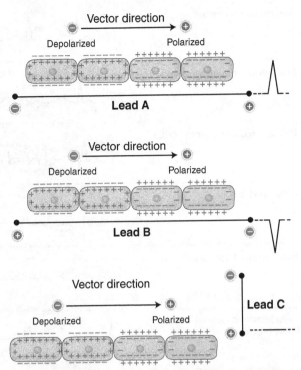

Figure 4-12: An electrical vector recorded by different electrocar leads. Adjacent areas of cells at different potentials produce a vector. A large positive recording in lead A is seen because the vector is parallel to lead A and directed at its positive terminal. A large negative recording is seen in lead B because the vector is parallel to lead B but directed at its negative terminal. No net signal is recorded in lead C because it is perpendicular to the vector.

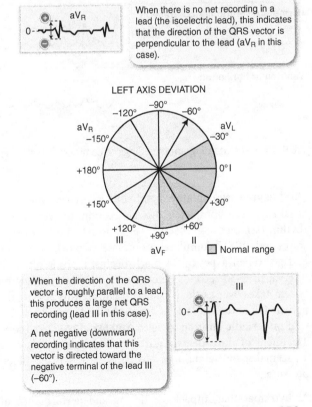

Figure 4-13: Inspection method to assess the mean QRS axis (mean electrical axis of the heart).

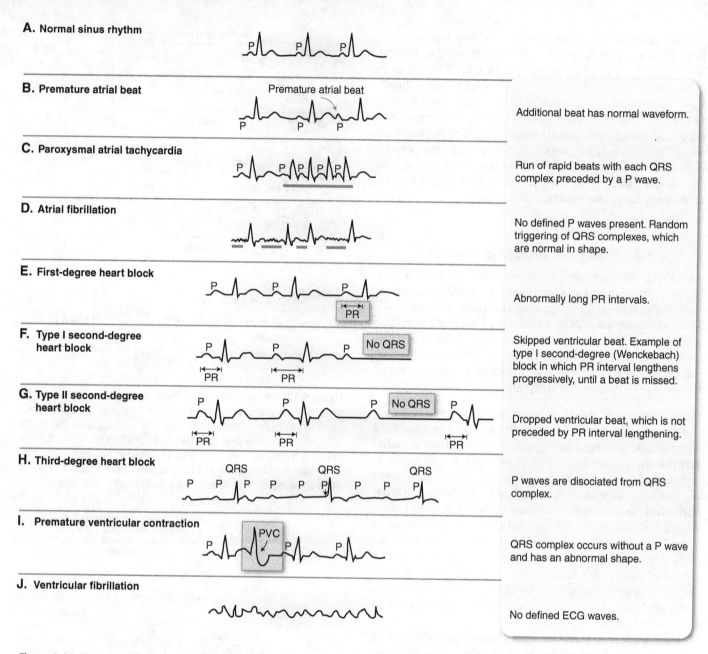

A. Normal sinus rhythm

B. Premature atrial beat

Premature atrial beat

Additional beat has normal waveform.

C. Paroxysmal atrial tachycardia

Run of rapid beats with each QRS complex preceded by a P wave.

D. Atrial fibrillation

No defined P waves present. Random triggering of QRS complexes, which are normal in shape.

E. First-degree heart block

Abnormally long PR intervals.

F. Type I second-degree heart block

No QRS

Skipped ventricular beat. Example of type I second-degree (Wenckebach) block in which PR interval lengthens progressively, until a beat is missed.

G. Type II second-degree heart block

No QRS

Dropped ventricular beat, which is not preceded by PR interval lengthening.

H. Third-degree heart block

P waves are disociated from QRS complex.

I. Premature ventricular contraction

QRS complex occurs without a P wave and has an abnormal shape.

J. Ventricular fibrillation

No defined ECG waves.

Figure 4-14: Electrocardiogram recordings of common arrhythmias.

Third-degree (complete) heart block occurs when the atrial rhythm is completely dissociated from the ventricular rhythm (see Figure 4-14H). There is no relation between P waves and QRS-T complexes. Complete AV block may come and go. When a period of block begins, there is often an interval of 5–30 seconds before the ventricular conducting system takes over as the pacemaker. During this period, the patient faints due to lack of cerebral blood flow. This pattern of periodic fainting is called **Stokes-Adams syndrome.** Treatment of third-degree heart block includes implanting a pacemaker to maintain an adequate heart rate and blood pressure.

Arrhythmias that impact the timing and performance of ventricular contraction may arise from within the ventricles rather than being the result of abnormalities of atrial rhythm or AV node. **Premature ventricular contractions (PVCs)** occur with no preceding P wave (see Figure 4-14I). The origin of the ventricular excitation is within the ventricular conducting system or from a ventricular muscle focus. The QRS complex is often an irregular shape, reflecting a pattern of electrical spread that differs from a normal pacemaker source. *Abnormal ventricular pacemakers, which are often damaged or unstable areas of ventricular myocardium, can drive ventricular tachycardia.* This is a dangerous type of arrhythmia because the beating frequency may be too high to allow adequate ventricular filling. Ventricular tachycardia may degenerate into **ventricular fibrillation** associated with random chaotic electrical activity (see Figure 4-14J). *Ventricular fibrillation is fatal within a short period of time due to lack of coordinated ventricular contraction.*

PVCs are either asymptomatic or are sensed as palpitations. They occur in most of the normal population and are benign. However, in the setting of a current or past **myocardial infarction (MI),** PVCs may become more frequent. Two episodes of PVCs coupled together are known as couplets; three or more episodes of PVCs coupled together are known as ventricular tachycardia and are associated with increased mortality. *The most common cause of death during an MI is fatal arrhythmia (ventricular fibrillation or ventricular tachycardia).*

Arrhythmias are often caused by electrolyte abnormalities. For example, as plasma K^+ concentration increases, hyperkalemia produces the following sequence of cardiotoxic effects: peaked T waves, prolonged PR interval, widening of the QRS complex, blockage of the AV node, loss of P waves, and eventual merging of the QRS complex with the T wave, which produces a "sine wave" pattern that can degenerate into ventricular fibrillation or asystole. ▼

THE CARDIAC CYCLE

The cardiac cycle is described as the repetitive electrical and mechanical events that occur with each beat of the heart. Electrical events precede mechanical events, which result from the entry of Ca^{2+} into the myocytes during cardiac action potentials. ECG waves can be correlated with mechanical events. The P wave precedes atrial contraction. During the PR segment, there is no apparent electrical activity in the ECG. During this time, there is conduction through the AV node and the ventricular conducting system. The QRS complex precedes contraction of the ventricle. The T wave of ventricular repolarization precedes ventricular relaxation.

Blood is pressurized by ventricular contraction and then ejected into the circulation during systole. Muscle relaxation is followed by ventricular filling during diastole. Mechanical events of the cardiac cycle occur in five phases (Figure 4-15):

1. **Ventricular diastole.** Throughout most of ventricular diastole, the atria and ventricles are relaxed. The AV valves are open, and the ventricles fill passively.

2. **Atrial systole.** During atrial systole, a small amount of additional blood is pumped into the ventricles.

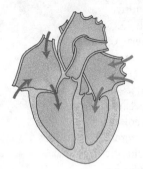

① MID-DIASTOLE: Atrioventricular valves open, ventricles are relaxed, filling passively.

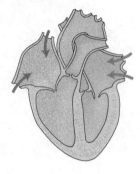

⑤ ISOVOLUMIC RELAXATION

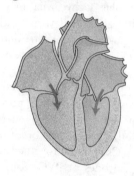

② ATRIAL SYSTOLE

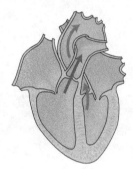

④ VENTRICULAR EJECTION (systole)

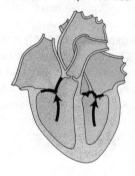

③ ISOVOLUMIC CONTRACTION: Atrioventricular valves close; blood is pressurized.

Figure 4-15: Major phases of the cardiac cycle.

3. **Isovolumic ventricular contraction.** Initial contraction increases ventricular pressure, closing the AV valves. Blood is pressurized during isovolumic ventricular contraction.

4. **Ventricular ejection.** The semilunar valves open when ventricular pressures exceed pressures in the aorta and pulmonary artery. Ventricular ejection (systole) of blood follows.

5. **Isovolumic relaxation.** The semilunar valves close when the ventricles relax and pressure in the ventricles decreases. The AV valves open when pressure in the ventricles decreases below atrial pressure. Atria fill with blood throughout ventricular systole, allowing rapid ventricular filling at the start of the next diastolic period.

WIGGERS DIAGRAM

Several variables can be measured to assess the electrical and mechanical events that occur with each beat of the heart. Electrical events can be followed using an ECG. Pressure changes in each chamber of the heart and in the central blood vessels can be measured by cardiac catheterization. Volume changes can be derived by echocardiography. Heart sounds can be recorded as a phonocardiogram. The Wiggers diagram,

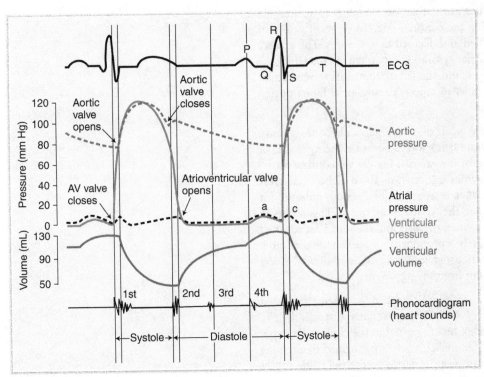

Figure 4-16: Wiggers diagram, a correlation of electrical and mechanical events during the cardiac cycle. A phonocardiogram records heart sounds.

shown in Figure 4-16, integrates all of these variables and allows correlation of the following **electrical and mechanical events during the cardiac cycle:**

- **Left ventricular pressure** is normally 0–10 mm Hg at the end of diastole but increases rapidly as the ventricles contract. The mitral valve closes when the left ventricular pressure exceeds left atrial pressure. The mitral and tricuspid valves are not forced back into the atria during ventricular contraction because they are anchored to the papillary muscles via the fibrous chordae tendineae. The aortic valve opens when the left ventricular pressure increases to a value just higher than the aortic diastolic pressure, typically about 80 mm Hg. Forceful contraction during early ventricular ejection increases the left ventricular pressure to a peak value of about 120 mm Hg, corresponding to the aortic systolic blood pressure. As the ventricular contraction weakens, the left ventricular pressure decreases. When the left ventricular pressure decreases just below the aortic blood pressure, the aortic valve closes. Left ventricular pressure decreases rapidly as the muscle relaxes; when the pressure decreases just below the left atrial pressure, the mitral valve opens. Ventricular filling occurs at low pressures, reflecting the left atrial pressure.

- **Aortic pressure** increases in concert with the left ventricular pressure during ventricular ejection. Vibration caused by closure of the aortic valve causes a deviation in the aortic pressure, called the **dicrotic notch.** The aortic pressure decreases between ventricular beats as blood continues to flow from the aorta into the circulation. Diastolic blood pressure is the aortic pressure minimum recorded just before the next ventricular ejection.

Left atrial pressure normally is no greater than 10 mm Hg at any time during the cardiac cycle. Three small peaks, or waves, are identified and denoted as a, c, and v. The **a wave** is produced by atrial systole. The **c wave** occurs when the mitral valve bulges into the left atrium during ventricular contraction. The **v wave** reflects passive atrial filling during ventricular systole.

▼ Although the Wiggers diagram includes left-sided events, similar **atrial pressure waves** occur on the right side of the heart. Inspection of the external jugular vein during physical examination provides information about right atrial pressure. A **"cannon" a wave** is seen in jugular venous pulsations if the atria contract when the AV valves are closed. This occurs in complete heart block when the atria and the ventricles contract independently. Similarly, a prominent v wave can be seen in the jugular vein during tricuspid regurgitation as additional blood enters the right atrium from the right ventricle. ▼

▼ Right-sided heart failure results in increased right-sided heart pressures and jugular venous distention. The **abdominojugular reflux test** can assist in the clinical diagnosis of right-sided heart failure. This test is performed by pressing on the liver to increase venous return to the right side of the heart while observing jugular venous distention. In a healthy patient, there is a slight rise in jugular distention that quickly returns to its previous level. In a patient with right-sided heart failure, jugular distention is pronounced and remains pronounced because the failing right ventricle is unable to accommodate increased venous return. ▼

The Wiggers diagram includes changes in left ventricular volume during the cardiac cycle. **Left ventricular end-diastolic volume** is about 140 mL in a normal heart at rest. *Ventricular systole ejects about half of the end-diastolic volume at rest,* producing a typical **end-systolic volume** of about 70 mL. Ventricular filling is rapid in early diastole. Ventricular volume reaches a plateau during passive filling, called **diastasis,** because ventricular compliance decreases as the chamber fills. Atrial systole produces a final boost to achieve end-diastolic volume. The stroke volume ejected during ventricular systole is the difference between end-diastolic volume and end-systolic volume.

▼ Atrial systole normally contributes about 10% of ventricular filling at rest. As the heart rate increases, the amount of time necessary for passive ventricular filling decreases, and the contribution of atrial systole can increase to over 30% of end-diastolic volume. Patients with atrial fibrillation lack this "**atrial kick**" and may have inadequate ventricular filling, particularly during physical activity. Patients with cardiovascular disease may rely on the atrial kick to maintain adequate cardiac output; without it, they may develop heart failure. ▼

The Wiggers diagram includes a **phonocardiogram,** which is a recording of sounds that occur during the cardiac cycle. The first heart sound (S_1) is caused by closure of the atrioventricular valves, and the second heart sound (S_2) is caused by closure of the pulmonic and aortic valves. The third

(S_3) and fourth (S_4) heart sounds may be normal sounds associated with ventricular filling. *Abnormal heart sounds are most commonly recorded when the heart valves are defective.*

NORMAL HEART SOUNDS

Heart valves prevent reverse blood flow. AV valves prevent backflow of blood into the atria during ventricular contraction, and semilunar valves prevent backflow of blood from the aorta and pulmonary artery to the ventricles during diastole. Heart valves open and close passively in response to pressure differences across the valves. *Valve opening is silent in the normal heart.* Closure of the valves produces vibrations that are heard as heart sounds. Figure 4-17 shows timing of the heart sounds in relation to events seen on an ECG.

The **first heart sound (S_1),** a "lub," is generated by the closing of the mitral (M_1) and tricuspid (T_1) valves. Closure of the tricuspid valve follows so closely after mitral valve closure that these sounds are perceived as a single sound. The larger diameter of the AV valves produces a low-pitched sound that is best heard with the bell of a stethoscope. The anatomic complexity of the AV valve apparatus contributes to the longer duration of the first heart sound compared to the second.

The **second heart sound (S_2),** a "dup," occurs when the semilunar valves snap closed at the onset of diastole. The S_2 has a crisper, higher pitch and shorter duration, and is best heard with the diaphragm of a stethoscope because the pressure gradients producing valve closure are larger. The second sound is composed of aortic (A_2) and pulmonic (P_2) valve closures. During inspiration, A_2 and P_2 are often heard as separate sounds (Figure 4-17). The **splitting of S_2** is caused by delayed closure of the pulmonic valve and earlier closure of the aortic valve. Decreased intrathoracic pressure on inspiration allows the distensible pulmonary circulation to receive a greater stroke volume from the right ventricle, prolonging right ventricular systole and delaying the P_2 sound. Increased pulmonary vascular capacitance during inspiration also reduces venous return to the left atrium, which shortens left ventricular systole and produces an earlier A_2 sound.

▽ **Paradoxical splitting of S_2** occurs when closure of the aortic valve is delayed, causing P_2 to occur first, followed by A_2. The most notable causes are **aortic stenosis** (which prolongs left ventricular systole) and **left bundle branch block** (which delays the onset of left ventricular contraction). ▼

A **third heart sound (S_3)** is sometimes heard in normal persons. It is a low-pitched, early diastolic sound heard best at the apex of the heart, and is caused by vibrations due to rapid ventricular filling. S_3 may be normal in children and in adults after exercise.

▽ A **fourth heart sound (S_4)** can be caused by atrial systole. It is a low-pitched, late diastolic or presystolic sound. S_4 may be heard normally in young children but is usually associated with cardiovascular pathology in adults. In atrial fibrillation, there is no atrial kick; these patients, therefore, cannot have an S_4. In patients with **tachycardia**, S_4 may be fused with an S_3 sound, producing a **summation gallop.** ▼

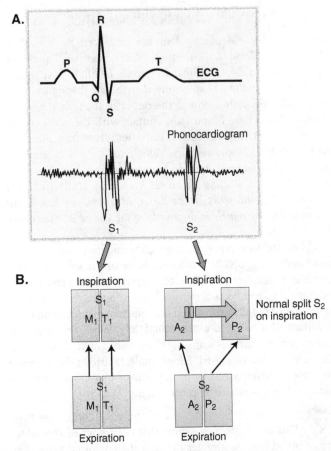

Figure 4-17: A. First (S_1) and second (S_2) heart sounds. **B.** Physiologic splitting of S_2. S_1 is caused by the closure of the atrioventricular valves; S_2 is caused by the closure of the semilunar valves. Physiologic splitting mainly results from the delayed closure of the pulmonic valve on inspiration. M_1, mitral valve closure; T_1, tricuspid valve closure; A_2, aortic valve closure; P_2, pulmonic valve closure.

COMMON VALVULAR ABNORMALITIES

Sounds in the vascular system are produced by turbulent blood flow. Blood flow through blood vessels is normally silent because flow is laminar in nature. **Laminar flow** means that the blood flow is smoothly distributed throughout the vessel, with the fastest flow in the center of the lumen and the slowest flow where blood is in contact with the walls of the blood vessel. The likelihood of noisy **turbulent flow** increases with high blood flow velocity. Velocity of flow is accelerated across narrow areas of blood vessels or heart valves. This creates turbulence, leading to noises known as **bruits** in blood vessels and as **murmurs** in the heart. *Murmurs are best heard "downstream" from their origin along the course of the turbulent blood flow.*

There are two types of valve abnormalities that produce heart murmurs. **Stenosis** is a narrowing of the valve that creates higher velocity blood flow through the partially constricted opening and produces a murmur when the valve is normally open. **Insufficiency** (also called incompetence or regurgitation) is **failure of a valve to close completely.** When valves do not close properly, there is some backflow of blood at a time when the valve should be closed. For example, failure of the AV valve to close completely results in the flow of blood back into the atrium during ventricular contraction.

▽   Figure 4-18 illustrates the murmur of **aortic stenosis.** This is a systolic murmur that occurs when the velocity of blood flow accelerates through the narrowed valve. The murmur is loudest in the middle of systole when the pressure gradient across the valve is greatest. Aortic stenosis leads to reduced stroke volume and a decrease in systolic pressure in the aorta. Pressure in the left ventricle is increased above normal to eject the stroke volume. Aortic stenosis is most common in elderly patients and is caused by calcification of the valve. Three cardinal symptoms of aortic stenosis are **angina, syncope,** and **congestive heart failure.**

Figure 4-19 illustrates the murmur of **mitral insufficiency.** This is a systolic murmur produced by blood flowing backward through the valve when it is normally closed. This produces a soft, **holosystolic (throughout systole) murmur.** Mitral insufficiency results in an increased volume load to the left atrium and ventricle. Forward flow into the aorta usually does not change significantly unless congestive heart failure occurs late in the course of the disease. Increased left atrial pressure and large atrial v waves should be predicted due to the backflow of blood from the left ventricle during systole, but they often are absent due to increasing compliance of the left atrium during the course of the disease.

Mitral valve prolapse is billowing of floppy, redundant mitral leaflets back into the left atrium during ventricular systole. Sudden tensing of floppy leaflets produces the classic auscultatory finding of **midsystolic click.** Mitral valve prolapse can be accompanied by mitral insufficiency. If the prolapsing leaflets do not come together properly, then a late systolic murmur can be heard, corresponding to regurgitant flow back into the atrium.

Figure 4-20 illustrates the murmur of **aortic insufficiency.** A normal aortic valve controls the large pressure difference

Aortic Stenosis

A. Phonocardiogram: paradoxical split S_2

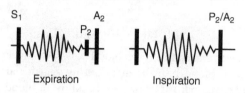

B. Elevated left ventricular pressure

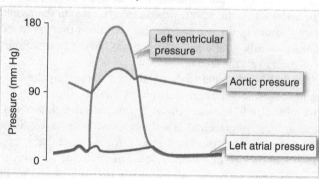

Note high left ventricular pressure to maintain cardiac output through narrow aortic valve.

Figure 4-18: Systolic murmur of aortic stenosis. **A.** Paradoxical splitting of the second (S_2) heart sound occurs because the aortic valve (A_2) closes later than the pulmonic valve (P_2) due to prolonged left ventricular systole. **B.** Pressure gradient across the narrowed aortic valve.

Mitral Insufficiency

A. Holosystolic murmur, early aortic valve closure

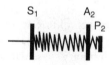

B. Possible elevated left atrial pressure

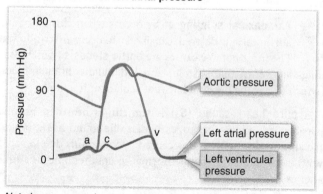

Note large v wave due to regurgitation of blood from left ventricle to left atrium.

Figure 4-19: Systolic murmur of mitral insufficiency. **A.** The early aortic valve (A_2) sound indicates the shortened systole due to retrograde blood flow into the left atrium. **B.** The large atrial v wave due to regurgitation of blood from the left ventricle into the left atrium during systole.

between the aortic diastolic blood pressure and the left ventricular diastolic pressure. A leaking aortic valve allows regurgitation of flow backward through the valve during diastole, when it should normally be closed. The murmur decreases in intensity as the pressure gradient across the valve decreases in late diastole. Retrograde flow from the aorta into the left ventricle during diastole increases the ventricular end-diastolic volume. This subsequently increases the stroke volume and the aortic systolic blood pressure. An abnormal blood flow from the aorta into the ventricle during diastole causes the aortic diastolic pressure to decrease. *Increased systolic pressure and decreased diastolic pressure produce a large arterial pulse* that is the basis of several physical findings, including (1) **Corrigan's pulse,** the "water-hammer pulse" that collapses rapidly; (2) **Quincke's pulse,** when pulsations are noted in the root of the fingernail bed while lightly pinching the tip of the fingernail; and (3) **de Musset's sign,** when the head bobs with each pulsation. Aortic insufficiency may result from valve disease (e.g., rheumatic heart disease) or aortic root dilation (e.g., syphilis or Marfan's syndrome).

Figure 4-21 illustrates the murmur of **mitral stenosis.** High resistance across the mitral valve produces turbulent blood flow into the left ventricle, causing a **soft crescendo murmur.** There may also be an "**opening snap,**" created by rapid movement of the contracted mitral valve apparatus and heard as a sharp sound immediately after S_2. Systemic blood pressure may be reduced in mitral stenosis because of decreased filling of the left ventricle, resulting in a decrease in stroke volume. *Left atrial pressure is often elevated, causing pulmonary congestion.*

Mitral stenosis is the most common valvular lesion caused by rheumatic heart disease. However, proper treatment of streptococcal pharyngitis with penicillin can prevent the valvular complications of rheumatic fever.

Patent ductus arteriosus produces a characteristic continuous **murmur in neonates.** The ductus arteriosus is a normal fetal connection between the aorta and the pulmonary artery, which normally closes near the time of birth. When this connection remains open, blood flows from the high pressure in the aorta to the lower pressure in the pulmonary artery. The murmur is continuous because there is a pressure gradient from the aorta to the pulmonary artery throughout the entire cardiac cycle. *The incidence of patent ductus arteriosus is high in premature infants.*

Patent ductus arteriosus produces increased pulmonary blood flow and greater filling of the left atrium and ventricle. A large stroke volume increases systolic aortic blood pressure. Runoff of blood from the aorta through a patent ductus during diastole accounts for reduced aortic diastolic blood pressure. There is a large arterial pulse wave similar to that seen in aortic insufficiency in the adult. Prostaglandin E and low arterial partial pressure of O_2 (P_aO_2) maintain patency of the ductus, so that *administering O_2 and prostaglandin inhibitors (e.g., indomethacin) promotes closure of the patent ductus arteriosus.*

Flow murmurs can occur in a structurally normal vascular system. Anemia causes flow murmurs because cardiac output is

Aortic Insufficiency

A. Decrescendo murmur

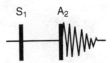

B. "Water-hammer" pulse: increased systolic blood pressure and decreased diastolic blood pressure

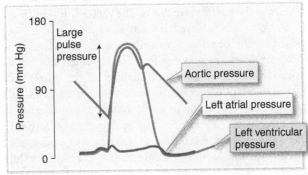

Figure 4-20: Diastolic murmur of aortic insufficiency. **A.** Sound intensity of the murmur decreases during diastole as a function of aortic blood pressure. S_1 is the first heart sound; A_2 indicates timing of the closure of the aortic valve. **B.** Pathologic runoff of blood from the aorta into the left ventricle decreases aortic diastolic blood pressure and increases left ventricular filling, increasing stroke volume and systolic blood pressure.

Mitral Stenosis

A. Presystolic murmur (PSM) and opening snap (OS)

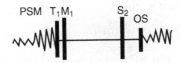

B. Continually elevated left atrial pressure

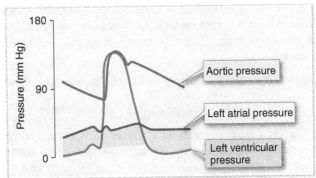

Note high left atrial pressure due to obstructed flow through mitral valve.

Figure 4-21: Diastolic murmur of mitral stenosis. **A.** An opening snap (OS) is a unique sound that is characteristic of mitral stenosis. The sound produced by obstructed flow through the mitral valve is described as a presystolic murmur (PSM). Obstructed ventricular filling may delay closure of the mitral valve (M_1) relative to closure of the tricuspid valve (T_1). **B.** Obstruction of the mitral valve causes a sustained increase in left atrial pressure.

increased to maintain delivery of O_2 to the tissues. There is increased velocity of blood flow and decreased blood viscosity in anemia, which can result in turbulent flow and cause vibrations. Turbulent flow occurs mostly at the cardiac valves and at bifurcations of the large and the medium-sized arteries. ▼

PRESSURE-VOLUME LOOPS

Figure 4-22 shows the cardiac cycle of the left ventricle, represented by plotting pressure against volume to produce a loop. At point A, the ventricle contains the end-systolic blood volume, and the mitral valve opens. The ventricle fills until end-diastolic volume is achieved at point B, where the mitral valve is closed by the onset of ventricular contraction. Isovolumic contraction increases pressure to point C, which corresponds to diastolic blood pressure and opening of the aortic valve. Ventricular ejection propels pressure through its peak value at point D, corresponding to aortic systolic pressure, until the aortic valve closes at point E. Pressure decreases back to point A during isovolumic relaxation, completing one cardiac cycle. The width of the pressure-volume loop is the stroke volume (the difference between end-diastolic volume and end-systolic volume). The area within a pressure-volume loop is an index of **stroke work.**

CARDIAC OUTPUT

Cardiac output is the volume of blood pumped by each ventricle per minute. Cardiac output (Q_T) is regulated by autonomic nerves and hormones through changes in heart rate (HR) or stroke volume (SV). In adults, cardiac output is usually expressed in liters per minute:

$$Q_T = (SV \times HR)/1000 \qquad \textbf{Equation 4-4}$$

Q_T = Cardiac output (L/min)
SV = Stroke volume (mL/min)
HR = Heart rate (beats/min)

HR is measured by feeling a pulse in an artery that is close to the skin or it is seen on an ECG. SV can be estimated from an echocardiogram. Cardiac output is then calculated using Equation 4-4.

Example If resting SV is 70 mL and HR is 70 beats/min, then

$$Q_T = (70 \text{ mL} \times 70 \text{ beats/min})/1000 = 4.9 L/min$$

Cardiac output can also be measured clinically in the cardiac catheterization laboratory, using a **thermodilution method** whereby a cold saline solution of known temperature and volume is injected into the right atrium. The reduction in blood temperature measured downstream in the pulmonary artery is a function of cardiac output.

THE FICK PRINCIPLE

A traditional physiologic method for calculating cardiac output applies the Fick principle, which derives blood flow from variables related to O_2 consumption. The O_2 consumption (Vo_2) of

A. Left ventricular pressure and volume

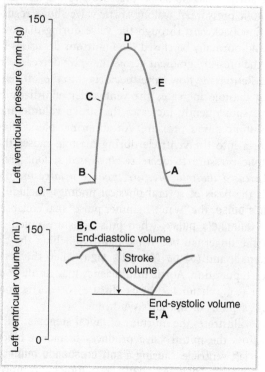

B. Pressure-volume loop

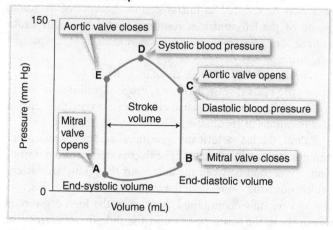

Figure 4-22: Left ventricular pressure-volume loop. **A.** Correlation between changes in left ventricular pressure (*upper panel*) and left ventricular volume (*lower panel*) during a single cardiac cycle. **B.** Left ventricular pressure is plotted as a function of left ventricular volume. Landmark events of valve opening and closure and the point where peak systolic blood pressure occurs are noted in both figures at points A–E.

a specific organ is the product of blood flow and the decrease in O_2 content between the artery and the vein ($CaO_2 - CvO_2$). In the Fick equation (Equation 4-5), these terms are rearranged to determine blood flow. Cardiac output can be calculated by applying the Fick concept to the entire body, relating total body O_2 consumption to the difference in O_2 content between blood in the systemic arteries and the mixed venous blood sampled from the pulmonary artery or the right ventricle:

$$Q_T = Vo_2 / (CaO_2 - CvO_2)$$ **Equation 4-5**

Q_T = Cardiac output
Vo_2 = O_2 consumption
CaO_2 = Arterial O_2 content
CvO_2 = Mixed venous O_2 content

Example A person consumes 250 mL of O_2 per min. Arterial O_2 content is 20 mL of O_2 per dL of blood, and the O_2 content of mixed venous blood is 15 mL of O_2 per dL of blood:

$$Q_T = 250 \ (mL/min) \div (20 \ mL/dL - 15 \ mL/dL) = 50 \ dL/min$$

Q_T = 50 dL/min = 5 L/min

▽ **Hypovolemic and cardiogenic shock** are classic examples of low cardiac output, which results in inadequate tissue perfusion (shock). Paradoxically, low cardiac output is not a universal finding in patients in shock. In **septic shock,** for example, there is inadequate tissue perfusion with high cardiac output. **Release of inflammatory cytokines** during sepsis, which results from an overwhelming systemic infection, has many effects, which together may cause shock:

▪ **Decreased systemic vascular resistance** (decreased afterload) to the point where increasing cardiac output cannot maintain blood pressure.

▪ **Increased capillary permeability,** causing edema and loss of effective circulating volume (decreased preload).

▪ **Reduced cardiac contractility,** caused by the release of myocardial depressant factors. ▽

EJECTION FRACTION Ejection fraction is a simple measurement of ventricular performance and describes the fraction of end-diastolic volume ejected from the ventricle during systole:

$$EF = SV \div EDV$$ **Equation 4-6**

EF = Ejection fraction
SV = Stroke volume
EDV = End-diastolic volume

Example A healthy man of average size is found to have a resting end-diastolic volume of 140 mL and a resting SV of 70 mL:

EF = 70/140 = 0.5 (50%)

▽ **Congestive heart failure** is classified as either systolic dysfunction (loss of contractility) or diastolic dysfunction (impaired compliance). *The ejection fraction is decreased in patients with systolic dysfunction due to the loss of contractility, but it is maintained in patients with diastolic dysfunction.* ▽

CARDIAC INDEX The adequacy of cardiac output should be considered in relation to tissue metabolic demand, which varies by body size and activity. Therefore, cardiac output is expressed relative to the body surface area (BSA) as the cardiac index (CI):

$$CI = Q_T / BSA \qquad \text{Equation 4-7}$$

CI = Cardiac index (L/min/m²)
Q_T = Cardiac output (L/min)
BSA = Body surface area (m²)

Example A 24-year-old woman is found to have a resting cardiac output of 4.0 L/min. Her body surface area is 1.40 m²:

$$CI = 4.0 / 1.40 = 2.86 \text{ L/min/m}^2$$

THE FRANK-STARLING PRINCIPLE

The **Frank-Starling principle,** illustrated in Figure 4-23, describes the relationship between SV and end-diastolic volume. Increased diastolic filling produces greater stretch of heart muscle, resulting in a larger SV. The mechanism involves more optimal overlap between the thin and thick muscle filaments as preload increases and increased sensitivity of troponin C to Ca^{2+} as cardiac muscle is stretched. *End-diastolic volume is the most important determinant of SV.* Outputs from the left and right sides of the heart are also equalized as a result of the Frank-Starling principle because the output of one side becomes the venous return of the other side.

ASSESSMENT OF VENTRICULAR FUNCTION

SV is determined by three factors: preload, afterload, and contractility. Ventricular **preload** is the end-diastolic volume created by venous return. Ventricular **afterload** is the sum of factors that oppose ejection of blood during systole. **Contractility** is the intrinsic vigor of muscle contraction related to the biochemical state of the cell.

PRELOAD Preload is enhanced by several factors, including:

- Increased circulating blood volume.
- Rhythmic skeletal muscle contraction, which propels blood toward the heart due to the presence of one-way valves in veins.
- Deep inspiration, which decreases intrathoracic pressure and increases abdominal pressure, promoting venous return to the thorax.
- Atrial systole.
- Venoconstriction, which reduces venous pooling and promotes the return of blood to the central circulation.

Figure 4-24 shows representations of the effect of increased preload on SV, using either the Frank-Starling curve or a pressure-volume loop.

▼ Preload can be quickly increased at the bedside by placing the patient in the **Trendelenburg position** (supine with the head lower than the feet), as well as by using drugs and intravenous fluids. **Interventions that increase preload** are often used to improve cardiac output, but this is

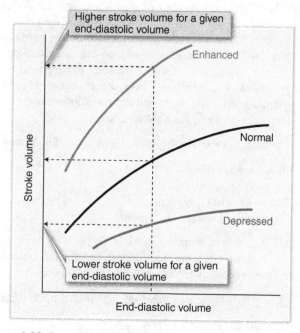

Figure 4-23: Frank-Starling relationship. End-diastolic volume is the most important determinant of stroke volume. Increased contractility of ventricular muscle produces a left shift in the Frank-Starling relationship; decreased contractility produces a right shift.

not always beneficial. For example, during an acute MI, the O_2 supply to the myocardium is disrupted, and treatments that reduce myocardial O_2 consumption are desirable. Nitrates can be used to reduce preload, decreasing the ventricular wall tension and, as a result, decreasing the myocardial O_2 consumption. ▼

AFTERLOAD The second factor that determines SV is afterload. The major component of afterload is resistance to blood flow created by the circulation, with the small muscular arteries and arterioles offering the most vascular resistance. *Blood pressure is used as an index of afterload because it is created by blood flow through vascular resistance.*

Vascular resistance is only one source of ventricular afterload. Another source is low compliance of the ventricle or great vessels, which impedes the ejection of blood. Stenosis of the semilunar valves is a pathologic example of increased afterload. Afterload is represented using a pressure-volume loop, as shown in Figure 4-25 by a line drawn from the end-diastolic pressure-volume point (B) to the end-systolic pressure-volume point (E). *The slope of this line represents all factors opposing the volume change that occurs in systole.* If the slope of the line is increased, there is higher systolic pressure and/or reduced SV.

▼   **Afterload reduction** is an important therapeutic approach in the treatment of heart failure to allow higher SV without increasing myocardial O_2 consumption. One of the main categories of the afterload-reducing drugs used in congestive heart failure is **angiotensin-converting enzyme (ACE) inhibitors** or **angiotensin-receptor blockers.** The effects of these drugs go beyond afterload reduction to include inhibiting the maladaptive neurohormonal effects of angiotensin II on cardiac remodeling in congestive heart failure. ▼

CONTRACTILITY Contractility is the third factor that determines SV and is the intrinsic vigor of muscle contraction under defined loading conditions. Several graphic representations of altered contractility are shown in Figure 4-26. In isolated muscle, altered contractility is indicated as a change in the maximal velocity of shortening (V_{max}) (see Figure 4-26A). V_{max} is obtained by extrapolating the load-velocity relation to a theoretic zero load. *An increase in V_{max} implies faster myosin cross-bridge cycling.*

Contractility is more difficult to define in the intact heart than in isolated muscle. The rate of pressure change in the left ventricle at the onset of isovolumic contraction is one indicator of contractility (see Figure 4-26B). *A left shift in the Frank-Starling relation also indicates greater contractility,* whereas a right shift indicates depression of function (see Figure 4-26C).

Contractility can be assessed using a pressure-volume loop by examining the rate at which the end of systole is reached. *The slope of a line drawn from a zero pressure point to the end-systolic pressure-volume point (E) is an index of contractility* (see Figure 4-26D). For a given preload and afterload, an increase in the slope of this line yields greater SV and higher systolic pressure, indicating increased contractility.

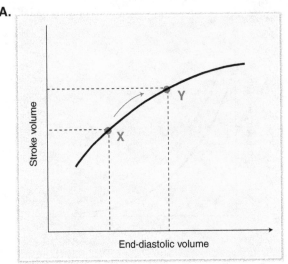

A.

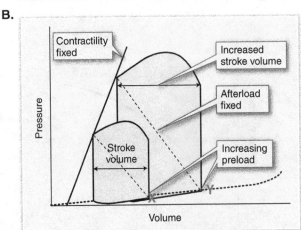

B.

Figure 4-24: Effect of increased preload on ventricular performance. **A.** Increase in the end-diastolic volume from point X to point Y increases stroke volume due to greater force of ventricular contraction via the Frank-Starling mechanism. **B.** Higher preload moves the end-diastolic pressure-volume point to the right from point X to point Y. The increased left ventricular systolic pressure and stroke volume result from greater force of ventricular contraction.

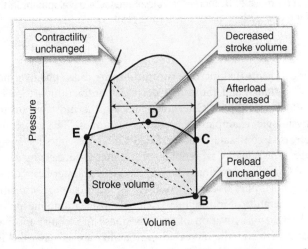

Figure 4-25: Effect of increased afterload on ventricular performance. Dashed lines indicate the afterload slope, which becomes steeper when the ventricle develops more pressure but delivers a smaller stroke volume, reflecting higher impedance opposing blood flow (increased afterload).

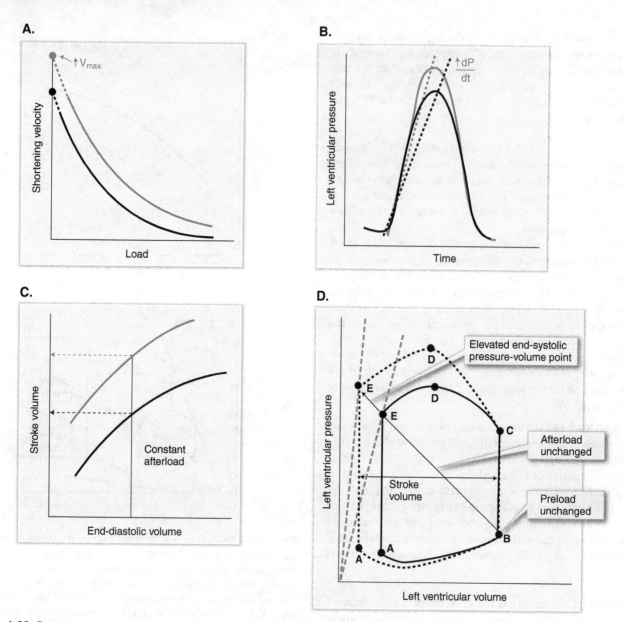

Figure 4-26: Representations of increased ventricular contractility. **A.** Increased velocity of muscle shortening at zero muscle load (V_{max}) in isolated muscle. **B.** Increased rate of pressure development in the left ventricle (dP/dt). **C.** Left shift of Frank-Starling relation. **D.** Elevation of the end-systolic pressure-volume point.

Agents that increase contractility are called **positive inotropes,** and those that decrease contractility are called **negative inotropes.** Catecholamines are the most important physiologic examples of positive inotropes. The basis for increased contractility is increased Ca^{2+} entry into the myocytes. The rate of Ca^{2+} reuptake is also increased, causing more rapid muscle relaxation, which is necessary at faster heart rates. Catecholamines occupy myocardial β_1-adrenoceptors, causing the generation of intracellular cyclic adenosine monophosphate (cAMP) and activation of protein kinase A. Cellular mechanisms that underlie increased contractility are summarized in Table 4-4. "Sympathomimetic" drugs that are positive inotropes include dobutamine, dopamine, and isoproterenol. *Using positive inotropes to treat heart failure increases mortality; therefore, these drugs must be used with caution.* ▼

TABLE 4-4. Mechanisms of Increased Myocardial Contractility Following β-Adrenergic Stimulation

Cellular Mechanism	Effect
L-type Ca^{2+} channel activation	↑ Ca^{2+} entry in phase 2 of action potential → ↑ Ca^{2+}-induced Ca^{2+}-release → ↑contractility
Phosphorylation of phospholamban (Ca^{2+}-ATPase suppressor protein)	↓ Phospholamban → ↑ Ca^{2+}-ATPase → ↑ Ca^{2+} reuptake into sarcoplasmic reticulum → ↑ Rate of muscle relaxation
Phosphorylation of troponin I	↑ Rate of Ca^{2+} dissociation from troponin C → ↑ Rate of muscle relaxation

LEFT VENTRICULAR FAILURE

Ventricular failure can result from systolic or diastolic dysfunction, illustrated in Figure 4-27 using pressure-volume loops. **Systolic dysfunction** occurs when myocardial contraction is weak, most commonly following a **MI**. Patients have reduced SV despite normal preload; contractility is reduced (see Figure 4-27A) and tachycardia is present to maintain cardiac output. *Treatment is aimed at afterload reduction to increase SV.*

In **diastolic dysfunction**, there is low cardiac muscle compliance and poor filling. Patients have a right shift of the end-diastolic pressure-volume point (see Figure 4-27B). Increased ventricular diastolic pressure at any given volume indicates low compliance. Common causes include **ischemic heart disease** and **ventricular hypertrophy** from longstanding hypertension. *Treatment is aimed at reducing blood volume and preload and promoting ventricular relaxation.*

VASCULAR FUNCTION

Blood flows through a **circuit of vessels** consisting of, in sequence, arteries, arterioles, capillaries, venules, and veins. Each of these vascular segments has different attributes and functions within the circulation.

- **Large arteries** (e.g., the aorta) are **high pressure reservoirs** that store energy in their elastic walls during ventricular ejection and release it during diastole to maintain blood flow.

- **Small muscular arteries and arterioles** are the *site of greatest vascular resistance in the circulation.* This accounts for the large decrease in blood pressure that occurs across this segment of the circulation (Figure 4-28). Neurohumoral regulation of arteriolar tone controls vascular resistance and has a major effect on arterial blood pressure.

- **Capillaries** are thin-walled vessels that provide a large surface area for the **exchange** of gases, nutrients, and wastes. Imbalances of hydrostatic and osmotic pressure gradients across the capillary walls are the most common causes of edema (swelling due to excess interstitial fluid volume).

- **Venules and veins** present little resistance to flow. The venous system is a high capacitance, **low pressure reservoir.**

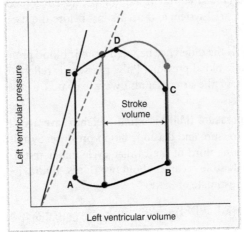

A. Systolic dysfunction

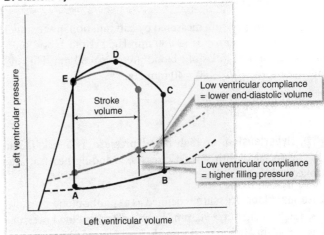

B. Diastolic dysfunction

Low ventricular compliance = lower end-diastolic volume

Low ventricular compliance = higher filling pressure

Figure 4-27: Reduced ventricular performance. **A.** Low stroke volume at a given preload and afterload shows lower ventricular contractility and defines systolic dysfunction. **B.** Low ventricular compliance in diastolic dysfunction reduces end-diastolic volume and increases end-diastolic pressure.

The largest blood volume in the cardiovascular system is in the systemic veins (the second largest blood volume is in the pulmonary vasculature). Small muscular veins assist in the regulation of venous return. *Increased venous tone reduces the capacitance of veins, causing increased venous return.* Larger cardiac preload results in increased cardiac output via the Frank-Starling mechanism.

SYSTEMIC ARTERIAL BLOOD PRESSURE

The pressure difference across the circulation from the arteries to the veins drives blood flow. An adequate arterial blood pressure is necessary to sustain cardiac output. Arterial blood pressure is a major physiologic controlled variable subject to short-term and long-term negative feedback regulation. Several **arterial pressure indices** are discussed below (Figure 4-29):

- **Systolic blood pressure** is the peak pressure recorded in the central arterial system and occurs during ventricular ejection.

- **Diastolic blood pressure** is the minimum pressure recorded in the central arterial system and occurs just before the start of ventricular systole.

- **Pulse pressure** is the difference between systolic blood pressure and diastolic blood pressure. Pulse pressure is reflected by the strength of the arterial pulse wave palpated in the peripheral arteries.

- **Mean arterial pressure (MAP)** is a time-weighted average of systolic blood pressure and diastolic blood pressure. Systole occupies about one third of the cardiac cycle under resting conditions and diastole occupies about two thirds, giving rise to the following estimate of MAP:

$$MAP = DBP + \frac{1}{3}PP \qquad \textbf{Equation 4-8}$$

MAP = Mean arterial blood pressure
DBP = Diastolic blood pressure
PP = Pulse pressure

Example Blood pressure measured by cuff inflation in the upper arm of a healthy person is 120/80 mm Hg. Systolic blood pressure = 120 mm Hg; diastolic blood pressure = 80 mm Hg; and pulse pressure = 120 − 80 = 40 mm Hg.

MAP = 80 + 1/3 (40)
    = 93.3 mm Hg

▽ **Hypertension,** or high blood pressure, is a risk factor associated with several diseases, including heart attack, stroke, and renal failure.

- **Normal blood pressure** is defined as a systolic blood pressure < 120 mm Hg but > 90 mm Hg, and diastolic blood pressure is < 80 mm Hg but > 60 mm Hg.

- Systolic blood pressure between 120–139 mm Hg and diastolic blood pressure between 80–89 mm Hg is considered **prehypertension.**

- Hypertension is defined as systolic blood pressure > 140 mm Hg or diastolic blood pressure > 90 mm Hg.

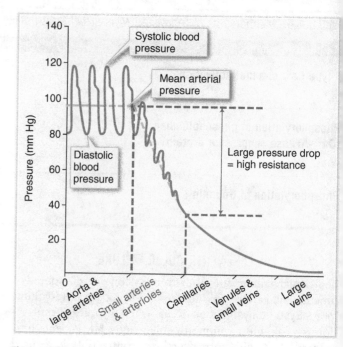

Figure 4-28: Blood pressures throughout the systemic vasculature. Pressure is highest in the central arteries and lowest in the central veins. The largest pressure decrease occurs across the arterioles, indicating that they are the site of highest vascular resistance.

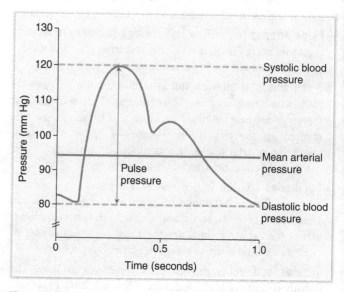

Figure 4-29: Indices of arterial blood pressure.

Hypertension causes end-organ damage and may be an asymptomatic disease for many years before being diagnosed. To assess the severity and duration of hypertension, the physician can examine the interior of the eye using an ophthalmoscope to assess the extent of retinal artery damage. ▼

DETERMINANTS OF SYSTEMIC BLOOD PRESSURE MAP is proportional to cardiac output and vascular resistance. Factors that increase cardiac output or vascular resistance increase MAP. To understand specific determinants of blood pressure indices, it is necessary to interpret a patient's vital signs. **Systolic blood pressure has three determinants:**

1. **SV.** Increased SV increases systolic blood pressure and pulse pressure.

2. **Aortic compliance.** If compliance is low, the SV produces a large systolic blood pressure. Aortic compliance is not physiologically regulated but declines gradually in older persons. *Systolic blood pressure typically increases 1 mm Hg for each year after age 60.* This increase results from the loss of tissue elasticity in the aorta and atherosclerotic change in arterial walls.

3. **Diastolic blood pressure.** The absolute value of systolic blood pressure must be interpreted with respect to diastolic blood pressure because this is the baseline pressure before systole. For this reason, pulse pressure is also observed to assess SV.

Similar to systolic blood pressure, **diastolic blood pressure has three determinants:**

1. **Vascular resistance** is the main determinant of diastolic blood pressure. Blood flow through the circulation continues throughout diastole, although ventricular ejection is over. Flow is sustained because the arterial pressure exceeds the venous pressure. In addition, the elastic aorta stores energy during systole that is imparted to arterial blood during diastole. Diastolic blood pressure is determined by the size of arteriolar resistance encountered by blood flow. Higher arteriolar resistance (vasoconstriction) increases diastolic blood pressure.

2. **Runoff of blood from the aorta.** Diastolic blood pressure decreases if blood flow into the circulation during diastole is reduced. In aortic valve insufficiency, the aortic pressure rapidly decreases during diastole because backflow of blood into the left ventricle reduces forward flow into the circulation. This also occurs when a patent ductus arteriosus is present.

3. **Diastolic time interval.** Aortic pressure decreases with time between heart beats because blood continues to flow into the circulation from the aorta throughout diastole. The measured diastolic blood pressure is lower when the HR is slow because more time elapses between beats. Diastolic blood pressure is higher at faster HRs because there is less time for a decline in aortic pressure between beats. Figure 4-30 illustrates the effect of altered HR on diastolic blood pressure.

 Isolated systolic hypertension is mainly a disease of elderly patients. It occurs because of a gradual decline in arterial compliance (a component of systolic blood pressure, not diastolic blood pressure), so that systolic blood pressure increases and diastolic blood pressure decreases. Treatment adds an additional challenge because reducing diastolic blood pressure further may increase cardiovascular events, which occur because *most coronary perfusion occurs during diastole, not systole.* ▼

REGULATION OF SYSTEMIC VASCULAR RESISTANCE

The collective resistance to blood flow presented by the systemic vasculature is called systemic vascular resistance, or **total peripheral resistance.** Systemic vascular resistance is mainly determined by changes in the diameter of the arterioles. These vessels exhibit partial constriction under normal physiologic conditions, called **vascular tone,** and are the sites of active regulation of blood flow in the circulation. Arteriolar tone is affected by many factors, including sympathetic tone and hormones and endothelial and metabolic factors. Systemic vascular resistance is increased by vasoconstriction and reduced by vasodilatation.

VENOUS RETURN

Venous return is the volume of blood returning to the central venous compartment (thoracic venae cavae and right atrium) per minute (i.e., it is a flow rate). It is helpful to think about properties of the venous circulation in isolation to understand processes that influence venous return, such as altered posture, ventilation, and skeletal muscle activity. **Central venous pressure** is the pressure of venous blood in the thoracic vena cava and the right atrium. Low central venous pressure promotes venous return into the central venous compartment, whereas *high central venous pressure reduces venous return.* Central venous pressure has a strong influence on cardiac preload and, through the Frank-Starling mechanism, determines ventricular SV.

▼ Measuring or estimating **central venous pressure** in the hemodynamically unstable patient guides management. For example, in hypovolemia, a low central venous pressure indicates the need for aggressive intravenous fluid resuscitation prior to using drugs. Intravenous fluid replacement will increase preload, thereby increasing cardiac output, blood pressure, and tissue perfusion. Drugs such as phenylephrine, which is a potent arterial vasoconstrictor, will increase blood pressure at the expense of decreasing blood flow to certain tissues and organs. These drugs are used as a last line attempt to maintain blood pressure in a decompensating patient. ▼

A **change in posture** from a supine to a standing position causes an initial decrease in central venous pressure because gravity causes an accumulation of blood in the veins of the lower limbs. Reduced thoracic venous blood volume results in a decrease in venous return and, therefore, in a decrease in the cardiac output and systemic arterial pressure. Blood pressure normally is restored by baroreceptor reflexes that mediate vasoconstriction and cardiac stimulation (see Neurohumoral Control of the Cardiovascular System).

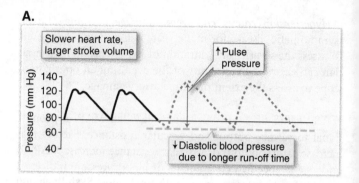

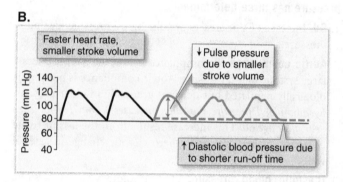

Figure 4-30: Effect of heart rate on diastolic blood pressure. **A.** Decrease in diastolic blood pressure at a reduced heart rate due to increased run-off time. **B.** Increase in diastolic blood pressure at a faster heart rate due to reduced run-off time. Cardiac output is the same in A and B, but there is a faster heart rate and a smaller stroke volume in B compared to A.

During dynamic exercise, mechanisms to support venous return are essential because ventricular diastolic filling time is reduced by rapid HRs. **Rhythmic contraction of skeletal muscles** is one mechanism that promotes venous return during exercise by compressing veins in the limbs, forcing venous return back toward the thorax. *Retrograde flow is prevented by one-way valves in the veins.* The increased **rate and depth of ventilation** during exercise is another mechanism that causes greater venous return. Forceful inspiration causes intrathoracic pressure to become more negative to expand the lungs and achieve deeper inhalation. Figure 4-31 shows that the decrease in intrathoracic pressure acts as an external force on the venae cavae and the right atrium, causing them to distend. As more blood is drawn into the thoracic vena cava from the abdomen, more blood enters the right atrium. Effects such as these are often described in terms of transmural pressure changes.

Transmural pressure is the pressure exerted across the wall of a structure and is calculated by subtracting the external pressure from the internal pressure. *Transmural pressure can be thought of as the pressure acting to distend or dilate a structure.* In the example of deep inspiration increasing venous return, transmural pressure across the wall of the vena cava and right atrium increases because the external pressure becomes more negative during inspiration.

▽ **Kussmaul's sign** occurs when there is an increase (instead of the normal decrease) in jugular venous distention during an inspiration, and is a sign of right-sided heart failure. In the healthy heart, a deep inspiration (i.e., more negative intrathoracic pressure) will collapse the jugular veins as the blood is pulled into the right side of the heart. However, in right-sided heart failure, the pressures on the right side of the heart are high and are unable to accommodate the increased volume coming from the venae cavae. This is detected clinically as increased jugular venous distention. ▼

CARDIAC AND SYSTEMIC VASCULAR FUNCTION CURVES

The factors discussed previously that affect venous return are important because in a closed system, such as the cardiovascular system, cardiac output must equal venous return. Blood flow through the system depends on both cardiac and vascular function. Viewing the systemic circulation as a whole, flow is indicated by the pressure difference between the aorta and the right atrium, divided by systemic vascular resistance. Factors such as cardiac excitation, blood volume, and vascular compliance and resistance all influence total blood flow. The effects of changes in these variables are often described using systemic vascular function curves and cardiac function curves.

Figure 4-32A illustrates a systemic vascular function curve showing venous return as a function of right atrial pressure. Venous return increases as the right atrial pressure is reduced because there is a larger pressure gradient favoring venous return into the atrium. At the point where venous return (flow) becomes zero, the right atrial pressure is typically between 6 mm Hg and 12 mm Hg. If blood flow in the circulation stops, the arterial pressure decreases and the venous pressure increases until the pressure equalizes at all points in the

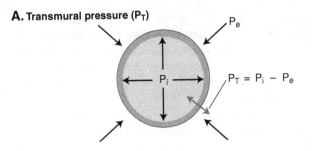

A. Transmural pressure (P_T)

$$P_T = P_i - P_e$$

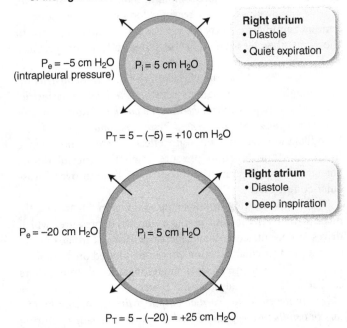

B. Example of the change in transmural pressure across the wall of the right atrium during deep inspiration

$P_e = -5$ cm H_2O (intrapleural pressure) $P_i = 5$ cm H_2O

Right atrium
- Diastole
- Quiet expiration

$$P_T = 5 - (-5) = +10 \text{ cm } H_2O$$

$P_e = -20$ cm H_2O $P_i = 5$ cm H_2O

Right atrium
- Diastole
- Deep inspiration

$$P_T = 5 - (-20) = +25 \text{ cm } H_2O$$

Figure 4-31: A. Transmural pressure difference (P_T). **B.** Worked example of altered transmural pressure difference across the right atrium during deep inspiration.

cardiovascular system. This pressure is called **systemic function pressure (P_SF), or mean circulatory filling pressure,** and is obtained from a systemic vascular function curve. *Systemic function pressure is not measured clinically, but can be thought of as the amount of pressure in the vascular system that drives venous return.*

Systemic function pressure is determined by the relationship between blood volume and vascular compliance. Systemic function pressure increases if blood volume is high or if vascular compliance is low. *The overall compliance of the vascular system is determined by venous tone because the venous system is 10–20 times more compliant than the arterial system.* Figure 4-32B shows that increasing blood volume or reducing venous compliance shifts the venous return curve upward to the right, thereby increasing the systemic function pressure and venous return.

Figure 4-32C shows the effect of arteriolar vasoconstriction and vasodilatation on venous return. *Arteriolar vasoconstriction reduces venous return because blood flow into the microcirculation, and into the venous system beyond it, is reduced. Vasodilatation has the opposite effect.* There is no change in the systemic function pressure when the arteriolar tone changes because the arterioles contribute little to overall vascular compliance.

The **Frank-Starling relationship,** shown in Figure 4-33A, dictates that an increase in the right atrial pressure, which drives more ventricular filling, increases SV and cardiac output. Cardiac and vascular function curves are plotted on a graph in Figure 4-33B, which reveals a single operational point where cardiac output is equal to venous return.

In physiologic states, cardiac output is limited mostly by factors that influence vascular function and venous return. During exercise, for example, there is activation of the sympathetic nervous system, resulting in simultaneous enhancement of cardiac function as well as venoconstriction. In dynamic exercise, systemic vascular resistance decreases due to arteriolar dilation in working muscles. In Figure 4-34A, a combination of vascular and cardiac function curves are used to show how increased cardiac output and venous return occurs during dynamic exercise.

Figure 4-34B illustrates how **compensation** occurs in patients with **heart failure.** There is increased blood volume and reduced venous compliance, which increases venous return and cardiac output. However, this occurs at the expense of higher right atrial pressure, which in turn increases the venous blood pressure. *The risk of edema formation is increased when venous blood pressure increases* (see Capillary Microcirculation).

NEUROHUMORAL REGULATION OF THE CARDIOVASCULAR SYSTEM

The main homeostatic goal in cardiovascular regulation is to maintain adequate cardiac output. Wall stretch is determined at strategic locations in the cardiovascular system to provide **information about blood pressures** as an index of blood flow:

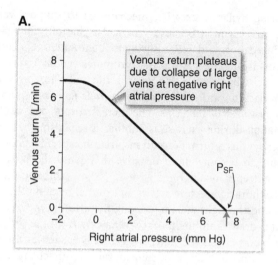
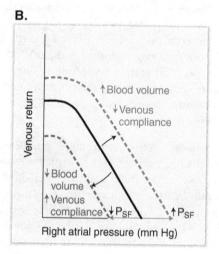
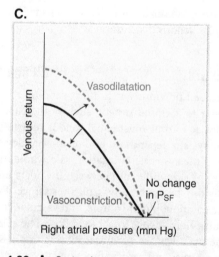

Figure 4-32: A. Systemic vascular function curve indicating the determination of mean circulatory filling pressure (P_SF) at zero blood flow. **B.** Changes in the mean circulatory filling pressure (P_SF) and venous return caused by altered blood volume or venous tone. **C.** Effects of changes in the arteriolar tone on venous return.

- **Carotid sinus baroreceptors** provide momentary feedback about arterial blood pressure.
- The **renal juxtaglomerular apparatus** senses effective circulating blood volume.
- **Low pressure baroreceptors** in the venous system and cardiac atria provide further information about blood volume.

The collective input from these sensors is coupled to changes in autonomic nervous tone and endocrine axes such as **renin-angiotensin-aldosterone, atrial natriuretic peptide,** and **vasopressin** (see Chapters 6 and 8). Changes in vascular resistance and compliance, cardiac performance, and renal handling of sodium and water are integrated to maintain normal blood pressure and blood flow. Integrated responses to blood volume and pressure changes are discussed in more detail in Chapter 6.

THE AUTONOMIC NERVOUS SYSTEM

The primary site of cardiovascular control within the central nervous system is the medulla oblongata. Sensory inputs enter the **nucleus tractus solitarius.** Inhibitory interneurons project to networks of sympathetic nerve cell bodies, and excitatory interneurons project to parasympathetic nerve cell bodies. As a consequence, *basal baroreceptor input results in tonic activation of parasympathetic outflow and suppression of sympathetic outflow.*

Parasympathetic (vagal) fibers innervate the SA and AV nodes, the conduction pathways, and the cardiac myocytes. The principal neurotransmitter released is acetylcholine, which in most cases acts via the muscarinic (M_2) receptors. *The main cardiovascular effects of the parasympathetic nerves are to slow HR and conduction velocity and to reduce the force of atrial contraction,* with minor direct effect on ventricular function. Parasympathetic activation causes vasodilatation in erectile tissue but has no significant overall effect on systemic vascular resistance.

Extensive sympathetic innervation occurs in the heart and vasculature. The primary neurotransmitter released during sympathetic innervation is **norepinephrine,** which mediates responses through several different adrenergic receptors. Increased HR, increased conduction velocity, and increased contractility are all mediated via the β_1 receptors. Generalized vasoconstriction and venoconstriction are mediated via the α_1 receptors. Vascular beds such as skeletal muscle also express β_2 receptors, which mediate vasodilatation. The α_1 receptors are more widely expressed in vascular smooth muscle than the β_2 receptors, and norepinephrine has a higher affinity for α receptors; therefore, *the net effect of sympathetic nerve stimulation is vasoconstriction and an increase in systemic vascular resistance.*

Activation of the sympathetic nervous system causes simultaneous secretion of catecholamine hormones from the adrenal medulla. **Epinephrine** is the primary hormone secreted, which has actions similar to norepinephrine but produces less change in systemic vascular resistance. This difference is because epinephrine has a higher affinity for β_2 receptors and, at low doses, produces a mixture of vasoconstriction and vasodilatation in different parts of the circulation.

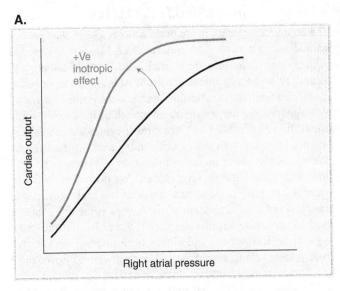

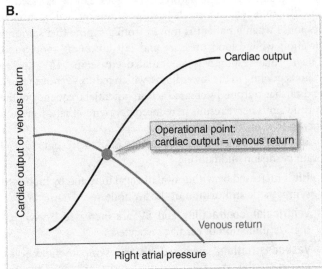

Figure 4-33: A. Frank-Starling curve representing cardiac function. A left shift indicates increased ventricular contractility. **B.** The cardiac function curve and the systemic vascular function curve, plotted together, showing a single operational point where cardiac output equals venous return.

THE BARORECEPTOR REFLEX

The baroreceptor reflex is the main acute response that protects against changes in the systemic arterial blood pressure. The primary stretch sensors are located in the **carotid sinus,** with secondary sensors in the **aortic arch.** Afferent nerve impulses are carried from the carotid sinus nerve to the brainstem via the glossopharyngeal nerves. Increased stretch of the carotid sinus, caused by a rise in MAP or pulse pressure, increases the action potential frequency in the carotid sinus nerve. In the medulla oblongata, this input increases inhibition of sympathetic outflow and stimulates parasympathetic outflow. The opposite occurs when MAP or pulse pressure decreases and carotid sinus stretch is reduced. Activation of the baroreceptor reflex can be used to terminate supraventricular tachycardia. **Carotid massage** or an intravenous fluid bolus both increase wall stretch in the carotid sinus, activating parasympathetic outflow, which can terminate supraventricular tachycardia.

The adequacy of the baroreceptor reflex can be assessed by the **tilt-table test.** Figure 4-35 shows the expected baroreflex response when a patient is moved from a supine to a standing position while blood pressure and HR are being monitored. The normal response is an initial decrease in MAP due to venous pooling in the lower limbs, which reduces venous return and cardiac output. Decreased action potential frequency in the carotid sinus nerve results in reduced parasympathetic tone and increased sympathetic tone.

Several **effector mechanisms restore MAP** to prevent reduced brain perfusion and fainting:

▪ **HR** is increased by withdrawal of vagal tone and by increased sympathetic stimulation of the SA node.

▪ **Ventricular contractility** and SV are increased by sympathetic stimulation of cardiac myocytes.

▪ **Vasoconstriction,** mediated by the sympathetic nerves, increases the systemic vascular resistance and thereby increases the diastolic blood pressure and MAP.

▪ **Venoconstriction,** due to sympathetic stimulation, reduces vascular compliance, increasing venous return and restoring cardiac preload.

▽ Patients with poor vascular or neural tone or low blood volume may sustain a decrease in MAP of more than 20 mm Hg when moving to a standing position; this is defined as **postural (orthostatic) hypotension.** Patients with diabetes mellitus may develop neuropathy, causing autonomic nervous system dysfunction. When moving from a supine to a standing position, these patients do not combat postural hypotension with reflex tachycardia—they will have a decrease in blood pressure and a slow to normal HR. ▼

REGIONAL BLOOD FLOW

Blood flow is not distributed equally to all organs and tissues and depends on the control of relative vascular resistance between organs. In some organs, there is considerable variation in blood flow; this occurs, for example, in the gastrointestinal tract during digestion of a meal or in muscle during exercise. In other organs, such as the brain and the kidney, blood flow

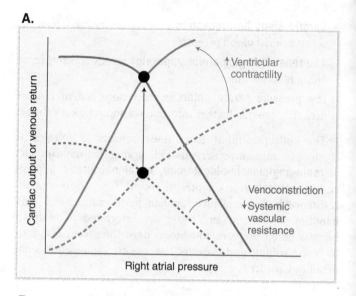

A.

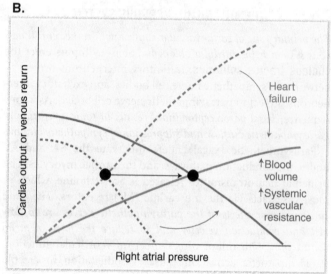

B.

Figure 4-34: A. Increased cardiac output and venous return in dynamic exercise. The sympathetic nervous system activation increases ventricular contractility, producing a left shift in the cardiac function curve. Venoconstriction causes a right shift in the vascular function curve, with increased mean circulatory filling pressure and venous return. Vasodilatation in working muscle causes systemic vascular resistance to decrease, increasing the slope of the venous return curve. A new operating point at higher venous return and cardiac output is achieved. **B.** Cardiac output and venous return in compensated heart failure. Decreased ventricular performance causes a right shift in the cardiac function curve. Mean circulatory filling pressure is increased by fluid retention but venous return is restricted by increased systemic vascular resistance. Cardiac output and venous return are almost maintained in this patient, but at the cost of high right atrial pressure.

is relatively constant. Table 4-5 summarizes the distribution of blood flow to various organs at rest.

CORONARY BLOOD FLOW

Unlike blood flow to other organs, *blood flow to the myocardium is higher during diastole than during systole* (Figure 4-36). The higher rate of flow to the myocardium occurs because contraction of the myocardium during systole compresses coronary blood vessels, limiting coronary blood flow. Tachycardia may present a problem for coronary perfusion because most blood flow occurs during the diastolic period, which becomes shorter as HR increases.

Coronary perfusion pressure is estimated clinically as the difference between diastolic blood pressure and left ventricular end-diastolic pressure. *Therefore, patients with low diastolic blood pressure or high filling pressures in the heart have a reduced driving force for coronary perfusion.*

The extraction of O_2 from arterial blood in the myocardium is maximal at rest. Increased O_2 demand in other organs is supplied by a combination of increased blood flow and increased O_2 extraction. *The only means of increasing O_2 supply to the heart is to increase coronary blood flow.* This can only be achieved by increasing coronary perfusion pressure or by reducing coronary vascular resistance. Coronary arteriolar resistance is affected most by metabolic demand of myocytes. An increase in myocardial metabolism causes a local release of vasodilator metabolites such as adenosine and CO_2, K^+, and H^+ into the interstitial fluid.

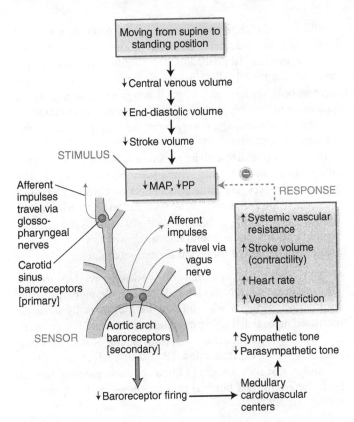

Figure 4-35: Baroreceptor reflex response to a decrease in mean arterial blood pressure. MAP, mean arterial pressure; PP, pulse pressure.

TABLE 4-5. Regional Control of Systemic Blood Flow

Organ	% Cardiac Output at Rest	Blood Flow (per min/100 g)	Major Vascular Resistance Control Mechanism
Heart	15	55 mL	• Local metabolic control • Nitric oxide • Autoregulation
Brain	4	70 mL	• Autoregulation • Arterial blood gases • Local metabolic control
Splanchnic organs	26	100 mL	• Sympathetic control (α_1-mediated vaso- and venoconstriction)
Kidneys	20	400 mL	• Autoregulation • Sympathetic control (α_1-mediated vasoconstriction)
Skeletal muscle	20	6 mL	• Local metabolic control (active muscle) • Sympathetic control (synaptic norepinephrine release mediates α_1-mediated vasoconstriction)
Skin	5	10 mL	• Sympathetic control • Medullary cardiovascular centers: α_1-mediated vasoconstriction • Hypothalamic thermoregulation: sweating and vasodilatation via cholinergic sympathetic nerves
Other	10	-	-

When cardiac activity increases, **nitric oxide** is produced by the vascular endothelial cells. The stimulus for nitric oxide release is mechanical distortion (shearing forces) acting on the vascular endothelial cells. Nitric oxide diffuses into nearby vascular smooth muscle cells, where it acts through soluble cyclic guanosine monophosphate (cGMP) to produce vasodilatation. *Nitric oxide donors (e.g., nitroglycerin) are used to provide relief from* **angina pectoris.**

Increases in cardiac activity are often associated with stimulation of the heart by the sympathetic nervous system. The autonomic nerves have little direct effect on coronary vascular resistance. However, sympathetic stimulation (e.g., injection of epinephrine) results in coronary vasodilatation. The mechanism is indirect and is due to increased cardiac work, causing greater production of local vasodilator metabolites.

▽ Cardiac O_2 consumption is closely related to the amount of ventricular wall tension developed during contraction. Patients with **dilated cardiomyopathy** have an increased myocardial O_2 demand because a dilated heart must develop more wall tension to pressurize the blood. This is a consequence of **Laplace's law (P = 2T/r),** which states that the amount of wall tension (T) in a sphere is proportional to both the amount of luminal pressure developed (P) and the radius (r). ▽

▽ CORONARY ARTERY DISEASE Patients with **atherosclerotic coronary artery disease** have maximal arteriolar dilation at rest and are unable to further increase coronary blood flow. These patients are at risk of developing cardiac ischemia when local O_2 demand increases. Myocardial O_2 consumption is increased by increased HR, increased contractility, and increased afterload (aortic blood pressure). The severity of coronary artery disease can be assessed using a **treadmill stress test,** which may produce angina pectoris and changes that can be seen on an ECG that indicate coronary ischemia. The phenomenon of "**coronary steal**" can be used to show coronary ischemia in some patients by administering a vasodilator such as dipyridamole. The vessel distal to the stenosis is already maximally dilated; vasodilatation of collateral coronary vessels "steals" blood flow from the stenotic segment, causing it to become hypoperfused. ▽

CEREBRAL BLOOD FLOW

The brain requires a constant supply of O_2, and its blood flow is relatively independent of MAP and autonomic nervous system activity. *Cerebral blood flow is mainly determined by* **myogenic autoregulation,** *in which blood flow is relatively constant over a wide range of MAP,* from approximately 60 mm Hg to 130 mm Hg, as shown in Figure 4-37A. Cerebral arterioles respond directly to the degree of distention by varying smooth muscle tone. When MAP decreases, there is less wall distention on arterioles; thus, smooth muscle relaxes and increases vessel diameter, which reduces resistance and restores blood flow.

▽ In patients with **chronic hypertension,** the autoregulation curve shifts to the right. When these patients are treated with antihypertensive drugs to restore blood pressure

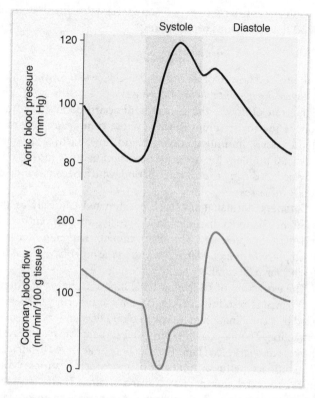

Figure 4-36: Variation in coronary blood flow throughout the cardiac cycle.

to normal, the corrected blood pressure may be below their range of autoregulation, in which case cerebral blood flow decreases, causing dizziness or altered cognitive function (see Figure 4-37A). ▼

Cerebral blood flow responds to changes in local metabolic demand. Increased neuronal activity and O_2 consumption cause local vasodilation. *Blood gases, particularly the arterial CO_2 partial pressure ($PaCO_2$), strongly influence cerebral blood flow* (see Figure 4-37B). For example, dizziness associated with hyperventilation is caused by cerebral vasoconstriction resulting from increased CO_2 excretion and reduced $PaCO_2$. Conversely, increased $PaCO_2$ causes cerebral vasodilatation. Variations in PaO_2 have little effect unless severe hypoxemia (low PaO_2) occurs, resulting in pronounced cerebral vasodilatation.

The brain is the only circulation encased in bone, which limits the total volume of brain tissue, cerebrospinal fluid, and blood. **Intracranial pressure** increases if there is a tumor, bleeding, or cerebral edema, in which case compression of the blood vessels increases vascular resistance and reduces blood flow. Cerebral perfusion pressure is estimated as the difference between MAP and intracranial pressure. Reducing intracranial pressure in the patient with a head injury is critical. Hyperventilation reduces intracranial pressure by decreasing $PaCO_2$, causing reflexive cerebral vasoconstriction and reducing cerebral blood volume and pressure.

RENAL BLOOD FLOW

Among the major organs, the kidneys have one of the highest rates of blood flow, which is necessary to supply enough plasma for glomerular filtration. Despite high O_2 consumption rates per gram of kidney tissue, usually renal perfusion far exceeds the needs of local cellular metabolism. As a result, the kidney has the lowest O_2 extraction of the major organs. Unlike cerebral blood flow, blood flow to the kidneys is not controlled by metabolic factors.

Renal perfusion pressure is the difference between MAP and venous pressure and is therefore similar to most other organs. High renal blood flow is achieved with normal perfusion pressure because vascular resistance is low. Vascular resistance is shared equally by afferent and efferent glomerular arterioles (see Chapter 6).

Renal blood flow is most strongly influenced by **autoregulation** *and* **sympathetic tone.** Under most circumstances, renal blood flow is relatively constant because myogenic autoregulation operates over a MAP range of 60 mm Hg to 160 mm Hg. Increases in sympathetic tone occur during exercise or if the baroreceptor reflex is stimulated by reduced MAP, resulting in renal vasoconstriction. *The kidney is susceptible to ischemic damage (e.g., acute tubular necrosis) in states of shock associated with profound sympathetic vasoconstriction.*

SPLANCHNIC BLOOD FLOW

The splanchnic circulation receives the highest proportion of cardiac output at rest and is shared among the liver, the spleen, and the digestive organs (see Chapter 7). *The sympathetic nervous system exerts dominant control over splanchnic blood flow,* causing vasoconstriction and venoconstriction. Local metabolism increases blood flow after a meal. Parasympathetic

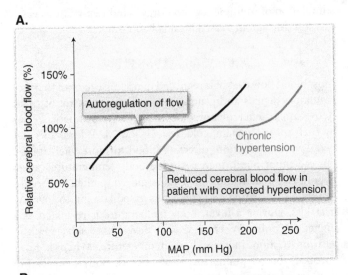

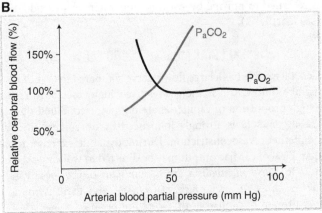

Figure 4-37: Autoregulation of cerebral blood flow. **A.** The red curve shows adaptation in the autoregulatory range in a patient with chronic hypertension. If the normal mean arterial pressure (MAP) is below the patient's autoregulatory range, a correction of hypertension may reduce the cerebral blood flow. **B.** The effect of arterial blood gases on cerebral blood flow.

stimulation of multiple digestive organs indirectly causes vaso-dilation through increased local metabolism.

CUTANEOUS BLOOD FLOW

Most blood flow to skin is regulated in response to both thermo-regulatory signals and general cardiovascular control of MAP. Activation of efferent norepinephrinergic sympathetic nerves by such means as pain, cold, fear, or low MAP leads to cuta-neous vasoconstriction, directing blood to more vital organs. On the other hand, increased core body temperature causes hypothalamic activation of cholinergic sympathetic efferents, resulting in sweating and cutaneous vasodilatation to increase heat loss. During a **fever,** body temperature is regulated at a higher set point. When a fever is developing, shivering and vasoconstriction increase body temperature. When a fever "breaks," the set point returns to normal. Body temperature is returned to normal by sweating and cutaneous vasodilation (see Chapter 2).

SKELETAL MUSCLE BLOOD FLOW

Skeletal muscle has a large flow reserve compared to that of rest-ing blood flow. At rest, there is relatively high vascular tone and a high proportion of capillaries are not perfused. **Blood flow to resting muscle** is strongly influenced by norepinephrinergic sympathetic vasoconstriction. During dynamic exercise, more than 75% of cardiac output may be directed to working skeletal muscle. *Local metabolism exerts dominant control over vascu-lar resistance in working skeletal muscle,* and there is marked recruitment of capillaries that were not perfused at rest.

THE CAPILLARY MICROCIRCULATION

Capillaries have the largest collective surface area for the exchange of nutrients and wastes. **Diffusion** is the most important mechanism for exchange across capillary walls. Lipid-soluble substances and gases diffuse readily. Lipid-insoluble substances such as peptides have low permeability and are restricted to openings between adjacent endothelial cells or transport through cells using vesicular pathways. The time available for diffusion as blood flows through the microcirculation is maximized by slow velocity of blood flow. The velocity of flow is least in the capillaries because blood flow is shared among many parallel vessels, with a large collec-tive cross-sectional area.

TRANSCAPILLARY FLUID FLUX

Bulk fluid flow occurs between plasma and interstitium. Understanding factors that determine **transcapillary fluid movement** is clinically important as the basis for understanding edema formation (tissue swelling caused by excessive accumula-tion of interstitial fluid). For example, brain edema is dangerous because it increases intracranial pressure, leading to brain com-pression. Pulmonary edema is dangerous because it presents a diffusion barrier for O_2 uptake into the blood. In almost all other organs, a large amount of edema fluid can accumulate before organ function is compromised.

Fluid moves readily across the capillary walls of most tissues by filtration. Net fluid movement is a function of the driving pressure for filtration and the capillary permeability. The net driving force for filtration consists of a gradient of hydrostatic pressure that pushes fluid out of plasma and is opposed by a gradient of oncotic pressure:

$$J_v = K_f\,[(P_c - P_i) - \sigma\,(\pi_c - \pi_i)]$$ **Equation 4-9**

J_v = Net fluid flux
K_f = Filtration coefficient
P_c = Capillary hydrostatic pressure
P_i = Interstitial fluid hydrostatic pressure
π_c = Capillary oncotic pressure
π_i = Interstitial fluid oncotic pressure
σ = Protein reflection coefficient

Equation 4-9 is known as the Starling equation, and the individual components of the net driving pressure are referred to as **Starling's forces:**

■ **Capillary hydrostatic pressure (P_c)** is a force pushing fluid out of the capillaries. Hydrostatic pressure is usually about 35 mm Hg at the arteriolar end of a capillary, decreasing to about 15 mm Hg at the venous end of a capillary.

■ **Interstitial fluid hydrostatic pressure (P_i)** is usually near zero or is slightly subatmospheric, favoring fluid movement into the interstitial space.

■ **Capillary oncotic pressure (π_c)** is an osmotic force exerted by plasma proteins, and pulls fluid into the plasma from the interstitium and is approximately 25 mm Hg.

■ **Interstitial fluid oncotic pressure (π_i)** is normally low because proteins have reflection coefficients of 0.8–1.0 and interstitial protein concentration is low (see Chapter 1 for a discussion of reflection coefficient).

Example The following Starling forces were measured in a systemic capillary:

■ Capillary hydrostatic pressure = 30 mm Hg
■ Interstitial hydrostatic pressure = 1 mm Hg
■ Capillary oncotic pressure = 25 mm Hg
■ Interstitial oncotic pressure = 2 mm Hg

$$\begin{aligned}
\text{Net pressure} &= (P_c - P_i) - (\pi_c - \pi_i)\ \text{mm Hg} \\
&= (30 - 1) - (25 - 2)\ \text{mm Hg} \\
&= +2\ \text{mm Hg (favors net filtration)}
\end{aligned}$$

Figure 4-38 shows that the balance of forces changes along the length of a typical capillary as capillary hydrostatic pressure decreases. Net fluid filtration out of plasma occurs at the arterial end of capillary beds, and net fluid reabsorption into plasma occurs toward the venous end.

LYMPHATICS

Blind-ended lymphatic capillaries consisting of single-layered endothelial plates are found in all tissues except the brain and the heart. These capillaries are permeable to fluid and to protein. There is net formation of 3–4 L daily of interstitial fluid, which enters the lymphatic capillaries and is delivered back to

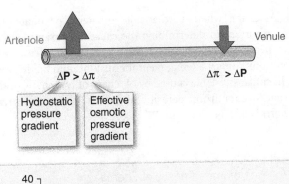

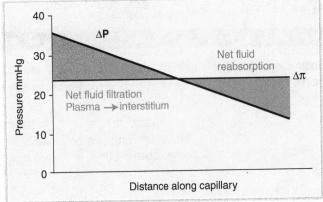

Figure 4-38: Balance of Starling's forces along a normal systemic blood capillary.

the venous system through larger lymph vessels, lymph nodes, and lymphatic ducts. Uptake of lymphatic fluid resists edema formation and can increase as interstitial fluid hydrostatic pressure (P_i) increases. *Proteins that enter the interstitium from plasma are removed by the lymphatic system.*

CAUSES OF EDEMA Most causes of edema can be explained in terms of changes in one or more of the variables noted in Equation 4-9 and are described as follows:

- The most common causes of edema result from **increased venous pressure** due to heart failure or venous obstruction (Table 4-6).

- **Generalized edema** may also result from low serum protein concentration due to reduced capillary oncotic pressure (π_c). This can occur in liver failure when insufficient albumin is synthesized and in nephrotic syndrome when plasma protein is excreted in the urine.

- In **inflammation or sepsis,** generalized edema may occur because inflammatory mediators reduce protein reflection coefficient (σ) and proteins leak into the interstitium, thereby increasing interstitial fluid oncotic pressure.

- **Lymphatic blockage** causes edema because the tissue fluid that has formed is trapped in the interstitium when the outflow pathway is blocked.

▽ Pulmonary capillaries are normally surrounded by negative intrathoracic pressures, which promote net filtration. Patients with **acute respiratory distress syndrome** may develop pulmonary edema. The edema occurs because the patient must inspire forcefully to breathe, causing intrathoracic pressure and interstitial fluid oncotic pressure to become more negative. ▽

▽ Assessing whether edema is unilateral or bilateral is important in determining the cause. For example, congestive heart failure typically results in bilateral edema (e.g., bilateral pulmonary edema, pleural effusions, and ankle swelling). In contrast, edema caused by blockage of lymphatic drainage that occurs from parasitic infection (e.g., *Wuchereria bancrofti*) is often unilateral. ▽

TABLE 4-6. Common Causes of Edema

Mechanism of Edema	↑ P_c	↓ π_c	↓ σ	Lymphatic Blockage
Some conditions that cause edema	Heart failure	Malnutrition	Sepsis	Tumor
	Hypervolemia	Liver disease	Inflammation	Surgery
	Venous thrombosis or other obstruction	Nephrotic syndrome (renal protein loss)	Burns	Inflammation
	Gravity			Parasite (e.g., filariasis)
	Sustained vasodilation			

STUDY QUESTIONS

Directions: Each numbered item is followed by lettered options. Some options may be partially correct, but there is only *ONE BEST* answer.

1. A 14-year-old boy with sickle cell disease received a blood transfusion that caused his blood volume to increase significantly above normal. What changes in cardiac contractility and total peripheral resistance (TPR) would occur within a few minutes of receiving this transfusion?

   A. Increased contractility and increased TPR
   B. Increased contractility and decreased TPR
   C. Decreased contractility and increased TPR
   D. Decreased contractility and decreased TPR

2. A 29-year-old elite endurance athlete completes a medical examination as part of her registration for a triathlon event. Her resting HR is measured at 36 beats/min. Compared with untrained individuals, what change in the cardiac conduction system or autonomic nervous tone is most responsible for this woman's low resting HR?

   A. Decreased automatic rate of (SA) node discharge
   B. Decreased sympathetic neural tone
   C. Decreased vagal tone
   D. Increased automatic rate of SA node discharge
   E. Increased sympathetic neural tone
   F. Increased vagal tone

3. Paramedics were called to attend to a 74-year-old man who fainted while watching a baseball game. When they arrived, the man was conscious but confused. He was noticeably short of breath, had profound bradycardia (HR 25 beats/min) and appeared to be complaining of chest pain. An ECG showed normal P waves that were regularly spaced. QRS complexes were wide and regularly spaced but were dissociated from P waves. What is the most likely origin for electrical stimulation of this patient's ventricles?

   A. (SA) node
   B. Atrial internodal conduction pathways
   C. AV node
   D. Bundle of His
   E. Purkinje fibers

4. A 40-year-old woman from a remote rural area is transferred to a city hospital for treatment of a longstanding heart valve abnormality. Her chief current complaint is the inability to perform any physical work, although she also reports waking several times each night with severe shortness of breath. Auscultation reveals a long rumbling diastolic murmur and an opening snap. Which valve abnormality does this patient most likely have?

   A. Aortic stenosis
   B. Aortic insufficiency
   C. Mitral stenosis
   D. Mitral insufficiency

5. An 80-year-old man visits a new family physician. He has not visited a physician for 15 years, but is presently having trouble sleeping and is seeking a prescription for sleeping pills. Upon physical examination, the man seems in good physical health but his blood pressure is 160/80 mm Hg, and his HR is 66 beats/min. The patient has never been treated for hypertension and recalls no previous blood pressure problems. What is the most likely cause of elevated blood pressure in this patient?

   A. Decreased aortic compliance
   B. Decreased parasympathetic nerve activity
   C. Increased sympathetic nerve activity
   D. Increased vascular smooth muscle tone

6. A 64-year-old woman with hypertension (blood pressure of 160/110 mm Hg) and coronary artery disease was treated with angiotensin-converting enzyme (ACE) inhibitors. After a period when the treatment was no longer effective, the dose of ACE inhibitors was abruptly increased. Although this successfully reduced her blood pressure to 130/80 mm Hg, she complained that the medications now made her very dizzy. Reduced cerebral perfusion, resulting in dizziness, is most likely to be explained in this case by

   A. decreased brain angiotensin II levels
   B. decreased sympathetic tone
   C. inadequate blood flow autoregulation
   D. increased intracranial pressure
   E. increased parasympathetic tone

7. A 41-year-old woman has a routine physical examination as part of a well-woman initiative by her family physician. She is an office worker with a sedentary lifestyle and is concerned about being overweight, but reports no recent illness. Her blood pressure is 140/100 mm Hg, and her HR is 80 beats/min. The most likely reason for her increased systolic blood pressure is an increased

   A. baroreceptor sensitivity
   B. diastolic blood pressure
   C. HR
   D. SV
   E. vascular tone

8. A 40-year-old man with a history of rheumatic fever as a child is awaiting valve replacement surgery to treat chronic mitral valve stenosis. He is severely short of breath, with rales and crackles clearly audible over both lungs. There is pitting edema of the lower extremities and ascites in his abdomen. Which of the following changes in Starling's forces is the most likely cause of edema in this patient?

   A. Decreased capillary hydrostatic pressure
   B. Decreased capillary oncotic pressure
   C. Decreased interstitial hydrostatic pressure
   D. Decreased interstitial oncotic pressure
   E. Increased capillary hydrostatic pressure
   F. Increased capillary oncotic pressure
   G. Increased interstitial hydrostatic pressure
   H. Increased interstitial oncotic pressure

9. A 52-year-old man with a history of alcoholism has recently developed generalized edema. Abnormal liver function tests include increased serum levels of transaminase enzymes. His blood clotting time is increased, and he is unresponsive to vitamin K treatment. What is the most likely cause of edema in this patient?

   A. Decreased capillary hydrostatic pressure
   B. Decreased capillary oncotic pressure
   C. Decreased interstitial hydrostatic pressure
   D. Decreased interstitial oncotic pressure
   E. Increased capillary hydrostatic pressure
   F. Increased capillary oncotic pressure
   G. Increased interstitial hydrostatic pressure
   H. Increased interstitial oncotic pressure

10. A 14-year-old girl from the southern Caribbean was rescued after a major hurricane. She was initially treated for minor injuries and dehydration but was referred for further investigations due to a persistently low blood pressure (95/40 mm Hg). A continuous machinery-like murmur was heard upon auscultation of her chest. An ECG and an echocardiogram revealed left ventricular hypertrophy. Which of the following cardiac abnormalities is most likely to be present?

   A. Aortic valve insufficiency
   B. Aortic valve stenosis
   C. Mitral valve prolapse
   D. Mitral valve stenosis
   E. Patent ductus arteriosus

ANSWERS

1—D. The baroreceptor reflex would cause a decrease in sympathetic nervous tone as a result of this sudden blood volume expansion. The intrinsic contractility of the heart would decrease due to less norepinephrinergic stimulation (*note: "contractility" refers to intrinsic contraction strength for a given preload; in this case, SV may be increased due to high preload but contractility is reduced*). Reduced vasoconstrictor tone causes decreased TPR.

2—F. A decrease in resting HR and an increase in SV is a characteristic of endurance training that allows a greater increase in cardiac output during exercise. This adaptation of training results from increased vagal tone to the SA node.

3—E. The results of this patient's ECG are consistent with complete heart block. In the normal hierarchy of pacemakers, the AV node would be next to initiate ventricular beating at about 40 beats/min, when the SA node is unable to excite the ventricles. A pacemaker originating in the AV node or bundle of His would produce normally shaped QRS complexes. Excitation that spreads from a bundle branch or Purkinje fiber takes longer to reach all parts of the ventricles, producing wide QRS complexes. Purkinje fibers have a slow rate of spontaneous depolarization, consistent with a HR of 25 beats/min.

4—C. Diastolic murmurs include mitral stenosis and aortic insufficiency; an opening snap is characteristic of mitral stenosis. Dyspnea on exertion and paroxysmal nocturnal dyspnea suggest pulmonary edema. Pulmonary edema is consistent with increased left atrial (and therefore pulmonary capillary) pressure, which results from impedance of blood flow through the mitral valve.

5—A. The patient has isolated systolic hypertension. Vascular tone appears to be normal because diastolic pressure is most affected by changes in peripheral resistance. Sympathetic stimulation would cause increases in both systolic pressure and diastolic pressure; parasympathetic tone has little impact on blood pressure. In any case, the patient's HR is normal, indicating that there is no abnormal autonomic nervous system activity. Low aortic compliance produces high systolic pressure in response to the ejection of a normal SV.

6—C. Autoregulation is the dominant mechanism of blood flow control in the cerebral circulation. Autoregulation is reset in chronic hypertension to regulate cerebral blood flow around higher than normal blood pressures. In this case, treatment of hypertension reduces blood pressure to a value below the autoregulatory range, causing cerebral blood flow to decrease.

7—B. Systolic pressure is primarily determined by SV, aortic compliance, and the diastolic pressure. In this case, diastolic pressure is increased, causing systolic pressure to be higher; pulse pressure is normal (40 mm Hg), suggesting that SV and aortic compliance are normal.

8—E. Mitral stenosis causes increased left atrial pressure, which results in increased pulmonary capillary pressure, thereby accounting for the signs of pulmonary edema. Systemic edema is present, most likely resulting from failure of the right ventricle, which developed over time due to high pulmonary vascular resistance; right ventricular failure increases venous and capillary pressures in the systemic circulation. Increased capillary hydrostatic pressure increases the formation of interstitial fluid.

9—B. The patient has liver failure and is therefore unlikely to synthesize enough albumin to maintain a normal plasma oncotic pressure. Capillary oncotic pressure is the major force opposing filtration of plasma out of capillaries; low capillary oncotic pressure therefore results in edema.

10—E. A patent ductus arteriosus is a communication between the aorta and the pulmonary artery, which normally closes shortly after birth. In most cases, this disorder becomes apparent in infants. A continuous murmur is produced because turbulent blood flow occurs along the ductus throughout the cardiac cycle (because pressure is always higher in the aorta than in the pulmonary artery). Increased pulmonary blood flow and venous filling to the left side of the heart have, over time, resulted in left ventricular hypertrophy. Low diastolic blood pressure results from pathologic runoff of blood along the patent ductus. The increased pulse pressure reflects the large left ventricular SV, which is the result of increased venous filling on the left side.

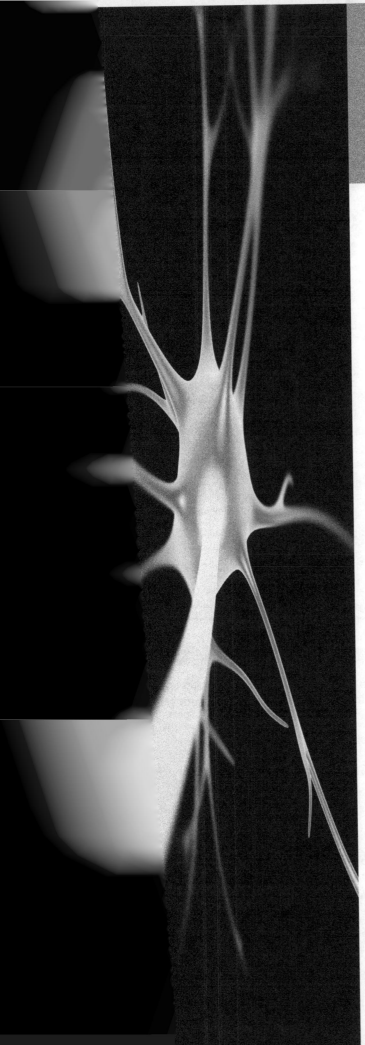

PULMONARY PHYSIOLOGY

THE RESPIRATORY SYSTEM

OVERVIEW OF THE RESPIRATORY SYSTEM

The primary function of the respiratory (pulmonary) system is to maintain systemic arterial blood gas levels within normal range. To achieve this, the rates of O_2 uptake and CO_2 excretion at the lungs must match the respective rates of O_2 use and CO_2 production by cellular respiration. The main components of the respiratory system are the lungs, the chest wall, and the pulmonary blood vessels. Muscles of the chest wall power the movement of air into the lungs during inspiration. Distribution of the pulmonary blood flow, to match ventilation, ensures the proper gas exchange. The levels of systemic O_2 and CO_2 are monitored by chemoreceptors, allowing the pulmonary system to respond to changes in cellular respiration. Treatment of respiratory disorders requires an understanding of factors that govern **ventilation** (gas flow), **diffusion** of gases, and **perfusion** (blood flow) in the lungs.

BLOOD-GAS INTERFACE

The lung is specialized for gas diffusion and has an internal surface area of 50–100 m^2. The large surface area is produced by repeated branching of the airways, which begins at the trachea and terminates in over 300 million closed air sacs called

175

alveoli. Ventilation is the process whereby air enters the lungs and comes into contact with alveoli, which are the sites of gas exchange. Each alveolus is surrounded by a dense network of pulmonary capillaries. The blood gas interface is less than 1-µm thick and consists of the following **four elements in series** (Figure 5-1):

1. Thin layer of surface liquid.
2. Alveolar lining cells (**type 1 pneumocytes**), plus associated basement membrane.
3. Thin layer of interstitial fluid.
4. Pulmonary capillary endothelial cells, plus associated basement membrane.

GAS LAWS

The volume, pressure, and temperature of gases are all closely related by physical laws (Table 5-1). These laws can be applied to help explain the mechanics of air movement into and out of alveoli as well as the diffusion of gases across the blood-gas interface.

According to **Boyle's law,** the volume of a gas varies inversely with its pressure at a constant temperature. For example, a gas can be compressed to a smaller volume at higher pressure. Boyle's law explains the mechanism of air flow into the lung on inspiration—lung volume is first increased when contraction of the inspiratory muscles expands the chest, which reduces the alveolar pressure below atmospheric pressure and draws air into the lung.

Dalton's law states that each gas in a mixture of gases exerts a **partial pressure** that is proportional to its concentration. The sum of partial pressures equals the total pressure

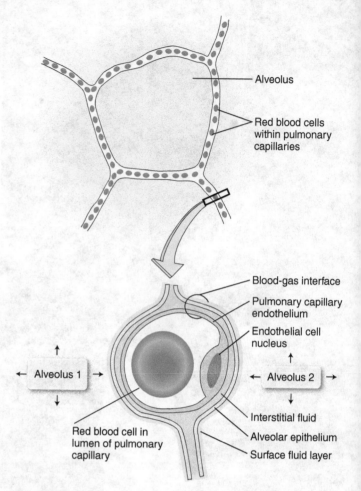

Figure 5-1: Alveolar blood gas barrier.

TABLE 5-1. Gas Laws and Applications in Respiratory Physiology

Law	Formula	Application
Boyle's law	$P_1V_1 = P_2V_2$	• Basis of gas flow during ventilation: mechanical events change lung volume, resulting in pressure gradients that drive gas flow. • Derivation of residual volume using whole-body plethysmography.
Charles' law	$V_1/V_2 = T_1/T_2$	• Gas volume varies in proportion to temperature; air expands as it is warmed during inspiration.
Dalton's law	$P_{total} = \sum\limits_{x=1}^{n} P_{gas}(x)$	• For atmospheric air: $P_B \approx P_{N_2} + P_{O_2}$ • Estimate of inspired O_2: $P_{IO_2} = P_B - P_{H_2O} - P_{N_2}$ or $P_{IO_2} = (P_B - P_{H_2O}) \times F_{IO_2}$
Henry's law	$C_x = KP_x$	• Volume of dissolved gas is proportional to partial pressure. If arterial blood $P_{CO_2} = 40$ mm Hg and K (solubility constant) = 0.06 mL CO_2 per dL blood per mm Hg CO_2: $C_{CO_2} = 0.06 \times 40 = 2.4$ mL/dL *(note: total blood CO_2 content includes bicarbonate ions and carbamino compounds; this calculation is only dissolved CO_2 molecules).*

P, pressure; V, volume; T, temperature; C, gas concentration; F, gas fraction.

(Figure 5-2). Dalton's law is used frequently to estimate alveolar O_2 partial pressure (PO_2) when investigating the basis of low arterial O_2 content. The term **"gas tension"** is used interchangeably with partial pressure.

Henry's law states that the volume of gas dissolved in a liquid is directly proportional to its partial pressure. In clinical medicine, partial pressures are reported for gases in blood as well as in air. Partial pressure in a liquid refers to gas molecules that are free in solution rather than bound to hemoglobin. At the alveolus, respiratory gases diffuse to equilibrium so that *the partial pressures of O_2 (PO_2) and CO_2 (PCO_2) are the same in alveolar air and in end-pulmonary capillary blood plasma.*

UNITS AND TERMINOLOGY USED IN RESPIRATORY PHYSIOLOGY

When describing mechanisms of gas exchange in respiratory physiology, gas quantities at various sites (e.g., inspired air, alveolar gas, and arterial blood) are referred to using standard notations (Table 5-2). Gas pressures are traditionally reported based on the height of a column of liquid; for example, mm Hg (also called **Torr**) or cm H_2O (1 mm Hg = 1.36 cm H_2O). The **Pascal** is the international unit of pressure: 1 kPa (kilopascal) = 7.5 mm Hg. **Barometric pressure (P_B)** is the total gas

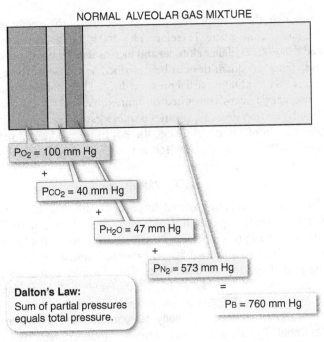

NORMAL ALVEOLAR GAS MIXTURE

PO_2 = 100 mm Hg
+
PCO_2 = 40 mm Hg
+
PH_2O = 47 mm Hg
+
PN_2 = 573 mm Hg
=
P_B = 760 mm Hg

Dalton's Law:
Sum of partial pressures equals total pressure.

Figure 5-2: Dalton's law of partial pressures applied to normal alveolar gas composition.

TABLE 5-2. Standard Notations Used for Gas Quantities and Locations

Symbol	Definition	Example
Px	Partial pressure of gas x	PCO_2: partial pressure of carbon dioxide
Fx	Fractional volume or pressure $F_x = P_x/P_{total}$	FN_2: nitrogen fraction of gas mixture
Sx	Saturation (usually of hemoglobin with O_2), expressed as decimal fraction or %	SO_2: % saturation of hemoglobin with oxygen
Cx	Concentration (content) of gas; blood content for O_2 and CO_2 includes several forms of the gas (e.g., some O_2 is carried as dissolved molecules but most is bound to hemoglobin)	CO_2: total oxygen content
Locations		
a	Arterial blood	$PaCO_2$: carbon dioxide partial pressure of arterial blood
v	Mixed venous blood	$PvCO_2$: carbon dioxide partial pressure of mixed venous blood
c	Pulmonary capillary blood	PcO_2: oxygen partial pressure of pulmonary capillary blood
A	Alveolar gas	PAO_2: alveolar oxygen partial pressure
I	Inspired air	FIO_2: oxygen fraction of inspired gas
E	Mixed expired air	$PECO_2$: carbon dioxide partial pressure in mixed expired air.

pressure in the atmosphere, and arises because of the weight of the earth's atmosphere. Therefore, $P_B = 760$ mm Hg at sea level and decreases at higher altitudes and increases at greater depths. Individual gas quantities can be described as fractions; therefore, a **gas fraction** is partial pressure divided by total pressure. Atmospheric gas is comprised of approximately 21% O_2 and 78% N_2 and very small quantities of other gases. Knowing that the fraction of O_2 in air is 21%, the P_{O_2} in inspired air at sea level is 21% of 760 mm Hg = 160 mm Hg.

WATER VAPOR

The composition of air is altered during inspiration because air is humidified in the upper respiratory tract. The water vapor pressure, or partial pressure of water (P_{H_2O}) in inspired air, is 47 mm Hg at 37°C. The addition of water vapor to inspired air reduces the partial pressure of other gases. For example, at sea level, inspired O_2 (P_{IO_2}) is reduced from 160 mm Hg to 150 mm Hg [$0.21 \times (760 - 47)$]. When gas volume is reported clinically, the standard condition of **body temperature and pressure, saturated (BTPS)**, is used and assumes a body temperature of 37°C (310 K), a barometric pressure of 760 mm Hg, and a water vapor pressure of 47 mm Hg.

MECHANICS OF BREATHING

Airflow into and out of the lungs requires pressure gradients between the mouth and the alveolus, which are created by mechanical changes in lung volume. Breathing becomes difficult if the lung or the chest wall is stiff (there is low compliance) or if the resistance to gas flow along the airway is high. **Resistance is a dynamic property** determined during gas flow. **Compliance** is referred to as an **elastic property** and is measured without gas flow.

LUNG VOLUMES

A **spirometer** is an instrument that is used during **pulmonary function testing** to measure lung volumes and gas flow rates. A patient breathes normally for a given period, and then inspires maximally before forcefully expiring as much air as possible. Figure 5-3 illustrates primary lung volumes and capacities and lists essential terminology necessary for describing and understanding respiratory function.

Tidal volume (V_T) is the amount breathed in and out during normal breathing.

Vital capacity (VC) is the maximum possible volume that can be expired following the largest breath inspired.

Residual volume (RV) is the volume of gas remaining in the lung at the end of forceful expiration and cannot be expelled without collapsing the lung.

Functional residual capacity (FRC) is the resting lung volume at the end of quiet expiration.

Normal FRC is approximately 40% of **total lung capacity (TLC)**. *Many variables are optimized at normal FRC, including work of breathing, vascular resistance, and ventilation/perfusion ($\dot{V}/\dot{Q}$) matching.* Mechanical ventilation of patients

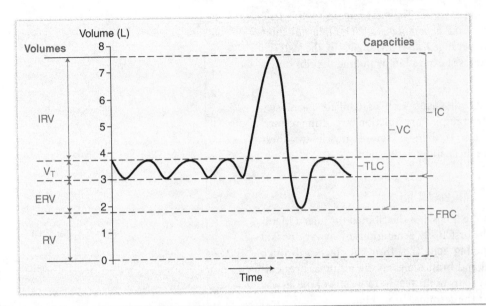

Figure 5-3: Normal spirogram showing four primary lung volumes and four capacities.

Primary Lung Volume	Definition
Tidal volume (V_T)	Volume of a quiet breath.
Inspiratory reserve volume (IRV)	Volume that can be inspired above V_T.
Expiratory reserve volume (ERV)	Volume that can be expired from the end of a tidal expiration.
Residual volume (RV)*	Volume remaining in the lung after maximal expiration.
Primary Lung Capacity	
Total lung capacity (TLC)*	(IRV + V_T + ERV + RV): Total volume of gas in the lung after maximal inspiration.
Vital capacity (VC)	(IRV + V_T + ERV): Volume of maximal expiration from a maximal inspiration.
Inspiratory capacity (IC)	(IRV + V_T): Maximal inspiration from the end of tidal expiration.
Functional residual capacity (FRC)*	(ERV + RV): Volume of gas in the lungs at the end of tidal expiration *(reflects equilibrium between lung and chest wall recoil forces).*

*These capacities cannot be measured directly by spirometry because they include residual volume.

is often used to correct an abnormal FRC to help restore normal respiratory function.

▽ Certain pulmonary conditions can be divided into restrictive versus obstructive lung disease. **Restrictive lung diseases** (e.g., pulmonary fibrosis and acute respiratory distress syndrome) are characterized by reduced lung volumes. In contrast, **obstructive lung diseases** (e.g., asthma, emphysema, and chronic bronchitis) are characterized by obstruction to airflow. ▽

MUSCLES OF VENTILATION

*The **diaphragm** is the most important muscle of inspiration.* Its contraction increases the vertical height of the thoracic cavity due to flattening of the domes of the diaphragm. The **external intercostal muscles** slope downward and forward between the adjacent ribs, which produces a "bucket-handle" movement of the ribs and increases the lateral and anteroposterior diameter of the chest. Expiration is passive during quiet breathing but becomes active during exercise. *The most important muscles of expiration are those of the abdominal wall.* The **internal intercostal muscles** are arranged at right angles to the external oblique muscles and assist expiration by pulling the ribs downward and inward.

▽ **Neuromuscular diseases** such as Guillain-Barré syndrome can affect respiratory function by causing respiratory muscle weakness. If there is severe muscle weakness, patients may require mechanical ventilation. ▼

AIRWAY ANATOMY

As air is drawn into the lungs, it is distributed through a highly branched airway. The first 16–17 generations of airway division comprise the **conducting zone** (i.e., from the trachea through the various bronchi and bronchioles to the terminal bronchioles). Gas exchange occurs in the **respiratory zone** of the airway and begins distal to the terminal bronchioles (Figure 5-4). A **lung acinus** is a functional unit formed by the division of a terminal bronchiole into the respiratory bronchioles, the alveolar ducts, and the terminal alveoli. Gas moves by diffusion within lung acini because the cross-sectional area of the respiratory zone is so large that bulk gas flow approaches zero.

▽ When describing certain lung pathologies, it is helpful to visualize the concept of a lung acinus. Alveolar damage in patients with **emphysema** is either centriacinar (most common) or panacinar. In centriacinar emphysema, the primary site of damage is the respiratory bronchioles, with sparing of the distal alveoli. This type of emphysema is associated with smoking, and most damage is seen in the apical regions of the upper lobes. In panacinar emphysema, the entire acinus is damaged. Panacinar emphysema is associated with α_1-**antitrypsin disease.** α_1-Antitrypsin is a serum protein produced by the liver and combats damaging protease activity, particularly in the lung. α_1-**Antitrypsin disease** is a genetic condition in which α_1-antitrypsin accumulates in the liver (resulting in cirrhosis), causing the protein to be systemically unavailable. The panacinar emphysema that develops typically involves the entire lung, with the lung bases being most diseased. ▼

LUNG AND CHEST WALL RECOIL

The presence of subatmospheric pressure within the chest accounts for a person's ability to draw air into the airway during inspiration. *Subatmospheric pressure in the intrapleural space is created by the opposing recoil of the lungs and chest wall.* When all the respiratory muscles are relaxed, the lung is at its resting lung volume (FRC), and there is equilibrium between the recoil of the lung and the chest wall. At this point, the lung tends to collapse and the chest wall tends to expand, with the two being held together by a thin layer of pleural fluid. By acting to pull the lung and chest wall apart, the opposing recoil forces create negative pressure in the intrapleural space. If the chest wall is punctured, air will flow into the pleural space (**pneumothorax**) until intrapleural pressure (PIP) equals atmospheric pressure; the lung will then collapse and the chest wall will spring outward (Figure 5-5).

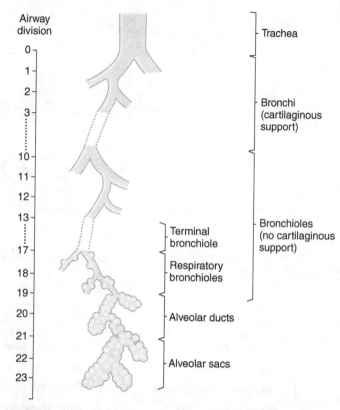

Figure 5-4: Airway divisions. The first 16–17 generations are conducting airways only. Gas exchange only occurs in the respiratory zone from generations 17–23. A lung acinus is formed from the divisions of a terminal bronchiole. A lung unit includes a lung acinus and associated blood vessels.

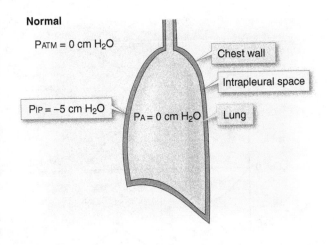
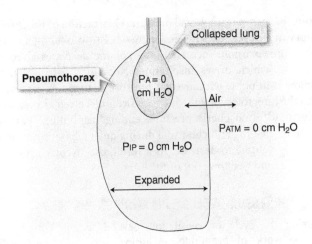

Figure 5-5: Effect of pneumothorax on lung volume and thoracic volume.

▽ **Pneumothorax** can be spontaneous or traumatic in origin. In either case, the intrapleural air must be evacuated and is usually achieved by connecting a chest tube to suction, which restores negative intrapleural pressures and reexpands the collapsed lung. ▽

The force acting across the wall of the lung to expand it is a transmural pressure called the **transpulmonary pressure** (P_{TP}). P_{TP} is calculated as the difference in pressure between the alveoli (P_A) and the intrapleural space (P_{IP}):

$$P_{TP} = P_A - P_{IP}$$ **Equation 5-1**

P_{TP} = Transpulmonary pressure

P_A = Alveolar pressure

P_{IP} = Intrapleural pressure

Example When the respiratory muscles are relaxed, the alveolar pressure is the same as the atmospheric pressure (given a relative value of 0 cm H_2O) and the intrapleural pressure (P_{IP}) is about −5 cm H_2O:

At rest: $P_{TP} = 0 - (-5) = +5$ cm H_2O

The force between the lung and the chest wall increases when the inspiratory muscles contract, causing P_{IP} to become more negative; for example, P_{IP} is −10 cm H_2O during normal quiet inspiration. The lung expands because P_{TP} is increased:

Inspiration: $P_{TP} = 0 - (-10) = +10$ cm H_2O

It is a general convention in physiology to calculate transmural pressures as the inside pressure minus the outside pressure. In the case of transpulmonary pressure, a positive value indicates a distending force for lung expansion (inspiration). A negative P_{TP} is a compression force on the airway as would be observed, for example, during forced expiration.

THE VENTILATION CYCLE

Air flows into or out of the lung when there is a difference in pressure along the airway between the mouth and alveoli. Airflow is driven by changes in alveolar pressure, which in turn result from changes in intrapleural pressure. Contraction of the inspiratory muscles reduces PIP and increases PTP, providing a force for lung expansion. Increased lung volume decreases alveolar pressure, which drives inspiration. Note in Figure 5-6 that airflow is in phase with alveolar pressure changes. As air flows into the lung to occupy the increased volume, alveolar pressure returns to atmospheric pressure, ending inspiration. Passive recoil of the lung and chest wall during quiet expiration causes the lung volume to decrease. As a result, the alveolar pressure increases and gas flows out of the lung.

PRESSURE-VOLUME RELATION OF THE LUNG

During the cycle of ventilation, several factors contribute to the **work of breathing,** including lung and chest wall compliance and resistance to gas flow. Compliance is a pressure-volume relation, and is defined as the transpulmonary pressure change that is required to produce a unit change in lung volume. If measurements are recorded at the start and end of a tidal breath when gas flow has stopped, **static compliance** is determined as:

$$C_{STAT} = V_T / \Delta P_{TP} \qquad \textbf{Equation 5-2}$$

C_{STAT} = Static compliance (mL / cm H_2O)

V_T = Tidal volume (mL)

P_{TP} = Transpulmonary pressure (cm H_2O)

▽ Patients with **pulmonary fibrosis** or **lung edema** have reduced lung compliance and, therefore, have increased the work of breathing, which is sensed as dyspnea or shortness of breath. These patients tend to take small tidal breaths to minimize the change in PTP needed to inspire. On the other hand, patients with **pulmonary emphysema** have increased lung compliance. They do not have difficulty breathing in but experience airway obstruction on expiration (see Dynamic Airway Compression). ▼

Figure 5-7 shows a pressure-volume relationship of a healthy person inspiring and expiring from RV to TLC, revealing several **important features of lung mechanics:**

Lung compliance is low at both high and low lung volumes.

- At high volume, lung tissue is already stretched and further distension requires more force.
- At low volume, many lung acini are collapsed and more force is needed to initiate inspiration.

The steepest part of the pressure-volume relation, where compliance is largest, is at the point of FRC. This explains why it is easier for a person to breathe around FRC and uncomfortable to breathe at high or low lung volume.

SURFACTANTS Figure 5-7 shows that the pressure-volume relation for expiration is positioned to the left of that of inspiration. This phenomenon is called **hysteresis** and exists because of the action of lung surfactants. Surfactants are phospholipids, mainly dipalmitoyl phosphatidylcholine, secreted by **type 2 pneumocytes** in the alveolar walls. The surfactant molecules line up on the inner surface of the alveoli. As the lung volume decreases during expiration, adjacent surfactant molecules are

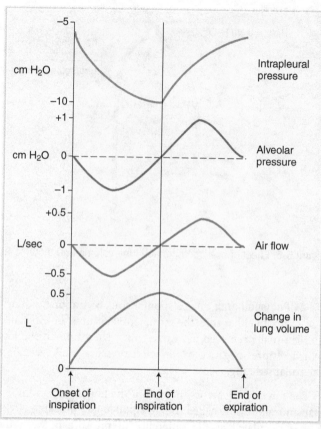

Figure 5-6: Ventilation cycle. Lung volume changes due to airflow into or out of the lung. Gas flow depends on a gradient of pressure from the mouth to the alveolus; alveolar pressure change occurs in response to altered intrapleural pressure.

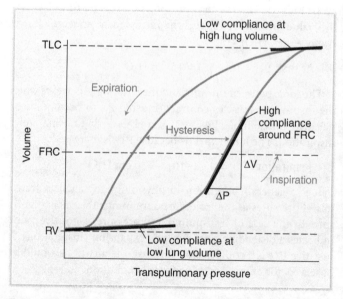

Figure 5-7: Pressure-volume (compliance) curve for a maximal breath. Compliance is low at both high and low lung volumes. Hysteresis is the phenomenon of the different path of the expiration curve compared to inspiration. TLC, total lung capacity; FRC, functional residual capacity; RV, residual volume.

forced closer together. *Surfactant molecules repel each other and resist the tendency of alveoli to become smaller.* The left shift of the pressure-volume relation on expiration, compared to inspiration (hysteresis), is explained by the action of surfactant to maintain alveoli open during expiration. An advantage of this phenomenon is that there is more time for gases to diffuse across the alveolar membranes.

Surface tension acts at the air-liquid interface of alveoli and tends to reduce the area of the alveolus and to generate pressure within it. Surfactants are required to counteract surface tension, which is the main reason that the lung tends to collapse. The presence of the detergent-like surfactant molecules at the air-liquid interface of the alveoli reduces surface tension, thereby maintaining normal lung compliance and preventing alveolar atelectasis (collapse).

▽ **Atelectasis** is an area of collapsed lung, and is often considered the culprit that causes the mild fever that can occur within the first 24–48 hours after surgery. Atelectasis predisposes the patient to pneumonia, but can be reversed or prevented by having the patient cough or perform breathing exercises. ▼

The **law of Laplace** (Equation 5-3) predicts another problem caused by surface tension (as well as the collapse of alveoli)—alveoli with small radii (r) will have higher internal pressure (P) for a given surface tension (T) than will larger alveoli. As a consequence, small alveoli will empty into larger alveoli unless lung surfactants maintain a low surface tension.

$$P = \frac{2T}{r}$$ **Equation 5-3**

P = Pressure

T = Surface tension

r = Radius of sphere

▽ **Respiratory distress syndrome of the newborn (hyaline membrane disease)** is caused by a deficiency of surfactant and is associated with prematurity and with infants of diabetic mothers. Without surfactant, the infant's lungs undergo widespread alveolar collapse, producing low lung compliance. A collection of debris consisting of damaged cells, exudative necrosis, and proteins lines the alveoli and is referred to as the **hyaline membrane.** Treating the mother with corticosteroids 48 hours prior to the delivery of the premature infant has been shown to increase surfactant production and decrease the incidence of respiratory distress syndrome of the newborn. ▼

ELASTIC PROPERTIES OF THE LUNG AND CHEST WALL

Examination of the pressure-volume relation of the lung shows that compliance is optimal (largest) around FRC. A normal FRC is therefore associated with the smallest work of breathing. FRC is controlled by the relative strength of the lung and the chest wall recoil forces. Normally, there is opposition of the elastic forces of the lung and chest wall, and the lung tends to collapse and the chest wall tends to expand, as illustrated in Figure 5-8. The figure shows relaxation pressures in the airway if a patient is asked to take several breaths of different

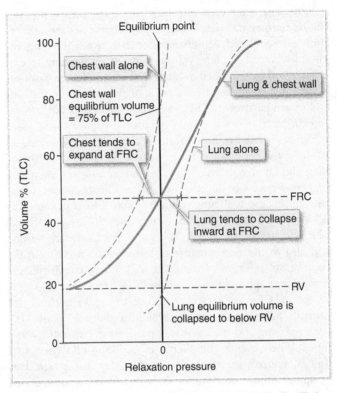

Figure 5-8: Control of functional residual capacity (FRC). Equilibrium between opposing lung and chest wall recoil forces determines FRC. In general, lungs tend to collapse and the chest wall tends to expand. TLC, total lung capacity; RV, residual volume.

volume, and after each inspiration to then completely relax the respiratory muscles. When airway pressure is zero and all muscles are relaxed, equilibrium occurs between the lung and chest wall recoil and lung volume is at FRC. If the lung volume is increased or decreased away from this equilibrium position, effort must be applied by the respiratory muscles but the lung will return passively to FRC. In normal, quiet breathing, therefore, inspiration is active and expiration is passive.

Figure 5-8 shows how the individual elastic properties of the lung and chest wall compare to properties of the combined lung and chest wall unit (*note: individual lung and chest wall properties cannot be directly measured in a living person*). Lungs tend to collapse at all lung volumes from RV to TLC, shown by positive recoil pressures in the airway after the lung is inflated. The tendency of the lung to collapse is due to surface tension and also to the elastic nature of lung tissue. In contrast, the equilibrium position of the chest wall, where recoil pressure is zero, is at approximately 75% of TLC. At all volumes below 75% of TLC, recoil pressures are negative and the chest wall expands passively. At thoracic volumes above 75% of TLC, both the lung and the chest wall passively decrease their volumes. When overall compliance of the lung and chest wall unit is reduced, greater force is needed for inspiration. **Low compliance** has many causes, some of which are summarized in Table 5-3.

▽ **Interstitial lung disease** is a general term used for many diseases that involve the lung parenchyma and cause the lung to be stiff and fibrotic with low compliance. Regardless of the cause, patients with interstitial lung disease typically present with similar manifestations of progressive exertional dyspnea, nonproductive cough, fatigue, and weight loss. ▽

AIRWAY RESISTANCE

Mechanical work required for gas flow into and out of the lung requires overcoming airway resistance and the elastic properties of the lung and the chest wall. **Airway resistance** is referred to as a **dynamic property** because it is only apparent during gas flow. Airway resistance (R) determines the rate of gas flow ($\dot{V}$) for a given pressure gradient from the alveolus to the mouth (ΔP). According to **Ohm's law,**

$$\dot{V} = \Delta P / R \qquad \textbf{Equation 5-4}$$

$\dot{V}$ = Gas flow rate
ΔP = Pressure gradient mouth to alveolus
R = Airway resistance

There are three major **factors that affect resistance to air flow:**

1. **Airway radius** is the main component of airway resistance. Figure 5-9 illustrates the resistance changes along the airway. The upper airway offers significant fixed resistance, which then declines rapidly from the fifth through the tenth generation of airway division. Because the collective cross-sectional area of lung acini is enormous, the respiratory zone of the lung has very low resistance. Bronchi and **bronchioles** contain smooth muscle and, therefore, are sites of **variable resistance.** Parasympathetic nerves release acetylcholine and

TABLE 5-3. Causes and Effects of Low Thoracic Compliance

Cause	Effect
Pulmonary fibrosis	Lung tissue is difficult to distend; lung compliance is low.
Pulmonary edema	Lung is difficult to distend; lung compliance is low.
Pleural effusion	Increased fluid in pleural space resists lung expansion.
Thoracic musculoskeletal pain	Patient avoids deep inspiration due to pain.
Rib fracture	Example of musculoskeletal pain but with reflex spasm of intercostal muscles to produce rigid chest wall.
Morbid obesity	Especially in supine position, weight of tissue on the chest wall and abdomen resists thoracic expansion.
Increased abdominal pressure (e.g., ascites, bowel distension)	The diaphragm is normally the most compliant part of the chest wall; pressure from below resists descent of the diaphragm during inspiration.

cause **bronchoconstriction.** Catecholamines relax bronchial smooth muscle through β_2 receptors. Selective β_2-receptor agonists are used to induce **bronchodilation** and reduce airway resistance in patients with asthma.

▽ **Asthma** is a classic, obstructive lung disease whose key differentiating feature demonstrated on spirometry is reversible bronchoconstriction following treatment with a β_2 agonist such as albuterol. Asthma is characterized by inflammatory hyperreactive airways, and triggers can include allergens (most common), infections (often viral), exercise, cold air, and drugs such as aspirin. When attempting to diagnose airway hyperreactivity, methacholine (a parasympathomimetic agent) can be given during pulmonary function testing to provoke bronchospasm. ▼

2. **Lung volume** is an important determinant of airway resistance because the overall cross-sectional area of airways varies with lung volume, causing global changes in airway radius (Figure 5-10). At low lung volume, the cross-sectional area is reduced and airway resistance increases. For example, patients with pulmonary fibrosis have low lung compliance and low resting lung volume; high airway resistance contributes to their increased work of breathing.

▽ **Idiopathic pulmonary fibrosis** is a specific type of interstitial lung disease. It is the most common cause of idiopathic interstitial pneumonia and has a poor prognosis. The histologic hallmark of idiopathic pulmonary fibrosis is alternating areas of a normal lung with areas of inflammation and fibrosis with architectural changes known as honeycombing. These patients have a restrictive pattern of lung disease (see Clinical Spirometry). ▼

3. **Turbulent gas flow** increases airway resistance. Turbulent flow occurs in the larger central airways, where flow velocity is high, and at branch points along the conducting airways. Disorganization of the gas stream requires more pressure to drive flow and effectively increases resistance. Bronchoconstriction reduces the airway diameter and increases the velocity of flow. High velocity causes turbulent flow, which generates a **wheezing** sound (e.g., in asthma). Table 5-4 describes different breath sounds (including wheezing) and the common causes of these sounds.

DYNAMIC AIRWAY COMPRESSION

Airway resistance increases during **forced expiration** because intrapleural pressure becomes positive and the airways are compressed. Figure 5-11A shows the normal state at the end of inspiration, in which there is a positive PTP that tends to maintain airways open. Figure 5-11B shows transmural pressures acting to compress airways during forced expiration. Forceful contraction of the expiratory muscles increases both intrapleural pressure and alveolar pressure to positive values. A positive pressure gradient between the alveolus and the mouth drives the expiratory gas flow. Notice that there is a roughly linear decline in airway pressure from the alveolus to the mouth. Because the same positive intrapleural pressure now surrounds all the airways, the transmural pressure gradient compressing

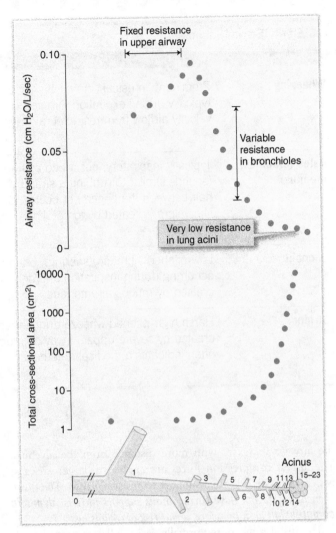

Figure 5-9: Location of airway resistance. The upper airway offers high fixed resistance. Bronchiolar resistance is variable and depends on smooth muscle tone. Resistance is very low in the respiratory zone due to the large total cross-sectional area of the airway at this location.

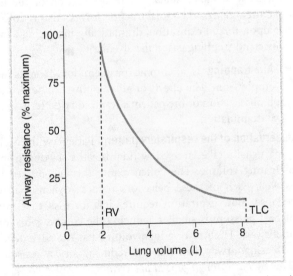

Figure 5-10: Effect of lung volume on airway resistance. Low lung volume increases airway resistance due to reduced airway diameter. RV, residual volume; TLC, total lung capacity.

TABLE 5-4. Breath Sounds

Breath Sound	Description	Occurrence
Wheezing	Prominent "musical" or whistling sound, typically during expiration, created by high velocity airflow from restricted airways	Commonly occurs during bronchospasm (asthma), airway edema (allergic reaction/anaphylaxis), or airway partial obstruction (neoplasm, secretions, foreign object)
Rales (crackles, crepitus)	Typically inspiratory; described as fine (sounds similar to rubbing a strand of hair between the fingers) or coarse (sounds like Velcro), created by forceful opening of alveoli	Commonly occurs in pulmonary edema, atelectasis, and interstitial lung disease
Rhonchi	Low-pitched vibration (snoring), often rattling, occurring during inspiration and/or expiration; created by mucus-air interface	Commonly occurs in bronchitis or chronic obstructive pulmonary disease (COPD)
Stridor	Harsh high-pitched wheeze during inspiration created by severe upper-airway obstruction; often indicates a medical emergency	Commonly occurs in infants with croup (laryngotracheobronchitis), foreign body obstruction at the level of the larynx, epiglottitis, or laryngeal tumor or edema

the airways increases with more distance from the alveolus. The largest compression forces are applied to larger airways, which have cartilaginous support to resist collapse. *The distal bronchioles do not have cartilaginous support to resist* **dynamic compression** *and, therefore, are at risk of collapsing.*

The distal lung units normally resist collapse because each unit is connected to several neighboring units; therefore, if one unit collapses, other units are distorted. This mutual support is called **radial traction force.** Nevertheless, normal airways are compressed in forced expiration and airway resistance rises. Dynamic airway compression is a particular problem in patients with **emphysema,** where destruction of the lung architecture weakens the radial traction forces. Airway collapse occurs upon forced expiration, dramatically increasing airway resistance and trapping gas in the alveoli.

▽ **Air trapping** is a chronic problem for patients with emphysema. The effects of air trapping can be detected through observation of the patient's respiratory pattern and by physical examination.

Observation of the respiratory pattern. Patients with emphysema usually take large, slow tidal breaths starting from a high lung volume. They often expire through pursed lips as well. Each of these behaviors reduces dynamic airway collapse. Slow expiration requires less force so that intrapleural pressure is smaller, reducing the compression force on airways. High resting lung volume has the advantage of increasing airway diameter and reducing airway resistance. *Blowing out through pursed lips creates a positive pressure in the mouth, which increases pressure inside the airways.* As a result, the transmural pressure that compresses the airways is reduced.

A. End-inspiration

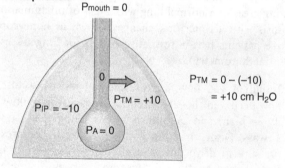

$P_{mouth} = 0$

$P_{IP} = -10$

$P_{TM} = +10$

$P_A = 0$

$P_{TM} = 0 - (-10)$
$= +10$ cm H_2O

B. Forced expiration

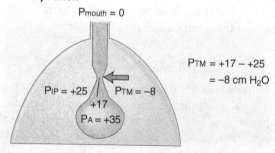

$P_{mouth} = 0$

$P_{IP} = +25$ $P_{TM} = -8$
+17
$P_A = +35$

$P_{TM} = +17 - +25$
$= -8$ cm H_2O

Figure 5-11: Dynamic airway compression. At the end of deep inspiration **(A),** A positive transmural pressure maintains open airways. In the example of forced expiration, shown in **(B),** 35 cm H_2O is added to both alveolar pressure and intrapleural pressure ($P_{IP} = -10 + 35 = +25$; $P_A = 0 + 35 = +35$). Airways are compressed by high intrapleural pressure. The transmural pressure compressing the airways increases with distance from the alveolus because pressure inside the airway decreases from the alveolus to the mouth. Small airways only have radial traction forces to prevent airway collapse.

Clinical examination findings associated with air trapping include:

- **Physical examination.** Increased anterior to posterior diameter, known as **barrel chest.**
- **Percussion.** Hyperresonance.
- **Auscultation.** Decreased breath sounds.
- **Chest radiography.** Large, hyperlucent lung fields, flattened diaphragm, and increased retrosternal airspace. ▼

EXPIRATORY FLOW LIMITATION

Maximal expiratory flow rate is achieved with relatively little expiratory effort due to the existence of dynamic airway compression. Figure 5-12A shows plots of expiratory flow rate as a function of lung volume when a patient uses different degrees of effort to breathe out from TLC to RV. In forced expiration from TLC, there is a rapid initial increase in flow rate to a peak, and then a steady decline in flow rate as RV is approached. The remarkable feature shown in Figure 5-12A is that, *regardless of effort, the descending limb of the flow-volume loop follows the same curve.*

Figure 5-12B shows that expiratory flow becomes independent of effort (measured as the size of alveolar pressure). At medium to low lung volumes, maximal expiratory flow rate is established with modest effort. Increases in voluntary force do not increase expiratory flow. Although alveolar pressure increases with effort, it cannot drive more gas flow because intrapleural pressure also becomes progressively larger. Thus, the force driving expiratory gas flow (alveolar pressure) and the force compressing the airway (intrapleural pressure) increase in parallel, and the net effect is that there is no change in expiratory flow rate. *Patients with emphysema may experience expiratory flow limitation during normal quiet breathing;* they attempt to breathe at even higher lung volumes, which usually lead to dyspnea, coughing, and discomfort.

STATIC AND DYNAMIC COMPLIANCE

When patients are mechanically ventilated, positive pressure is used to push gas into the lung. If airway pressure is too high, there is a risk that the lung will rupture. The peak airway pressure reached when a VT is delivered includes the pressure required to overcome both elastic forces (**static compliance**) and airway resistance. When static compliance is calculated, using Equation 5-2, pressure measurements are recorded at the beginning and end of inspiration, after gas flow has stopped. If measurements are recorded during gas flow, an additional component of airway pressure is present due to air flowing through a resistance (Equation 5-4). **Dynamic compliance** includes the pressure component due to airway resistance.

Figure 5-13A shows a protocol to determine if development of high airway pressure in a mechanically ventilated patient is due to low static compliance (e.g., the patient has developed pulmonary edema) or to increased airway resistance (e.g., bronchoconstriction). The respirator applies a positive end-expiratory pressure (PEEP) between breaths to help maintain open airways, which will reduce atelectasis in the mechanically

A. Expiratory flow-volume curve

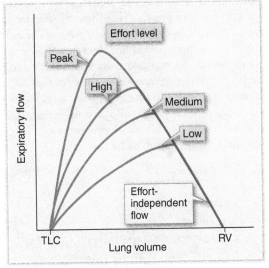

B. Isovolume pressure-flow curve

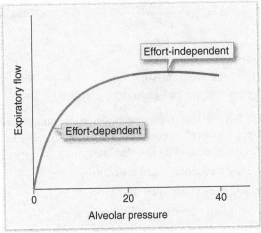

Figure 5-12: Expiratory flow limitation. A series of expirations from total lung capacity are measured with varying degrees of effort. Curves converge at mid and low lung volumes (**A**), showing that expiratory rate is independent of effort in this region. If alveolar pressure is measured as an index of effort (**B**), expiratory flow rate plateaus, demonstrating expiratory flow limitation. TLC, total lung capacity; RV, residual volume.

ventilated patient. A known V_T is pushed into the lung and airway pressure is recorded. The highest pressure recorded is called peak inspiratory pressure (PIP) (*note: PIP is distinct from intrapleural pressure, which is notated by P_{IP}*). The respirator then pauses for a short period but does not allow expiration. During this pause, airway pressure decreases to a stable plateau pressure (P_{PLAT}). *Pressure decreases because gas flow has stopped and the component of airway pressure caused by gas flow through resistance is no longer present.* P_{PLAT} only reflects the force needed to overcome elastic (static) properties of the lung and chest wall. Static compliance can be calculated as:

$$C_{STAT} = \frac{V_T}{P_{PLAT} - PEEP}$$ **Equation 5-5**

C_{STAT} = Static compliance
V_T = Tidal volume
P_{PLAT} = Plateau (pause) pressure
PEEP = Positive end-expiratory pressure

Effective dynamic compliance (C_{DYN}) is then calculated, taking into account all components of airway pressure:

$$C_{DYN} = \frac{V_T}{PIP - PEEP}$$ **Equation 5-6**

C_{DYN} = Dynamic compliance
V_T = Tidal volume
PIP = Peak inspiratory pressure
PEEP = Positive end-expiratory pressure

Example 1 A patient receiving positive pressure mechanical ventilatory support has been stable for 24 hours. The following variables have been set by the ventilator:

Breathing frequency = 12 breaths/min

Tidal volume (V_T) = 1000 mL

End-expiratory pressure (PEEP) = 5 cm H_2O

Peak inspiratory airway pressure (PIP) = 25 cm H_2O

End-inspiratory plateau pressure (P_{PLAT}) = 20 cm H_2O (determined periodically)

Static compliance: $C_{STAT} = \dfrac{V_T}{P_{PLAT} - PEEP}$

$$= 1000/(20 - 5) \text{ mL/cm } H_2O$$
$$= 66.7 \text{ mL/cm } H_2O$$

Dynamic compliance: $C_{DYN} = \dfrac{V_T}{PIP - PEEP}$

$$= 1000 / (25 - 5) \text{ mL/cm } H_2O$$
$$= 50 \text{ mL/cm } H_2O$$

Calculations of static and dynamic compliance are helpful to reveal the cause of high airway pressure in a mechanically ventilated patient. Compliance is inversely proportional to pressure; thus *increased airway pressures are associated with reduced compliance.*

Example 2 The patient in Example 1 has abruptly developed an increase in airway pressure due to bronchospasm. The results of his pulmonary function tests are:

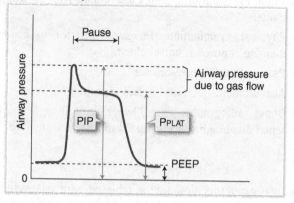

A. Normal response

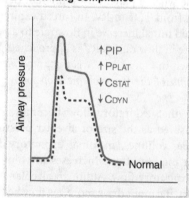

B. Low lung compliance

↑ PIP
↑ P_{PLAT}
↓ C_{STAT}
↓ C_{DYN}

Normal

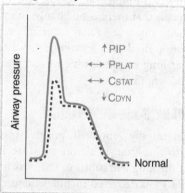

C. High airway resistance

↑ PIP
↔ P_{PLAT}
↔ C_{STAT}
↓ C_{DYN}

Normal

Figure 5-13: Measurement of static and dynamic compliance during mechanical ventilation. A tidal volume is delivered, causing a peak in airway pressure; dynamic compliance is calculated at the peak inspiratory pressure (PIP). A short pause is applied before expiration to eliminate airway pressure caused by gas flow, and airway pressure decreases to a plateau (P_{PLAT}). Static compliance is calculated during the plateau. **A.** Normal response. **B.** Low lung compliance causes a global increase in airway pressure and a decrease in both static and dynamic compliance. **C.** High airway resistance increases peak airway pressure but does not change the plateau pressure; dynamic compliance is decreased but static compliance is unchanged.

Breathing frequency = 12 breaths/min (set by respirator)

Tidal volume (V_T) = 1000 mL (set by respirator)

End-expiratory pressure (PEEP) = 5 cm H_2O (set by respirator)

Peak inspiratory airway pressure (PIP) = 45 cm H_2O

End-inspiratory plateau pressure (PPLAT) = 20 cm H_2O

Static compliance: $C_{STAT} = \dfrac{V_T}{P_{PLAT} - PEEP}$

$$= 1000/(20 - 5) \text{ mL/cm } H_2O$$
$$= 66.7 \text{ mL / cm } H_2O \text{ (unchanged)}$$

Dynamic compliance: $C_{DYN} = \dfrac{V_T}{PIP - PEEP}$

$$= 1000/(45 - 5) \text{ mL/cm } H_2O$$
$$= 25 \text{ mL/cm } H_2O \text{ (reduced)}$$

Figures 5-13B and 5-13C compare the two general causes of increased airway pressure in a mechanically ventilated patient. Figure 5-13B is an example of reduced static lung compliance in which both PIP and PPLAT are increased (both static and dynamic compliance are reduced). Figure 5-13C is an example of high airway resistance in which PIP increases but PPLAT does not change (dynamic compliance is reduced but static compliance is unchanged). In Example 2, the patient developed bronchospasms, the pattern shown in Figure 5-13C, and would benefit from treatment with a bronchodilator to reduce peak airway pressure when the respirator delivers a tidal breath.

CLINICAL SPIROMETRY

Figure 5-14A shows the results of a forced expiration test using a spirometer, in which the patient inspires and expires maximally.

The volume expired in the first second is called the **forced expiratory volume (FEV) in 1 sec ($FEV_{1.0}$).**

The total volume expired under maximum effort is the **forced vital capacity (FVC).**

$FEV_{1.0}$ is normally about 80% of FVC ($FEV_{1.0}$:FVC ratio = 0.8). $FEV_{1.0}$ represents forced expiration from high lung volume and is effort-dependent.

Expiratory flow through the middle 50% of the expired breath (FEF_{25-75}) is also determined. FEF_{25-75} is useful in patients who do not use maximal effort, recalling that expiratory flow becomes effort-independent at lower lung volumes (see Figure 5-12).

Two general patterns of disease can be distinguished using spirometry: obstructive and restrictive disease. ***Obstructive lung diseases*** *(e.g., emphysema, chronic bronchitis, and asthma) are characterized by difficulty in moving gas out of the lung due to high airway resistance* (Figure 5-14B). The $FEV_{1.0}$ and the $FEV_{1.0}$: FVC ratios are both reduced. *In **restrictive lung diseases** (e.g., pulmonary fibrosis), it is difficult to move gas into the lung due to low lung compliance* (Figure 5-14C). Virtually all lung volumes, particularly TLC and FVC, are decreased. Expiration is not impeded because lung recoil forces are

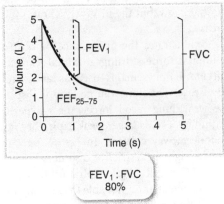

A. Normal

FEV$_1$: FVC
80%

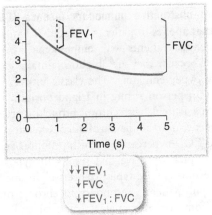

B. Obstructive

↓↓FEV$_1$
↓FVC
↓FEV$_1$: FVC

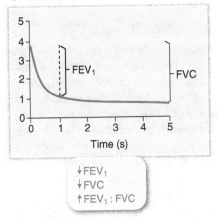

C. Restrictive

↓FEV$_1$
↓FVC
↑FEV$_1$: FVC

Figure 5-14: Spirograms showing a normal lung **(A)** and obstructive **(B)** and restrictive **(C)** lung diseases. Obstructive and restrictive lung diseases are associated with smaller forced vital capacity (FVC) and forced expired volume in the first second ($FEV_{1.0}$). In obstructive lung disease, the $FEV_{1.0}$:FVC ratio is significantly decreased, whereas in restrictive lung disease, the $FEV_{1.0}$:FVC ratio is normal or increased.

increased. The absolute value of $FEV_{1.0}$ is low because inspired volume is initially low, but the $FEV_{1.0}:FVC$ ratio is either normal or increased.

Figure 5-15 illustrates the appearance of obstructive and restrictive lung disorders using maximal expiratory **flow-volume curves.** Emphysema is used as an example of an obstructive disease. The flow-volume loop is displaced to the left because weak lung recoil force causes hyperinflation of the lung. Although TLC is larger, peak expiratory flow is small due to dynamic airway collapse. In Figure 5-15, the loop is displaced to the right in restrictive disorders because patients have reduced TLC and RV. Peak expiratory flow is lower than normal because the patient is not able to reach high inspiratory volumes, where flow rate is effort-dependent. The slope of the descending part of the curve may be steeper, reflecting higher lung recoil forces.

▼ **Chronic obstructive pulmonary disease (COPD)** is a term that applies to patients with either emphysema or chronic bronchitis. Patients with emphysema are known as "pink puffers" because they are able to maintain adequate O_2 saturation by hyperventilating. The classic profile of a "pink puffer" is a thin person sitting in tripod position, breathing with pursed lips. Patients with chronic bronchitis are known as "blue bloaters" because they have a blunted respiratory response to high blood CO_2 (hypercarbia), which produces an inappropriately low respiratory drive that results in hypoxemia and cyanosis. Blue bloaters are typically overweight and have red faces due to polycythemia secondary to chronic hypoxemia. They suffer from cor pulmonale (structural and functional changes in the right ventricle caused by chronic pulmonary hypertension). ▼

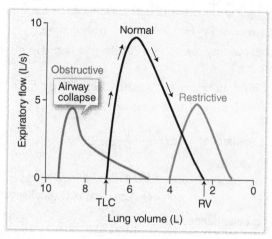

Figure 5-15: Flow-volume curves in obstructive and restrictive lung disease. TLC, total lung capacity; RV, residual volume.

WORK OF BREATHING

Work of breathing has two major components: "**elastic work**" to overcome static compliance, and "**resistive work**" to overcome airway and tissue resistance. Patients usually adopt a pattern of breathing that minimizes work. In restrictive disease, small tidal breaths are taken more rapidly because a large amount of elastic work is needed to inflate the lungs. Patients with obstructive lung disease often expire slowly, which reduces dynamic airway collapse and resistive work of breathing.

VENTILATION AND CARBON DIOXIDE ELIMINATION

Ventilation can be defined as mechanical events producing gas movement in the lung, which results in CO_2 elimination from the body. During this process, CO_2 diffuses readily from the pulmonary capillaries into the alveoli. CO_2 elimination depends solely on how well the alveoli are ventilated. Alveolar ventilation is reduced by the volume of dead space (wasted) ventilation. The conducting airways contribute fixed "anatomic" dead space. Alveoli that are ventilated but not perfused ("**alveolar" dead space**) also contribute to **total "physiologic" dead space**. In disease states, this space can be large, resulting in inadequate CO_2 excretion. **Hypoventilation** is defined as *inadequate CO_2 excretion, which results in an increase in arterial PCO_2.* Key terminology used in the discussion of ventilation is summarized in Table 5-5.

▼ **Pulmonary embolism** is a potentially fatal condition that occurs when a thromboembolism lodges in a pulmonary artery, stopping all blood flow distal to the blockage. A pulmonary embolism is a classic example of a large, total ("physiologic") dead space in which the affected lung segment continues to have alveolar ventilation but lacks blood flow. ▼

THE ALVEOLAR VENTILATION EQUATION

The rate of alveolar ventilation is the sole determinant of the rate of CO_2 excretion. Because all CO_2 excretion is derived from alveolar gas, the following relationship can be written as:

$$\dot{V}_{CO_2} = \dot{V}_A \times F_{ACO_2} \qquad \textbf{Equation 5-7}$$

$\dot{V}_{CO_2}$ = Rate of CO_2 excretion

$\dot{V}_A$ = Alveolar ventilation rate

F_{ACO_2} = Fraction of alveolar CO_2

The gas fraction is proportional to partial pressure, so F_{ACO_2} can be replaced by P_{ACO_2} multiplied by a constant (k) to produce the **alveolar ventilation equation:**

$$\dot{V}_{CO_2} = \dot{V}_A \times P_{ACO_2} \times k \qquad \textbf{Equation 5-8}$$

$\dot{V}_{CO_2}$ = Rate of CO_2 elimination or production

$\dot{V}_A$ = Alveolar ventilation rate

P_{ACO_2} = Partial pressure of CO_2 in alveolar gas

k = Constant

The blood entering the left side of the heart has equilibrated with alveolar gas. As a result, P_{ACO_2} can be replaced by Pa_{CO_2}, as shown in Equation 5-8. In addition, if CO_2 production is understood to be constant, Equation 5-8 reduces to:

$$Pa_{CO_2} \propto \frac{1}{\dot{V}_A} \qquad \textbf{Equation 5-9}$$

Pa_{CO_2} = Partial pressure of CO_2 in alveolar gas

$\dot{V}_A$ = Alveolar ventilation rate

This equation demonstrates a fundamentally important concept that arterial PCO_2 varies inversely with alveolar ventilation; for example, if $\dot{V}_A$ is doubled, arterial PCO_2 is halved. Arterial PCO_2 is influenced by the balance between CO_2 production and excretion. However, changes in CO_2 production will only change arterial PCO_2 if pulmonary function is impaired and $\dot{V}_A$ cannot be adjusted appropriately. For example, patients with **acute respiratory depression** or those with COPD are at risk of having inadequate alveolar ventilation for the rate of CO_2 production, which results in increased arterial PCO_2.

VENTILATION OF DEAD SPACE

The alveolar ventilation rate is less than the expired ventilation rate because a proportion of each breath moves to areas of dead

TABLE 5-5. Terminology Related to Ventilation

Term	Description
Apnea	No breathing; breathing frequency is zero
Bradypnea (hypopnea)	Low breathing frequency (<10 per min)
Eupnea	Normal breathing frequency (10–20 per min)
Tachypnea (hyperpnea)	High breathing frequency (>20 per min)
Hypoventilation[*]	Functionally inadequate ventilation produces increased arterial PCO_2 (hypercarbia, hypercapnia) >45 mm Hg
Hyperventilation[*]	Excessive ventilation produces decreased arterial PCO_2 (hypocarbia, hypocapnea) <35 mm Hg
Dyspnea	Subjective sensation of shortness of breath or difficulty breathing; indicates physiologic demand for ventilation is greater than the patient's ability to respond

[*] *Note.* Hypo- and hyperventilation should *not* be used to describe abnormal respiratory rate.

space. **Expired minute ventilation** is the product of tidal volume (V_T) and breathing frequency (f):

$$\dot{V}_E = V_T \times f \qquad \text{Equation 5-10}$$

$\dot{V}_E$ = Expired minute ventilation rate

V_T = Tidal volume

f = Breathing frequency

For each breath, about 150 mL of air remains in the anatomic dead space; there is very little additional alveolar dead space in the lungs of a healthy person. $\dot{V}_E$ can be divided into two functional quantities, alveolar ventilation ($\dot{V}_A$) and dead space ventilation ($\dot{V}_D$):

$$\dot{V}_E = \dot{V}_A + \dot{V}_D \qquad \text{Equation 5-11}$$

$\dot{V}_E$ = Expired minute ventilation rate

$\dot{V}_A$ = Alveolar ventilation rate

$\dot{V}_D$ = Dead space ventilation rate

Patients who have a large total physiologic dead space waste an excessive fraction of each tidal breath to regions of the lung that do not exchange gas. There are two possible outcomes: either the patient increases $\dot{V}_E$ to restore $\dot{V}_A$, or $\dot{V}_A$ is inadequate and arterial P_{CO_2} increases (hypoventilation). *Patients with severe COPD are unable to increase $\dot{V}_E$ sufficiently and often have a chronically elevated arterial P_{CO_2}.*

▽ Symptoms associated with **chronic hypercapnia** (elevated arterial P_{CO_2}) differ from those associated with **acute hypercapnia.** Clinical manifestations of the patient with chronic hypercapnia include sleep disturbance, daytime somnolence, tremor, myoclonic jerks, and asterixis. Conversely, clinical manifestations of acute hypercapnia include anxiety, dyspnea, confusion, psychosis, and coma. ▼

QUANTIFYING DEAD SPACE Figure 5-16 shows P_{O_2} and P_{CO_2} in inspired air, in alveolar gas, and in mixed expired air. The composition of alveolar gas is fairly constant throughout the ventilatory cycle; there is a steady state between CO_2 diffusion from pulmonary capillary blood into the alveoli and from CO_2 removal by alveolar ventilation. On inspiration, the dead space is filled with inspired gas, which contains only a minimal amount of CO_2. However, the highest concentration of CO_2 is in the alveoli. On expiration, alveolar gas mixes with fresh air in the dead space, causing dilution of CO_2. Thus, the P_{CO_2} in mixed expired gas (P_{ECO_2}) is lower than the P_{CO_2} in alveolar gas (P_{ACO_2}). As dead space becomes larger, P_{ECO_2} is reduced. The **Bohr equation** applies the idea that the difference between alveolar P_{CO_2} and expired P_{CO_2} is a function of the dead space volume:

$$\frac{V_D}{V_T} = \frac{P_{ACO_2} - P_{ECO_2}}{P_{ACO_2}} \qquad \text{Equation 5-12}$$

V_D/V_T = Ratio of dead space to tidal volume

P_{ACO_2} = Alveolar partial pressure of CO_2

P_{ECO_2} = Partial pressure of CO_2 in mixed expired air

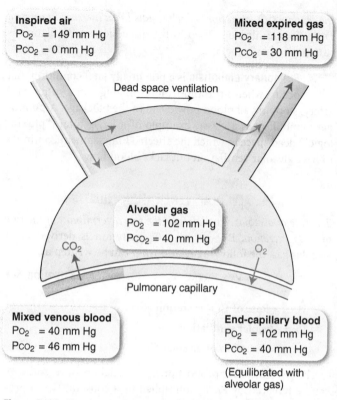

Figure 5-16: Normal profile of P_{O_2} and P_{CO_2} in inspired air, mixed venous blood, alveolar gas, end-pulmonary capillary blood, and mixed expired gas. Alveolar gas composition is intermediate between inspired air and mixed venous blood, reflecting CO_2 excretion and O_2 uptake. End-pulmonary capillary blood is in equilibrium with alveolar gas. Expired gas has a lower CO_2 and a higher O_2 than alveolar gas, because alveolar gas mixes with inspired air in anatomic dead space during expiration.

In clinical practice, P_{ACO_2} is estimated as Pa_{CO_2} and can be measured from an arterial blood sample. Equation 5-12 now becomes:

$$\frac{V_D}{V_T} = \frac{Pa_{CO_2} - P_{ECO_2}}{Pa_{CO_2}} \qquad \textbf{Equation 5-13}$$

V_D/V_T = Ratio of dead space to tidal volume

Pa_{CO_2} = Partial pressure of CO_2 in arterial blood

P_{ECO_2} = Partial pressure of CO_2 in mixed expired air

Dead space ventilation ($\dot{V}_D$) is the product of expired minute ventilation ($\dot{V}_E$) and the ratio of dead space to tidal volume $\left(\frac{V_D}{V_T}\right)$, and because $\dot{V}_D$ subtracted from $\dot{V}_E$ equals the alveolar ventilation ($\dot{V}_A$):

$$\dot{V}_A = \dot{V}_E - \left(\dot{V}_E \times \frac{V_D}{V_T}\right) \qquad \textbf{Equation 5-14}$$

$\dot{V}_A$ = Alveolar ventilation rate

$\dot{V}_E$ = Expired minute ventilation rate

V_D/V_T = Ratio of dead space to tidal volume

Example 1 The following results of pulmonary function testing were obtained in a healthy man:

Tidal volume (V_T) = 600 mL

Breathing frequency = 12 breaths/min

Pa_{CO_2} (arterial) = 40 mm Hg

P_{ECO_2} (expired air) = 30 mm Hg

Minute ventilation: $\dot{V} = V_T \times f$

$$= 600 \times 12$$

$$= \textbf{7200 mL/min}$$

Dead space/tidal volume ratio: $\dfrac{V_D}{V_T} = \dfrac{Pa_{CO_2} - P_{ECO_2}}{Pa_{CO_2}}$

$$\frac{V_D}{V_T} = \frac{40 - 30}{40}$$

$$= \textbf{0.25 (25\%)}$$

Alveolar ventilation: $\dot{V}_A = \dot{V}_E - \left(\dot{V}_E \times \dfrac{V_D}{V_T}\right)$

$$\dot{V}_A = 7200 - (7200 \times 0.25)$$

$$= \textbf{5400 mL/min}$$

Example 2 The following results of pulmonary function testing were obtained in a patient with severe emphysema who had smoked two packs of cigarettes a day for 30 years:

Tidal volume (V_T) = 1400 mL

Breathing frequency = 8 breaths/min

Pa_{CO_2} (arterial) = 60 mm Hg

P_{ECO_2} (expired air) = 20 mm Hg

Minute ventilation: $\dot{V}_E = V_T \times f$

$$= 1400 \times 8$$

$$= \mathbf{11200 \ mL/min}$$

Dead space/tidal volume ratio: $\dfrac{V_D}{V_T} = \dfrac{P_{ACO_2} - P_{ECO_2}}{P_{ACO_2}}$

$$\frac{V_D}{V_T} = \frac{60 - 20}{60}$$

$$= \mathbf{0.67 \ (67\%)}$$

Alveolar ventilation: $\dot{V}_A = \dot{V}_E - \left(\dot{V}_E \times \dfrac{V_D}{V_T} \right)$

$$\dot{V}_A = 11200 - (11200 \times 0.67)$$

$$= \mathbf{3733 \ mL/min}$$

Despite a large expired minute ventilation rate, the patient has chronic hypercapnia (excess blood CO_2) resulting from the large dead space/tidal volume ratio of 0.67, which causes a low alveolar ventilation rate.

CO_2 PRODUCTION

Blood-CO_2 concentration is determined by a balance between CO_2 production from cellular metabolism and excretion via the process of alveolar ventilation. Metabolic rate is defined by O_2 consumption, and CO_2 production is related to O_2 consumption by calculating the **respiratory quotient** using the following equation:

$$RQ = \frac{\dot{V}_{CO_2}}{\dot{V}_{O_2}}$$

Equation 5-15

RQ = Respiratory quotient

$\dot{V}_{CO_2}$ = Rate of CO_2 production

$\dot{V}_{O_2}$ = Rate of O_2 consumption

The respiratory quotient is determined by the nutrients that are metabolized; for carbohydrates (RQ = 1.0); for proteins (RQ = 0.8); and for lipids (RQ = 0.7). For example, more O_2 is required to metabolize lipids because fat molecules have less O_2 atoms than do carbohydrates, and more gaseous O_2 is needed to produce CO_2 and H_2O. Under basal conditions, the average respiratory quotient is about 0.8 because more CO_2 is produced than O_2 is consumed. *The respiratory quotient may change during trauma or infection, which in turn affects the rate of CO_2 production.* For example, in patients with sepsis, the respiratory quotient decreases due to increased fat oxidation.

CO_2 TRANSPORT IN BLOOD

Figure 5-17 summarizes the fate of CO_2 produced by metabolism. The figure illustrates how CO_2 diffuses as a dissolved gas along a gradient of partial pressure from cells to interstitium to systemic capillary blood plasma. CO_2 enters the red blood cells and combines with H_2O to produce H_2CO_3 in a reaction catalyzed by **carbonic anhydrase.** H_2CO_3 then dissociates to produce HCO_3^- ions inside red blood cells, which are delivered into plasma via the Cl/HCO_3 exchange (known as the "**chloride shift**"). The total CO_2 content of arterial blood is about 48 mL of CO_2 per dL of blood. CO_2 is **carried in three forms:**

1. 90% of CO_2 is carried as HCO_3^- **ions in plasma.**

2. 5% is carried as **dissolved CO_2 molecules.** CO_2 is 20 times more soluble than O_2 at body temperature, and about 2.4 mL of CO_2 is dissolved per liter of blood at a normal arterial P_{CO_2} of 40 mm Hg.

3. 5% of CO_2 is carried as **carbamino compounds,** which consist of CO_2 bound to plasma proteins or to hemoglobin within red blood cells.

Mixed venous blood contains about 52 mL of CO_2 per dL of blood, or approximately 88% HCO_3^-, 7% carbamino compounds, and 5% dissolved CO_2. The arterial-to-venous difference in CO_2 content is small compared to that of O_2 (*note: this is important for understanding the effects of the $\dot{V}/\dot{Q}$ mismatch on arterial blood gases*) (see Oxygenation).

CO_2 **CONTENT CURVE** Figure 5-18 compares the CO_2 and O_2 content ("dissociation") curves, which describe the total amount of each gas present in blood as a function of its partial pressure. The O_2 content curve (see Oxygenation) plateaus because hemoglobin becomes saturated with O_2. Further increases in arterial P_{O_2} have little effect on total O_2 content of blood. In contrast, the CO_2 content curve is roughly linear. As a consequence, CO_2 excretion can continue to increase as a function of the alveolar ventilation rate. This explains why a patient with a large area of lung that fails to excrete CO_2 can still have a normal arterial P_{CO_2}. *Alveolar ventilation in other areas of the functional lung can increase to excrete more CO_2 and compensate for the dysfunctional areas.* The same cannot occur for O_2. If poorly oxygenated blood leaves a region of the lung, other areas cannot take up more O_2 to compensate because blood from these areas is already saturated with O_2.

▽ **Pneumonia** is an infection of the airspaces and results in pus-filled alveoli, which effectively reduces alveolar ventilation in the affected areas. Other healthy areas of the lung can compensate to eliminate CO_2, but patients can become hypoxemic (low arterial P_{O_2}) and require supplemental O_2. ▽

THE HALDANE EFFECT

The Haldane effect refers to changes in the position of the CO_2 content curve that occur with oxygenation of the blood and which affect diffusion gradients for CO_2. *The only form of CO_2 that can diffuse from cells to plasma at the tissues and from plasma to alveolar gas at the lung is free CO_2 molecules.*

Gases obey **Fick's law of diffusion** (see Chapter 1). The rate of diffusion is proportional to the surface area and inversely proportional to the thickness of the diffusion barrier, making the lung ideally suited for gas diffusion. The rate of diffusion is proportional to the diffusion constant. CO_2 has a high diffusion constant and diffuses about 20 times more rapidly than O_2. For this reason, *CO_2 diffusion is almost never a clinical concern.*

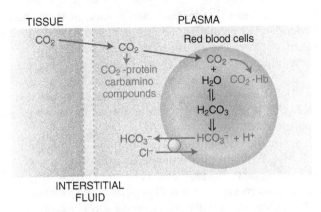

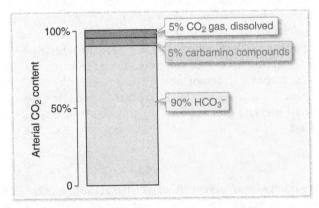

Figure 5-17: CO_2 transport in blood. CO_2 generated by tissues diffuses into blood. Most CO_2 is converted to HCO_3^- ions inside erythrocytes, via carbonic anhydrase, and is delivered into plasma via the Cl/HCO_3 exchange.

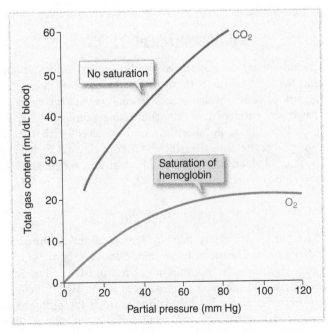

Figure 5-18: CO_2 and O_2 dissociation (content) curves. Hb, hemoglobin.

However, diseases that increase the thickness of the diffusion barrier, such as pulmonary fibrosis or pulmonary edema, can affect O_2 uptake. The diffusion rate is also proportional to the partial pressure gradient. CO_2 excretion at the lung occurs because P_{CO_2} is higher in mixed venous blood than in alveolar gas. The partial pressure gradient is reversed in the tissues, where CO_2 is generated by cells and diffuses into the systemic capillary blood.

The Haldane effect describes variations in plasma P_{CO_2} with oxygenation, which promote CO_2 diffusion at both the lung and tissues. *The basis of the Haldane effect is redistribution of CO_2 between carbamino hemoglobin and dissolved CO_2.* In the pulmonary capillaries, O_2 binding to hemoglobin liberates free CO_2 from carbamino hemoglobin. As a result, the pulmonary capillary partial pressure of CO_2 (P_{CcO_2}) increases (shown by a right shift in the CO_2 dissociation curve), resulting in more CO_2 excretion (Figure 5-19). The reverse process occurs at the tissues—O_2 unloading from hemoglobin allows more carbamino hemoglobin to form. This decreases the plasma P_{CO_2} in the systemic capillaries and increases the partial pressure gradient for CO_2 diffusion from tissues into blood.

REGIONAL DIFFERENCES IN VENTILATION

As a result of gravity, ventilation is higher at the base of the lung than at the apex in a person who is standing (Figure 5-20). The weight of the lung compresses alveoli at the base of the lung. *When the lung is at FRC, alveoli at the base of the lung have optimal compliance and are more easily ventilated,* whereas alveoli at the apex have a high resting volume and are more difficult to ventilate due to lower compliance. In addition, *basal alveoli have a larger range of volume through which they can expand during inspiration.* It is important to consider the effects of gravity on the distribution of ventilation and perfusion when considering $\dot{V}/\dot{Q}$ matching (see Oxygenation).

PULMONARY BLOOD FLOW

The pulmonary circulation receives the entire cardiac output from the right ventricle. Deoxygenated blood flows through a network of vessels, which branch in concert with the airways. Alveoli are enveloped by interconnecting pulmonary capillaries. Blood flows in "sheets" around the alveoli rather than through discrete capillaries, thereby maximizing gas exchange. Oxygenated blood is returned to the left atrium via the pulmonary venous system.

PULMONARY BLOOD PRESSURE

Mean pulmonary artery pressure is only about 10 mm Hg, and systolic and diastolic pressures are about 25 mm Hg and 8 mm Hg, respectively. Outlet pressure from the pulmonary circulation into the left atrium is about 5 mm Hg. Therefore, the driving pressure for blood flow through the pulmonary circulation is only about 10% to that of the systemic circulation. The lower blood pressure in the pulmonary circulation is reflected in the thin walls of the right ventricle and pulmonary

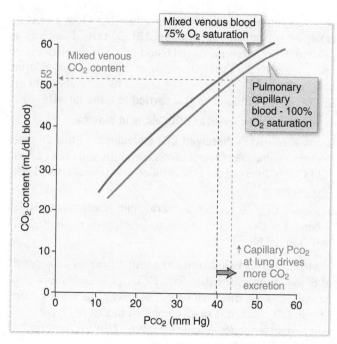

Figure 5-19: The Haldane effect. Formation of oxyhemoglobin in the pulmonary capillary blood reduces the affinity of hemoglobin for CO_2, thereby increasing the concentration of freely dissolved CO_2 (P_{CO_2}). Increased P_{CO_2} in blood drives more CO_2 diffusion into the alveolus.

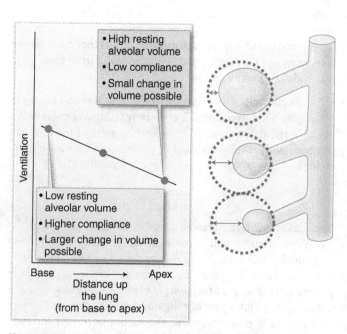

Figure 5-20: Gradient of ventilation in the lung when a person is standing. Gravity compresses alveoli at the base of the lung compared to the apex of the lung. Lung acini at the base have more optimal compliance and a larger range of volume change available during inspiration.

arteries. A lower pressure blood circulation has the advantage of reducing workload on the right ventricle and also reduces the risk of excessive interstitial fluid formation, which would interfere with O_2 diffusion.

▽ **Cor pulmonale** is right ventricular failure due to excessively high pulmonary artery pressures that can arise from pulmonary emboli (either massive or multiple emboli), pulmonary vascular disease (e.g., collagen vascular disease such as scleroderma), or parenchymal disease (e.g., COPD; pulmonary fibrosis). ▽

PULMONARY VASCULAR RESISTANCE

Low perfusion pressure is able to drive the entire cardiac output through the pulmonary circulation because pulmonary vascular resistance is very low. In the systemic circulation, arterioles offer most vascular resistance. In the pulmonary circulation, resistance is shared between arterioles, capillaries, and venules. The behavior of capillaries and larger vessels is very different, giving rise to the concept of **alveolar and extraalveolar vessels.** *Alveolar vessels are influenced by alveolar pressure and are compressed if the alveolar pressure increases above the vascular pressure. Extraalveolar vessels are affected most by lung volume.* As the lungs expand, radial forces increase. The increased radial traction causes the extraalveolar vessels to open, which reduces their resistance. When lung volume decreases, extraalveolar vessels are compressed.

The pulmonary circulation is forced to accommodate large increases in blood flow whenever cardiac output increases (e.g., exercise). Increased cardiac output through the pulmonary circulation can be accommodated because pulmonary vascular resistance decreases as cardiac output increases (Figure 5-21A). The decrease in pulmonary vascular resistance that is observed when cardiac output increases occurs because of the **distention** of the pulmonary capillaries and by **recruitment** of capillaries that were not perfused at rest. In contrast, most systemic vascular beds actively autoregulate blood flow in response to increased blood pressure.

Lung volume is an important passive determinant of pulmonary vascular resistance. Figure 5-21B shows that pulmonary vascular resistance is optimal around FRC. *Vascular resistance increases at either high or low lung volume.* At low lung volumes (patients with restrictive lung disease), compression of the extraalveolar vessels predominates to increase resistance. At high lung volumes (e.g., patients with emphysema), the pulmonary capillaries are stretched, resulting in reduced capillary diameter and increased pulmonary vascular resistance.

▽ **Smoking** destroys the alveolar membranes and their corresponding pulmonary capillaries, significantly decreasing the pulmonary capillary cross-sectional area and therefore contributing to **increased pulmonary artery pressure.** ▽

HYPOXIC PULMONARY VASOCONSTRICTION Active control of pulmonary vascular resistance occurs in response to **alveolar hypoxia** (low Po_2). Figure 5-22 shows decreased pulmonary blood flow when the alveolar Po_2 decreases below 60 mm Hg. A rapid ascent to a high altitude, where atmospheric Po_2 is low,

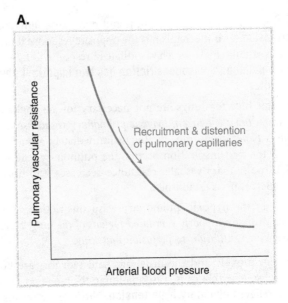

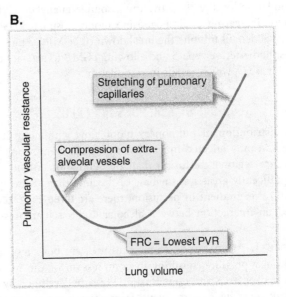

Figure 5-21: Effects of pulmonary blood pressure (or cardiac output) **(A)** and lung volume **(B)** on pulmonary vascular resistance. FRC, functional residual capacity; PVR, pulmonary vascular resistance.

causes pulmonary vasoconstriction and may cause **pulmonary hypertension**. This mechanism is the opposite response to most systemic vascular beds, which vasodilate in response to hypoxia. **Hypoxic pulmonary vasoconstriction has two important physiologic roles:**

1. In **fetal life,** the lungs are not necessary for gas exchange. *Before a breath is taken, hypoxic pulmonary vasoconstriction shunts blood away from the lungs.* Immediately after birth, when the first inspiration occurs, the pulmonary arterioles dilate, pulmonary vascular resistance decreases, and normal lung perfusion is established.

2. After birth, hypoxic pulmonary vasoconstriction *shunts blood away from poorly ventilated regions of the lung, thereby improving ventilation-to-perfusion matching.*

▽ Nitric oxide and the drug sildenafil (Viagra) are both substances that cause vasodilation in the lung and can be used to relieve **pulmonary hypertension.** Nitric oxide results in vasodilation by directly activating a soluble guanylate cyclase, thereby increasing cyclic guanosine monophosphate (cGMP) levels. Sildenafil inhibits the breakdown of cGMP by blocking phosphodiesterase type-5 and allowing cGMP to activate protein kinase G, which results in vasodilation. ▽

REGIONAL DIFFERENCES IN PERFUSION

The distribution of pulmonary blood flow within the lungs is significantly affected by gravity, which has a more marked effect on regional perfusion than on ventilation. Blood flow is significantly greater at the base of the lung than at the apex. Within this gradient of perfusion, there are **three lung zones** based on interaction between alveolar and vascular pressure (Figure 5-23):

Zone 1. Arterial and venous pressures are both less than alveolar pressure, resulting in compression of the pulmonary capillaries and no perfusion. Pressure developed by the right ventricle is normally just large enough to prevent zone 1 from occurring at the apex of the lung. Zone 1 is alveolar dead space, which is ventilated but not perfused. *If blood pressure decreases (e.g., hemorrhage) or if alveolar pressure increases (e.g., mechanical ventilation), zone 1 may become a significant fraction of total perfusion.*

Zone 2. Alveolar pressure is between arterial and venous pressure. The perfusion pressure in zone 2 is the difference between arterial and alveolar pressure. Vessels are partially constricted, and blood flow is more limited.

Zone 3. Arterial and venous pressures both exceed alveolar pressure. Perfusion pressure is the arterial-to-venous pressure difference. *Zone 3 represents the areas of the lung with the largest rate of blood flow (i.e., the base of the upright lung).*

▽ A Swan-Ganz catheter is used to obtain **pulmonary capillary wedge pressure,** an estimate of left atrial pressure and left ventricular end-diastolic pressure. The balloon-tipped catheter is inserted into a central vein and allowed to float along the path through the right atrium, the right ventricle, the pulmonary artery, and down to a pulmonary capillary. The inflated balloon will "wedge" into place, occluding the small pulmonary

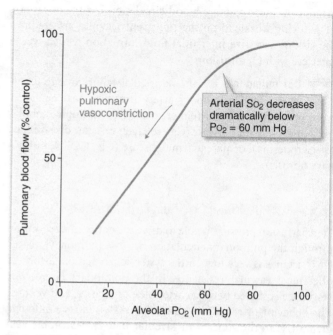

Figure 5-22: Hypoxic pulmonary vasoconstriction. Low alveolar P_{O_2} causes pulmonary vasoconstriction. The effect is marked at alveolar P_{O_2} lower than 60 mm Hg, where arterial S_{O_2} begins to sharply decrease on the oxyhemoglobin dissociation curve.

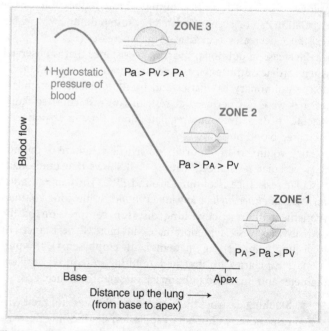

Figure 5-23: Gradient of perfusion in the lung when a person is standing. Perfusion is prevented if alveolar pressure exceeds arterial and venous pressure (zone 1). Blood flow is impeded when alveolar pressure exceeds venous pressure but not arterial pressure (zone 2) and perfusion depends on the arterial-to-alveolar pressure gradient. Blood flow is not impeded by alveolar pressure if both arterial and venous pressures are higher than alveolar pressure (zone 3). The base of the lung has the highest perfusion because gravity increases arterial and venous pressure, creating zone 3 perfusion.

vessel. To estimate the left atrial and left ventricular pressures, the sensor on the tip of the catheter must have a continuous column of blood from the pulmonary capillary to the left atrium and ventricle. To achieve this, *the catheter must be placed in lung zone 3 because capillary collapse is present in zones 1 and 2, which prevents direct connection with the left atrium.* ▼

OXYGENATION

Delivery of O_2 from the atmosphere to cells involves several steps. **Successful oxygenation requires:**

Ventilation of perfused alveoli with atmospheric O_2.

Diffusion of O_2 across the blood-gas barrier and **binding of O_2 to hemoglobin** in the erythrocytes.

A balance between ventilation and perfusion to prevent desaturated venous blood from entering the systemic arterial circulation (i.e., **venous admixture**).

Adequate blood flow to the tissues in relation to metabolic demand.

Unloading of O_2 from hemoglobin at the tissues.

O_2 diffuses down a cascade of partial pressure from atmospheric gas (which has a P_{O_2} of about 150 mm Hg at sea level) to mitochondria (which can have a P_{O_2} of less than 5 mm Hg) (Figure 5-24). The gradient for O_2 diffusion along this cascade can be varied by the external conditions applied. For example, the P_{O_2} of inspired air for a patient at sea level on 100% O_2, via non-rebreather face mask, is approximately 700 mm Hg, whereas the inspired P_{O_2} at the top of Mt. Everest is about 40 mm Hg!

TISSUE O_2 DELIVERY AND CONSUMPTION

The body has very limited stores of O_2; therefore interruptions to cardiac output or pulmonary oxygenation are fatal within a few minutes. To avoid cellular hypoxia, matching between tissue O_2 consumption and O_2 delivery in arterial blood must be continuous. The rate of O_2 delivery is the product of cardiac output and arterial O_2 content:

$$D_{O_2} = \dot{Q}_T \times C_{a O_2} \times 10 \qquad \textbf{Equation 5-16A}$$

D_{O_2} = O_2 delivery (mL O_2/min)
$\dot{Q}_T$ = Cardiac output (L blood/min)
$C_{a O_2}$ = O_2 content of arterial blood (mL O_2/dL blood)

The rate of O_2 consumption is the product of cardiac output and the arteriovenous difference in O_2 content:

$$\dot{V}_{O_2} = \dot{Q}_T \times (C_{a O_2} - C_{v O_2}) \times 10 \qquad \textbf{Equation 5-16B}$$

$\dot{V}_{O_2}$ = O_2 consumption (mL O_2/min)
$\dot{Q}_T$ = Cardiac output (l blood/min)
$C_{a O_2}$ = O_2 content of arterial blood (mL of O_2/dL of blood)
$C_{v O_2}$ = O_2 content of venous blood (mL of O_2/dL of blood)

Typical values for a resting adult are $\dot{Q}_T$ = 5 L/min, $C_{a O_2}$ = 20 mL/dL, and $C_{v O_2}$ = 15 mL/dL. From Equation 5-16B, basal $\dot{V}_{O_2}$ = 250 mL/min.

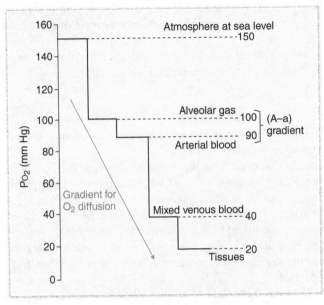

Figure 5-24: Cascade of P_{O_2} from the atmosphere at sea level to tissues.

▽ $V_{O_2 max}$ is a measure of peak O_2 consumption at maximal aerobic exercise and is used as a measure of aerobic fitness. As such, it can vary from 20 mL/kg/min for a sedentary person, to 40 mL/kg/min for the average untrained person, to 85 mL/kg/min for an elite trained athlete. ▽

O_2 TRANSPORT IN BLOOD

Despite the relatively low solubility of O_2 in plasma, the volume of gaseous O_2 per liter of blood remarkably is almost the same as that in air. This is possible because red blood cells contain a large quantity of the O_2-binding protein **hemoglobin.** Only 2% of O_2 in arterial blood is present as dissolved O_2. At an arterial P_{O_2} of 100 mm Hg, only 0.3 mL of O_2 is dissolved in every 100 mL of blood. *Ninety-eight percent of O_2 in blood is carried bound to hemoglobin within red blood cells.* One gram of hemoglobin carries approximately 1.35 mL of O_2 when 100% saturated.

The **total O_2 content of arterial blood** is calculated as:

$$Ca_{O_2} = (1.35 \times [Hb] \times Sa_{O_2}) + (k_{O_2} \times Pa_{O_2})$$

Equation 5-17

Ca_{O_2} = O_2 content (mL O_2/dL blood)

[Hb] = Hemoglobin concentration (g/dL)

Sa_{O_2} = O_2 saturation of hemoglobin (0–1.0)

k_{O_2} = O_2 solubility constant (0.0031 mL O_2/dL blood)

The function of the pulmonary system is to provide an adequate arterial P_{O_2}. This pressure is crucial because hemoglobin saturation depends on adequate arterial P_{O_2}, and oxyhemoglobin is the primary O_2 carrier in blood. As illustrated by Equation 5-17, *O_2 content will be inadequate if hemoglobin concentration is low (anemia) or if Sa_{O_2} is low.* Low Sa_{O_2} results from hypoxemia (low arterial P_{O_2}). Potential causes of hypoxemia include inadequate ventilation, diffusion, and $\dot{V}/\dot{Q}$ mismatch.

▽ When caring for a **critically ill patient** (e.g., shock from significant trauma), it is imperative to maximize O_2 content. This can be accomplished by careful assessment and correction of the hemoglobin concentration, the arterial P_{O_2}, and the Sa_{O_2}. ▽

THE OXYHEMOGLOBIN DISSOCIATION CURVE

Figure 5-25 shows the normal relationship between percent hemoglobin saturation and P_{O_2}. Each hemoglobin molecule can bind four O_2 molecules. There is cooperative binding of O_2 so that each additional O_2 binds more easily, producing the sigmoidal shape of the O_2 dissociation curve. In healthy lungs with an alveolar partial pressure of O_2 of 100 mm Hg, pulmonary capillary blood is 100% saturated with O_2. *When P_{O_2} decreases below 60 mm Hg, there is a rapid decline in hemoglobin saturation.* Mechanisms that control breathing strongly increase ventilation if arterial P_{O_2} decreases below 60 mm Hg.

▽ A **general rule of thumb concerning oxygenation** is the "4-5-6:7-8-9" rule. An arterial P_{O_2} of 40 mm Hg, 50 mm Hg, or 60 mm Hg roughly corresponds to Sa_{O_2} of 70%, 80%,

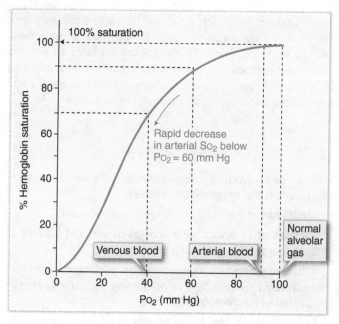

Figure 5-25: Oxyhemoglobin dissociation curve. Hemoglobin (Hb) is saturated at normal arterial P_{O_2} values at sea level. Arterial hypoxemia below 60 mm Hg threatens the arterial O_2 content due to the loss of O_2-Hb saturation.

or 90%, respectively. Due to the rapid decline in hemoglobin saturation at an arterial P_{O_2} <60 mm Hg (or Sa_{O_2} <90%), *the therapeutic goals for oxygenation (with a few exceptions) are typically arterial P_{O_2} >60 mm Hg (or Sa_{O_2} >90%), which corresponds with the flat portion of the O_2 dissociation curve.* ▼

Figure 5-26 shows that the position of the O_2 dissociation curve can shift, affecting the ability to take up O_2 at the lung and alter the amount of O_2 unloaded from hemoglobin at the tissues. The O_2 affinity of hemoglobin is described using a P_{50} value, which is the P_{O_2} resulting in 50% saturation. A normal P_{50} is about 27 mm Hg; lower P_{50} indicates an increase in O_2 affinity and a left shift in the dissociation curve, whereas a higher P_{50} indicates a decrease in O_2 affinity and a right shift in the dissociation curve.

A left shift in the oxyhemoglobin dissociation curve causes hemoglobin to become saturated at lower P_{O_2}. Therefore, loading O_2 into blood at the lung is easier, but it is more difficult to unload O_2 at the tissues. The O_2 dissociation curve for **fetal hemoglobin** lies to the left of the curve for adult (maternal) hemoglobin; *higher O_2 affinity of fetal hemoglobin aids in O_2 transfer across the placenta.* If the curve shifts right, O_2 loading at the lungs is reduced and the proportion of hemoglobin saturated with O_2 (Sa_{O_2}) may be reduced, but O_2 is unloaded more readily at the tissues.

▼ In **clinical management of acutely ill patients,** it is preferable to retain some right shift in the curve to increase O_2 availability at the tissues. This can be achieved by accepting a slightly lower blood pH because an acidic environment will cause a right shift, enhancing O_2 delivery to the tissues. ▼

Several factors cause a right shift in the O_2 dissociation curve, including:

Increased temperature (e.g., exercise). Higher temperature increases O_2 unloading in working muscle.

Increased CO_2. High levels of CO_2 in metabolically active tissues indicate high O_2 demand, and more O_2 unloading is desirable.

Increased $[H^+]$. Buffering of H^+ by hemoglobin reduces its O_2 affinity (known as the **Bohr effect**). For example, anaerobic metabolism produces lactic acid, indicating that more O_2 delivery to the tissue is needed.

Increased concentration of 2,3-bisphosphoglycerate (BPG) in erythrocytes. BPG is an end product of metabolism in erythrocytes. Hypoxemia increases BPG formation, causing more unloading of O_2 from hemoglobin. If blood is stored in blood banks for a long period, BPG levels are reduced. *A transfusion with blood that has been stored for a long period causes an unwanted left shift in the O_2 dissociation curve.*

Carbon monoxide (CO) is a product of incomplete combustion and is a colorless, odorless, tasteless, nonirritating gas. CO is a poisonous gas because it binds irreversibly to hemoglobin and prevents O_2 binding. It binds to hemoglobin with very high affinity to produce carboxyhemoglobin. Figure 5-27 shows the effect of CO poisoning on the O_2 dissociation curve. In the

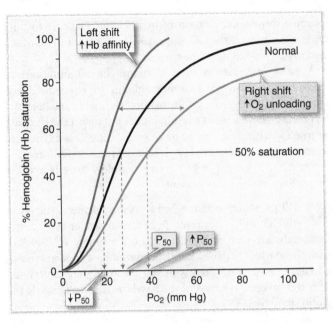

Figure 5-26: Effect of left and right shift of oxyhemoglobin dissociation curve on P_{50} values. A left shift increases Sa_{O_2} but reduces O_2 unloading at the tissues. A right shift has the opposite effect.

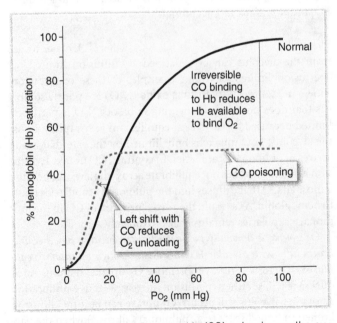

Figure 5-27: Effect of carbon monoxide (CO) poisoning on the oxyhemoglobin dissociation curve. CO binds irreversibly to hemoglobin, decreasing the fraction of total hemoglobin available for O_2 saturation. CO binding also causes a left shift in the curve, reducing O_2 unloading from the remaining oxyhemoglobin.

example shown, the amount of hemoglobin available to bind O_2 is reduced by 50%. CO also causes a decrease in P_{50}, which reduces O_2 unloading at the tissues.

A **pulse oximeter** is used in many clinical situations to measure the ratio of deoxyhemoglobin to oxyhemoglobin (functional saturation). A pulse oximeter is unable to detect carboxyhemoglobin and, as a result, it does not detect the decrease in true O_2 saturation caused by CO poisoning. It is a common misconception that arterial PO_2 is reduced in CO poisoning. *The arterial PO_2 is normal in CO poisoning* unless there is another pulmonary abnormality present.

▽ **CO poisoning** occurs when a person inspires toxic levels of CO, which can result in brain damage or even death. Symptoms are very nonspecific and often mimic viral illness, with headache, malaise, nausea, vomiting, and drowsiness. Classic findings associated with CO poisoning are cherry-red skin and bilateral necrosis of the basal ganglia, particularly the globus pallidus. ▽

ALVEOLAR O_2 TRANSFER

Before O_2 can bind to hemoglobin, it must first diffuse across the blood-gas barrier. A red blood cell is in transit only 0.75 seconds through a pulmonary capillary at rest. In extreme exercise, when cardiac output is increased, the transit time may be less than 0.25 seconds. In healthy persons, the equilibration of the partial pressure of O_2 occurs between alveolar gas and pulmonary capillary blood in this brief amount of time (Figure 5-28A). Patients with lung disease (e.g., pulmonary fibrosis) may have reduced diffusion capacity, and equilibration of O_2 across the alveolus may be incomplete. *Diffusion defects are unmasked when the blood transit time is low (e.g., exercise) or if the driving force for O_2 diffusion is reduced (e.g., low inspired O_2 partial pressure at high altitude).*

DIFFUSION AND PERFUSION LIMITED GAS TRANSFER
Uptake of gas from the alveolus can be described as "diffusion limited" or "perfusion limited." Extreme examples of these concepts are shown in Figure 5-28B. **Nitrous oxide** (N_2O) is a poorly soluble gas that does not bind to anything in blood. N_2O is perfusion limited because PN_2O arrives at equilibrium very rapidly across the alveolus; N_2O uptake is only limited by the rate that blood arrives in pulmonary capillaries. In contrast, CO uptake is diffusion limited. PCO does not equilibrate across the alveolus because almost all CO that diffuses into the pulmonary capillaries binds to hemoglobin. As a result, the partial pressure of CO in the pulmonary capillaries remains at approximately zero.

O_2 uptake is normally perfusion limited because blood equilibrates fully with alveolar PO_2 in transit through pulmonary capillaries. There is a reserve for more O_2 uptake, demonstrated during exercise when perfusion increases and equilibration across the alveolus still occurs. O_2 uptake can become diffusion limited in lung disease (e.g., pulmonary fibrosis) when the partial pressure of O_2 is unable to equilibrate between the alveoli and the pulmonary capillary blood. In healthy individuals, this is also possible under extreme conditions such as heavy exercise at a high altitude.

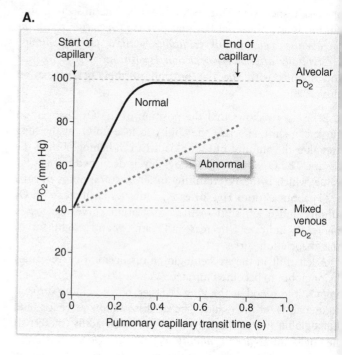

A.

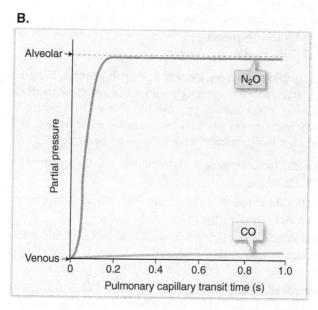

B.

Figure 5-28: Gas uptake kinetics across the blood-gas barrier for O_2 **(A)** compared to nitrous oxide (N_2O) and carbon monoxide (CO) **(B)** N_2O equilibrates almost immediately between blood and alveolar gas and uptake is perfusion limited. Alveolar PCO never equilibrates with pulmonary capillary PCO because blood has such a large capacity for the irreversible binding of CO to hemoglobin. CO uptake is diffusion limited.

LUNG DIFFUSION CAPACITY Small nontoxic doses of CO can be administered to measure lung diffusion capacity. Even at low blood flow rates, the capacity for CO binding is so large that its uptake is only limited by the rate of diffusion:

$$D_L = \dot{V}_{CO} \div P_{ACO}$$ **Equation 5-18**

D_L = Lung diffusion capacity

$\dot{V}_{CO}$ = Rate of CO uptake

P_{ACO} = Alveolar partial pressure of CO

▽ Diffusion capacity can be measured to assess for **diseases that impair the alveolar-capillary membrane.** Decreased diffusion capacity can be seen in interstitial lung disease, emphysema, and pulmonary vascular disease. (*Note: diffusion capacity is normal in patients with asthma.*) ▼

V̇/Q̇ MATCHING

The most common cause of hypoxemia (low arterial O₂ partial pressure) is mismatch between the distribution of ventilation and pulmonary blood flow. Expired minute ventilation and cardiac output are both about 5–6 L/min at rest, yielding an overall $\dot{V}/\dot{Q}$ ratio of about 1. Even when overall $\dot{V}/\dot{Q} = 1$, abnormalities in gas exchange result if there are regional differences in the distribution of ventilation and perfusion. The two most extreme situations are **intrapulmonary shunt** ($\dot{V}/\dot{Q} = 0$), where lung units are perfused with blood but receive no ventilation (e.g., complete airway obstruction), and **dead space** ($\dot{V}/\dot{Q} = \infty$), where lung units are ventilated but not perfused (e.g., pulmonary embolism). Figure 5-29 shows the spectrum of alveolar P_{O_2} and P_{CO_2} as $\dot{V}/\dot{Q}$ deviates from normal toward these extreme positions. *Perfusion without ventilation results in an alveolar gas composition in equilibrium with mixed venous blood. Ventilation without perfusion results in alveoli containing inspired air.*

▽ A $\dot{V}/\dot{Q}$ scan is a nuclear medicine study that can be used in the diagnosis of **pulmonary emboli** and illustrates the concept of matching ventilation to perfusion. Pulmonary emboli will show a reduced blood flow in an area of normal ventilation. In cases of multiple pulmonary emboli, the perfusion scan can show a "moth-eaten" appearance in areas of normal ventilation. ▼

CHARACTERISTICS OF HIGH V̇/Q̇

Regions of the lung that are ventilated but not perfused contribute to physiologic dead space. A patient with areas of high $\dot{V}/\dot{Q}$ will experience a decrease in useful alveolar ventilation unless total ventilation can be adequately increased. This decrease results in less CO₂ excretion and a buildup of the arterial partial pressure of CO₂, a common finding in patients with COPD. In acute situations when hypoxemia occurs, the arterial P_{CO_2} is often normal or may even be reduced. This occurs because lung units that are well perfused can increase CO₂ excretion if ventilation is increased. Similarly, *loss of CO₂ excretion in a region of high $\dot{V}/\dot{Q}$ can be compensated by increasing ventilation of well-perfused lung units. Oxygenation is not directly affected by high $\dot{V}/\dot{Q}$.*

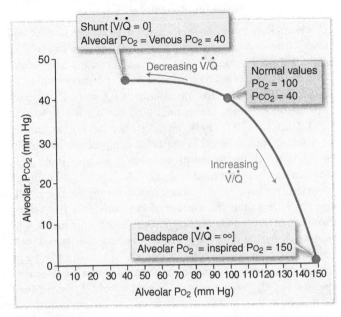

Figure 5-29: Spectrum of alveolar gas composition caused by ventilation/perfusion (V̇/Q̇) mismatch. Ventilation without perfusion represents pure inspired air only. In lung units with perfusion but no ventilation, alveolar gas equilibrates with mixed venous blood. Note the decrease in alveolar P_{O_2} as V̇/Q̇ decreases from normal toward zero, showing that low V̇/Q̇ areas will contribute to hypoxemia.

INTRAPULMONARY SHUNT

Intrapulmonary (right-to-left) shunt mixes deoxygenated blood directly into arterial blood and, as a result, the arterial P_{O_2} may be dramatically reduced. Figure 5-30 shows an example where 50% of blood delivered to the left atrium is from a normal lung and 50% is shunted blood flow ($\dot{V}/\dot{Q} = 0$). Pulmonary capillary blood from the normal lung has a partial pressure of O_2 (P_{CO_2}) = 100 mm Hg, yielding a hemoglobin saturation of 100%. Shunted blood is the same composition as venous blood, in which the partial pressure of O_2 is about 40 mm Hg and hemoglobin saturation is about 75%. When equal volumes of oxygenated and deoxygenated blood are mixed, the resulting P_{O_2} is less than the average of the individual P_{O_2} values. Nonlinearity of the O_2 dissociation curve accounts for the low arterial O_2 partial pressure produced by shunt. The law of mass conservation allows the total O_2 content of two samples to be averaged; therefore hemoglobin saturation can be averaged because the O_2 content is 98% oxyhemoglobin. P_{O_2} must then be read from the O_2 dissociation curve.

In contrast to the effect of shunt to produce hypoxemia, there is little direct change in the arterial partial pressure of CO_2 because the venous CO_2 content is not much larger than the arterial CO_2 content. *When mixed venous blood is combined with oxygenated blood, the resulting arterial P_{CO_2} is only slightly increased* (Figure 5-30). In contrast to O_2, partial pressures of CO_2 can be averaged because the CO_2 dissociation curve is linear and differences in P_{CO_2} reflect differences in total CO_2 content. The physiologic response to the hypoxemia caused by intrapulmonary shunt is to increase ventilation. Increased ventilation would increase CO_2 excretion, but would not add more O_2 because pulmonary capillary blood leaving ventilated lung units is already saturated with O_2.

Treatment of hypoxemia caused by an intrapulmonary shunt is difficult because the hypoxemia is refractory to supplemental O_2. Figure 5-31 shows the effect of breathing 100% O_2 using an example of 50% shunt. Because nonventilated areas cannot receive supplemental O_2, they continue to deliver deoxygenated blood to the arterial circulation. There is a large increase in the alveolar and pulmonary capillary P_{O_2} in well-ventilated alveoli. However, the O_2 content of blood from these lung units increases only minimally because hemoglobin is already saturated with O_2. Note that the amount of extra dissolved O_2 in pulmonary capillary blood is small, even at very high partial pressure of O_2.

QUANTIFYING RIGHT-TO-LEFT SHUNT The amount of right-to-left shunt, as a fraction of cardiac output, can be calculated using the principle of mass conservation. This calculation can be used clinically to determine the extent of right-to-left shunt in patients with arterial hypoxemia. The total amount of O_2 delivered to the systemic circulation is the product of cardiac output and arterial O_2 content ($\dot{Q}_T \times Ca_{O_2}$). This amount must equal the sum of O_2 from shunted blood ($\dot{Q}_S \times Cv_{O_2}$) and pulmonary capillary blood ($\dot{Q}_T$ $\dot{Q}_S) \times Cc_{O_2}$. Rearranging for the shunt fraction $\dot{Q}_S/\dot{Q}_T$:

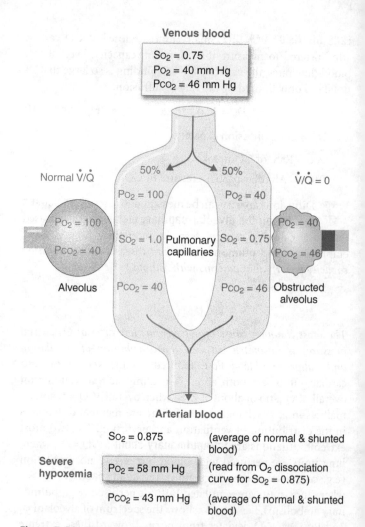

Venous blood

$S_{O_2} = 0.75$
$P_{O_2} = 40$ mm Hg
$P_{CO_2} = 46$ mm Hg

Normal $\dot{V}/\dot{Q}$ 50%   50% $\dot{V}/\dot{Q} = 0$

$P_{O_2} = 100$ $P_{O_2} = 40$

$P_{O_2} = 100$ $P_{O_2} = 40$

$S_{O_2} = 1.0$ Pulmonary $S_{O_2} = 0.75$
$P_{CO_2} = 40$ capillaries $P_{CO_2} = 46$

Alveolus $P_{CO_2} = 40$ $P_{CO_2} = 46$ Obstructed alveolus

Arterial blood

Severe hypoxemia

$S_{O_2} = 0.875$ (average of normal & shunted blood)

$P_{O_2} = 58$ mm Hg   (read from O_2 dissociation curve for $S_{O_2} = 0.875$)

$P_{CO_2} = 43$ mm Hg   (average of normal & shunted blood)

Figure 5-30: Effect of 50% intrapulmonary (right-to-left) shunt on arterial blood gases. Note the severe hypoxemia caused by mixing arterial and venous blood.

$$\frac{\dot{Q}_S}{\dot{Q}_T} = \frac{Cc_{O_2} - Ca_{O_2}}{Cc_{O_2} - Cv_{O_2}}$$

Equation 5-19

$\dot{Q}_S$ = Shunt blood flow

$\dot{Q}_T$ = Cardiac output

C_{CO_2} = Pulmonary capillary blood O_2 content

C_{aO_2} = Systemic arterial blood O_2 content

C_{vO_2} = Mixed venous blood O_2 content

Example A 36-year-old man has severe viral pneumonia and is admitted to the hospital. The results of his arterial blood gas analysis show hypoxemia with an arterial P_{O_2} of 58 mm Hg and hemoglobin saturation (S_{aO_2}) of 88%:

C_{CO_2} = 19.2 mL O_2/dL of blood

C_{aO_2} = 16.8 mL O_2/dL of blood

C_{vO_2} = 15.0 mL O_2/dL of blood

Shunt fraction $\dot{Q}_S/\dot{Q}_T$ = (19.2 − 16.8) / (19.2 − 15.0)

$\qquad\qquad$ = 0.57 = 57% (normal 2–5%)

▽ A high shunt ratio ($\dot{Q}_S/\dot{Q}_T$) can result from either **intracardiac or intrapulmonary shunting.** Intracardiac shunting is an example of a cyanotic congenital heart disease caused by a ventriculoseptal defect, with pulmonary hypertension causing a right to left shunt (**Eisenmenger syndrome**). Intrapulmonary shunting can occur as a result of atelectasis, pulmonary edema, or pneumonia. ▼

ALVEOLAR-ARTERIAL P_{O_2} GRADIENT

Despite equilibration between alveolar gas and pulmonary capillary blood (alveolar P_{O_2} = pulmonary capillary P_{O_2}), arterial P_{O_2} is always less than alveolar P_{O_2}. This *$P_{(A-a)O_2}$ gradient is calculated clinically to identify the cause of hypoxemia* (Figure 5-32). Diffusion abnormality and intrapulmonary shunt are examples where the $P_{(A-a)O_2}$ gradient is increased. To calculate a $P_{(A-a)O_2}$ gradient, the alveolar P_{O_2} must first be calculated, using the **alveolar gas equation:**

$$P_{AO_2} = P_{IO_2} - \frac{P_{ACO_2}}{RQ} \qquad \textbf{Equation 5-20}$$

P_{AO_2} = Alveolar O_2 partial pressure

P_{IO_2} = O_2 partial pressure of inspired gas

RQ = Respiratory quotient

Another form of the alveolar gas equation that is used clinically:

$$P_{AO_2} = F_{IO_2}(P_B - P_{H_2O}) - \frac{P_{ACO_2}}{RQ} \qquad \textbf{Equation 5-21}$$

P_{AO_2} = Alveolar O_2 partial pressure

F_{IO_2} = O_2 fraction of inspired gas

P_B = Barometric pressure

$\dot{P}_{H_2O}$ = Water vapor pressure of inspired gas

P_{aCO_2} = Arterial CO_2 partial pressure

RQ = Respiratory quotient

After alveolar P_{O_2} is calculated using Equation 5-21, and arterial P_{O_2} is measured in an arterial blood sample, the $P_{(A-a)O_2}$

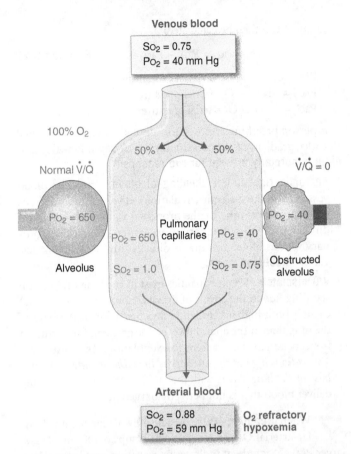

Figure 5-31: Effect of breathing 100% O_2 in a patient with 50% intrapulmonary shunt. Note that supplemental O_2 does not reach unventilated regions and has almost no effect on arterial S_{O_2} of mixed arterial blood. Very high P_{O_2} of blood exposed to 100% O_2 has little effect on total O_2 of blood because hemoglobin is already saturated and dissolved O_2 is a minor component of total O_2.

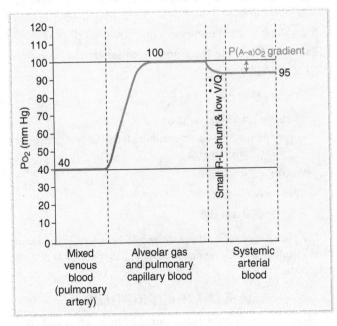

Figure 5-32: Normal A-a gradient.

gradient can then be calculated:

$$P(A\text{-}a)O_2 = PAO_2 - PaO_2 \qquad \textbf{Equation 5-22}$$

$P(A\text{-}a)O_2$ = Alveolar-arterial O_2 tension gradient
PAO_2 = Alveolar O_2 partial pressure
PaO_2 = Arterial O_2 partial pressure

A person breathing atmospheric air at sea level has a normal $P(A\text{-}a)O_2$ gradient of about 5–10 mm Hg. **A small $P(A\text{-}a)O_2$ gradient is normally present for two reasons:**

1. **Anatomic right-to-left shunting of blood.** Bronchial blood vessels from the systemic circulation deliver O_2 and nutrients to lung tissue. Some of the bronchial venous blood drains directly into the pulmonary vein. A small amount of coronary venous blood also drains directly into the left ventricle via the **thebesian veins.**

2. **V̇/Q̇ mismatch.** V̇/Q̇ inequalities exist in the lung of a person standing due to the effects of gravity. Figure 5-33 shows that there is both higher ventilation and perfusion at the base of the lung than at the apex; however, the gradient for perfusion is steeper than the gradient for ventilation. As a result, *the V̇/Q̇ ratio is high at the apex of the lung and slightly low at the base of the lung.* Areas with low V̇/Q̇ at the base of the lung deliver blood that is not perfectly oxygenated.

▽ When **breathing 100% O_2,** a healthy person has an alveolar-arterial O_2 tension gradient of up to 100 mm Hg. A larger $P(A\text{-}a)O_2$ gradient indicates oxygenation problems. ▼

Example A patient with pneumonia was breathing 100% O_2 at sea level via a non-rebreather oxygen mask. This information, together with the results of an arterial blood gas analysis, provided the following data to calculate alveolar PO_2:

   FIO_2 = 100% (1.0)

   PB = 760 mm Hg

   PH_2O = 47 mm Hg

   $PaCO_2$ = 36 mm Hg (measured from an arterial blood gas sample)

   RQ = 0.8 (standard respiratory quotient used clinically)

   PaO_2 = 168 mm Hg (measured from an arterial blood gas sample)

$$PAO_2 = FIO_2(PB - PH_2O) - \frac{PaCO_2}{RQ}$$

$$= 1.0\,(760 - 47) - (36/0.8)$$

$$= 668 \text{ mm Hg } (\textit{note: breathing 100\% } O_2 \textit{ produces a very large alveolar } PO_2)$$

$$P(A\text{-}a)O_2 = PAO_2 - PaO_2$$

$$= 668 - 168$$

$$= \textbf{500 mm Hg!}$$

The presence of such a large difference between O_2 tension in alveoli compared to O_2 tension in arterial blood indicates a severe oxygenation defect.

CAUSES OF ARTERIAL HYPOXEMIA

Table 5-6 summarizes the major causes of hypoxemia and characterizes the $P(A\text{-}a)O_2$ gradient and response to supplemental O_2

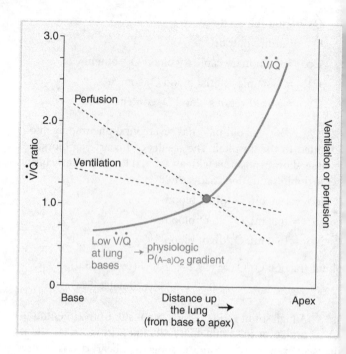

Figure 5-33: Ventilation/perfusion (V̇/Q̇) inequalities in the lung of a healthy person who is standing. High V̇/Q̇ areas at the lung apex excrete only a minimal amount of CO_2, but this is easily compensated by other areas of the lung. Slightly low V̇/Q̇ at the bases of the lung cannot be compensated by other areas and contributes to the normal $P(A\text{-}a)O_2$ gradient.

TABLE 5-6. Major Causes of Arterial Hypoxemia and Response to Supplemental Oxygen

Cause	$P(A\text{-}a)O_2$ Gradient	Responds to Supplemental O_2
Low PIO_2	Normal	Yes
Global hypoventilation	Normal	Yes
Diffusion abnormality	Increased	Yes
V̇/Q̇ mismatch (low V̇/Q̇)	Increased	Yes
Intrapulmonary shunt	Increased	No

for each. An interpretation of low arterial P_{O_2} requires a calculation of the $P(A-a)_{O_2}$ gradient and measurement of arterial P_{CO_2}.

Low P_{IO_2} is an effect of high altitude but can also result from incorrect air mixtures used in scuba diving. Low alveolar P_{O_2} is the cause of low arterial P_{O_2}. The $P(A-a)_{O_2}$ gradient is normal, and the treatment is to restore alveolar P_{O_2} with supplemental O_2.

Global hypoventilation occurs when total minute ventilation is low. This condition may be due to defective central control of breathing, such as narcotic overdose or from paralysis of ventilatory muscles. High arterial P_{CO_2} is always present. High alveolar P_{CO_2} develops because the venous blood P_{CO_2} is increased, and CO_2 diffuses readily into alveoli. CO_2 displaces O_2 in the alveolus, decreasing the alveolar P_{O_2}. The $P(A-a)_{O_2}$ gradient is normal. Low arterial P_{O_2} responds to supplemental O_2; ventilatory support is needed to restore alveolar ventilation.

Diffusion abnormality (e.g., pulmonary fibrosis) is a rare cause of hypoxemia. Alveolar P_{O_2} is normal, but a $P(A-a)_{O_2}$ gradient develops. Supplemental O_2 is an effective treatment because it increases the driving force of O_2 diffusion.

Regional $\dot{V}/\dot{Q}$ imbalance (e.g., pneumonia) is the most common cause of hypoxemia. Unlike global hypoventilation, arterial P_{CO_2} is not increased because total alveolar ventilation is normal, or it may even be increased. Regions of the lung with low $\dot{V}/\dot{Q}$ deliver poorly oxygenated blood and cause the development of a $P(A-a)_{O_2}$ gradient. Hypoxemia responds to supplemental O_2 because affected lung units have some ventilation that can be enriched with O_2.

Intrapulmonary shunt is the most dangerous cause of hypoxemia because, as shown in Figure 5-31, no compensation is possible by normal lung units, even when 100% O_2 is given. The effect of shunt is magnified if venous desaturation (low S_{VO_2}) develops. The S_{VO_2} is determined by the balance between O_2 delivery and consumption. O_2 delivery is too low in conditions such as low cardiac output or severe anemia. The causes of shunt and low S_{VO_2} must be addressed to treat these causes of hypoxemia (e.g., acute respiratory distress syndrome).

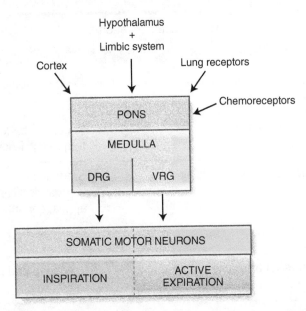

Figure 5-34: Components of the central nervous system controller for ventilation. DRG, dorsal respiratory group; VRG, ventral respiratory group.

CONTROL OF BREATHING

A **central pattern generator in the medulla and pons** initiates the basic rhythmic pattern of breathing, which proceeds without the need for conscious control (e.g., during sleep). There are many **inputs to the central pattern generator that influence breathing;** for example:

Negative feedback responses to maintain the **arterial P_{CO_2} and P_{O_2} and pH.**

Sensory feedback relating to the **mechanical state of the lung and chest wall to** minimize work of breathing, to prevent overinflation of the lung, and to respond to irritants.

Sensory feedback from **receptors in the joints and muscles** to increase ventilation in response to exercise.

TABLE 5-7. Abnormal Breathing Patterns

Breathing Pattern	Description	Comments
Apneustic breathing (apneusis)	Deep inspiration with bradypnea	Rare condition caused by damage to the pons
Biot's breathing	Recurring pattern with fixed V_T and frequency, followed by period of apnea	Central nervous system damage (e.g., meningitis)
Cheyne–Stokes breathing	Gradual increase in V_T followed by gradual decrease, then a period of apnea; continues in cycles	Benign pattern; seen in healthy persons with hypoxemia and hypocapnia at high altitude; also seen in patients with bilateral cortical disease and heart failure
Kussmaul breathing	Very deep and rapid breathing	Characteristic of severe metabolic acidosis (e.g., diabetic ketoacidosis)

Integration with the **sympathetic nervous system** to increase ventilation during "fight or flight" responses, and with other stress responses such as a high body temperature or a low arterial blood pressure.

Integration to allow **speech and swallowing.**

Conscious control to allow hyperventilation or breath holding.

THE CENTRAL NERVOUS SYSTEM NEURAL CONTROLLER

Figure 5-34 illustrates the main components of the central nervous system controller for ventilation. The basic rhythm of breathing is controlled by groups of neurons in the medulla and pons. The medullary center has a **dorsal respiratory group** of neurons in the nucleus of the tractus solitarius and a **ventral respiratory group** in the nucleus ambiguous and nucleus retroambiguus. *The dorsal respiratory group generates the basic inspiratory pattern. Stimulation of the ventral respiratory group increases the breathing rate and causes active expiration.* Outflow from the medullary centers reaches the muscles of ventilation via somatic motor neurons. Control of the diaphragm via the **phrenic nerves** (C3–C5) is most important. Two pontine centers provide fine-tuning to the dorsal respiratory group—*the* **apneustic center** *promotes inspiration, and the* **pneumotaxic center** *inhibits inspiration.*

▽ **Hangman's fracture** results in a spinal cord injury at the level of C2. The fracture causes apnea (cessation of breathing) because the spinal cord is interrupted proximal to the origin of the phrenic nerve roots. In contrast, a spinal cord injury at the level of C4 will result in quadriplegia (motor dysfunction of the upper and lower extremities) but only weakened ventilatory muscles because part of the phrenic nerve remains functional. ▽

Table 5-7 summarizes some abnormal breathing patterns and their causes. **The activity of the central pattern generator is modified by multiple inputs:**

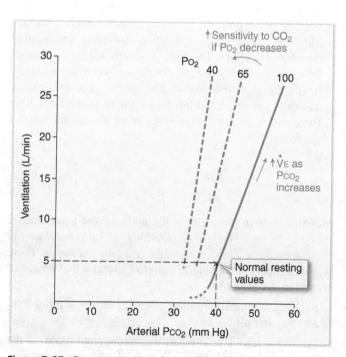

Figure 5-35: Regulation of ventilation by arterial P_{CO_2}. The steep increase in ventilation as arterial P_{CO_2} increases reflects dominant control of ventilation by CO_2. Low arterial P_{O_2} has a synergistic effect with high arterial P_{CO_2}.

Descending cortical inputs allow voluntary control of breathing.

Hypothalamic and limbic system inputs account for breathing patterns seen in emotional states such as rage or fear.

Input from neural receptors in the lung and chest wall is conveyed to the central nervous system via the vagus nerves. Changes in the mechanical state of the lung and chest wall can cause reflex changes in the breathing pattern. For example, stretch receptors in the airway initiate the **Hering-Breuer reflex,** which increases breathing frequency and prevents hyperinflation of the lungs. **Pulmonary J receptors** surround blood vessels and initiate increased ventilation associated with edema in the lung.

Ascending spinal inputs from neural receptors in working muscles and joints provide information about the workload of exercise. Ventilation is stimulated as a function of workload to match O_2 demand. Ventilation also matches increased cardiac output during exercise to ensure $\dot{V}/\dot{Q}$ matching and preservation of normal arterial blood gas tensions.

NEGATIVE FEEDBACK CONTROL OF VENTILATION BY CO₂, O₂, AND PH

Ventilation is increased if the arterial Pco_2 increases or if the arterial Po_2 decreases. These negative feedback responses assist in maintaining blood gases within a normal range. Under normal conditions, maintenance of arterial Pco_2 predominates. Ventilation is also stimulated by **reduced arterial blood pH,** representing the pulmonary contribution to acid-base balance (see Chapter 6).

Figure 5-35 shows increased ventilation in response to high arterial Pco_2, which represents a negative feedback response to increase CO_2 excretion and thereby to restore the arterial Pco_2 to normal. The **predominance of arterial Pco_2** in control of ventilation is indicated by the steepness of the curves shown in Figure 5-35, although the ventilatory response to hypercapnia is blunted by increased arterial Po_2 and stimulated by a coexisting hypoxemia.

Figure 5-36 shows increased ventilation in response to reduced arterial Po_2. *This response accounts for a presentation of low arterial Pco_2 in patients with hypoxemia.* A marked increase in ventilation does not occur until arterial Po_2 is below 60 mm Hg, corresponding with the region of steep decline in oxyhemoglobin saturation on the O_2 dissociation curve. The response to hypoxemia is blunted if arterial Pco_2 is reduced, but stimulated if arterial Pco_2 is increased. Many patients with COPD have hypercapnia; they often adapt to tolerate high arterial Pco_2 but rely on hypoxemia to drive ventilation. *Treatment with supplemental O_2 may cause these patients to stop breathing because arterial Po_2 is increased abruptly, removing their drive to breathe.*

Patients with acidemia (e.g., lactic acidosis) usually have reduced arterial Pco_2 due to the stimulation of ventilation by low pH (Figure 5-37). The equilibrium $CO_2 + H_2O \leftrightarrow H_2CO_3 \leftrightarrow H^+ + HCO_3^-$ shifts to the left when the arterial Pco_2 is reduced, which reduces $[H^+]$ and moves pH back toward the normal range. Ventilation is affected only slightly by alkalemia. If ventilation were to be reduced to return pH to normal, it

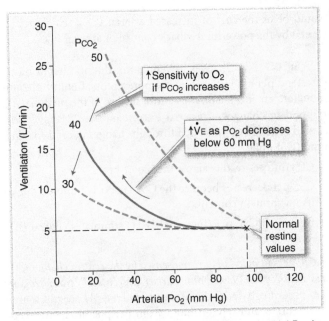

Figure 5-36: Regulation of ventilation by arterial Po_2. Arterial Po_2 less than 60 mm Hg causes a large increase in ventilation. High arterial Pco_2 has a synergistic effect with low arterial Po_2.

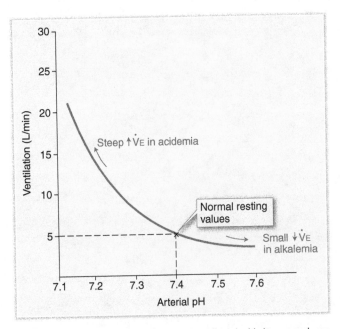

Figure 5-37: Regulation of ventilation by arterial pH. Increased ventilation due to acidemia reflects pulmonary compensation for metabolic acidosis. The response to alkalemia is weak because control of arterial Pco_2 prevents decreased ventilation.

would be at the cost of increased arterial P_{CO_2}, which is prevented by the powerful feedback control of arterial P_{CO_2}.

CHEMORECEPTORS Changes in ventilation due to altered blood gases and pH are initiated by chemoreceptors. **Central chemoreceptors** are located on the ventral surface of the medulla and respond to changes in arterial P_{CO_2}. Figure 5-38 shows how altered arterial P_{CO_2} is sensed through changes in cerebrospinal fluid (CSF) pH:

CO₂ diffuses readily across the blood-brain barrier.

CSF pH decreases because the CSF is poorly buffered due to its low protein content.

Decreased CSF pH (increased [H⁺]) stimulates central chemoreceptors.

Changes in blood pH are not sensed by the central chemoreceptors because the blood-brain barrier prevents H⁺ from crossing into the brain. Arterial P_{O_2} as well as arterial pH are not sensed by the brain and rely on input from peripheral chemoreceptors.

Peripheral chemoreceptors are located in the carotid bodies at the bifurcation of the common carotid arteries and in the aortic bodies in the aortic arch. Glomus cells within the carotid body are able to sense changes in O₂, H⁺, and CO₂, and relay signals to the central pattern generator via the glossopharyngeal and vagus nerves. *The control of ventilation by O_2 and pH is initiated in peripheral chemoreceptors. Control of ventilation by CO_2 is mainly through central chemoreceptors* (Figure 5-39).

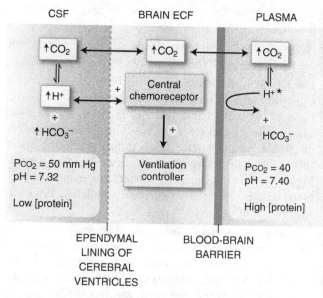

*No effect of plasma H⁺ on central receptor

Figure 5-38: Measurement of arterial CO₂ by central chemoreceptors. Central nervous system chemoreceptors sense [H⁺] in extracellular fluid (ECF) in the brain as an index of arterial P_{CO_2}. CO₂ diffuses readily across the blood-brain barrier. Levels of CO₂ in the brain reflect changes in arterial P_{CO_2} due to the high rate of blood flow in the brain. CO₂ is converted to H⁺ + HCO₃⁻ via carbonic anhydrase. The low buffering power of cerebrospinal fluid (CSF), due to low protein concentration, allows larger changes in [H⁺] in the CSF than occur in plasma. Central chemoreceptors are isolated from changes in blood [H⁺] by the blood-brain barrier.

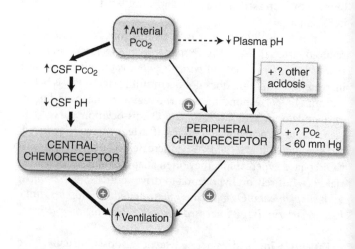

Figure 5-39: Integrated feedback control of ventilation by blood gases and pH. The CO₂ response of central chemoreceptors dominates control under normal circumstances. Central chemoreceptors are set to respond most strongly to an increase in arterial P_{CO_2}. Patients with metabolic acidosis or hypoxemia often have low arterial P_{CO_2} due to peripheral chemoreceptor activation. CSF, cerebrospinal fluid.

STUDY QUESTIONS

Directions: Each numbered item is followed by lettered options. Some options may be partially correct, but there is only ONE BEST answer.

1. A 50-year-old man with a persistent cough and difficulty breathing is referred by his family physician for pulmonary function tests. The test results show that the forced vital capacity (FVC), forced expired volume in 1 s (FEV_1), and functional residual capacity (FRC) are all significantly below normal. Which of the following diagnosis is consistent with these pulmonary function test results?

   A. Asthma

   B. Chronic bronchitis

   C. Emphysema

   D. Pulmonary fibrosis

2. A 19-year-old man is taken to the emergency department after being stabbed in the right side of the chest. The entry of air through the wound resulted in a pneumothorax on the right side of his chest. What difference between the right and left sides of the chest would be apparent on a plain chest x-ray?

   A. The lung volume on the right would be larger

   B. The position of the diaphragm on the right would be higher

   C. The thoracic volume on the right would be larger

   D. There would be no differences in thoracic geometry

3. A 28-year-old man is involved in a high speed motor vehicle accident in which he suffers multiple rib fractures. On arrival at the emergency department, he is conscious but in severe pain. His respiratory rate is 34 breaths/min, and his breathing is labored. His blood pressure is 110/95 mm Hg, and his pulse is 140 beats/min. His arterial Po_2 is 50 mm Hg, and he is unresponsive to supplemental O_2. His arterial Pco_2 is 28 mm Hg. What is the most likely cause of this patient's hypoxemia?

   A. Alveolar hypoventilation

   B. High ventilation/perfusion $(\dot{V}/\dot{Q})$ ratio

   C. Increased dead space ventilation

   D. Intrapulmonary shunt

   E. Low $\dot{V}/\dot{Q}$ ratio

4. A 16-year-old girl is found unconscious in the street. She has no visible injuries but is cold and is taking shallow breaths at a rate of 6–8 per minute. An arterial blood gas analysis recorded in the emergency department shows that her Po_2 is 55 mm Hg and her Pco_2 is 75 mm Hg. What is the most likely cause of hypoxemia in this patient?

   A. Alveolar hypoventilation

   B. High ventilation/perfusion $(\dot{V}/\dot{Q})$ ratio

   C. Increased dead space ventilation

   D. Intrapulmonary shunt

   E. Low $\dot{V}/\dot{Q}$ ratio

5. A 62-year-old man with a history of COPD is admitted to the hospital due to acute deterioration in lung function as a result of a viral chest infection. An arterial blood gases analysis shows that his Po_2 is 60 mm Hg and his Pco_2 is 70 mm Hg. His exhaled minute ventilation rate is two times higher than that of a normal individual of the same age and body size. He has hypercapnea, despite having an increased exhaled minute ventilation rate because his

   A. alveolar ventilation is increased

   B. dead space ventilation is increased

   C. V_T is increased

   D. ventilation/perfusion $(\dot{V}/\dot{Q})$ ratio is decreased

   E. intrapulmonary shunt is increased

6. A 40-year-old woman presented with dyspnea, hematuria, and right flank pain. CT scans revealed a renal tumor, with an extensive venous thrombus that had invaded the inferior vena cava. Fragments of the thrombus had entered the lungs and were blocking several major branches of the pulmonary arteries. Assuming that there was no change in V_T or respiratory rate, what effect would these pulmonary emboli have on arterial blood gases within the first few minutes of their occurrence?

   A. Decreased Pco_2 and decreased Po_2

   B. Decreased Pco_2 and increased Po_2

   C. Increased Pco_2 and decreased Po_2

   D. Increased Pco_2 and increased Po_2

   E. No change in Pco_2 or Po_2

7. A 9-year-old boy decided to find out for how long he could continue to breathe into and out of a paper bag. After approximately 2 minutes, his friends noticed that he was breathing very rapidly so they forced him to stop the experiment. What change in arterial blood gas composition was the most potent stimulus for this boy's hyperventilation?

   A. Decreased Pco_2

   B. Decreased Po_2

   C. Decreased pH

   D. Increased Pco_2

   E. Increased Po_2

   F. Increased pH

8. A 54-year-old woman with advanced emphysema due to many years of cigarette smoking is admitted to the hospital because of severe peripheral edema and shortness of breath. On physical examination, there is jugular venous distension and a widely split second heart sound with a loud pulmonic sound. A differential diagnosis of right heart failure and pulmonary hypertension is confirmed by cardiac catheterization. The results of her arterial blood gas analysis show $P_{O_2} = 55$ mm Hg, $P_{CO_2} = 75$ mm Hg, and pH = 7.30. What is the most likely cause of pulmonary hypertension in this patient?

A. Decreased alveolar P_{O_2}

B. Decreased lung compliance

C. Decreased parasympathetic neural tone

D. Increased alveolar P_{CO_2}

E. Increased thoracic volume

F. Increased sympathetic neural tone

9. A group of medical students is experimenting with a peak flow meter in the respiratory physiology laboratory. Two students decide to compete to see which of them can blow the hardest into the device. Which of the following muscles is most effective at producing a maximal expiratory effort such as this?

A. Diaphragm

B. External intercostal muscles

C. Internal intercostal muscles

D. Rectus abdominus

E. Sternocleidomastoid

10. A 22-year-old man was involved in a fight in which he received a severe blow to the head. On arrival at the emergency department, he was unconscious and initially received assisted ventilation via a manual bag-valve device. An analysis of his arterial blood gases shows:

$P_{O_2} = 45$ mm Hg

$P_{CO_2} = 80$ mm Hg

pH = 7.05

$HCO_3^- = 27$ mM

In what form was most CO_2 being transported in his arterial blood?

A. Bicarbonate ions

B. Carbaminohemoglobin compounds

C. Dissolved CO_2 molecules

ANSWERS

1—D. FVC and FEV_1 are expected to be reduced in all these conditions. The coexistence of low FRC indicates reduced resting lung volume and is consistent with the low static lung compliance found in patients with pulmonary fibrosis.

2—C. A pneumothorax interrupts the pleural fluid between the lung and chest wall, allowing each structure to assume its equilibrium position. Therefore, the lung collapses to a small volume and the chest wall expands; the diaphragm is part of the chest wall and also moves outward (i.e., flattens to a lower position compared to the unaffected side).

3—D. Severe O_2 refractory hypoxemia results from right-to-left intrapulmonary shunting of blood. This patient is hyperventilating, indicated by his low arterial PCO_2. A high respiratory rate results from pain and splinting as a result of rib fractures. A severe reduction in pulse pressure suggests low cardiac output. The source of intrapulmonary shunt in this case is a tension pneumothorax, with a collapsed lung that is perfused but not ventilated.

4—A. The patient is hypoventilating, causing CO_2 retention and hypercapnia. As a result, alveolar CO_2 is increased and O_2 is decreased.

5—B. The patient has a decreased alveolar ventilation rate, evidenced by the increased arterial PCO_2. Decreased alveolar ventilation in the presence of increased total exhaled minute ventilation can only be explained if dead space ventilation is increased.

6—C. Pulmonary emboli create areas of the lung that are ventilated but not perfused, thereby increasing dead space, reducing alveolar ventilation, and decreasing CO_2 excretion. Blood is forced to flow to other areas of the lung, some of which are not ventilated, creating a degree of intrapulmonary shunt, which decreases oxygenation.

7—D. Breathing into and out of a paper bag will result in accumulation of CO_2 and depletion of O_2 in the bag. The same changes will, therefore, be reflected in alveolar air and in arterial blood. Accumulation of CO_2 will also result in a decrease in the blood pH. However, in normal subjects, the most potent drive to breathe is the arterial PCO_2, acting through central chemoreceptors.

8—A Chronic pulmonary hypertension is caused by a sustained increase in pulmonary vascular resistance. In patients with alveolar hypoxia, active vasoconstriction increases the vascular resistance. High lung volume contributes to the increased vascular resistance to a lesser degree. Vascular resistance is at a minimum at the FRC. Patients with emphysema have an increased resting lung volume, which causes compression of pulmonary capillaries and therefore increases vascular resistance. Pulmonary vascular resistance is not significantly affected by autonomic nerves.

9—D. The abdominal muscles are the most powerful expiratory muscles; the internal intercostal muscles are weak expiratory muscles. The diaphragm is the primary inspiratory muscle, supported by the external intercostal muscles; the sternocleidomastoid is an accessory muscle of inspiration.

10—A. Even in the presence of elevated PCO_2 levels, bicarbonate ions convey the majority (approximately 90%) of the CO_2 in blood.

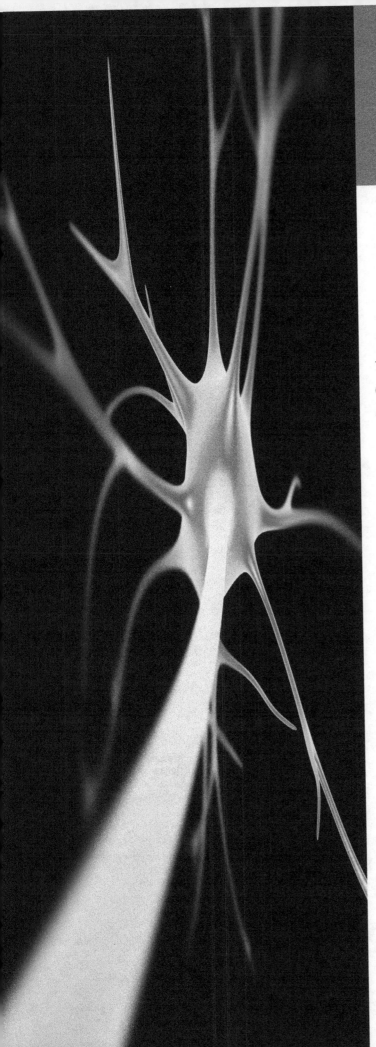

CHAPTER 6

RENAL PHYSIOLOGY AND ACID-BASE BALANCE

THE RENAL SYSTEM

OVERVIEW

The kidney is a homeostatic organ that varies the excretion of water, electrolytes, and other hydrophilic molecules to maintain constancy of the composition of the extracellular fluid (ECF). This organ plays the most important role in the long-term regulation of blood pressure through its control of ECF volume. The kidney is also the major effector that varies excretion of metabolic acids and many electrolytes, including K^+, Ca^{2+}, and Mg^{2+}.

ANATOMY OF THE KIDNEY

The paired kidneys are bean-shaped retroperitoneal organs, each about 12-cm long and located on the posterior abdominal wall. Figure 6-1 shows the structures that pass through the **renal hilus,** including the renal artery, the renal vein, and the renal pelvis (the renal nerves and lymphatic vessels are associated with the renal blood vessels). The cut surface of the kidney has a pale outer region, the **cortex,** and a darker inner region, the **medulla.** The medulla is further divided into several conical areas called renal pyramids. The apex of each pyramid tapers toward the renal pelvis, forming the **renal papillae.** The renal pelvis has a funnel-shaped upper end and is continuous with the ureter below it, which conveys urine to the bladder.

▽ **Renal colic** is pain in the flank that radiates toward the groin. Colicky pain is pain that comes and goes and is often accompanied by nausea, vomiting, diaphoresis, and hematuria. Renal colic occurs with sudden acute onset and is often severely painful. The most common cause of renal colic is **renal calculi** ("kidney stones"), which make their way from the renal pelvis down the ureter to the bladder. The three common **sites of obstruction** leading to the clinical presentation of renal colic are:

1. At the junction of the renal pelvis and ureter.

2. At the site where the ureter passes over the pelvic brim.

3. At the uterovesicular junction. ▽

Papillary necrosis is another condition that can result in renal colic. Necrosis of the renal papillae is associated with the use of analgesics (e.g., nonsteroidal anti-inflammatory drugs). The necrotic papillae can slough off, resulting in obstruction and symptoms of renal colic.

STRUCTURE OF THE NEPHRON

The functional unit of the kidney is a nephron, a tube that consists of different transporting epithelia in sequence. Each kidney has between 500,000 and 800,000 nephrons. A nephron has several functionally and histologically distinct segments (Figure 6-2). The **glomerulus** is the site of primary urine formation where blood plasma is filtered into the nephron. The glomerular capillaries are enveloped by the blind-ended upper part of the nephron, known as Bowman's capsule. Filtrate flows from Bowman's space into the **proximal tubule,** which consists of convoluted and straight portions. The proximal tubule is continuous with the **loop of Henle,** which is a U-shaped tubule that descends variable distances into the medulla before turning back toward the cortex. The loop of Henle has three functionally distinct parts: the thin descending limb, the thin ascending limb, and the thick ascending limb. The **macula densa** is a short segment that passes close to the glomerulus and connects the thick ascending limb to the **distal tubule** in the cortex. Distal tubules from approximately six nephrons converge with a single **collecting duct.** As the collecting ducts descend through the renal medulla, toward the papilla, they converge to form the larger ducts of Bellini, which deliver final urine into the **renal calyces.** Urine proceeds to the **renal pelvis** and then to the lower urinary tract.

TYPES OF NEPHRONS There are two types of nephrons: about 85% are **cortical nephrons** and 15% are **juxtamedullary nephrons** (Figure 6-3). The glomeruli of cortical nephrons are located in

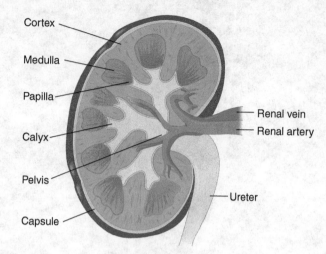

Figure 6-1: Gross anatomy of the kidney.

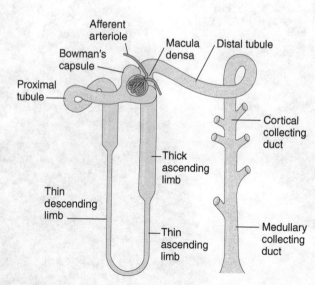

Figure 6-2: The nephron.

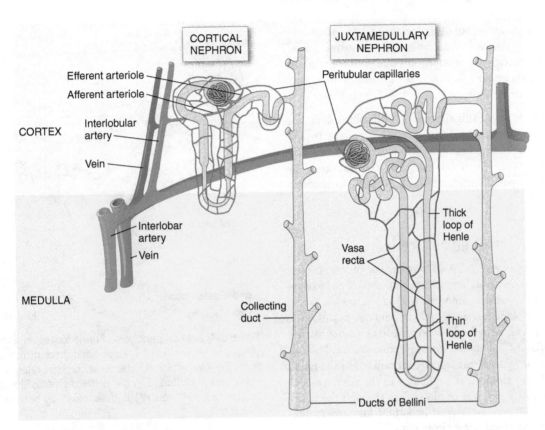

Figure 6-3: The cortical and juxtamedullary nephrons.

the outer cortex and the loops of Henle are short. In contrast, the juxtamedullary nephrons have glomeruli located deep in the cortex and the loops of Henle are long, with many extending all the way to the tip of the renal papilla. *The juxtamedullary nephrons are important for urine concentration.* They also reabsorb a higher proportion of glomerular filtrate than cortical nephrons and are said to be "salt-conserving." In states where effective circulating blood volume is reduced, a higher proportion of **renal blood flow (RBF)** is directed to the juxtamedullary nephrons, helping to conserve extracellular fluid volume.

GENERAL PRINCIPLES OF URINE FORMATION

Urine formation begins with glomerular filtration of plasma at a rate of about 150–200 L daily. The **glomerular filtration rate (GFR)** is a **controlled variable** and in most circumstances is fairly constant (see Chapter 1). **Renal insufficiency** occurs when GFR is low, however. A progressive decline in GFR indicates the **stages of chronic kidney disease** as mild (60–89 mL/min/1.73m^2), moderate (30–59 mL/min/1.73m^2), and severe (15–29 mL/min/1.73m^2).

Glomerular filtrate is modified by epithelial transport as it flows along the nephron. For water and many solutes, 98–99% of the filtrate is reabsorbed back into the blood during passage along the renal tubules. A variation of excretion rates in final urine usually reflects changes in renal tubular reabsorption. The rate of reabsorption for most substances is highest in the proximal tubule and is reduced as the flow becomes more distal. Fine control of excretion usually occurs in the distal parts of the renal tubule, which receive a fairly constant fraction of the filtrate (about 10%). The model of filtration–reabsorption applies to most substances. For others, such as K^+, H^+, and some organic molecules, the rate of secretion into the urine across the nephron epithelia is more important than reabsorption in determining the excretion rate. Figure 6-4 illustrates these general principles of urine formation.

▽   **Penicillin** is an antibiotic that is both filtered at the glomerulus and secreted into the tubular urine by the proximal tubule. The secretion of penicillin can be inhibited by the drug **probenecid,** which can be given concomitantly to reduce the rate of penicillin excretion and thereby to increase serum penicillin levels. ▼

RENAL BLOOD FLOW

The kidneys normally receive 20–25% of cardiac output; a very high rate of RBF is needed to supply enough plasma for glomerular filtration. RBF is usually autoregulated across a wide range of mean arterial blood pressures, which helps to maintain a stable GFR. RBF can be reduced by sympathetic vasoconstriction if extracellular fluid volume must be conserved. All blood entering the kidney passes through larger branches of the renal artery to reach the glomerular capillaries in the renal cortex. Figure 6-4 shows the pathway of blood flow through the renal microvasculature. There are several **important features in the organization of the renal microcirculation:**

1. The **glomerular capillary bed** is supplied by an afferent arteriole and drained via an efferent arteriole rather than by a venule. A resistance vessel at each end of the glomerular capillary maintains the large capillary blood pressure that drives filtration.

2. The **peritubular capillary bed** surrounding the nephrons receives reabsorbed water and solutes; it is supplied from the efferent arterioles and is in series with the glomerular capillaries. Filtration of protein-free fluid from the glomerular capillaries increases the osmolarity of blood entering the peritubular capillaries. This provides a driving force to assist in water reabsorption into the peritubular capillaries from the nephron.

3. Some of the peritubular capillaries give off long capillary loops called **vasa recta,** which travel with the loops of Henle and are involved in the urine-concentrating mechanism. Less than 10% of RBF follows a course through the vasa recta to the renal medulla and only about 1% reaches the renal papilla. *Low blood flow in the renal medulla helps to preserve the medullary hypertonicity necessary for the concentration of urine but causes it to be susceptible to ischemia in the setting of hypotension or renal vasoconstriction.*

Renal perfusion is achieved with a typical systemic arterial perfusion pressure of about 90–100 mm Hg. High rates of RBF are possible because renal vascular resistance is low. Figure 6-5 shows sites of pressure decreases between the renal artery and vein. The large pressure decreases across the afferent and efferent arterioles demonstrate that vascular resistance is shared somewhat equally between the arterioles. There is very little pressure decrease in the glomerular capillaries, facilitating glomerular filtration.

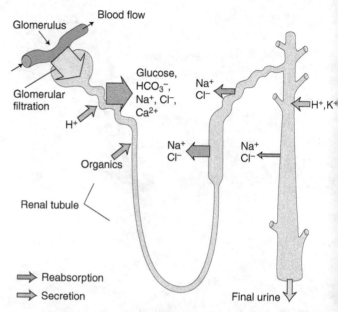

Figure 6-4: General principles of urine formation. Excretion of most solutes is determined by varying the amount that is reabsorbed from the glomerular filtrate. Reabsorption rates are high proximally and finely tuned in the distal segments. Excretion of some solutes (e.g., H^+ and K^+) is determined by secretion rather than reabsorption.

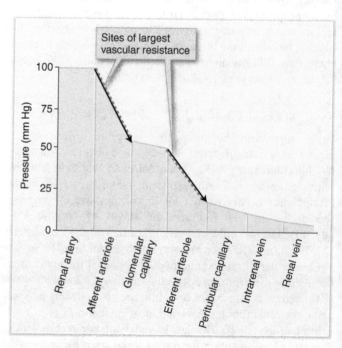

Figure 6-5: Vascular resistance is shared between the afferent and efferent arterioles. Glomerular capillary pressure is higher than in other systemic vascular beds due to the presence of an efferent arteriole at the glomerular outlet. Greater capillary pressure facilitates glomerular filtration.

The normally high rates of renal perfusion provide a large excess of O_2 for tissue metabolism. However, the kidney is readily injured in states of shock, where RBF decreases because renal tissue has a high rate of O_2 use. *Persistently low renal perfusion may result in* **acute renal failure (ARF).**

▽ The terms ARF versus chronic renal failure merely describe a different time course.

▪ **ARF** is defined as a decrease in GFR that occurs over hours to days.

▪ **Chronic renal failure** is present if GFR remains impaired for more than 3 months.

ARF is often asymptomatic and completely reversible and incorporates a vast array of conditions and diseases. For diagnostic and management purposes, **ARF is organized into the following three categories:**

1. **Prerenal ARF** is most common and is caused by any condition that results in renal hypoperfusion without impairing the renal parenchyma (e.g., hypovolemia).

2. **Renal ARF** describes diseases that directly result in damage to the renal parenchyma (e.g., glomerular nephritis).

3. **Postrenal ARF** occurs in diseases that cause obstruction of the urinary tract (e.g., tumors or benign prostatic hyperplasia).

(Note: severe prerenal ARF can progress to renal ARF if hypoperfusion is severe enough to cause ischemic injury to the renal parenchyma. This results in **acute tubular necrosis,** *which is the most common cause of renal ARF.)* ▽

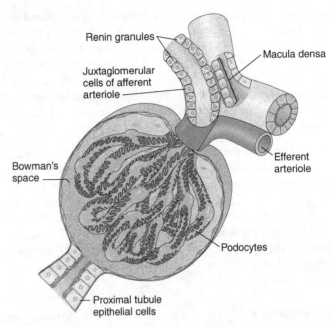

Figure 6-6: Juxtaglomerular apparatus. The juxtaglomerular apparatus comprises the granular renin-secreting cells in the wall of the afferent arteriole plus the macula densa segment of the nephron. Paracrine signaling from the macula densa to the afferent arteriole influences glomerular filtration and renin secretion.

ENDOCRINE FUNCTIONS OF THE KIDNEY

The kidney is a target organ for several hormones, including antidiuretic hormone (ADH), angiotensin II, aldosterone, atrial natriuretic peptide (ANP), and parathyroid hormone (PTH). The kidney is also an endocrine organ that secretes renin, erythropoietin (EPO), and the active form of vitamin D_3, 1,25-dihydroxycholecalciferol (1,25-$(OH)_2$ vitamin D).

RENIN SECRETION Renin is an enzyme released by the **juxtaglomerular apparatus** of the kidney in response to a decrease in effective circulating blood volume. Figure 6-6 shows the juxtaglomerular apparatus, which is formed from the close association between the vascular and tubular structures where the distal nephron comes in contact with its own glomerulus. Renin is released from the juxtaglomerular cells lining the afferent arterioles, which respond to reduced renal perfusion, and initiates a cascade of events that result in the production of the hormones angiotensin II and aldosterone (see Chapter 8). *The* **renin-angiotensin-aldosterone system** *is the most important endocrine axis in control of the extracellular fluid volume.* A second key regulatory function of the juxtaglomerular apparatus is the feedback regulation of GFR resulting from interaction between the macula densa and the afferent arteriole (see Tubuloglomerular Feedback).

EPO SECRETION EPO is a glycoprotein hormone produced by fibroblasts in the renal interstitium. Local PO_2 in renal tissue is used as an indicator of the systemic arterial O_2 content. *EPO* *is released in response to low renal interstitial P_{O_2}.* It stimulates red blood cell formation in the bone marrow to restore the O_2-carrying capacity of blood (Figure 6-7). About 80% of plasma EPO is produced in the kidney and the remainder is secreted by the liver. The mechanism coupling low P_{O_2} to EPO secretion involves increased local production of **prostaglandins.** *Patients with renal failure do not secrete sufficient amounts of EPO and, therefore, they usually develop anemia.*

▽ Clinically, the main uses of EPO are related to treating **anemia** associated with chronic renal failure or to cancer chemotherapy. However, EPO has also gained notoriety in the lay press as a "**blood-doping**" agent that is used illegally by endurance athletes. In healthy individuals, injection of EPO will lead to supraphysiologic levels of red blood cells (increased hematocrit) and consequently an increase in O_2-carrying capacity, a result that boosts aerobic output in athletes during competition. ▽

ACTIVATION OF VITAMIN D Vitamin D is a steroid derived from precursors that are either ingested or produced by the action of ultraviolet light on the skin. The active form of vitamin D is 1,25-dihydroxycholecalciferol (1,25-(OH)$_2$ vitamin D). *The liver produces 25-hydroxycholecalciferol (25-OH vitamin D), which is converted to 1,25-(OH)$_2$ vitamin D in the kidney under the control of parathyroid hormone.* Vitamin D$_3$ promotes Ca^{2+} conservation in the body by increasing intestinal Ca^{2+} absorption and also by reducing urinary Ca^{2+} loss (Figure 6-8).

▽ Manifestations of chronic renal failure plague many of the body's systems, including bone. **Osteitis fibrosa cystica (renal osteodystrophy)** is the classic bone disease related to chronic renal failure. The **pathophysiologic cascade begins in the kidneys and ends in the bones:**

1. As the kidneys fail, so does the function of **1α-hydroxylase,** the enzyme that converts inactive 25-OH vitamin D to active 1,25-OH vitamin D, resulting in vitamin D deficiency.

2. **Vitamin D deficiency** results in low serum Ca^{2+} due to impaired dietary absorption.

3. Low serum Ca^{2+} stimulates the parathyroid glands to increase PTH production (**secondary hyperparathyroidism**) (see Chapter 8).

4. PTH acts on bone to cause a **high rate of bone turnover,** which releases Ca^{2+} back into the serum.

The end result of this cascade is that near normal plasma Ca^{2+} concentration is maintained at the expense of chronic bone resorption resulting from hyperparathyroidism. *Osteitis fibrosa cystica is a condition characterized by fibrous replacement of the marrow and cystic trabecular bone, which renders the bones fragile and, therefore, increases the risk of fracture.* ▼

GLOMERULAR FILTRATION

A large GFR provides the potential to excrete multiple solutes that may be present at low concentrations in plasma. *The glomerular filter should not allow passage of blood cells or plasma*

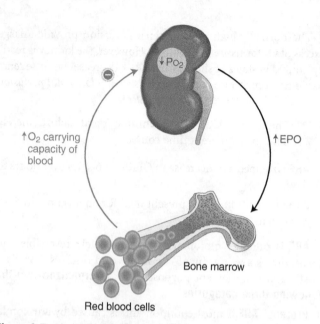

Figure 6-7: Negative feedback regulation of blood-O_2 content via erythropoietin (EPO) secretion.

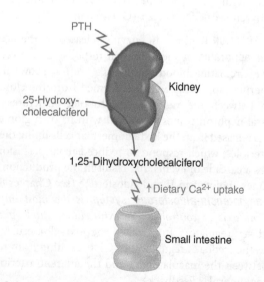

Figure 6-8: Renal activation of vitamin D. Parathyroid hormone (PTH) activates the mitochondrial enzyme 1α-hydroxylase in the proximal tubule to produce activated vitamin D$_3$ (1,25-dihydroxycholecalciferol).

proteins. **Starling's forces** are responsible for the net filtration pressure across the glomerular capillaries. GFR is generally stable due to autoregulation but can be varied by active changes in afferent and efferent arteriolar tone.

▽ The term **glomerulonephritis** is used to denote glomerular injury. In virtually all cases, GFR is impaired and protein or blood cells can be seen in the urine. Diseases that affect the glomeruli can be classified according to the syndrome of symptoms produced.

■ **Nephrotic syndrome** is characterized by severe proteinuria (>3.5 g/d), hypoalbuminemia (<3 g/L), generalized edema, and hyperlipidemia.

■ **Nephritic syndrome** is characterized by hematuria, hypertension, oliguria (<400 mL/d urine output), and azotemia (increased blood urea nitrogen [BUN] and plasma creatinine concentration). ▽

GLOMERULAR FILTRATION BARRIER

Molecular size and electric charge are two determinants of solute **filterability.** Substances with a molecular weight of about 10 kDa are freely filtered; as molecular weight increases from 10 kDa to 70 kDa, there is a roughly linear decline in the amount of solute filtered (Figure 6-9A). **Albumin,** with a molecular weight of 70 kDa, is almost small enough to be filtered. *It is essential that albumin is not lost in the urine because the plasma albumin concentration is the largest contributor to plasma oncotic pressure.* The electrical charge on a macromolecule also determines its filterability (see Figure 6-9B). There is less filtration of negatively charged macromolecules compared to neutral molecules of the same size. At a physiologic extracellular fluid pH of 7.4, proteins carry net negative charges, which reduce their filtration.

The **three anatomic structures that a solute passes through during filtration** are described as follows (Figure 6-10):

1. The **glomerular capillary endothelial cell layer.** The large fenestrations between glomerular capillary endothelial cells only exclude blood cells.

2. The **glomerular basement membrane** consists of a fiber meshwork and offers significant resistance to the sieving of macromolecules.

3. **Podocytes** are a layer of specialized epithelial cells that coat the glomerular capillaries. Podocytes bear finger-like projections that interlock around the glomerular capillaries. Narrow filtration that slits between these projections are bridged by a membrane protein called **nephrin,** which also contributes significantly to the filtration barrier.

Fixed negative charges are present in the basement membrane and the filtration slits, and account for electrical repulsion of negatively charged macromolecules by the filtration barrier.

▽ **Loss of nephrin,** such as occurs in **minimal change disease,** allows for selective loss of albumin resulting in a nephrotic syndrome. Minimal change disease (or nil disease) is most common in children. The name is derived from the lack

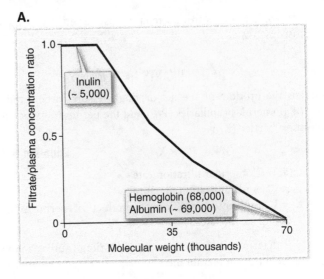

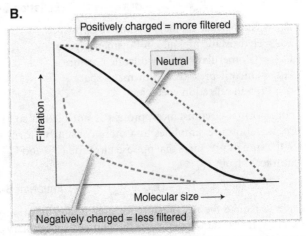

Figure 6-9: Properties of the glomerular filtration barrier. **A.** Effect of molecular size on the glomerular filtration of macromolecules: hemoglobin and albumin are just large enough to avoid filtration at normal glomeruli on the basis of their size. **B.** Effect of electrical charge on glomerular filtration of macromolecules: filtration of negatively charged macromolecules (but not small anions) is reduced.

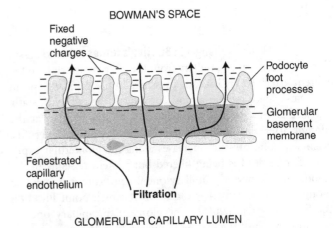

Figure 6-10: The glomerular filtration membrane. Filtered water and solutes must pass through the glomerular capillary endothelium, the glomerular basement membrane, and through the filtration slits between podocytes.

of pathologic findings from a renal biopsy examined by light microscopy. ▼

DETERMINANTS OF GFR

GFR is the product of the net driving pressure forcing fluid out of glomerular capillaries (P_{UF}) and the permeability of the filtration barrier (K_f):

$$GFR = P_{UF} \times K_f \qquad \text{Equation 6-1}$$

GFR = Glomerular filtration rate

P_{UF} = Net ultrafiltration pressure

K_f = Ultrafiltration coefficient (product of permeability and surface area)

P_{UF} is determined by the balance of Starling's forces acting across the filtration membrane:

$$P_{UF} = (P_{GC} - P_{BS}) - \sigma(\pi_{GC} - \pi_{BS}) \qquad \text{Equation 6-2}$$

P_{GC} = Glomerular capillary hydrostatic pressure

P_{BS} = Hydrostatic pressure in Bowman's space

Π_{GC} = Glomerular capillary oncotic pressure

Π_{BS} = Oncotic pressure in Bowman's space

σ = Protein reflection coefficient

Under normal circumstances, protein is not filtered so Π_{BS} is zero. Equation 6-2 simplifies to a more convenient form in which the sum of pressures that oppose filtration (P_{BS} and Π_{GC}) are subtracted from P_{GC}:

$$P_{UF} = P_{GC} - (\pi_{GC} + P_{BS}) \qquad \text{Equation 6-3}$$

Example Calculate the net pressure for glomerular filtration if the average hydrostatic pressure in the glomerular capillary is 58 mm Hg, the oncotic pressure in the glomerular capillary is 32 mm Hg, and the hydrostatic pressure in Bowman's space is 10 mm Hg.

The net ultrafiltration pressure is:

$$P_{UF} = P_{GC} - (\pi_{GC} + P_{BS})$$

In this example, P_{GC} = 58 mm Hg, π_{GC} = 32 mm Hg, and P_{BS} = 10 mm Hg:

$$P_{UF} = 58 - (32 + 10)$$
$$= 14 \text{ mm Hg}$$

Figure 6-11 shows changes in **Starling's forces** as blood passes along the glomerular capillary from the afferent arteriole to the efferent arteriole. Hydrostatic pressures in the capillary and in Bowman's space remain almost constant, although hydrostatic pressure at the afferent arteriole must be higher than at the efferent arteriole for blood to flow through the glomerulus. Plasma oncotic pressure increases along the glomerular capillary because fluid is being filtered but protein remains in the blood. The glomerular capillary oncotic pressure may increase enough to prevent further filtration, at which point **filtration equilibrium** is reached. Plotting glomerular capillary oncotic pressure on top of the hydrostatic pressure in Bowman's space, as shown in Figure 6-11, yields a curve describing the sum of forces that oppose filtration; the yellow area indicates net ultrafiltration pressure.

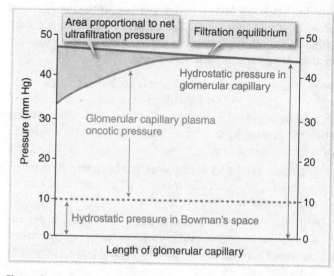

Figure 6-11: Starling's forces in glomerular filtration. The π_{GC} rises along the glomerular capillary due to filtration of protein-free fluid. Filtration stops if the sum of π_{GC} and P_{BS} increases to equal P_{GC} (filtration equilibrium).

AFFERENT AND EFFERENT ARTERIOLAR RESISTANCE

Changes in the afferent or efferent arteriolar tone alter both vascular resistance and the glomerular capillary hydrostatic pressure, resulting in changes in renal blood flow and glomerular filtration. Constriction of either arteriole increases vascular resistance and reduces RBF. Afferent arteriolar constriction also reduces GFR because blood flow into the glomerular capillary decreases, reducing the capillary hydrostatic pressure. In contrast, efferent arteriolar constriction increases outflow resistance from the glomerular capillary, increasing the capillary hydrostatic pressure and GFR. The **filtration fraction** is the proportion of RBF that is filtered and is **normally about 20%.** *Constriction of the afferent arteriole reduces both the RBF and the GFR, leaving the filtration fraction unchanged. Efferent arteriole constriction reduces RBF but conserves GFR, causing an increase in the filtration fraction.*

Changes in the filtration fraction affect the Starling's forces in the peritubular capillary network, which is immediately downstream of the glomerulus. Changes in these physical forces within the peritubular capillaries in turn influence fluid reabsorption from the nephron. This is called **glomerulotubular balance.** In the case of efferent arteriolar constriction, the filtration fraction increases, causing an increase in the peritubular capillary oncotic pressure and a decrease in the peritubular capillary hydrostatic pressure. This causes more fluid to be reabsorbed from the proximal nephron, which prevents a significant change in fluid delivery to the distal nephron. Selective changes in efferent arteriole tone, therefore, have minimal effect on excretion. In contrast, afferent arteriolar constriction does not change the filtration fraction; therefore, a decrease in GFR translates into reduced fluid delivery to the later portions of the renal tubule. Table 6-1 summarizes the changes to RBF, GFR, and the filtration fraction, which result from an altered arteriolar tone. **Norepinephrine,** a neurotransmitter released by the sympathetic nerves, preferentially **constricts the afferent arteriole** and reduces RBF, GFR, and Na^+ excretion. The hormone **angiotensin II** preferentially **constricts the efferent arteriole,** which reduces RBF but maintains GFR.

TABLE 6-1. Effects of Changes in Afferent and Efferent Arteriolar Tone

Stimulus	RBF	P_{GC}	GFR	FF	End-proximal Fluid Delivery
Afferent arteriole constriction (e.g., norepinephrine, NSAIDs)	↓	↓	↓	↔	↓
Efferent arteriole constriction (e.g., angiotensin II)	↓	↑	↑	↑	↔
Afferent arteriole dilation (e.g., prostaglandins)	↑	↑	↑	↔	↑
Efferent arteriole dilation (e.g., ACE inhibitors)	↑	↓	↓	↓	↔

RBF, renal blood flow; P_{GC}, glomerular capillary hydrostatic pressure; GFR, glomerular filtration rate; FF, filtration fraction; NSAID, nonsteroidal anti-inflammatory drug; ACE, angiotensin-converting enzyme.

▼ **Renal insufficiency** can be caused by commonly used drugs that interfere with renal vascular resistance; for example:

■ **Nonsteroidal anti-inflammatory drugs** (NSAIDs) such as ibuprofen inhibit **prostaglandins,** which are the primary endogenous vasodilators of the afferent arteriole. *Reduced local prostaglandin levels cause vasoconstriction of the afferent arteriole and a decrease in GFR.*

■ **Angiotensin-converting enzyme (ACE) inhibitors** or *angiotensin II receptor blockers may cause a decrease in GFR due to vasodilation of the efferent arteriole.* ▼

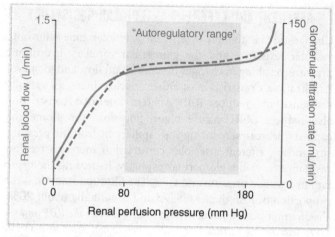

Figure 6-12: Autoregulation of renal blood flow (RBF) and the glomerular filtration rate (GFR).

AUTOREGULATION OF RBF AND GFR

RBF and GFR are autoregulated across a wide range of arterial blood pressures (Figure 6-12) (see Chapter 4). Renal vascular resistance varies in direct proportion to renal arterial pressure so that RBF remains almost constant. Control of afferent arteriolar resistance is the basis of autoregulation and occurs by a **myogenic mechanism.** If blood flow increases, the wall of the afferent arteriole distends. Stretching vascular smooth muscle causes it to contract, which increases vascular resistance and normalizes blood flow.

The myogenic mechanism is assisted by **tubuloglomerular feedback.** In every nephron, the macula densa senses changes in GFR by measuring the tubular fluid flow rate. If the tubular fluid flow rate increases, the macula densa signals to the afferent arteriole to contract, thereby reducing GFR and normalizing flow past the macula densa (Figure 6-13). The paracrine signaling molecule that passes from the macula densa to the afferent arteriole is thought to be **adenosine** or **adenosine triphosphate (ATP).** *The autoregulation mechanism can be overridden by sympathetic vasoconstriction to reduce RBF and GFR;* for example, a **hemorrhage** that is severe enough to reduce the mean arterial blood pressure and to activate the sympathetic nervous system via the baroreceptor reflex (see Chapter 4).

CLEARANCE

Clearance is defined as the volume of plasma rendered free of a given substance in 1 minute. Clearance is calculated as the ratio of urinary excretion rate to plasma concentration:

$$C_x = (U_x \times \dot{V}) \div P_x \qquad \textbf{Equation 6-4}$$

C_x = Renal clearance of solute x
U_x = Urine concentration of solute x
$\dot{V}$ = Urine flow rate
P_x = Plasma concentration of solute x

Example If the *plasma* [urea] is 0.25 mg/mL, the *urinary* [urea] is 10 mg/mL, and the urine flow rate is 1 mL/min, calculate the excretion rate and the clearance of urea.

$$\begin{aligned} Excretion &= U_{urea} \times \dot{V} \\ &= 10\ mg/mL \times 1\ mL/min \\ &= 10\ mg/min \end{aligned}$$

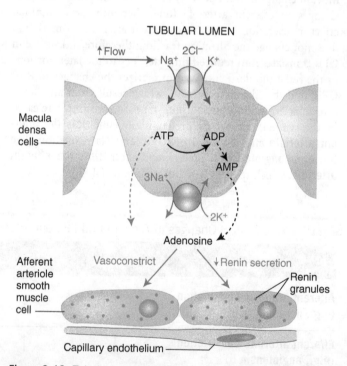

Figure 6-13: Tubuloglomerular feedback mechanism. The macula densa senses the glomerular filtration rate (GFR) through changes in fluid delivery to the distal nephron. Paracrine release of adenosine and adenosine triphosphate (ATP) by the macula densa is metabolically coupled to NaCl uptake. At the single nephron level, tubuloglomerular feedback (TGF) autoregulates GFR; global changes in GFR reflect altered circulating volume and are linked to changes in renin secretion. ADP, adenosine diphosphate; AMP, adenosine monophosphate.

$$Clearance = 10 \text{ mg/min} \div 0.25 \text{ mg/mL}$$
$$= 40 \text{ mL/min}$$

Clearance is a volume of plasma "cleaned" per unit time (mL/min), not the amount of solute excreted in urine per unit time (mg/min). A clearance of 40 mL/min means that 40 mL of plasma is required to supply the urea lost in urine every minute. Although renal clearance can be calculated for any solute, the method is often applied to specific marker molecules as a means of estimating the RBF and GFR.

USING CLEARANCE TO ESTIMATE GFR

Inulin clearance can be used to estimate GFR. Inulin is a low-molecular-weight polysaccharide that is small enough to pass freely through the glomerular filtration barrier. Inulin is neither reabsorbed nor secreted by the nephron and cannot be metabolized. As shown in Figure 6-14, the rate of inulin filtration equals the rate of inulin excretion in urine so the volume of plasma cleared per minute equals GFR. Inulin usually is not used clinically because it must be intravenously infused.

Creatinine is a product of muscle metabolism and is a suitable endogenous alternative to inulin. The rate of creatinine production in the body is quite constant because it is a function of muscle mass. Creatinine clearance overestimates GFR by about 10% because, in addition to free filtration, there is some secretion into the proximal tubule. Plasma [creatinine] is determined by the balance between the production rate and the excretion rate. *Because the creatinine production rate is constant, and the excretion rate varies with GFR, plasma [creatinine] is a direct index of GFR. When GFR is low, plasma [creatinine] is increased.*

▼ *Calculation of GFR defines the stages of renal failure. A knowledge of GFR is vital in determining the proper dosage of drugs that are excreted via the kidney, because the half-life of a drug can be significantly increased in the setting of renal failure. Creatinine clearance can be estimated clinically using the* **Cockcroft-Gault equation:**

$$C_{CR} = \frac{(140 - age) \times (W)}{(P_{CR}) \times (72)} (\times\, 0.85 \text{ for women})$$ **Equation 6-5**

C_{CR} = Creatinine clearance (mL/min)
W = Body weight (kg)
P_{CR} = Plasma [creatinine] (mg/dL) ▼

USING CLEARANCE TO ESTIMATE RBF

The principle of clearance can also be used to estimate the **renal plasma flow (RPF) rate** using the marker **para-aminohippuric acid (PAH)**, which is a derivative of glycine. *PAH clearance provides an estimate of the renal plasma flow rate because all of the PAH entering the renal artery is excreted into the urine in a single pass through the kidney.* Therefore, the volume of plasma cleared of PAH is the total volume of plasma passing through the kidney per minute. Figure 6-15 illustrates renal PAH handling; at low plasma concentrations, all of the PAH that escapes filtration and enters the peritubular capillaries is secreted by organic anion transporters in the proximal tubule. The term

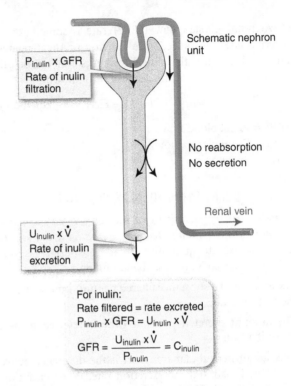

Figure 6-14: Use of inulin clearance to measure the glomerular filtration rate (GFR).

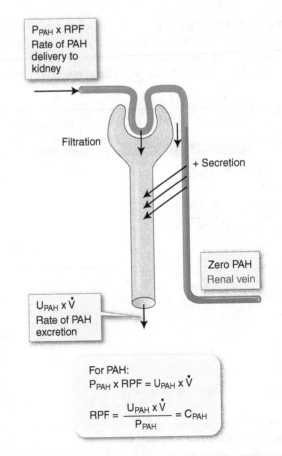

Figure 6-15: Using para-aminohippuric acid (PAH) clearance to measure the renal plasma flow (RPF).

effective renal plasma flow (ERPF) rate is sometimes used to describe PAH clearance, since the measurement relates to plasma flowing to functional nephron units. **RBF** can be calculated from the RPF rate if the hematocrit is known:

$$RBF = RPF \div (1 - Hct) \qquad \textbf{Equation 6-6}$$

RBF = Renal blood flow
RPF = Renal plasma flow
Hct = Hematocrit

QUANTIFYING TUBULAR FUNCTION

The rate of urinary excretion of a substance can be affected by glomerular filtration, tubular reabsorption, and tubular secretion. Calculations used to quantify tubular transport are summarized in Table 6-2 and are described as follows:

- The amount of a substance filtered per unit time is known as the **filtered load.**

- The amount excreted per unit time is referred to as the **excretion rate.**

- The rate of net tubular transport is the difference between the filtered load and the excretion rate. When excretion is less than the filtered load, there is net tubular **reabsorption.** When the excretion rate is more than the filtered load, there is net tubular **secretion.** Solutes with net reabsorption have clearance values less than GFR (i.e., less than creatinine clearance). If there is net tubular secretion, solute clearance is greater than GFR.

- **Fractional excretion (FE)** expresses solute excretion as a percentage of its filtered load. FE is useful because changes reflect altered tubular transport rather than simply changes in GFR. FE is also known as the **clearance ratio** because it

TABLE 6-2. Formulae Used to Quantify Renal Tubular Function

Quantity	Expression	Calculation	Abbreviations
Filtered load (of solute z)	FL_z	$FL_z = GFR \times P_z$	GFR = glomerular filtration rate; P_z = plasma concentration of solute z
Excretion rate (of solute z)	E_z	$E_z = \dot{V} \times U_z$	$\dot{V}$ = urine flow rate; U_z = urine concentration of solute z
Fractional excretion (clearance ratio)	FE_z	$FE_z = \dfrac{(\dot{V} \times U_z)}{(GFR \times P_z)} \times 100$ OR $FE_z = \dfrac{C_z}{C_{creatinine}} \times 100$ OR $^*FE_z = \dfrac{(U_z \times P_{creatinine})}{(U_{creatinine} \times P_z)} \times 100$	C = clearance
Fractional reabsorption	FR_z	$FR_z = 100 \times FE_z$	

* This form of the fractional excretion equation is often used clinically because it applies values readily measured in the laboratory.

can be calculated as the ratio of solute clearance to creatinine clearance.

▼ Calculating the **fractional sodium excretion (FE$_{Na}$)** can be useful in the setting of **acute renal failure (ARF)** to help determine if ARF is due to prerenal (hypovolemia) versus renal (acute tubular necrosis) pathology. In the prerenal state, the FE$_{Na}$ will be low (<1%) as the renal tubules attempt to maintain intravascular volume by maximally reabsorbing Na$^+$ (and water). If ARF is caused by an intrinsic renal process (most commonly acute tubular necrosis), then FE$_{Na}$ will be large (>2%) due to the reduced ability of the damaged renal tubules to reabsorb Na$^+$. *(Note: diuretics interfere with tubular Na$^+$ reabsorption and, therefore, impair the ability to interpret FE$_{Na}$. In this setting, FE$_{urea}$ can be used.)* ▼

RELATIONSHIPS BETWEEN CLEARANCE AND PLASMA CONCENTRATION

The clearance of a solute may change as a function of plasma concentration if a **saturable transport process** is involved in its renal handling. Because there are no tubular transport processes for inulin, the filtered load and the excretion rate of inulin increase in parallel with plasma concentration. Clearance is the ratio of excretion rate to plasma concentration; therefore, *inulin clearance remains constant at all plasma inulin concentrations*. By contrast, PAH clearance decreases with increasing plasma PAH concentration (Figure 6-16). At low plasma PAH concentrations, all PAH is excreted and the PAH clearance represents the RPF rate. As the plasma PAH concentration increases, the tubular secretion mechanism becomes saturated and some PAH remains in the plasma. PAH clearance decreases because not all plasma is now being cleared of PAH. PAH clearance never decreases below GFR because there are no tubular reabsorption mechanisms for PAH.

Tubular glucose transport can be saturated. At normal plasma glucose concentrations, glucose normally is not found in the urine because the filtered glucose load is completely reabsorbed. If the plasma glucose concentration increases (e.g., as occurs in patients with **diabetes mellitus**), the filtered load of glucose increases and the reabsorption mechanism may be saturated. This explains why *glucose is excreted in the urine of diabetic patients when there is poor glycemic control*. The glucose clearance can never exceed the inulin clearance because there is no secretion mechanism for glucose.

RENAL TITRATION CURVES

Renal titration curves can be used to determine the maximum rate of solute transport (**transport maximum, T$_m$**) for solutes with saturable transport. Construction of a titration curve first requires calculation of the filtered solute load for a range of plasma solute concentrations. Excretion rates are measured from urine samples across the same range of plasma solute concentrations. The net tubular transport is calculated from the difference between the filtered load and the excretion rate. The renal titration curve for glucose is shown in Figure 6-17. The plasma solute concentration at which the solute first appears in urine is called the **renal threshold.** The

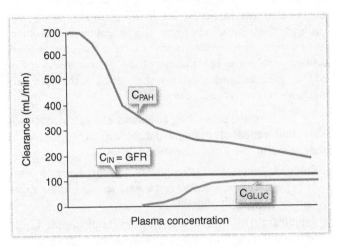

Figure 6-16: Relationships between clearance and plasma concentration. GFR, glomerular filtration rate.

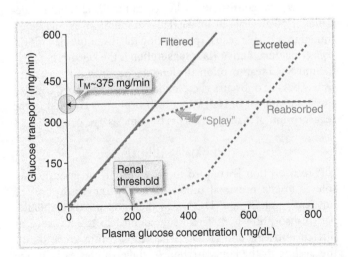

Figure 6-17: Renal titration curve for glucose. The renal threshold is the plasma glucose concentration at which glucose first appears in the urine. The plateau in the whole kidney reabsorption rate indicates the transport maximum (T$_m$) for glucose. The plateau is reached gradually as the filtered load increases (*splay*) due to differences in T$_m$ between individual nephrons.

glucose reabsorption curve levels off gradually rather than reaching the plateau abruptly. This phenomenon is called **splay** and is due to variability in the tubular transport maxima between nephrons. The plateau of the glucose reabsorption rate at glucose concentrations that saturate the transport mechanism reveals the T_m for glucose.

▽ Some of the **presenting symptoms of hyperglycemia in the untreated diabetic** patient can be explained by understanding the T_m for glucose as follows:

1. **Polyuria.** When the T_m for glucose is surpassed as a result of hyperglycemia, glucose (and water) remains in the urine, causing an **osmotic diuresis.**

2. **Polydipsia.** The osmotic diuresis from the glucosuria results in free water loss, which increases serum osmolarity, activating osmoreceptors in the hypothalamus, and provoking the sensation of thirst.

3. **Hypovolemia.** Polyuria and urinary free water loss can cause significant hypovolemia. ▼

RENAL SODIUM HANDLING AND DIURETICS

The daily filtered load of Na^+ is far greater than the daily requirement for Na^+ excretion; Na^+ balance is achieved with a FE_{Na} of 1–2%. *Filtration and reabsorption are the only significant processes affecting NaCl and water excretion.* If it is necessary to reduce the extracellular fluid volume in states such as **edema** or **hypertension, diuretic agents** can be given to increase urinary NaCl and water excretion. Most diuretics inhibit tubular Na^+ reabsorption.

OVERVIEW OF SEGMENTAL NA⁺ HANDLING

Figure 6-18 summarizes segmental Na^+ handling. The proximal tubule reabsorbs approximately 65% of filtered Na^+. The loop of Henle reabsorbs 20–25% of the filtered load, with about 10% of filtered Na^+ consistently delivered to the distal tubule, independent of dietary salt intake. Final excretion of Na^+ is determined by variable reabsorption along the distal tubule and the collecting duct. **Active Na^+ reabsorption** is the key driving force behind NaCl reabsorption all along the nephron. Cl^- reabsorption is passive or occurs via secondary active transport, coupled to the movement of Na^+. Water reabsorption is coupled to the reabsorption of NaCl and occurs by osmosis.

PROXIMAL TUBULE

Na^+ reabsorption is coupled to the transport of several other solutes in the proximal tubule, including the absorption of nutrients and Cl^- and HCO_3^-. In the **early proximal tubule,** Na^+ reabsorption is preferentially coupled to the recovery of filtered nutrients and HCO_3^-. This reabsorption accounts for the decline in the concentration of these solutes early in the proximal tubule, as shown in Figure 6-19A. In later portions of the proximal tubule, Na^+ reabsorption is coupled to Cl^- reabsorption. The osmolarity of tubular fluid does not change along the proximal tubule because the sum of all solute transport is **isosmotic** with plasma. The data in Figure 6-19A were

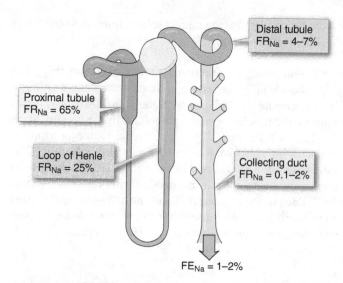

Figure 6-18: Overview of segmental sodium (Na^+) handling along the nephron. The fractional reabsorption (FR) is the percent of filtered Na^+ reabsorbed in each segment. The fractional excretion (FE) is the percent of filtered Na^+ excreted in final urine. FR_{Na}, fractional sodium reabsorption; FE_{Na}, fractional sodium excretion.

obtained after the administration of inulin; the extent of water reabsorption is demonstrated by the large increase in inulin concentration, which becomes concentrated in the lumen as water is reabsorbed.

Figure 6-19B shows mechanisms of cellular Na^+ uptake in the proximal tubule. Glucose and amino acids are recovered from the glomerular filtrate via Na^+-linked cotransporters. Nutrient uptake only requires a small proportion of filtered Na^+, and a much larger amount of Na^+ is reabsorbed via the Na^+/H^+ exchange. Secretion of H^+ into the lumen is then coupled indirectly to reabsorption of Cl^- or HCO_3^-. Approximately one third of Na^+ reabsorption in the proximal tubule occurs passively through the intercellular junctions via the paracellular pathway.

LOOP OF HENLE

There is no active Na^+ transport in the thin limbs of the loop of Henle. In contrast, the thick ascending limb is very metabolically active and Na^+ uptake occurs via cotransport with Cl^- and K^+ (Figure 6-20). This uptake mechanism is electrically neutral, with $1Na^+$, $2Cl^-$, and $1K^+$ carried across the apical cell membrane during each transport cycle. Na^+ is pumped out of the cell via the basolateral Na/K-ATPase. Cl^- leaves via a Cl^- channel in the basolateral membrane, and K^+ is recycled across the apical membrane via K^+ channels. The conjunction of an apical K^+ conductance and basolateral Cl^- conductance creates a **lumen-positive transepithelial electrical potential difference.** This voltage is important because it drives a significant paracellular flux of cations, particularly Ca^{2+} and Mg^{2+}. Loop diuretics (e.g., furosemide) induce natriuresis mainly by blocking the Na/2Cl/ K cotransporter; the transepithelial electrical potential is also decreased, resulting in the increased urinary loss of divalent cations.

▽ **Bartter's syndrome** is a salt-wasting disease caused by gene mutations in the Na/2Cl/K cotransporter, the luminal K^+ channel, or the basolateral Cl^- channel in the thick ascending limb. Loss of function in the thick ascending limb causes very large urinary losses of NaCl, reflecting the high proportion of the filtered load normally reabsorbed at this site. There is also urinary wasting of Ca^{2+} and Mg^{2+} due to the loss of the positive transepithelial potential difference in the thick ascending limb. ▽

DISTAL TUBULE AND CORTICAL COLLECTING DUCT

The distal tubule and the cortical collecting duct are important areas for fine regulation of Na^+ excretion. The hormone **aldosterone** increases the activity of the Na^+ transport proteins throughout this area to promote renal Na^+ conservation and maintain the extracellular fluid volume. In the early distal tubule, NaCl reabsorption is coupled via a **Na-Cl cotransporter** (Figure 6-21A). Na^+ exit at the basolateral membrane is via the Na/K-ATPase, and Cl^- exit is via the Cl^- channel.

The cortical collecting duct has two distinct cell types. The **principal cells** are the most abundant cells and are associated with NaCl reabsorption; the **intercalated cells** are involved with acid-base balance. Na^+ uptake in the principal cells occurs

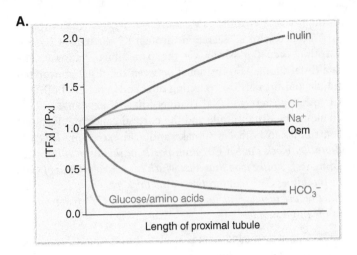

A.

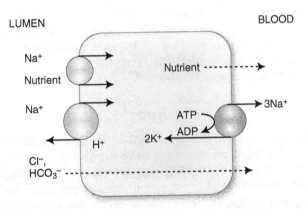

B.

Figure 6-19: Na^+ reabsorption in the proximal tubule. **A.** Solute reabsorption profile along the proximal tubule. The tubular fluid/plasma (TF/P) concentration ratio of inulin is an index of water reabsorption. If TF/P_{solute} is less than TF/P_{inulin}, there is net solute reabsorption. Preferential reabsorption of nutrients and HCO_3^- occur in the early proximal tubule. **B.** Cellular mechanisms of Na^+ reabsorption in the proximal tubule. Most Na^+ is reabsorbed via the Na^+/H^+ exchange. ATP, adenosine triphosphate; ADP, adenosine diphosphate.

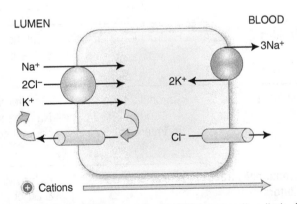

Figure 6-20: Na^+ reabsorption in the thick ascending limb. Na^+ uptake occurs via the $Na^+/K^+/2Cl^-$ cotransport. The combination of luminal K^+ channels and basolateral Cl^- channels creates a lumen-positive transepithelial potential difference, which drives paracellular cation reabsorption.

through a Na⁺ channel (see Figure 6-21B). Na⁺ reabsorption is associated with K⁺ secretion through K⁺ channels; Cl⁻ reabsorption occurs passively via the paracellular pathway. The late distal tubule is transitional between the distal convoluted tubule and the cortical collecting duct and expresses both Na-Cl cotransporters and Na⁺ channels. **Na⁺/H⁺ exchange** occurs all along the distal tubule and the cortical collecting duct and contributes to both Na⁺ uptake and acid excretion. *Thiazide diuretics block the Na-Cl cotransporter of the distal tubule (see Diuretics). Unlike loop diuretics, which cause urinary loss of Ca²⁺ by inhibiting Ca²⁺ reabsorption in the thick ascending limb, thiazides reduce urinary calcium loss by increasing Ca²⁺ reabsorption in the distal tubule.*

▽ **Gitelman's syndrome** is a salt-wasting condition caused by gene mutations in the Na-Cl cotransporter expressed in the distal tubule. The extent of salt wasting is milder than occurs in Bartter's syndrome and reflects the lower proportion of the filtered load that is normally reabsorbed in the distal tubule compared to the loop of Henle. *Hypocalciuria is a feature of Gitelman's syndrome and is the result of increased Ca²⁺ reabsorption in the distal nephron.* ▼

DIURETICS

Diuresis is defined as an increase in the urine flow rate; diuretics are agents that induce diuresis. Most diuretics used clinically are **organic acids** that are efficiently **secreted by the proximal tubule;** they act by inhibiting various luminal membrane Na⁺ transport proteins. Table 6-3 summarizes common agents, their sites of action, and their uses. Figure 6-22 illustrates sites of action for different classes of diuretics.

Loop diuretics (e.g., furosemide) inhibit the Na/2Cl/K cotransporter in the thick ascending limb. Explosive increases

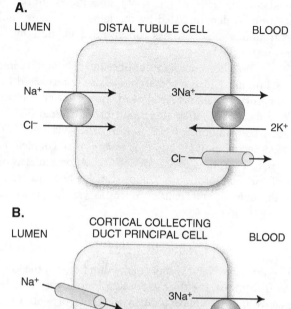

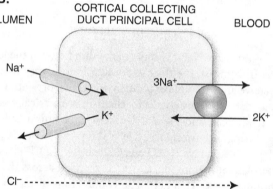

Figure 6-21: Mechanisms of Na⁺ reabsorption in the cortical collecting duct in the distal tubule.

TABLE 6-3. Sites of Diuretic Action and Clinical Uses

Class	Agents	Mechanism of Action	Examples of Use
Loop diuretics	Furosemide Bumetanide Torsemide	Inhibition of Na⁺/K⁺/2Cl⁻ cotransport in the thick ascending limb	• Pulmonary edema • Hypertension • Heart failure
Thiazides	Hydrochlorothiazide	Inhibition of Na/Cl cotransport in the distal tubule	• Hypertension • Heart failure (supplement to loop diuretics)
K⁺-sparing	Spironolactone Amiloride Triamterene	Aldosterone receptor antagonist Na⁺ channel inhibition in the cortical collecting duct	• Hypertension due to hyperaldosteronism • Supplement to loop or thiazide diuretics to reduce K⁺ wasting
Carbonic anhydrase inhibitors	Acetazolamide	Kidney: in the proximal tubule & other organs expressing carbonic anhydrase	• Rarely used to treat heart failure • Loss of HCO₃⁻ in urine useful in acute mountain sickness and in metabolic alkalosis • Glaucoma (eye) • Epilepsy (central nervous system)

in urine flow occur because this nephron segment normally reabsorbs 20–25% of filtered Na^+. *Because of their powerful diuretic effect, loop diuretics are particularly useful when rapid diuresis is needed (e.g., **pulmonary edema**).*

Thiazide diuretics (e.g., hydrochlorothiazide) inhibit Na-Cl cotransport in the distal tubule. Thiazides are less potent than loop diuretics because a lower proportion of the filtered NaCl load is reabsorbed in the distal tubule compared to the loop of Henle. *Thiazides are considered first-line agents in the treatment of **hypertension**, but they can also be used in a variety of other conditions, including **symptomatic relief of edema and hyper calciuria.***

Agents that act on the principal cells in the cortical collecting duct are called **K^+-sparing diuretics** because inhibition of Na^+ reabsorption at this site also inhibits K^+ secretion. **Amiloride** is an example of this class of diuretic, which acts by blocking apical Na^+ channels in the principal cells. **Aldosterone antagonists** (e.g., spironolactone) belong to the group of K^+-sparing diuretics and act by reducing the expression and activity of Na^+ transport proteins in the cortical collecting duct.

 K^+-sparing agents have a weak diuretic effect because less than 5% of filtered Na^+ is reabsorbed at this site. However, agents in this group can be helpful in the **treatment of certain specific disorders,** including:

Liddle's syndrome is caused by a genetic mutation that increases the function of the apical Na^+ channels in the principal cells. Patients have aggressive sodium retention and are at risk of developing **salt-sensitive hypertension.** The affected Na^+ channels are the same ones blocked by amiloride, which makes it the drug of choice for treating Liddle's syndrome.

Primary hyperaldosteronism (Conn's syndrome) most commonly occurs as a result of an aldosterone-secreting adenoma in the adrenal cortex (see Chapter 8). The classic clinical findings are hypertension, hypokalemia, and metabolic alkalosis. In addition to surgery, aldosterone antagonists (e.g., spironolactone) can be helpful in the treatment of Conn's syndrome. ▼

Carbonic anhydrase inhibitors (e.g., acetazolamide) dramatically reduce bicarbonate reabsorption in the early proximal tubule, producing a weak diuresis. Because of their weak diuretic effect, carbonic anhydrase inhibitors are rarely used for this purpose. *Acetazolamide is commonly used in the treatment or prophylaxis of **altitude sickness** and in reducing intraocular pressure associated with **glaucoma.***

Osmotic diuretics are nonreabsorbed solutes present in the tubule lumen; they cause water to remain in the lumen and to be passed into the urine. An example of osmotic diuresis discussed previously is untreated diabetes mellitus, when the glucose T_m is exceeded and glucose remains in the tubule lumen (see Renal Titration Curves). The proximal tubule and thin descending limb of the loop of Henle are the main sites of action because these areas have the highest membrane water permeability and are affected most by osmotic gradients.

▽ The inert sugar **mannitol** can be used to clinically induce an osmotic diuresis. *Mannitol can be helpful in the*

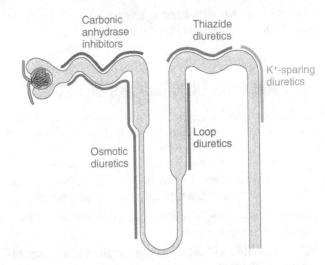

Figure 6-22: Sites of action of major classes of diuretics.

*treatment of patients with **head injuries** to reduce intracranial pressure by producing a fluid shift out of the brain.* ▼

URINE CONCENTRATION AND DILUTION

Body fluid osmolarity remains within narrow limits despite variations in water and solute intake or loss. The ability of the renal system to rapidly vary water excretion over a wide range in response to fluctuations in plasma osmolarity is the main reason that **water balance** exists. Three processes are required for the **renal system to vary urine concentration:**

1. **Adequate glomerular filtration** is needed to deliver NaCl and water to the loop of Henle.

2. **Na⁺ reabsorption without water reabsorption in the ascending limb of the loop of Henle** dilutes tubular fluid, providing the potential to excrete dilute urine. At the same time, the medullary interstitial fluid becomes hypertonic, providing the potential to concentrate urine in the collecting ducts.

3. **Water permeability in the collecting duct must be variable,** which is controlled via ADH.

ADH

Variation in water excretion in response to changes in plasma osmolarity is mediated through changes in ADH (vasopressin) secretion. Figure 6-23 shows a close correlation between plasma osmolarity and plasma ADH concentration. The normal set point for plasma osmolarity is 285–288 mOsm/L, which is associated with an ADH concentration of about 2–3 pg/mL. Large increases in ADH secretion occur if osmolarity increases and/or blood volume decreases. The combined effects of ADH at the kidney result in the formation of concentrated urine and retention of solute-free water in the body. ADH is called **vasopressin** because it is also a potent vasoconstrictor. ***V₁ receptors*** *mediate vasoconstriction;* ***V₂ receptors*** *mediate renal water retention.*

ADH is synthesized in the **supraoptic and paraventricular nuclei** of the hypothalamus and is secreted from nerve terminals in the posterior pituitary gland (see Chapter 8). ADH secretion is directed by neuronal osmoreceptors in the hypothalamus. A 1% deviation of plasma osmolarity is enough to vary ADH secretion. *Reductions in plasma volume of more than 10% are also a potent stimulus for ADH secretion.* Increased secretion of ADH in response to **low blood volume** is sensed by low pressure baroreceptors in the atria and lungs as well as by high pressure carotid baroreceptors. Commonly ingested agents that affect ADH are **nicotine,** which increases secretion, and **ethanol,** which inhibits secretion.

▽ Pathologic oversecretion of ADH results in the **syndrome of inappropriate antidiuretic hormone (SIADH).** SIADH is caused by various clinical conditions, including small cell carcinoma of the lung (most common), pneumonia, or head injury. Continuous ADH secretion leads to retention of solute-free water and eventually to hyponatremia; ***severe hyponatremia can be fatal.*** Treatment of SIADH revolves around identifying and treating the underlying condition. ▼

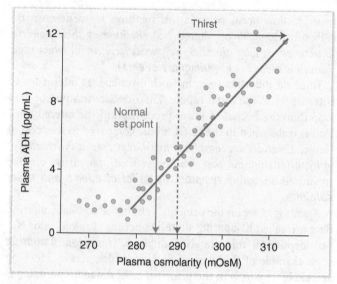

Figure 6-23: The relationship between plasma antidiuretic hormone (ADH) concentration and plasma osmolarity.

CONCENTRATING OR DILUTING URINE

An increase in plasma osmolarity results in the excretion of urine that is more concentrated than plasma; some solute-free water is returned to the extracellular fluid, and plasma osmolarity is reduced toward normal. A decrease in plasma osmolarity results in the excretion of urine that is more dilute than plasma; some **solute-free water** is excreted in the urine, increasing the body fluid osmolarity toward normal. These changes in urine osmolarity can occur without significant changes in GFR or total solute excretion. *Whether the kidney produces concentrated or dilute urine depends on ADH levels.*

Figure 6-24 compares the segmental osmolarity profile of tubular fluid when there is either a high or a low plasma ADH level. In either case, *fluid in the proximal tubule remains isosmotic with respect to plasma and makes no contribution to altering urine osmolarity.* In the descending thin limb of the loop of Henle, osmolarity reflects that of the surrounding medullary interstitium. There is always some degree of **hypertonicity in the medullary interstitium,** with a gradient of increasing osmolarity from the outer to the inner medulla. High ADH levels dramatically increase medullary osmolarity, which is reflected by increasing osmolarity along the descending thin limb of the loop of Henle (Figure 6-24). The ascending limb of the loop of Henle is called the **diluting segment** because it always reduces the tubular fluid osmolarity; in the ascending limb, NaCl is reabsorbed without water. *By the time fluid leaves the loop of Henle, it is hypotonic relative to plasma.* When ADH levels are low, the water permeability of the distal nephron and collecting duct is very low. Hypotonic fluid entering the distal nephron remains hypotonic during passage through the collecting duct when ADH is low and **dilute urine** is being produced. The maximal diluting capacity of the renal system is about five- to tenfold (i.e., urine osmolarity of 30–60 mOsm). In contrast, high ADH levels increase water permeability in the distal tubule and collecting duct. Osmotic water reabsorption into the hypertonic interstitium causes the osmolarity of the tubular fluid to increase along the collecting duct, emerging as **concentrated urine.**

COUNTERCURRENT MULTIPLICATION

The ability to concentrate urine depends on the generation of a **corticomedullary gradient** of increasing interstitial osmolarity. Formation of the corticomedullary gradient relies on the countercurrent arrangement of the descending and ascending limbs of the loop of Henle and their differing transport properties (Figure 6-25). The thin descending limb is characterized by high water permeability and the lack of active transport. Osmolarity of the luminal fluid simply reflects that of the surrounding interstitium. The ascending limb is characterized by very low water permeability. Salt reabsorption into the interstitium occurs in the ascending limb by active transport in the thick ascending limb (Figure 6-25, Step 1) and by diffusion in the salt-permeable thin ascending limb (see below). At any given horizontal level, the osmolarity of fluid in the descending limb and interstitium can be 200 mOsmole/L greater than in the ascending limb. This is known as the **single osmotic effect** and is due to salt reabsorption from the ascending limb.

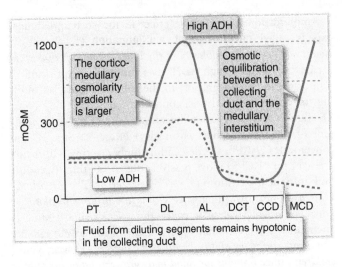

Figure 6-24: Effects of antidiuretic hormone (ADH) on tubular fluid osmolarity. PT, proximal tubule; DL, descending limb of the loop of Henle; AL, ascending limb of the loop of Henle; DCT, distal convoluted tubule; CCD, cortical collecting duct; MCD, medullary collecting duct.

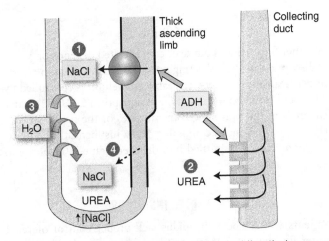

Figure 6-25: Countercurrent multiplication. Antidiuretic hormone (ADH) stimulates active NaCl reabsorption in the thick ascending limb (TAL) (*step 1*); passive countercurrent multiplication begins with ADH-stimulated reabsorption of urea from the medullary collecting duct (*step 2*). Water reabsorption in the descending limb (*step 3*) concentrates luminal NaCl and allows NaCl diffusion out of the thin ascending limb (*step 4*).

Amplification of the single effect in the corticomedullary axis is called **countercurrent multiplication** (Figure 6-25). *About 40% of total osmolarity in the inner medulla is due to the presence of urea.* A high ADH level causes the expression of uniporters for urea transport in the collecting duct, accounting for high interstitial urea concentration (Figure 6-25, Step 2). High urea concentration draws water out of the descending limb of the loop of Henle by osmosis (Figure 6-25, Step 3). This concentrates NaCl in the descending limb, creating a diffusion gradient for NaCl to move passively out of the thin ascending limb into the interstitium (Figure 6-25, Step 4). *The importance of urea is illustrated in patients with a low protein intake who have a reduced capacity to concentrate their urine because of lower urea levels. Children younger than 1 year have a reduced urine-concentrating ability because of lower urea levels; young children utilize proteins for rapid body growth and as a result do not produce much urea.*

COUNTERCURRENT EXCHANGE

In most organs, rapid diffusion between the capillary blood and the interstitium results in uniform composition of interstitial fluid. If rapid diffusion occurred in the renal medulla, the osmotic gradient would be dissipated. This does not occur because the **vasa recta capillaries** have a countercurrent loop configuration that tends to trap solutes in the medulla. As shown in Figure 6-26, blood flowing down the descending vasa recta receives solutes from the interstitium by diffusion and loses water by osmosis. Blood reaching the renal papilla is highly concentrated and, as it flows up the ascending vasa recta, solutes diffuse out and water enters by osmosis. This net effect of retaining high solute concentration in the medulla is known as countercurrent exchange. The **countercurrent exchange mechanism** depends on low medullary blood flow. *In states of low ADH, medullary blood flow increases, causing washout of medullary hypertonicity and reduced urine osmolarity.*

AQUAPORIN 2

Whether final urine is dilute or concentrated depends on water reabsorption in the collecting duct. The change from a water-impermeable to a water-permeable epithelium is controlled by ADH and is due to the insertion of aquaporin 2 (AQP2) water channels in the luminal cell membranes of the principal cells (Figure 6-27). Vesicles containing AQP2 just beneath the luminal membrane are shuttled into the membrane in response to ADH.

DIABETES INSIPIDUS

Patients with diabetes insipidus lack proper control of renal water flux by ADH. Water reabsorption under the control of ADH is called **facultative** reabsorption and is about 20–25 L/d. Water reabsorption that occurs in the more proximal nephron segments not under ADH control is called **obligatory reabsorption.** *Patients with diabetes insipidus may excrete as much as 20–25 L/d, and may require an equivalent water intake to maintain water balance.*

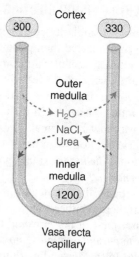

Figure 6-26: Countercurrent exchange. Numbers indicate typical osmolarity (mOsm/L) during maximal antidiuresis. Passive cycling of solutes from the ascending to the descending limbs of the vasa recta capillaries traps solutes in the medullary interstitium.

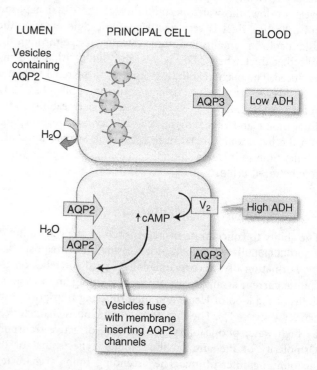

Figure 6-27: Aquaporin 2 (AQP 2) water channel expression in the collecting duct. In the absence of antidiuretic hormone (ADH), the water permeability in the collecting duct is low because water channels are not present in the apical membranes. AQP3 channels are expressed continually in the basolateral membrane. Binding of ADH to the V₂ receptors on the basolateral membrane of the principal cells causes insertion of vesicles containing AQP2 water channels into the apical cell membrane, completing the pathway for water flux.

There are **two types of diabetes insipidus:**

1. **Central diabetes insipidus** is the inability of the posterior pituitary gland to adequately secrete ADH. This type of diabetes insipidus may occur in patients with pituitary tumors that interfere with ADH secretion, or it may occur as a complication following surgical removal of a pituitary tumor.

2. **Nephrogenic diabetes insipidus** is failure of the kidney to respond to ADH. It can be caused by drugs such as **lithium** or by rare genetic mutations in AQP 2 or renal ADH receptors.

OSMOLAR CLEARANCE AND FREE WATER CLEARANCE

Free water clearance is calculated to determine if the ADH endocrine axis and the renal concentrating mechanism are functioning properly. It is the volume of solute-free water excreted per minute. Osmolar clearance must be calculated to derive free water clearance. Osmolar clearance is the volume of plasma cleared of total solute per minute and is calculated from the general **clearance equation:**

$$C_{osm} = (C_{osm} \times \dot{V}) \div P_{osm} \qquad \textbf{Equation 6-7}$$

P_{osm} = Plasma osmolarity
U_{osm} = Urine osmolarity
$\dot{V}$ = Urine flow rate

If urine and plasma osmolarity were equal ($U_{osm}/P_{osm} = 1$), Equation 6-7 would become ($C_{osm} = V$), and urine flow rate would represent the volume of plasma cleared of total solute per minute. If the same amount of solute were excreted in dilute urine, a volume of water would be "added" during urine formation, called **free water clearance (C_{H2O}):**

$$\dot{V} = C_{osm} + C_{H2O} \qquad \textbf{Equation 6-8}$$

Therefore, free water clearance is calculated by subtracting C_{osm} from V. When urine is dilute, C_{H2O} is a positive number, whereas a negative free water clearance reflects concentration of the urine. *Negative free water clearance should be present when a patient has elevated serum ADH levels; otherwise a renal defect is present.*

Example The following data were obtained over a period of several hours from a patient being monitored in the intensive care unit:

▨ Urine flow rate = 0.1 L/h

▨ Urine osmolarity = 330 mOsm/L

▨ Plasma osmolarity = 310 mOsm/L

Calculate free water clearance using the above information and interpret the result, given further information that the patient had a normal increase in the plasma ADH concentration in the setting of this greater than normal plasma osmolarity.

Osmolar clearance must first be calculated to proceed to calculate free water clearance:

$$C_{osm} = (U_{osm} \times \dot{V})/P_{osm}$$
$$= (330 \times 0.1)/310$$
$$= 0.1 \text{ L/h}$$

Free water clearance:

$$C_{H2O} = \overset{\bullet}{V} - C_{osm}$$
$$= 0.10 \text{ L/h} - 0.11 \text{ L/h}$$
$$= -0.01 \text{ L/h}$$

In the setting of increased plasma osmolality and increased plasma ADH, the patient is expected to concentrate the urine and therefore to generate a significant negative free water clearance. In this case, free water clearance is near zero, indicating a failure of urine concentration and therefore renal dysfunction.

REGULATION OF EXTRACELLULAR FLUID VOLUME

Long-term control of **blood pressure** requires maintenance of the normal extracellular fluid volume by the renal system. The vascular function curves presented in Chapter 4 (see Figure 4-32) showed that an increase in the extracellular fluid volume, through increased venous blood volume, will result in increased systemic function pressure (P_{SF}), increased venous return, increased cardiac output, and high mean arterial pressure. The extracellular fluid volume is a function of the total amount of Na^+ in extracellular fluid. Regulation of water balance should ensure that increased Na^+ content results in increased water retention and an increase in extracellular fluid volume. *Disorders of extracellular fluid volume (e.g., edema) reflect difficulties with Na^+ balance, whereas disorders of Na^+ concentration (i.e., **hypernatremia** or **hyponatremia**) indicate difficulties with water balance.*

EFFECTIVE CIRCULATING VOLUME

Negative feedback control of extracellular fluid volume operates through control of the effective circulating volume, which is related to the volume of blood in the circulation and the pressure within specific parts of the circulation. *The kidney is the main effective circulating volume sensor* and is well-suited to this role because of the high rate of renal perfusion. The juxtaglomerular apparatus measures changes in the afferent arteriolar wall tension as an index of renal perfusion. If perfusion decreases, there is less stretch of the afferent arteriolar wall, triggering renin release, which in turn activates the **angiotensin-aldosterone axis** (see Chapter 8). Other sensors of effective circulating volume include arterial baroreceptors and low pressure baroreceptors in the pulmonary system and the cardiac atria. Figure 6-28 shows a negative feedback loop in which changes in effective circulating volume result in altered renal Na^+ excretion to produce a change in the extracellular fluid Na^+ content and effective circulating volume. *Coupling between changes in the extracellular fluid Na^+ content and circulating volume occurs via changes in water excretion, which in turn are controlled by **ADH**.* For example, plasma osmolarity increases if more Na^+ is retained, resulting in ADH release, water retention, and, therefore, in an increase in extracellular fluid volume.

▼ Patients with **congestive heart failure** have low effective circulating volume because their cardiac performance is poor. Na^+ and fluid retention result, but effective circulating volume does not improve due to cardiac failure. Instead, **edema** results as venous and capillary hydrostatic pressures increase.

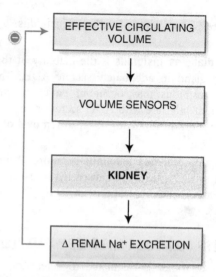

Figure 6-28: Feedback regulation of effective circulating volume (ECV). Changes in renal Na^+ excretion are linked to changes in ECV through altered extracellular fluid (ECF) osmolarity and resulting changes in water excretion. For example, increased Na^+ excretion reduces plasma osmolarity, which increases water excretion and reduces ECV.

Patients with heart failure continue to retain Na$^+$, increasing the extracellular fluid volume without correcting the effective circulating volume, which is why edema is a chronic problem in patients with congestive heart failure. This demonstrates that the effective circulating volume is the controlled physiologic variable, not absolute extracellular fluid volume. ▼

RESPONSES TO LOW EFFECTIVE CIRCULATING VOLUME

A **decrease in the effective circulating volume** is counteracted in four main ways (Figure 6-29):

1. Activation of the **renin-angiotensin-aldosterone axis.**
2. Stimulation of the **sympathetic nervous system** via the baroreceptor reflex.
3. Increased **ADH secretion.**
4. Increased renal fluid retention via altered **Starling's forces in the peritubular capillaries.**

The juxtaglomerular apparatus secretes renin in response to reduced renal perfusion, triggering a cascade that increases the serum levels of the hormones angiotensin II and aldosterone. **Angiotensin II** increases Na$^+$ reabsorption from the proximal tubule and causes generalized vasoconstriction to combat arterial hypotension. Angiotensin II supplements the stimulus from low pressure baroreceptors to increase ADH secretion, which increases renal water conservation. Aldosterone from the adrenal cortex acts to increase Na$^+$ reabsorption throughout the distal nephron and the cortical collecting duct.

If a decrease in the effective circulating volume is large enough to reduce the mean arterial blood pressure, the **baroreceptor reflex** activates the sympathetic nervous system. Cardiac output and blood pressure are supported by

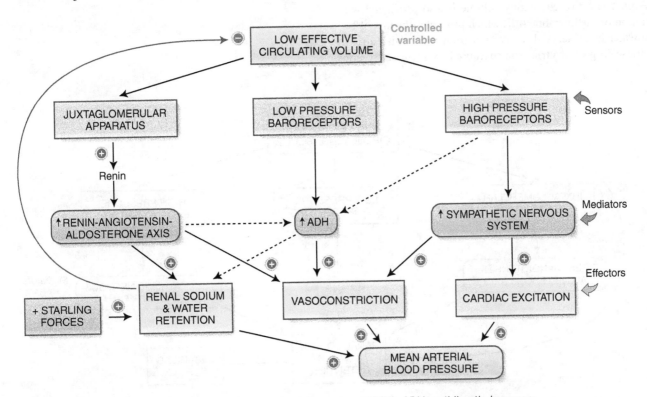

Figure 6-29: Negative feedback responses to low effective circulating volume (ECV). ADH, antidiuretic hormone.

vasoconstriction and venoconstriction and by increased heart rate and myocardial contractility. Renal sympathetic nerve activation constricts the afferent arterioles, reducing GFR and further stimulating renin release via the β_1 receptors on the juxtaglomerular cells. Norepinephrine also stimulates Na^+ reabsorption in the proximal tubule.

Low extracellular fluid volume causes a generalized decrease in the capillary hydrostatic pressure. If low effective circulating volume results from a loss of NaCl and water, there is also an increase in the plasma oncotic pressure because serum proteins are concentrated. These subtle changes in **Starling's forces** promote movement of fluid from the interstitial fluid to plasma. The peritubular capillaries are a site of very high fluid absorption from the renal cortical interstitial fluid to the plasma. Altered Starling forces in low effective circulating volume cause a significant increase in fluid reabsorption into the peritubular capillaries, which promotes fluid reabsorption from the nephron and contributes to renal Na^+ conservation.

RESPONSES TO HIGH EFFECTIVE CIRCULATING VOLUME

Figure 6-30 summarizes responses to high effective circulating volume. In persons with normal effective circulating volume and osmolarity, the activity of renin, angiotensin, aldosterone, ADH, and the sympathetic nerves is generally low. This limits the scope for further suppression of these systems when the effective circulating volume increases, and their role is less important than it is during low effective circulating volume. Changes in Starling forces continue to be significant because volume loading increases capillary hydrostatic pressure and decreases oncotic pressure. Reduced fluid reabsorption into the peritubular capillaries allows more fluid to be excreted by the renal tubule.

A high effective circulating volume is also associated with secretion of the hormone **ANP,** which promotes the loss of Na^+ and water in urine. ANP is secreted from the cardiac atria in response to greater atrial stretch caused by increased venous

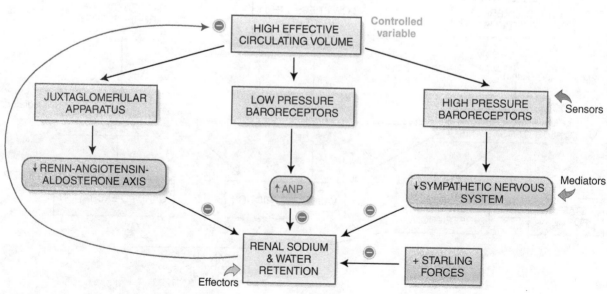

Figure 6-30: Negative feedback responses to high effective circulating volume (ECV). ANP, atrial natriuretic peptide.

blood volume. ANP promotes natriuresis (Na⁺ loss in urine) by increasing GFR and decreasing Na⁺ reabsorption in the collecting duct. ANP also inhibits the secretion of ADH, renin, and aldosterone.

▼ **Brain natriuretic peptide** is a peptide related to ANP and is named for the location where it was first isolated, the brain. However, it was later found to be produced in the ventricles of the heart. It is thought that the effects of brain natriuretic peptide are similar to ANP, but they may be more potent and longer lasting than the effects of ANP. With the use of recombinant DNA technology, brain natriuretic peptide (**nesiritide**) has been developed for use in the treatment of patients with **congestive heart failure.** ▼

PRESSURE NATRIURESIS

Increased arterial blood pressure causes increased renal Na⁺ excretion, known as pressure natriuresis, which is expected from the negative feedback control of effective circulating volume (Figure 6-31). However, pressure natriuresis persists in the absence of hormones or renal nerves, showing that there is also intrinsic control of renal Na⁺ excretion in response to altered renal perfusion. Pressure natriuresis occurs in concert with other mechanisms supporting Na⁺ balance and provides a feedback mechanism to maintain normal blood pressure. *In patients with* **hypertension,** *the pressure natriuresis curve shifts right* (Figure 6-31). These patients have insufficient Na⁺ excretion at normal blood pressure. A subset of hypertensive patients are **salt sensitive,** shown by a pressure-natriuresis curve that has both a right shift and a reduced gradient; in these patients, higher salt intake further increases the blood pressure.

DARROW-YANNET DIAGRAMS

Darrow-Yannet diagrams plot relative changes in the volume (*x*-axis) and osmolarity (*y*-axis) of extracellular fluid and intracellular fluid (Figure 6-32). The contraction or the expansion of body fluid volume can occur with low, normal, or high osmolarity. Note that the osmolarities of extracellular fluid and intracellular fluid are always the same at steady state because water moves freely by osmosis between extracellular fluid and intracellular fluid.

Secretory diarrhea (e.g., cholera) and **hemorrhage** are examples of **isosmotic volume contraction.** The loss of NaCl from the extracellular fluid in an isosmotic solution causes a decrease in the extracellular fluid volume. There is no change in the osmolarity of extracellular fluid; therefore, there is no osmotic driving force to cause water exchange with intracellular fluid, and intracellular fluid volume is unchanged. The mechanisms previously discussed for low effective circulating volume are activated, but salt and water ingestion or infusion are needed to restore normal conditions.

Sweating is an example of **hyperosmotic volume contraction.** NaCl is lost from extracellular fluid in a dilute solution, causing the extracellular fluid volume to decrease and the extracellular fluid osmolarity to increase. Water shifts out of intracellular fluid into extracellular fluid by osmosis. At steady

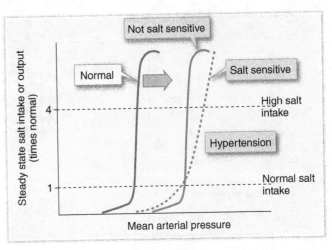

Figure 6-31: Pressure natriuresis. Acute increases in blood pressure induce renal Na⁺ excretion (natriuresis). Chronically hypertensive patients regulate the mean arterial pressure (MAP) around a higher set point value. Salt-sensitive patients have a weaker pressure natriuresis response during salt loading, causing the MAP to increase further.

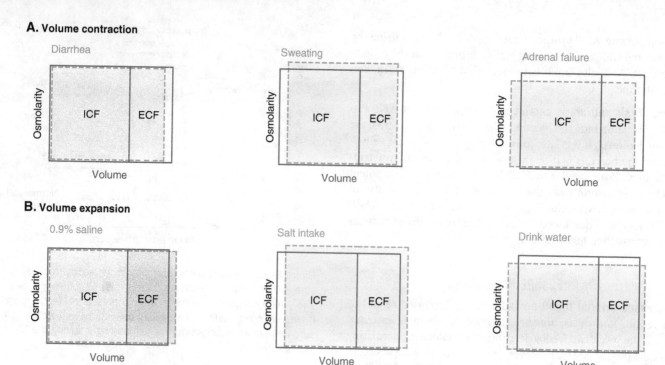

Figure 6-32: Darrow-Yannet diagrams. Volume contraction (**A**) and volume expansion (**B**) can be isosmotic (*left panels*), hyperosmotic (center panels), or hypoosmotic (*right panels*). ICF, intracellular fluid; ECF, extracellular fluid.

state, fluid loss from sweating reduces both extracellular fluid and intracellular fluid volumes, and body fluids have higher osmolarity. Mechanisms to correct low effective circulating volume are activated, particularly ADH secretion in response to high osmolarity.

Adrenocortical insufficiency (e.g., Addison's disease) is an example of **hyposmotic volume contraction.** Chronic loss of aldosterone results in renal NaCl loss in excess of water loss. Extracellular fluid volume and osmolarity are both reduced. Net water flux from the extracellular fluid into the intracellular fluid is driven by osmosis. At steady state, intracellular fluid volume is increased, and extracellular fluid volume and body fluid osmolarity are reduced. In this pathologic situation, restoration of the normal effective circulating volume is not possible due to the failure of aldosterone secretion. Low effective circulating volume stimulates ADH secretion despite low osmolarity, but the effective circulating volume cannot be restored without renal Na$^+$ retention.

Intravenous infusion of 0.9% saline is an example of **isosmotic volume expansion** of extracellular fluid. There is no change in osmolarity, so there is no fluid shift from the intracellular fluid. Following infusion, the extracellular fluid volume is larger, and the intracellular fluid volume and the body fluid osmolarity are unchanged. The mechanisms discussed previously for high effective circulating volume will restore normal conditions by promoting renal excretion of the volume load.

Ingestion of pure salt is an example of **hyperosmotic volume expansion.** Salt enters the extracellular fluid via the intestine, causing an increase in the extracellular fluid osmolarity. Water is absorbed from the intracellular fluid by osmosis. After salt absorption, the extracellular fluid volume is larger, the intracellular fluid volume is smaller, and body fluids have a higher osmolarity. Increased ADH secretion will result from high osmolarity and will initially cause further volume expansion due to water retention. The mechanisms discussed previously for high effective circulating volume will finally restore normal conditions by promoting renal Na^+ excretion.

▽ Patients with **congestive heart failure** have an expanded extracellular fluid volume, which greatly increases the likelihood of development of pulmonary edema. These patients must be cautious about the amount of salt they ingest because even small amounts can be enough to further expand their extracellular fluid volume, resulting in **florid pulmonary edema.** ▽

SIADH is an example of **hyposmotic volume expansion.** Renal water retention delivers excess free water to the extracellular fluid, which is distributed throughout the total body water. At equilibrium, both the extracellular fluid and intracellular fluid volumes are larger, and body fluid osmolarity is reduced. The normal response (e.g., following water ingestion) would be to suppress ADH secretion. In this case, however, abnormal ADH secretion is the cause of hyposmotic volume expansion and must be addressed to restore normal effective circulating volume.

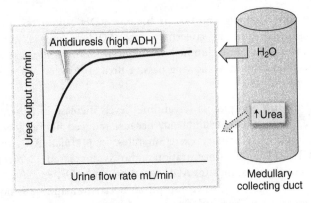

Figure 6-33: Dependence of urea excretion on urine flow rate. High plasma antidiuretic hormone (ADH) levels reduce urine flow rate. Urea excretion decreases during antidiuresis because urea reabsorption from the collecting duct increases. During antidiuresis, water reabsorption from the collecting duct concentrates urea in the lumen, creating a diffusion gradient for urea reabsorption. This mechanism accounts for increased blood urea nitrogen (BUN) in states of increased ADH.

MAGNESIUM HOMEOSTASIS

Mg^{2+} is an essential cofactor in many enzymatic reactions. Plasma $[Mg^{2+}]$ is homeostatically regulated by the balance between intestinal uptake and urinary excretion, although hormonal mechanisms are poorly defined. Only about 1% of the total Mg^{2+} in the body is in the extracellular fluid and the remainder is in the bone matrix or intracellular fluid. Dietary Mg^{2+} is reabsorbed mainly in the ileum. The **normal plasma $[Mg^{2+}]$ range** is from 1.3–2.1 mEq/L. **Mg is present in three forms in the plasma:**

1. **60**% of plasma Mg^{2+} is in the **free ionized form.**

2. **25**% of plasma Mg^{2+} is **bound to plasma protein.**

3. **15**% of plasma Mg^{2+} is **complexed to anions** such as phosphate.

Mg^{2+} has an unusual profile of segmental handling along the nephron: only 25% of filtered Mg^{2+} is reabsorbed in the proximal tubule, 65% in the thick ascending limb, and 1–5% in the distal tubule. The sites of regulation of Mg^{2+} reabsorption are the thick ascending limb and the distal tubule. *Loop diuretics cause urinary loss of divalent cations, including Mg^{2+} and Ca^{2+}* (see Diuretics).

RENAL UREA HANDLING

Urea is the end product of **nitrogen metabolism;** it is water soluble and has low toxicity. *Plasma urea concentration (BUN) ranges from 8 mg/dL to 25 mg/dL and is not subject to homeostatic regulation.* Figure 6-33 shows that FE_{urea} varies with a urine flow rate from about 30 to 60%. Lower rates of urea excretion are found during antidiuresis because ADH stimulates urea reabsorption in the collecting duct. ADH-dependent water reabsorption causes luminal urea concentration to increase in the collecting duct, allowing passive urea absorption via uniporters.

▽ **BUN** and plasma [creatinine] levels increase in patients with **renal insufficiency** because reduced filtered loads decrease their urinary excretion rates. In **prerenal** ARF, the BUN/creatinine concentration ratio is increased (>20:1). Hypovolemia stimulates ADH secretion, and ADH specifically increases tubular urea reabsorption. Because creatinine is not reabsorbed by the tubule, more urea (than creatinine) accumulates in plasma and the *BUN/creatinine concentration ratio is increased—a helpful biochemical clue in identifying patients with prerenal ARF.* ▽

RENAL CALCIUM HANDLING

Ca^{2+} homeostasis involves variable Ca^{2+} input from the gastrointestinal system and variable output by the renal system, plus exchanges of Ca^{2+} between the extracellular fluid and the bone matrix. PTH and vitamin D are the major hormones controlling Ca^{2+} balance (see Chapter 8). **Calcium exists in three forms in plasma** in approximately the following proportions:

1. **45%** exists as **free ionized Ca^{2+}**. The plasma concentration of free ionized Ca^{2+} is tightly regulated in the range of 1.0–1.3 mmol/L (4.0–5.2 mg/dL).

2. **45%** is bound to anionic sites on **plasma proteins.** Protein-bound Ca^{2+} does not enter the interstitial fluid and is not filtered at the glomerulus.

3. **10%** is complexed with **low-molecular-weight anions** such as citrate and oxalate.

SEGMENTAL CA²⁺ HANDLING

The filtered load of Ca^{2+} is the product of GFR and free plasma Ca^{2+} concentration. The pattern of segmental Ca^{2+} reabsorption is similar to that of Na^+ and results in a typical FE_{Ca} of 1–2%. A significant difference between Na^+ and Ca^{2+} is the absence of Ca^{2+} reabsorption in the collecting duct. Figure 6-34 shows mechanisms of Ca^{2+} reabsorption in the thick ascending limb and the distal tubule, which are sites of regulation. In the thick ascending limb, a lumen-positive transepithelial potential difference drives paracellular Ca^{2+} reabsorption. Epithelial cells in the thick ascending limb express the **extracellular Ca^{2+}-sensing receptor (CaR)** and are able to detect a decrease in free Ca^{2+} concentration in plasma. The response is increased Ca^{2+} uptake from the thick ascending limb due to a larger transepithelial potential difference (see Figure 6-34A). Regulation of Ca^{2+} reabsorption also occurs in the distal tubule. Ca^{2+} enters the cells of the distal tubule through Ca^{2+} channels. Ca^{2+}-binding proteins called **calbindins** keep the cytosolic Ca^{2+} concentration low, and it must be moved across the basolateral membrane by active transport. *PTH, vitamin D, and thiazide diuretics all stimulate Ca^{2+} reabsorption in the distal tubule* (see Figure 6-34B).

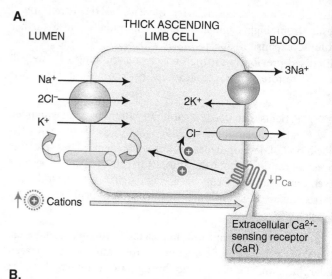

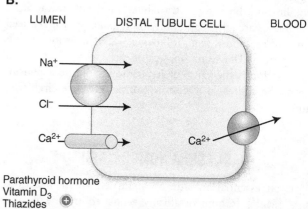

Figure 6-34: Sites of regulated Ca^{2+} reabsorption in the nephron. In the thick ascending limb (**A**), Ca^{2+} reabsorption depends on the size of a lumen-positive transepithelial potential difference. Stimulation of a Ca^{2+}-sensing receptor increases the voltage and Ca^{2+} reabsorption; loop diuretics reduce the voltage and Ca^{2+} reabsorption. In the distal tubule (**B**), Ca^{2+} uptake through the apical Ca^{2+} channel is stimulated by parathyroid hormone, vitamin D_3, and thiazide diuretics.

▽ **Urinary calculi** (stones) afflict many patients, causing painful renal colic. The most common chemical composition of the calculi is calcium oxalate. **Hypercalciuria** is the major risk factor for developing urinary calculi and is present in most patients who have calcium-based calculi. **Thiazide diuretics** used in the treatment of patients with hypercalciuria reduce stone formation by increasing distal tubular calcium reabsorption and therefore decreasing the urinary calcium load. This prevents supersaturation of the urine with insoluble calcium oxalate crystals and, therefore, reduces stone formation. ▽

RENAL PHOSPHATE HANDLING

The concentration of inorganic phosphate in the extracellular fluid is influenced by intestinal uptake, renal excretion, and exchanges with bone. Plasma inorganic phosphate concentration is regulated in the range of 0.8 mmol/L to 1.5 mmol/L (2.5–4.5 mg/dL). **Phosphate has two major forms in plasma:**

1. **80%** exists as **alkaline phosphate (HPO_4^{2-})** at a normal plasma pH of 7.4.

2. **20%** exists as **acid phosphate ($H_2PO_4^-$).**

Most phosphate is present in bone and intracellular fluid, with less than 1% in extracellular fluid. There is typically a daily dietary excess of phosphate, which is excreted from the kidney, with a fractional phosphate excretion of about 20%. Mechanisms of phosphate recovery from the filtrate are limited and restricted to Na/phosphate cotransport and are almost exclusively in the proximal tubule. *Phosphate excretion is therefore highly dependent on GFR, and renal insufficiency quickly results in inadequate phosphate excretion.* Increased plasma [phosphate] is a common feature of renal insufficiency. *PTH is the most important physiologic regulator of plasma [phosphate].* Increased plasma [phosphate] stimulates PTH secretion directly, which increases urinary phosphate excretion by inhibiting its reabsorption in the proximal tubule.

▽ **Hyperphosphatemia** is a persistent problem in patients who are in chronic renal failure due to a loss of renal excretory capacity for phosphate. **Oral phosphate binders** (e.g., calcium salts) are used to decrease intestinal phosphate absorption, thereby reducing plasma [phosphate]. ▽

POTASSIUM BALANCE

About 98% of K^+ in the body is in the intracellular fluid and is exchangeable with the extracellular fluid K^+. The extracellular fluid $[K^+]$ is controlled within the range of 3.5 mEq/L to 5.5 mEq/L. *Control of the extracellular fluid $[K^+]$ is essential to prevent membrane potential disruption because K^+ conductance determines the resting membrane potential of most cells.* The plasma K^+ is affected by shifts between the intracellular fluid and extracellular fluid (**internal K^+ homeostasis**) and by the balance between K^+ ingestion and excretion (**external potassium homeostasis**). *Aldosterone is the central hormone* controlling K⁺ balance and produces effects on both internal and external homeostasis. An increase in the extracellular fluid $[K^+]$ stimulates aldosterone secretion directly. Cellular uptake of K^+ in skeletal muscle is increased, which reduces extracellular fluid $[K^+]$, and renal K^+ excretion is stimulated to remove excess K^+. **Disturbances in plasma $[K^+]$** are a common clinical problem. For example:

Hypokalemia is defined as plasma $[K^+] < 3.5$ mEq/L. The most common causes of hypokalemia are from gastro-intestinal losses (e.g., diarrhea, vomiting, or gastric suctioning) or from a renal loss (e.g., caused by the use of a diuretic).

Hyperkalemia is defined as plasma $[K^+] > 5.5$ mEq/L.

▼ *In patients with chronic renal failure, hyperkalemia is an indication for hemodialysis treatment.* **Acute hyperkalemia** can be rapidly fatal as a result of **cardiac arrhythmia. Medical treatment of hyperkalemia** includes four approaches:

1. **Calcium gluconate infusion.** Increased plasma Ca^{2+} stabilizes cardiac membrane potential, decreasing the immediate risk of arrhythmia.

2. **Insulin and glucose infusion.** Insulin infusion drives K^+ back into the intracellular fluid, decreasing plasma levels; concomitant glucose infusion allows for continuous insulin administration without inducing hypoglycemia.

3. **Oral sodium polystyrene sulfonate (Kayexalate).** This intestinal K^+ chelator reduces K^+ absorption and increases fecal K^+ elimination.

4. **β_2 agonists (such as albuterol or epinephrine).** These drugs provide a short-acting mechanism to temporarily drive K^+ into the intracellular fluid. ▼

INTERNAL K⁺ HOMEOSTASIS

Figure 6-35 summarizes factors other than aldosterone that influence **K^+ distribution between the extracellular fluid and the intracellular fluid.**

Insulin stimulates K^+ movement from the extracellular fluid to the intracellular fluid. A single meal can contain as much K^+ as the entire extracellular fluid, so rapid sequestration of ingested K^+ into intracellular fluid is needed to prevent hyperkalemia after eating. Insulin causes K^+ uptake by the liver and skeletal muscle in addition to its effects on glucose homeostasis (see Chapter 8). *Insulin infusions can be used to control hyperkalemia.*

Epinephrine stimulates K^+ movement from the extracellular fluid to the intracellular fluid. An acute K^+ load is delivered into the extracellular fluid by exercising muscle. *Secretion of epinephrine during exercise stimulates K^+ reuptake into skeletal muscle cells through the activation of the β_2 receptors.*

Disturbances in acid-base balance also affect internal K^+ distribution. In **acidosis,** some H^+ is buffered by the intracellular fluid and is associated with K^+ efflux from the cells, thereby increasing plasma K^+. In **alkalosis,** H^+ exits the cells in exchange for K^+, thereby reducing plasma K^+.

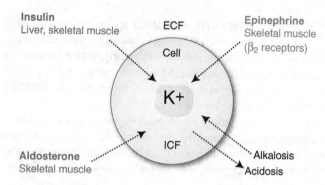

Figure 6-35: Factors affecting internal K^+ exchanges. Arrows indicate the net direction of K^+ flux between the extracellular fluid (ECF) and the intracellular fluid (ICF) in response to each stimulus.

RENAL K⁺ HANDLING

Urinary K^+ excretion varies with dietary K^+ intake. To achieve excretion of the moderate K^+ excess found in a normal diet, the *fractional K^+ excretion (FE_K) is typically 10–20%. FE_K can be 0% in states of K^+ deficiency, or it can reach 150–200% in states of K^+ excess.* Figure 6-36A summarizes segmental K^+ handling (external K^+ homeostasis). Seventy percent of filtered K^+ is reabsorbed in the proximal tubule, and an additional 25% is reabsorbed in the thick ascending limb. K^+ reabsorption at these proximal sites does not respond to changes in K^+ balance and are not physiologically regulated.

Secretion of K^+ from the principal cells in the late distal tubule and the cortical collecting duct is the most important determinant of urinary K^+ output. The mechanism of K^+ secretion by the principal cells is shown in Figure 6-36B. High intracellular K^+ activity is generated by the Na^+/K^+-ATPase in the basolateral membrane; K^+ secretion occurs through K^+ channels in the luminal cell membrane. **Aldosterone** simultaneously stimulates the principal cells to secrete K^+ while promoting Na^+ uptake. Aldosterone stimulates Na^+ influx via the Na^+ channels, causing depolarization of the luminal cell membrane and thereby increasing the driving force for K^+ secretion. Net reabsorption of K^+ is also possible in the collecting duct in states of K^+ depletion; α-intercalated cells reabsorb K^+ in exchange for H^+, via the H/K-ATPase.

An increase in Na^+ delivery to the cortical collecting duct causes an increase in K^+ secretion by the principal cells. For example, **thiazide and loop diuretics** inhibit Na^+ reabsorption upstream from the cortical collecting duct, causing high Na^+ delivery to the cortical collecting duct, which drives further K^+ secretion by the principal cells.

The presence of **luminal fixed anions,** normally not present in the cortical collecting duct, also stimulates K^+ secretion; for example, the large HCO_3^- load present in the tubule in **metabolic alkalosis.**

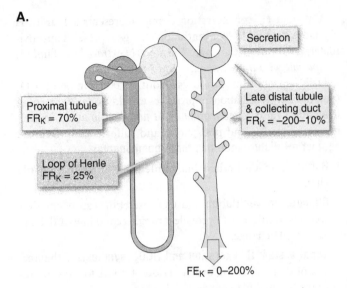

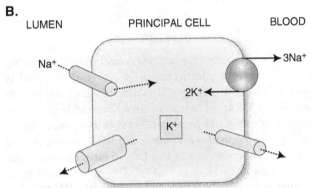

Figure 6-36: A. Segmental K^+ handling. K^+ excretion is mainly determined by secretion into the late distal tubule and the cortical collecting duct. **B.** Mechanism of K^+ secretion by the principal cells in the cortical collecting duct. K^+ enters the cell via the basolateral Na^+/K^+-ATPase and is secreted through K^+ channels into the lumen. Increased Na^+ reabsorption through Na^+ channels depolarizes the apical membrane and increases K^+ secretion.

ACID-BASE PHYSIOLOGY

Normal plasma pH is maintained within the range of 7.35 to 7.45. Regulation of pH occurs by varying CO_2 excretion from the lungs and by varying the rate of H^+ excretion and HCO_3^- production in the kidney. In most clinical acid-base problems, *the primary variables considered are pH, arterial P_{CO_2}, and $[HCO_3^-]$; the normal values are 7.40, 40 mm Hg, and 24 mmol/L, respectively.*

ACIDS AND BASES

Acids are molecules that release H^+ in solution; bases are ions or molecules that can accept H^+. Strong acids rapidly dissociate releasing large amounts of H^+; weak acids partially dissociate releasing less H^+. Strong bases react rapidly and strongly to neutralize H^+; weak bases bind less H^+. Most acids and bases encountered physiologically are "weak." The $[H^+]$ in extracellular fluid is only 0.00004 mmol/L = 40 nmol/L. The **logarithmic pH scale** is used to express these very small values:

$$pH = -\log_{10}[H^+]$$

Equation 6-8

A 10-fold H^+ concentration change represents a 1 unit pH change; a twofold H^+ concentration change represents approximately a 0.3 unit pH change. *The limits of extracellular fluid pH compatible with life are about 6.8 to 7.8.*

Daily metabolism produces about 15,000 mmol of CO_2 (**volatile acid**). Metabolism produces an additional 70 mmol of **fixed acids** (also called **metabolic or nonvolatile acid**), including organic acids and phosphoric and sulfuric acids. **Defense against pH disturbance has three components:**

1. **Buffers** provide limited but immediate limitations on pH change.

2. **Changes in ventilation** and CO_2 excretion can occur over seconds to minutes to provide a rapid second line of defense against pH change.

3. **Renal system H^+ excretion and HCO_3^- synthesis** is the final line of defense, acting over a period of hours to days to prevent sustained pH change.

BUFFERS

A buffer is a substance that can reversibly bind H^+. **Buffering power** expresses the effectiveness of a buffer system and is defined as "moles of strong acid added to 1 L of solution to reduce pH by 1 unit" or "moles of strong base added to 1 L of solution to increase pH by 1 unit." *The most important buffer in the extracellular fluid is the bicarbonate buffer system*, created by the reaction between water and CO_2 to form carbonic acid, which dissociates to H^+ and HCO_3^-. The pH resulting from this reaction is calculated from the **Henderson-Hasselbalch equation:**

$$pH = pKa + \log(HCO_3/s.Pa_{CO_2}) \qquad \textbf{Equation 6-9}$$

Ka = Dissociation constant for acid formation
    (pKa = 6.1)
s = Solubility of CO_2 (s = 0.03 mmole/mm Hg)

Example A healthy person in acid-base homeostasis has a plasma $[HCO_3^-]$ of 24 mmol/L, an arterial P_{CO_2} of 40 mm Hg, and a plasma pH of 7.4. Equation 6-9 correctly predicts this normal plasma pH:

$$pH = pKa + \log(HCO_3/s.Pa_{CO_2})$$
$$= 6.1 + \log(24/0.03 \times 40)$$
$$= 7.40$$

The Henderson-Hasselbalch equation predicts that plasma pH is a simple function of the ratio of HCO_3^- to Pa_{CO_2}. If the pH increases, it could be due to an increase in HCO_3^- (**metabolic alkalosis**) or a decrease in arterial P_{CO_2} (**respiratory alkalosis**). If the pH decreases, it could be due to a decrease in HCO_3^- (**metabolic acidosis**) or an increase in arterial P_{CO_2} (**respiratory acidosis**).

RESPIRATORY CONTRIBUTION TO ACID-BASE BALANCE

Normal pulmonary function balances CO_2 excretion with metabolic CO_2 production. Arterial P_{CO_2} is monitored primarily by central chemoreceptors (see Chapter 5); alveolar ventilation increases to excrete more CO_2 when the arterial P_{CO_2} increases and decreases when the arterial P_{CO_2} decreases.

Pulmonary pathology may result in defects in respiratory performance or control that cause acid-base disturbances. Hypoventilation results in high arterial P_{CO_2} (**respiratory acidosis**); hyperventilation results in low arterial P_{CO_2} (**respiratory alkalosis**).

Changes in CO_2 excretion can help to **compensate** for metabolic acid-base disturbances. Figure 6-37 shows that low plasma pH is a potent stimulus to increase alveolar ventilation, a response that is mediated through peripheral chemoreceptors (see Chapter 5). The resulting decrease in arterial P_{CO_2} increases the plasma pH back toward normal. An increase in plasma pH causes a smaller change in alveolar ventilation than an equivalent decrease in plasma pH. This is necessary because correction for increased pH would require low ventilation rates, which compromise oxygenation of the blood.

RENAL REGULATION OF ACID-BASE BALANCE

The kidney has two major functions related to acid-base homeostasis:

1. **Regulation of plasma [HCO$_3^-$]** in the range of 22 mmol/L to 28 mmol/L. The kidney can excrete HCO_3^-, and it can generate new HCO_3^-. Under most circumstances, the renal venous blood contains more HCO_3^- than the renal arterial blood, reflecting continuous renal HCO_3^- production. *The kidney generates just enough HCO_3^- to neutralize net acid production from metabolism.*

2. **Excretion of fixed metabolic acids.** Acid in the urine is mainly in the form of ammonium ions (NH_4^+) and phosphoric acid ($H_2PO_4^-$).

Recovery of filtered HCO_3^- and net acid excretion is usually required to maintain acid-base balance—almost all the filtered HCO_3^- must be recovered. Most HCO_3^- reabsorption occurs in the early proximal tubule via the mechanism shown in Figure 6-38. H^+ is secreted into the lumen via the Na/H exchange, where it combines with filtered HCO_3^- to form carbonic acid. The enzyme **carbonic anhydrase** is anchored to the brush-border membrane of the proximal tubular cells, where it generates CO_2 from carbonic acid. CO_2 diffuses into the proximal tubule cells, where cytoplasmic carbonic anhydrase facilitates carbonic acid formation again. H^+ and HCO_3^- are produced inside the cell from dissociation of carbonic acid. H^+ is recycled for secretion into the lumen, and HCO_3^- enters extracellular fluid via a Na/HCO_3^- cotransporter in the basolateral membrane.

▽ **Bicarbonaturia** (increased urinary HCO_3^- loss) is caused by carbonic anhydrase inhibitors such as **acetazolamide,** which disrupt tubular HCO_3^- reabsorption. **Renal tubular acidosis type 2** (or proximal renal tubular acidosis) is a condition in which HCO_3^- resorption in the proximal tubules is impaired, resulting in urinary HCO_3^- loss in the setting of systemic acidosis. ▽

Renal ammonia production accounts for approximately 75% of H^+ excretion and occurs in the form of ammonium ions (NH_4^+). The proximal and distal tubules produce ammonia (NH_3) from glutamate in the mitochondria. NH_3 consumes free H^+ and is converted to NH_4^+. Figure 6-39A shows that NH_4^+ is

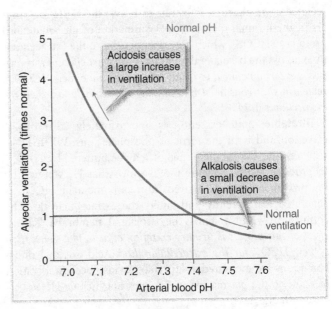

Figure 6-37: Respiratory response to altered blood pH.

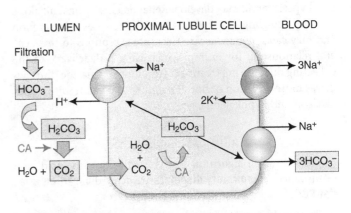

Figure 6-38: Mechanism of the proximal tubule HCO_3^- recovery. The pathway taken by filtered HCO_3^- is highlighted in yellow. The enzyme carbonic anhydrase (CA) catalyzes conversions of HCO_3^- to CO_2 via carbonic acid. Inhibition of CA by the diuretic acetazolamide causes bicarbonaturia.

secreted as an alternate substrate to H$^+$ via the Na/H exchangers in the luminal membrane. Deamination of glutamate also produces 2HCO$_3^-$, which are transported into the extracellular fluid across the basolateral membrane. *The net effect of this process is excretion of acid in urine, plus generation of new HCO$_3^-$ to replenish that consumed by buffering of metabolic acids in the extracellular fluid.*

Titratable acid excretion is approximately 25% of H$^+$ excretion and is in the form of phosphate ions. When H$^+$ is secreted into the tubule lumen, it may be buffered by HPO$_4^{2-}$ to produce H$_2$PO$_4^-$. Figure 6-39B shows that H$^+$ secreted by the proximal tubule is derived from carbonic acid; HCO$_3^-$ is generated concurrently and enters the extracellular fluid by cotransport with Na$^+$ across the basolateral membrane. *The net effect of this process is urinary excretion of acid, plus generation of new HCO$_3^-$ for the extracellular fluid.* Acid-excreted phosphate ions are measured as "titratable acids," because titration of urine to the plasma pH of 7.4 does not include H$^+$ associated with NH$_4^+$.

Acidification of urine occurs along the entire renal tubule. The proximal tubule secretes the most H$^+$, but the proximal tubular fluid pH usually does not decrease below 6.8 due to the large amount of HCO$_3^-$ and phosphate buffers present in the glomerular filtrate. The cells in the loop of Henle and the distal tubule and the principal cells in the cortical collecting duct all secrete H$^+$ via the Na/H exchange. The α-intercalated cells in the collecting duct use primary active H$^+$ secretion via the H$^+$-ATPase and H/K-ATPase.

Na/H exchange in the distal tubule and the principal cells of the cortical collecting duct is stimulated by aldosterone. ***Hyperaldosteronism** can be associated with metabolic alkalosis as a result of excessive H$^+$ secretion into the urine.*

H$^+$/K$^+$ INTERACTIONS

In many situations, there is a reciprocal relationship between the secretion of H$^+$ and K$^+$ in the collecting duct. This contributes to a general relationship in which *acidosis is associated with hyperkalemia and alkalosis is associated with hypokalemia.* For example, if the collecting duct is secreting a large amount of H$^+$ to combat a primary acidosis, then less K$^+$ is excreted and hyperkalemia may develop. Renal defense against alkalosis includes reducing H$^+$ secretion, which increases K$^+$ excretion and may cause hypokalemia. There are exceptions to this general relationship; for example, increasing Na$^+$ delivery to the collecting duct during treatment with loop or thiazide diuretics drives more secretion of both H$^+$ and K$^+$ and can result in both alkalosis and hypokalemia.

ACID-BASE DISORDERS

Figure 6-40 is an algorithm that is used to describe acid-base disturbances. **Respiratory disorders** are defined **based on arterial PCO$_2$**:

Paco$_2$ > 45 mm Hg defines respiratory acidosis.

Paco$_2$ < 35 mm Hg defines respiratory alkalosis.

Metabolic disorders can be defined **based on plasma HCO$_3^-$ concentration:**

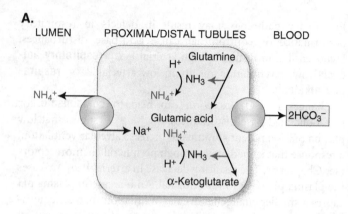

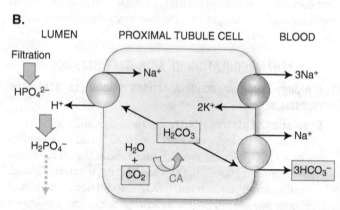

Figure 6-39: Mechanisms of H$^+$ excretion and HCO$_3^-$ generation. **A.** Renal ammoniagenesis results in the formation of NH$_4^+$ within cells because NH$_3$ readily combines with H$^+$ at physiologic pH. NH$_4^+$ is secreted via the Na/H exchangers. **B.** Titratable acid excretion as H$_2$PO$_4^-$ occurs when secreted H$^+$ combines with filtered HPO$_4^{2-}$. CA, carbonic anhydrase.

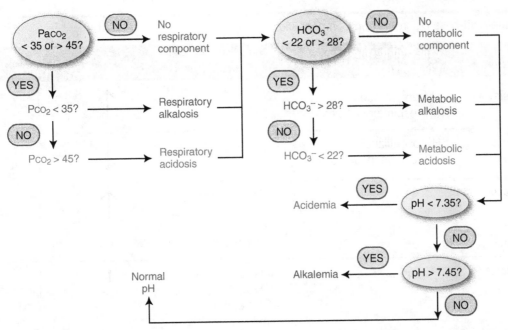

Figure 6-40: Algorithm used to describe acid-base disorders. Pa_{CO_2} defines the presence of respiratory disorders; plasma $[HCO_3^-]$ defines the presence of metabolic disorders.

- $HCO_3^- < 22$ *mEq/L defines metabolic acidosis.*
- $HCO_3^- > 28$ *mEq/L defines metabolic alkalosis.*

Base excess is another way of defining metabolic acid-base disturbances. Base excess is a calculated value that estimates the size of a metabolic disturbance independent of P_{CO_2}. It is defined as the amount of strong acid (or base), in mmol/L, needed to titrate the pH of 100% oxygenated blood to 7.4 at 37°C and at a P_{CO_2} of 40 mm Hg:

- *Base excess > 2 mmol/L defines metabolic alkalosis.*
- *A negative base excess (a base deficit) > 2 mmol/L defines metabolic acidosis.*

The most common clinical presentation is two opposing acid-base disorders in which a primary disorder is compensated by a secondary disorder. **Compensation** refers to responses that normalize plasma pH. Table 6-4 summarizes the four primary acid-base disorders and the expected pattern of physiologic compensation.

Metabolic acidosis can be caused by excess production or ingestion of fixed acids. Common examples include accumulation of **ketoacids** in diabetic patients or accumulation of **lactic acid** during hypoxia. Another common example is failure of the kidney to excrete metabolic acid in patients with **chronic renal failure.** Ingestion of poisons such as **methanol** and **ethylene glycol** or excessive ingestion of **aspirin** also results in the generation of excess fixed acids. Excess H^+ is buffered by plasma HCO_3^-, causing a decrease in plasma $[HCO_3^-]$, which defines metabolic acidosis. Elevated plasma H^+ stimulates ventilation via peripheral chemoreceptors. **Compensatory respiratory alkalosis** *is usually present, which reduces the arterial P_{CO_2} and increases the pH toward normal.* The resolution of metabolic acidosis without treatment requires increased renal generation of new HCO_3^- and increased H^+ excretion via NH_3 production and titratable acid excretion.

TABLE 6-4. Simple Acid-base Disorders and Compensation

Primary Disorder	Expected Respiratory Compensation	Expected Renal Compensation	$[H^+]$	$[HCO_3^-]$	Arterial P_{CO_2}
Metabolic acidosis	Hyperventilation (2° respiratory alkalosis)		↑	↓	↓
Metabolic alkalosis	Hypoventilation (2° respiratory acidosis)		↓	↑	↑
Respiratory acidosis		↑ H^+ excretion ↑ HCO_3^- generation (2° metabolic alkalosis)	↑	↑	↑
Respiratory alkalosis		↓ H^+ excretion ↓ HCO_3^- generation (2° metabolic acidosis)	↓	↓	↓

Red arrow, primary disorder; blue arrow, compensation; 2°, secondary.

*Metabolic acidosis can also be caused by the **loss of HCO_3^-**.* The most common example is gastrointestinal fluid loss due to **diarrhea;** however, renal HCO_3^- losses are also possible and may occur, for example, in patients with **renal tubular acidosis.** Calculation of the serum anion gap is used to help differentiate between metabolic acidosis caused by the addition of acid or the loss of HCO_3^-. **Anion gap** is calculated by subtracting the sum of serum Cl^- and HCO_3^- concentrations from serum Na^+ concentration:

$$AnionGap = [Na^+] - ([Cl^-] + [HCO_3^-]) \quad \textbf{Equation 6-10}$$

Extracellular fluid is an electroneutral solution in which the total number of anions and cations must be equal. Anion gap is normally in the range of 8–16 mEq/L, and indicates the concentration of unmeasured anions such as protein, phosphate, sulfate, and citrate. The addition of a metabolic acid consumes HCO_3^- and replaces it with a conjugate base anion (e.g., lactate ions in the case of lactic acid). This adds to the unmeasured anions, which increases the calculated anion gap. *When metabolic acidosis is caused by a loss of HCO_3^-, there is an increase in Cl^- (**hyperchloremic metabolic acidosis**) rather than the addition of other unmeasured anions, and the anion gap is normal.*

▼ Calculating the **anion gap** is helpful in approaching the differential diagnosis of **metabolic acidosis.**

1. The most common causes of **metabolic acidosis with *an increased anion gap*** are listed below. (*Note: MULEPAK can be a helpful mnemonic for remembering the causes of an anion gap metabolic acidosis.*)

Methanol ingestion

Uremia

Lactic acidosis

Ethylene glycol ingestion

- **P**araldehyde ingestion
- **A**spirin overdose
- **K**etoacidosis

2. The most common causes of **metabolic acidosis *without* an increased anion gap are:**

- Diarrhea
- Carbonic anhydrase inhibitors
- Renal tubular acidosis
- Hyperalimentation (intravenous feeding) ▼

Example A 16-year-old girl with diabetes mellitus was found unconscious and unresponsive. The results of arterial blood gas analysis showed the following abnormalities:

- P_{O_2} = 90 mm Hg
- P_{CO_2} = 36 mm Hg
- $[HCO_3^-]$ = 7 mEq/L (normal = 22–28 mEq/L)
- pH = 6.91 (normal = 7.35–7.45)
- Plasma $[Na^+]$ = 145 mEq/L
- Plasma $[Cl^-]$ = 110 mEq/L

The acid-base disorder described in the algorithm in Figure 6-40 is metabolic acidosis (low $[HCO_3^-]$) with no respiratory component (normal arterial P_{CO_2}), which is producing a severe acidemia (low plasma pH). The anion gap is calculated as follows:

$$Anion\ gap = [Na^+] - \left([Cl^-] + [HCO_3^-]\right)$$
$$= [145] - \left([110] + [7]\right)$$
$$= 28\ mEq\ /L\ (normal\ 8–16\ mEq/L)$$

Comment The patient has **diabetic ketoacidosis,** which produces an increased anion gap. A metabolic acidosis is present with no respiratory compensation, resulting in a severe life-threatening acidemia.

Metabolic alkalosis most commonly results from a loss of gastric H^+ due to **vomiting,** and results in excess HCO_3^- in the blood. A net gain of HCO_3^- by the renal system can also occur; an example is "**contraction alkalosis,**" when HCO_3^- retention occurs as a side-effect of responses to low effective circulating volume. HCO_3^- retention occurs with low effective circulating volume by a combination of a low GFR, which reduces filtered HCO_3^- load, and avid proximal tubular reabsorption. Aldosterone levels are also increased when the effective circulating volume is low, causing increased H^+ secretion by the distal nephron. Other causes of hyperaldosteronism may also cause metabolic alkalosis, including **Cushing's disease** (see Chapter 8).

Increased arterial blood pH (alkalemia) usually results in a degree of ***compensatory respiratory acidosis.*** Arterial P_{CO_2} increases as a result of reduced alveolar ventilation and decreases the pH toward normal. Physiologic correction of metabolic alkalosis requires increased renal excretion of HCO_3^-, with reduced rates of acid excretion and HCO_3^- retention.

 Metabolic alkalosis *may be either chloride sensitive or chloride resistant.* The presence of high plasma $[HCO_3^-]$

in metabolic alkalosis "displaces" Cl^- from the plasma. Patients with metabolic alkalosis are given intravenous saline solution (NaCl); if Cl^- is retained in the plasma, the $[HCO_3^-]$ is reduced and the metabolic alkalosis is Cl^- sensitive. Examples of Cl^--sensitive metabolic alkalosis include contraction alkalosis and vomiting or gastric suction. Cl^--resistant metabolic alkalosis occurs if urinary Cl^- excretion is persistently large; this occurs, for example, during active use of loop or thiazide diuretics or in tubular NaCl reabsorption disorders such as Bartter's or Gitelman's syndromes. ▼

Example A 2-year-old child who is lethargic and dehydrated has a 3-day history of vomiting. The results of arterial blood gas analysis show the following abnormalities:

- Po_2 = 90 mm Hg
- Pco_2 = 44 mm Hg
- $[HCO_3^-]$ = 37 mEq/L (normal = 22–28 mEq/L)
- pH = 7.56 (normal = 7.35–7.45)

The acid-base disorder described in the algorithm in Figure 6-40 is metabolic alkalosis (high $[HCO_3^-]$) with no respiratory component (normal arterial Pco_2), which is producing an alkalemia (high plasma pH). Treatment of the patient with saline infusion and an antiemetic agent will restore acid-base homeostasis.

Comment Metabolic alkalosis in this child was caused by a loss of HCl in gastric fluids. The alkalosis was Cl^- sensitive because fluid loss was stopped and the renal system was able to retain Cl^- and excrete HCO_3^-.

Respiratory acidosis *is caused by inadequate alveolar ventilation that results in CO_2 retention.* Inadequate ventilation may result from neuromuscular disorders, airway obstruction, or ingestion of agents that suppress breathing (e.g., narcotics). An increase in arterial Pco_2 defines respiratory acidosis, which increases plasma $[HCO_3^-]$ and $[H^+]$ through the Henderson-Hasselbalch equilibrium reaction. If respiratory acidosis occurs acutely, there is inadequate time for renal compensation. In chronic respiratory acidosis, the renal system normalizes the pH by excreting more acid and producing more HCO_3^-, which is added to extracellular fluid.

Example A 24-year-old man who is a known heroin addict was found unresponsive with a hypodermic needle in his arm. The results of arterial blood gas analysis showed the following abnormalities:

- Po_2 = 50 mm Hg (normal = 80–100 mm Hg)
- Pco_2 = 80 mm Hg
- $[HCO_3^-]$ = 23 mEq/L (normal = 22–28 mEq/L)
- pH = 7.08 (normal = 7.35–7.45)

The acid-base disorder described in the algorithm in Figure 6-40 is respiratory acidosis (high arterial Pco_2) with no metabolic component (normal $[HCO_3^-]$), which is producing a severe acidemia (low plasma pH).

Comment The patient overdosed on a narcotic that caused respiratory depression, alveolar hypoventilation, and respiratory acidosis.

Respiratory alkalosis is caused by excessive alveolar ventilation, resulting in greater CO_2 loss than production. Increased ventilation is most commonly a response to hypoxemia (e.g., ascent to high altitude; pulmonary embolism); another common cause is psychogenic hyperventilation. A low arterial P_{CO_2} decreases the plasma $[HCO_3^-]$ and $[H^+]$. If respiratory alkalosis occurs acutely, there is no time for renal compensation. In chronic respiratory alkalosis, the renal system normalizes the pH by excreting less acid and producing less "new" bicarbonate.

Example A 56-year-old man suffered a panic attack while awaiting surgery. The results of arterial blood gas analysis showed the following abnormalities:

- P_{O_2} = 112 mm Hg (normal 80–100 mm Hg)
- P_{CO_2} = 24 mm Hg
- $[HCO_3^-]$ = 23 mEq/L (normal = 22–28 mEq/L)
- pH = 7.60 (normal = 7.35–7.45)

The acid-base disorder described in the algorithm in Figure 6-40 is respiratory alkalosis (low arterial P_{CO_2}) with no metabolic component (normal plasma $[HCO_3^-]$), which is producing an alkalemia (high plasma pH).

Comment The patient's panic attack resulted in acute hyperventilation and respiratory alkalosis. The acid-base abnormality will be readily corrected when breathing returns to normal.

COMPENSATION OF PRIMARY ACID-BASE DISORDERS *Compensation refers to responses that normalize plasma pH.* Figure 6-41 illustrates compensatory responses and includes the expected size of changes in $[HCO_3^-]$ or arterial P_{CO_2}. Compensation usually is not complete, which allows the primary acid-base disorder to be recognized as the disorder that is consistent with plasma pH. For example, *if both alkalosis and acidosis are present and the pH is acidic, the acidosis must be considered the* **primary disorder,** *partially compensated by the alkalosis.*

Figure 6-41 also indicates expected changes in the arterial P_{CO_2} and $[HCO_3^-]$ during acute and chronic compensation. When $[H^+]$, $[HCO_3^-]$, and arterial P_{CO_2} differ from the expected compensatory range, the patient has a **complex acid-base**

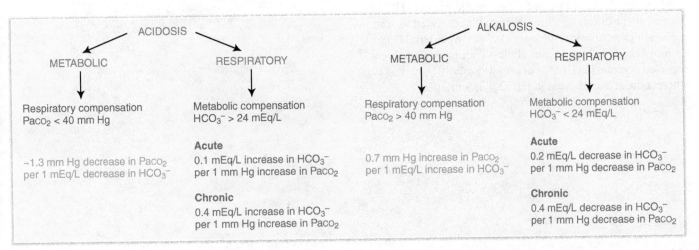

Figure 6-41: Compensatory acid-base changes. Primary acid-base disorders are usually consistent with plasma pH unless there is complete compensation. The expected degree of compensation for each primary disorder is shown.

disorder. This can arise if more than one acid-base disturbance is present with independent causes such as a trauma patient in shock, and respiratory failure can then result in primary lactic acidosis and a primary respiratory acidosis, or it can occur from prior clinical interventions such as intravenous infusion with fluids containing buffers.

▽ **Excessive aspirin ingestion** causes a mixed acid-base disorder. Aspirin uncouples oxidative phosphorylation, resulting in a primary metabolic lactic acidosis. Additionally, the direct effects of aspirin on the respiratory centers in the medulla cause the central chemoreceptors to be more sensitive to arterial P_{CO_2} levels, which results in a primary respiratory alkalosis. ▼

Example A 42-year-old man in chronic renal failure is being treated with hemodialysis. The results of arterial blood gas analysis showed the following abnormalities:

   P_{O_2} = 87 mm Hg

   P_{CO_2} = 28 mm Hg (normal = 35–45 mmHg)

   $[HCO_3^-]$ = 15 mEq/L (normal = 22–28 mEq/L)

   pH = 7.35

   Anion gap = 20 mEq/L

The acid-base disorder described in the algorithm in Figure 6-40 is metabolic acidosis (low $[HCO_3^-]$) with a respiratory alkalosis (decreased arterial P_{CO_2}) and a normal pH.

Comment The primary acid-base disorder is a chronic metabolic acidosis produced by renal failure and loss of urinary H^+ excretion. The expected respiratory compensation, as described in Figure 6-41, is approximately a 1.3-mm Hg decrease in arterial P_{CO_2} for every 1 mEq/L decrease in $[HCO_3^-]$. In this case, $[HCO_3^-]$ is 24–15 = 9 mEq/L below normal. The expected decrease in arterial P_{CO_2} is 9 × 1.3 = 11.7, which corresponds with the observed data (28 mm Hg is 12 mm Hg less than a normal average arterial P_{CO_2} of 40). The respiratory compensation is complete because pH is in the normal range. *Note: this is not a primary chronic respiratory alkalosis compensated by metabolic acidosis because the plasma pH is 7.35 and compensation never overshoots the normal pH of 7.40.* The same conclusion is indicated by the observation that the decrease in plasma $[HCO_3^-]$ in this patient differs significantly from that expected for compensation of a chronic respiratory alkalosis. An arterial P_{CO_2} of 28 mm Hg is 40–28 = 12 mm Hg less than normal, giving an expected decrease in $[HCO_3^-]$ of only 4–5 mEq/L (Figure 6-41), whereas the actual decrease in $[HCO_3^-]$ is 9 mEq/L.

STUDY QUESTIONS

Directions: Each numbered item is followed by lettered options. Some options may be partially correct, but there is only ONE BEST answer.

1. A 67-year-old woman involved in a motor vehicle accident lost 1 L of blood because of an open fracture of her left femur. Paramedics were able to prevent further bleeding. What changes to her intracellular fluid (ICF) and extracellular fluid (ECF) volumes would be observed 15 minutes after this blood loss?

    A. ECF volume smaller; ICF volume unchanged

    B. ECF volume smaller; ICF volume smaller

    C. ECF volume unchanged; ICF volume unchanged

    D. ECF volume unchanged; ICF volume smaller

2. The following pressure measurements were obtained from within the glomerulus of an experimental animal:

    Glomerular capillary hydrostatic pressure = 50 mm Hg

    Glomerular capillary oncotic pressure = 26 mm Hg

    Bowman's space hydrostatic pressure = 8 mm Hg

    Bowman's space oncotic pressure = 0 mm Hg

    Calculate the glomerular net ultrafiltration pressure (positive pressure favors filtration; negative pressure opposes filtration).

    A. +16 mm Hg

    B. +68 mm Hg

    C. +84 mm Hg

    D. 0 mm Hg

    E. −16 mm Hg

    F. −68 mm Hg

    G. −84 mm Hg

3. A novel drug aimed at treating heart failure was tested in experimental animals. The drug was rejected for testing in humans because it caused an unacceptable decrease in the glomerular filtration rate (GFR). Further analysis showed that the drug caused no change in mean arterial blood pressure but renal blood flow (RBF) was increased. The filtration fraction was decreased. What mechanism is most likely to explain the observed decrease in GFR?

    A. Afferent arteriole constriction

    B. Afferent arteriole dilation

    C. Efferent arteriole constriction

    D. Efferent arteriole dilation

4. A healthy 25-year-old woman was a subject in an approved research study. Her average urinary urea excretion rate was 12 mg/min, measured over a 24-hour period. Her average plasma urea concentration during the same period was 0.25 mg/mL. What is her calculated urea clearance?

    A. 0.25 mL/min

    B. 3 mL/min

    C. 48 mL/min

    D. 288 mL/min

5. A 54-year-old woman received a life-saving kidney transplant 6 months ago and had been well until the past few days. She now reports severe fatigue and dizziness upon standing. Urinalysis is positive for glucose, and there is excessive excretion of HCO_3^- and phosphate. In which segment of the nephron is function most likely to be abnormal?

    A. Proximal tubule

    B. Loop of Henle

    C. Distal tubule

    D. Collecting duct

6. A resident in internal medicine was called to the hospital room of an 85-year-old patient in the middle of night. The man was sitting up in bed coughing, and was severely short of breath. Crackles heard in both lungs suggested pulmonary edema. Which diuretic is most appropriate for this patient?

    A. Carbonic anhydrase inhibitor

    B. Loop diuretic

    C. Thiazide diuretic

    D. Potassium-sparing diuretic

7. A 46-year-old woman visited her family physician because she was urinating many times a day and was constantly thirsty. She was evaluated in the hospital to find out the cause of her severe polydipsia and polyuria. She was not given any fluids for 6 hours before testing, and no change in urine osmolarity was measured during this period. A nonpressor ADH agonist was then given, which produced a rapid increase in urine osmolarity. Which diagnosis is most likely to account for this patient's polydipsia and polyuria?

    A. Central diabetes insipidus

    B. Compulsive overconsumption of water

    C. Nephrogenic diabetes insipidus

    D. Type 1 diabetes mellitus

    E. Type 2 diabetes mellitus

8. A 61-year-old woman with moderate renal insufficiency ate a large amount of prunes in an effort to treat chronic constipation. She was unaware that prunes have high potassium content and the meal caused her serum potassium concentration to double. Which of the following short-term intravenous infusions would be most effective at reducing her serum potassium concentration?

A. α-Adrenoceptor agonist

B. Aldosterone antagonist

C. Dilute hydrochloric acid

D. Insulin/glucose

E. Parathyroid hormone

9. A 3-month-old infant presented with persistent vomiting and was lethargic. Arterial blood gas analysis showed the following results:

Pa_{O_2} = 88 mm Hg

Pa_{CO_2} = 44 mm Hg

pH = 7.60

$[HCO_3^-]$ = 36 mEq/L

Base excess = +12 mEq/L

Which of the following primary acid-base disturbances is present?

A. Respiratory alkalosis

B. Respiratory acidosis

C. Metabolic alkalosis

D. Metabolic acidosis

10. The results of an arterial blood gas analysis of a 56-year-old man with a history of heavy smoking are as follows:

Pa_{O_2} = 60 mm Hg

Pa_{CO_2} = 60 mm Hg

pH = 7.33

$[HCO_3^-]$ = 32 mEq/L

Base excess = +8 mEq/L

The patient has a partially compensated

A. respiratory alkalosis

B. respiratory acidosis

C. metabolic alkalosis

D. metabolic acidosis

ANSWERS

1—A. Acute blood loss is an example of isosmotic volume contraction. Volume loss is from the ECF. No change in ECF osmolarity occurs; therefore no fluid movement between the ECF and ICF occurs.

2—A. Using Equation 6-3 (in the text): $P_{UF} = P_{GC} - (\pi_{GC} + P_{GC})$. $P_{UF} = 50 - (26 + 8) = +16$ mm Hg (favoring filtration).

3—D. An increase in RBF without an increase in blood pressure indicates a decrease in renal vascular resistance. Dilation of the efferent arteriole increases glomerular capillary outflow and reduces P_{GC}, causing GFR to decrease. Filtration fraction decreases because GFR is smaller and RBF is larger.

4—C. Clearance is the ratio of excretion rate to plasma concentration. In this case, excretion rate is provided (often it must be calculated from the product of urine concentration and urine flow rate): $C_{urea} = 12$ mg/min / 0.25 mg/mL = 48 mL/min.

5—A. The patient has a condition called acquired Fanconi syndrome. The presence of high levels of glucose, HCO_3^-, and phosphate together in the urine suggest proximal tubule dysfunction because this is their main site of reabsorption.

6—B. A powerful diuretic is needed to remove fluids and reduce pulmonary edema. Inhibition of the thick ascending limb by loop diuretics provides the largest natriuresis and diuresis.

7—A. Removal of drinking water for 6 hours would increase urine osmolarity in cases of compulsive water drinking or in patients with diabetes mellitus. Restoration of urine concentration with exogenous ADH demonstrates a failure of endogenous ADH secretion and a diagnosis of central diabetes insipidus.

8—D. Acid infusion or aldosterone blockade would elevate serum potassium further. Insulin activates Na/K/ATPase and causes uptake of potassium by cells to alleviate the problem. α-Adrenoceptor agonists and PTH have no effect.

9—C. Plasma $[HCO_3^-]$ is high and base excess is elevated, defining metabolic alkalosis. There is alkalemia but no respiratory compensation.

10—B. The patient has high Pa_{CO_2} (respiratory acidosis) and high plasma HCO_3^- (metabolic alkalosis). The pH remains acidic, indicating that the primary disorder is the acidosis, which has been partially compensated. This is a chronic condition. The expected compensation for this condition is an increase of 0.4 mEq/L HCO_3^- for every 1 mm Hg increase in Pa_{CO_2}.

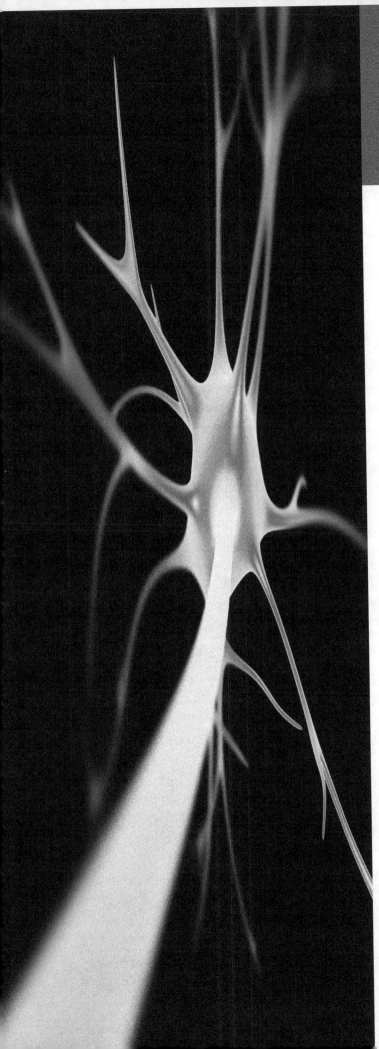

CHAPTER 7

GASTROINTESTINAL PHYSIOLOGY

THE GASTROINTESTINAL SYSTEM

OVERVIEW

The gastrointestinal system consists of the gastrointestinal tract and the accessory exocrine glands. The **gastrointestinal tract** includes the mouth, the esophagus, the stomach, the small intestine, and the large intestine. The major **accessory glands** are the salivary glands, the liver, the gallbladder, and the pancreas.

The major functions of the gastrointestinal system are **assimilation of nutrients** and **excretion** of waste products via the biliary system. Movement of food through the gastrointestinal system (**motility**) is carefully coordinated with the delivery of appropriate fluid and enzyme solutions (**secretion**) so that the macromolecules in food can be hydrolyzed (**digestion**) and the nutrient molecules, which are liberated, can be transported into the circulatory system (**absorption**). Coordinating multiple organs and physiologic processes is a significant challenge that must be solved to achieve the overall functions of the gastrointestinal system. Elaborate control mechanisms are provided by the **enteric**

259

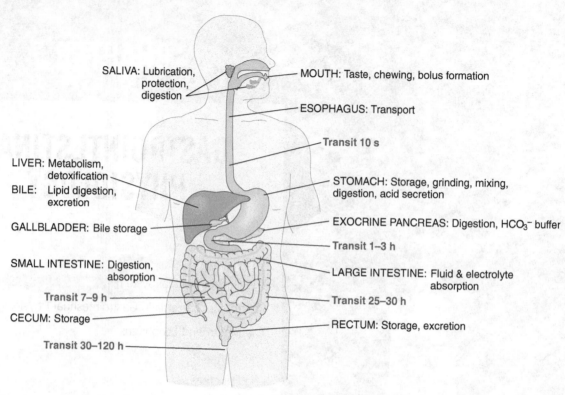

SALIVA: Lubrication, protection, digestion

MOUTH: Taste, chewing, bolus formation

ESOPHAGUS: Transport

Transit 10 s

LIVER: Metabolism, detoxification

BILE: Lipid digestion, excretion

STOMACH: Storage, grinding, mixing, digestion, acid secretion

GALLBLADDER: Bile storage

EXOCRINE PANCREAS: Digestion, HCO_3^- buffer

Transit 1–3 h

SMALL INTESTINE: Digestion, absorption

LARGE INTESTINE: Fluid & electrolyte absorption

Transit 7–9 h

Transit 25–30 h

CECUM: Storage

RECTUM: Storage, excretion

Transit 30–120 h

Figure 7-1: Functions of the gastrointestinal organs. Transit times shown are the length of time it takes food to reach each indicated point after ingestion.

nervous system (ENS), a large intrinsic network of neurons in the wall of the gastrointestinal tract, and by several hormones.

Figure 7-1 provides an overview of the main functions of each area of the gastrointestinal system during the passage of food. The following **sequence of events results in the efficient assimilation of nutrients from food:**

1. **Chewing** (mastication) of food breaks down the food to create a bolus that is suitable for swallowing. **Saliva** lubricates food and provides enzymes for digestion. It takes about 10 seconds for swallowed food to travel down the esophagus to the stomach.

2. Depending on its composition, food can remain in the **stomach** for about 1–4 hours. Stomach motility mixes and grinds food into small particles suitable for delivery to the small intestine via the pyloric sphincter. Exocrine secretions from the stomach mucosa help to dilute and dissolve food; **gastric acid** assists in dissolving and denaturing the components of food.

3. Entry of food into the small intestine is coordinated with the delivery of major **exocrine secretions** from the **biliary system** and the **pancreas.** *The pancreas is essential for digestion because it produces numerous enzymes.* The pancreas also secretes HCO_3^-, which neutralizes acid from the stomach. Contractions of the **gallbladder** deliver stored **bile** to the intestine. Bile acids are the major organic component of bile and are important for lipid assimilation.

4. Food moves through the **small intestine** within 7–10 hours. Motility patterns in the fed state mix food with digestive enzymes and distribute nutrients throughout the absorptive surface. *All significant absorption of nutrients occurs in the small intestine.*

▶. Transit through the **large intestine,** from the **cecum** to the **sigmoid colon,** usually occurs over a period of 12–24 hours. The functions of the large intestine include fluid and electrolyte transport and fermentation of undigested carbohydrates (e.g., cellulose). Storage of fecal waste occurs in the distal large intestine; elimination of fecal waste typically occurs within 1–3 days after ingestion of a meal.

▽   Gastric emptying is a key control point in the gastrointestinal tract to ensure the orderly delivery of nutrients in a form that can be digested and to give appropriate signals of fullness (satiety). **Gastroparesis ("weak stomach")** is a common complication of poorly controlled diabetes mellitus and significantly slows gastric emptying. *Gastroparesis causes early satiety and erratic stomach emptying, which can result in poor nutrient assimilation, making it more difficult to control blood glucose levels.* ▼

STRUCTURAL FEATURES OF THE GASTROINTESTINAL TRACT

There are **four major histologic layers** in the gastrointestinal tract, starting from the gut lumen and moving outward: mucosa, submucosa, muscularis externa, and serosa (Figure 7-2).

1. The **mucosa** is the most variable zone and consists of an epithelium, which is a single cell layer from the stomach to the anus. In most areas, the epithelium is highly folded to increase its surface area (e.g., for absorption) and is frequently invaginated to form the tubular exocrine glands. Exocrine secretions include mucus, electrolytes, water, and digestive enzymes. Numerous **endocrine cells** are also scattered among epithelial cells. Endocrine cells release **gastrointestinal hormones** into the blood in response to changes in the luminal environment; for example, the hormone **cholecystokinin** is released in response to fat and protein in the gut lumen. The epithelium is supported by a connective tissue lamina propria, which contains microvasculature and

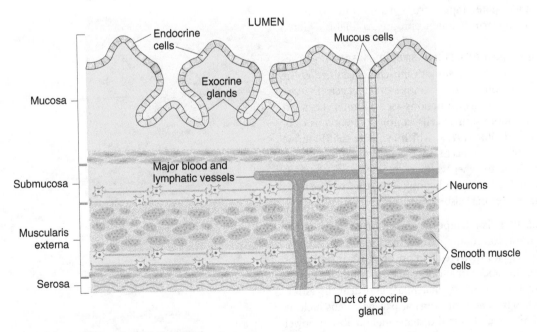

Figure 7-2: Structural features of the gastrointestinal tract.

nerves, and by a thin smooth muscle layer, the muscularis mucosae.

2. The **submucosa** is a layer of connective tissue that contains the major blood and lymphatic vessels that serve the gastrointestinal tract. This area also contains numerous ganglion cells organized to form the **submucosal (Meissner) nerve plexus.**

3. The **muscularis externa** contains the two major smooth muscle layers responsible for mixing and moving food along the gastrointestinal tract: the inner circular layer and the outer longitudinal layer. The **myenteric (Auerbach) nerve plexus** lies between the two layers of muscle.

4. The **serosa** is a thin connective tissue layer that is continuous with the peritoneal mesentery in most locations. Several major structures enter through the serosa, including blood vessels, extrinsic nerves, and the ducts of the large accessory exocrine glands.

▽ The peritoneal organs are covered by a serosa, whereas extraperitoneal or retroperitoneal organs are covered by an adventitia (loose connective tissue). The thoracic esophagus is an extraperitoneal structure and is therefore covered by an adventitia. *The lack of a serosal covering of the esophagus is thought to facilitate early spread of* **esophageal cancer.** ▽

CONTROL MECHANISMS IN GASTROINTESTINAL PHYSIOLOGY

Successful assimilation of nutrients requires the coordination of multiple organs, and is achieved by a series of overlapping controls that are applied through neural, hormonal, and paracrine mechanisms. The major regulated processes that can generate change (effectors) in the gastrointestinal physiology are **gut motility, epithelial secretion,** and **blood flow.** Each of these processes has a level of intrinsic activity, referred to as **gastrointestinal tone.** Inputs from nerves and hormones are integrated with intrinsic tone to produce a final integrated response.

The control of **gastrointestinal smooth muscle** underlies gut motility. Gastrointestinal smooth muscle is classified as the visceral type and is composed of bundles of small cells that are electrically coupled via gap junctions (see Chapter 1). Most gastrointestinal smooth muscle cells exhibit spontaneous electrical activity called **slow waves,** which facilitate the rhythmic muscle contractions that occur in the gastrointestinal tract. Action potentials occur when voltage-operated Ca^{2+} channels open, resulting in Ca^{2+} entry and contraction. Ca^{2+} release from the intracellular stores may also trigger contraction.

▽ **Paralytic ileus** is a temporary cessation of gut motility that is most commonly caused by abdominal surgery. Other common causes that result in an ileus are infection or inflammation in the abdominal cavity (e.g., appendicitis), electrolyte abnormalities (e.g., hypokalemia), and drug ingestion (e.g., narcotics). Signs and symptoms of paralytic ileus include nausea and vomiting, abdominal distension, and absent bowel sounds. ▽

ENTERIC NERVOUS SYSTEM

The ENS is a division of the autonomic nervous system (see Chapter 2). It is a large neural network located within the wall of the gastrointestinal tract, and can be viewed as a displaced part of the central nervous system (CNS) that is concerned with regulating gastrointestinal function. The ENS can be thought of as a "**minibrain**" with independent information processing capability. It contains a "**program library**" that initiates patterns of gastrointestinal activity (e.g., interdigestive, digestive, and emetic activity). *The ENS is responsible for much of the moment-to-moment control of gut motility and secretion.*

The ENS is arranged as myenteric and submucosal nerve plexuses (Figure 7-3A).

- The **myenteric plexus** is mainly involved with control of gut motility and innervates the longitudinal and circular smooth muscle layers.

- The **submucosal plexus** coordinates intestinal absorption and secretion through its innervation of the glandular epithelium, intestinal endocrine cells, and submucosal blood vessels.

▽ **Hirschsprung's disease** is a congenital absence of the myenteric plexus, usually involving a portion of the distal colon. The pathologic aganglionic section of large bowel lacks peristalsis and undergoes continuous spasm, leading to a functional obstruction. *The normally innervated proximal bowel dilates as a result of the obstruction and can lead to the most feared complication of Hirschsprung's disease,* **toxic megacolon!** ▽

In addition to its anatomic complexity, the ENS utilizes many different **neurotransmitters,** including acetylcholine, adenosine triphosphate (ATP), nitric oxide, and numerous peptides.

- *Acetylcholine is the primary neurotransmitter involved in the stimulation of secretion and motility.*

- ATP and nitric oxide function as inhibitory neurotransmitters.

- Numerous peptide neurotransmitters are found in both the ENS and the CNS and are referred to as **gut-brain peptides.** An example of a peptide neurotransmitter is **vasoactive intestinal polypeptide (VIP),** which is a potent stimulator of intestinal fluid and electrolyte secretion but inhibits motility.

▽ **Anticholinergic drugs** such as amitriptyline, a tricyclic antidepressant, inhibit the effects of acetylcholine systemically, resulting in a myriad of side effects. Gastrointestinal side effects include xerostomia (dry mouth), constipation, ileus, and nausea and vomiting. ▽

GUT-BRAIN AXIS Although the ENS can function without other connections, it is linked with the CNS via the parasympathetic and sympathetic nerves, giving rise to the concept of a **gut-brain axis** (see Figure 7-3B). The CNS may send "command signals" to the ENS, which link gastrointestinal activity with behavior; for example, salivation and gastric secretion occur in response to the thought or smell of food. *Emotions can also have a profound effect on gut physiology via the gut-brain axis (e.g., diarrhea induced by anxiety). The link between the gut and the brain also conveys sensory input to the CNS, giving rise to the conscious sensations of fullness, satiety, nausea, and pain.* The **link between**

A.

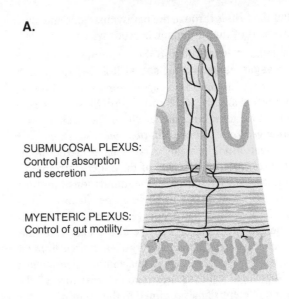

SUBMUCOSAL PLEXUS:
Control of absorption
and secretion

MYENTERIC PLEXUS:
Control of gut motility

B.

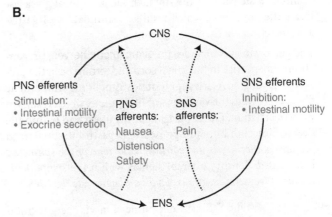

Figure 7-3: A. The enteric nervous system (ENS). The ENS is functionally organized as the submucosal plexus and the myenteric plexus. **B.** The gut-brain axis. The ENS is linked to the central nervous system (CNS) via the sensory and motor nerves of the parasympathetic nervous system (PNS) and the sympathetic nervous system (SNS).

the ENS and the CNS is through the parasympathetic and sympathetic divisions of the autonomic nervous system.

■ **Parasympathetic innervation** to the gastrointestinal system is via the **vagus nerve** and the **sacral (S2–S4) spinal outflow.** Long preganglionic axons arise from nerve cell bodies in the brainstem and the sacral spinal cord. Most fibers exert their effect by ending on ganglia within the ENS. *Efferent innervation generally causes* **excitation** *(more secretion, more propulsive motility).* The vagus nerve is particularly important in the control of the activity of the upper gastrointestinal tract during the fed state, with the stimulation of motility in the stomach and upper small intestine. It also stimulates gastric secretion, pancreatic secretion, and contraction of the gallbladder to deliver bile to the small intestine. *Parasympathetic nerves contain sensory afferent fibers from the gastrointestinal tract, which convey nonpainful distension and nausea.* **Vagovagal reflexes** are responses that involve the afferent and efferent signals confined to the vagus nerve; for example, distension of the stomach during a meal gives rise to an afferent signal, which results in stimulation of gastric acid secretion via the vagal efferents.

■ The gut-brain axis includes the **sympathetic nerves;** preganglionic fibers arise in the spinal cord and terminate in the prevertebral ganglia. A rich supply of postganglionic sympathetic fibers innervates the vascular smooth muscle, which results in vasoconstriction. Other postganglionic fibers end within the ENS to direct inhibitory responses in the gastrointestinal tract; *propulsive motility is decreased and the tone of the sphincters is increased.* Sensory afferent signals within the *sympathetic nerves convey the sensations of pain and nausea to the CNS.*

ROLE OF THE IMMUNE SYSTEM Communication via the gut-brain axis involves the immune system. Neuroimmune regulation in the intestines includes the **mast cells,** which are sensitive to a range of neurotransmitters and therefore can process information from the brain. The participation of mast cells in response to foreign antigens, through the release of mediators such as **histamine,** also provides a means of directly linking sensory information from the gut lumen to responses of the epithelial cells and smooth muscle.

GASTROINTESTINAL HORMONES Hormones play a prominent role in the control of gastrointestinal function, and in most cases these hormones are secreted by the gastrointestinal mucosa itself. Figure 7-4 summarizes the sites of secretion, the stimuli for secretion, and the actions of the major gastrointestinal hormones. Gastrointestinal hormones are peptides, most of which are also found as neurotransmitters in the ENS and CNS, giving rise to the term **gut-brain peptides.** The release of hormones is influenced by the chemical environment in the lumen of the gastrointestinal tract; **enteroendocrine cells** have microvilli-bearing receptors that "taste" the gut lumen, allowing the cells to secrete hormone at the appropriate time. The timing of hormone secretion is also guided by "crosstalk" with the ENS. Gastrointestinal hormones are first secreted into the capillary blood in the gastrointestinal tract and must pass through the portal venous system and liver before entering the systemic circulation, a process known as **first-pass metabolism.**

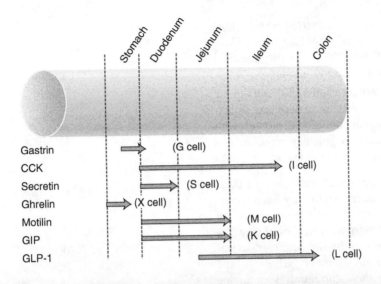

Hormone	Source	Stimulus for Secretion	Target Organ	Actions
Gastrin	G cells, antrum of stomach	• Amino acids in stomach • Distension of stomach • Vagus nerve (acetylcholine)	Stomach	↑ H⁺ secretion
CCK	I cells, duodenum and jejunum	Fat and protein digestion products in small intestine	Gallbladder Pancreas	↑ Contraction ↑ Enzyme secretion ↓ Gastric emptying
Secretin	S cells, duodenum	H⁺ in duodenum	Pancreas Stomach	↑ Pancreatic HCO_3^- secretion ↓ Gastric H⁺ secretion
Ghrelin	X cells, body of stomach	Hypoglycemia	CNS	↑ Food intake ↑ Growth hormone secretion
Motilin	M cells, duodenum and jejunum	ENS "clock"	Stomach Duodenum	↑ Contraction
GIP	K cells, duodenum and jejunum	Glucose and fats in small intestine	Pancreas	↑ Insulin secretion
GLP-1	L cell, jejunum and ileum	Glucose in small intenstine	Pancreas	↑ Insulin secretion

Figure 7-4: Gastrointestinal peptide hormones. Arrows indicate the areas of the gastrointestinal tract from which each hormone is secreted. Endocrine cells are scattered among the mucosal layer. The table summarizes the stimuli for hormone secretion and the major hormonal actions. CCK, cholecystokinin; GIP, glucose-dependent insulinotropic polypeptide (or gastric inhibitory peptide); GLP-1, glucagon-like peptide-1; CNS, central nervous system; ENS, enteric nervous system.

First-pass metabolism is an important concept that spans many topics, particularly pharmacology. Orally administered drugs that are absorbed in the gastrointestinal tract must enter the hepatic portal circulation prior to becoming systemically available to other areas of the body. The hepatic portal vein carries nutrients, gastrointestinal hormones, and absorbed drugs directly from the gut to the liver. *Many drugs are significantly metabolized by the liver enzymes, which reduces the amount of drug that is "bioavailable" to other areas of the body.*

PARACRINE CONTROL Paracrine control is exerted when a hormone diffuses locally to affect target cells (see Chapter 8). Three major examples of **paracrine mediators** in gastrointestinal physiology are serotonin, somatostatin, and histamine.

1. **Serotonin** is produced by **enterochromaffin (EC) cells** in the intestinal mucosa in response to distension of the gut wall. It exerts most of its effects indirectly through interactions with the ENS. *The effects of serotonin are generally excitatory and result in increased intestinal motility and secretion.*

▽ **Carcinoid tumors** arise from the EC cells. Because these cells originate as neuroendocrine cells, they often secrete hormones, most commonly serotonin. Systemic release of serotonin results in **carcinoid syndrome** with clinical manifestations of flushing, diarrhea, bronchospasm, and cardiac valvular disease. When carcinoid tumors arise in the gastrointestinal tract, they are most commonly seen in the ileum; the serotonin is secreted into the hepatic portal circulation, which undergoes first-pass metabolism. Serotonin is rapidly metabolized in the liver, resulting in very little systemic serotonin. *Carcinoid syndrome will manifest once the tumor has metastasized to the liver and can release serotonin directly into the systemic circulation.* ▽

2. *Somatostatin is a peptide produced by **D cells** and is a potent inhibitor substance in the gastrointestinal system.* It may be released both into the blood to act in an endocrine fashion and also as a paracrine mediator. Somatostatin inhibits pancreatic and gastric secretion, relaxes the stomach and gallbladder, and decreases nutrient absorption in the small intestine. These actions result partly from inhibition of several other stimulatory gut hormones, including gastrin, secretin, gastric inhibitory peptide (GIP), and motilin.

▽ **Ruptured esophageal varices** can cause severe bleeding into the gastrointestinal tract. Somatostatin analogues (e.g., octreotide) are used to reduce bleeding from ruptured esophageal varices, and are effective because somatostatin is a potent gastrointestinal vasoconstrictor. ▽

3. *Local release of **histamine** in the stomach has a potent stimulatory effect on acid secretion.* **Enterochromaffin-like (ECL) cells** are the source of histamine released as a paracrine mediator in the stomach.

▽ Cimetidine is a **histamine (H_2)-receptor blocker.** H_2-receptors are found on the parietal cells and stimulate gastric acid secretion. *When the H_2-receptors are blocked, the volume and acidity of gastric juice are reduced.* ▽

THE MOUTH AND ESOPHAGUS

MASTICATION

Chewing (mastication) reduces the particle size of food and increases its exposure to saliva. This process lubricates food for swallowing and also aids in carbohydrate digestion by the enzyme **salivary amylase.** The distribution of foodstuffs around the mouth during chewing stimulates the taste receptors.

Although chewing is a voluntary act, it is largely coordinated by the reflex centers in the brainstem.

SALIVARY SECRETION

Saliva secreted from each of several salivary glands is mixed together in the mouth to produce a composite juice that is mildly alkaline. The **volume of saliva** produced is approximately 1.5 L per day.

- **The submandibular glands** secrete approximately 70% of saliva.
- **The parotid glands** secrete 25%.
- **The sublingual glands** secrete 5%.

Although located at different sites, each of the salivary glands is histologically similar. A **salivon** is the functional unit of a salivary gland and consists of clusters of acinar cells that drain via a duct system (Figure 7-5A). Acinar cells secrete proteins (e.g., the enzyme salivary amylase) in an isotonic electrolyte solution. Duct cells modify the primary saliva by absorbing NaCl (see Figure 7-5B).

FUNCTIONS OF SALIVA The three major **functions of saliva** are lubrication, protection, and digestion.

1. **Lubrication** includes moistening the mouth as well as lubricating the food to aid swallowing. Saliva facilitates movements of the mouth and tongue for speech and helps to dissolve chemicals within food for its presentation to the taste receptors.

2. **Protection** relates to reducing the adverse effects of oral bacteria (e.g., dental caries). The alkalinity of fresh saliva neutralizes acid produced by oral bacteria; the flow of saliva across the teeth also helps to wash away bacteria. Saliva contains additional **substances that reduce bacterial growth.**

   - **Lysozyme** attacks bacterial cell walls.
   - **Lactoferrin** chelates iron, which is needed by many bacteria for replication.
   - **Immunoglobin A (IgA)-binding protein** is required for the immunologic activity of IgA.

3. The **digestive** function of saliva is to begin the breakdown of carbohydrates and fats via the enzymes α-amylase and lingual lipase.

   - **α-Amylase** hydrolyzes starches. *It has a pH optimum of 7, but remains active in the stomach because a high proportion of a meal remains unmixed for many minutes in the stomach.* α-Amylase can break down up to 75% of the starch in a meal before the enzyme is denatured by gastric acid.
   - **Lingual lipase** hydrolyzes triglycerides and is secreted by the small salivary glands present on the surface of the tongue. *It has an acidic pH optimum and remains active in the stomach.*

▽ **Sjögren's syndrome** is an autoimmune disease that destroys the exocrine glands and most commonly affects tear and saliva production. The hallmark manifestations of Sjögren's syndrome are dry eyes and dry mouth, known as **sicca symptoms.** Patients with **xerostomia** (dry mouth) lack

A.

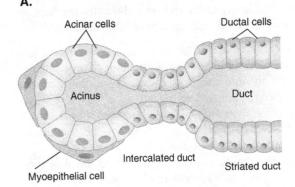

B.

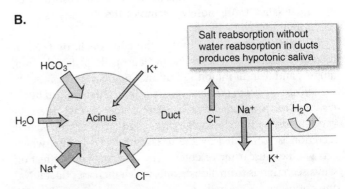

Salt reabsorption without water reabsorption in ducts produces hypotonic saliva

Figure 7-5: The salivon. **A.** The functional unit of the salivary gland consists of acinar cells, which secrete primary saliva into a duct system. **B.** Primary saliva secreted by the acinus is an isotonic solution resembling interstitial fluid; the duct reabsorbs NaCl (but not water), causing saliva to become hypotonic.

adequate saliva. They typically have dental caries and halitosis due to bacterial overgrowth and have difficulty speaking or swallowing solid food due to inadequate lubrication. ▼

MECHANISM OF SALIVA SECRETION An isotonic primary secretion is formed by **salivary acini.** The contraction of myoepithelial cells moves fluid into the striated ducts via a short, narrow structure called the intercalated duct.

Saliva becomes hypotonic because the striated duct cells reabsorb NaCl, but not water. Figure 7-6 shows the relationship between the composition of final saliva and the rate of saliva collection at the mouth (salivary flow rate). At low flow rates, the duct cells reduce saliva osmolarity to about 100 mOsm/L; at high flow rates, there is less time for the ducts to absorb NaCl, and final saliva more closely resembles the primary isotonic solution produced by the acini.

Salivation is stimulated by the thought, smell, or taste of food by conditioned reflexes and by nausea. Sleep, dehydration, fatigue, and fear all inhibit salivation. *Stimuli are integrated by the salivary nuclei in the pons, and salivation is determined by the resulting parasympathetic tone.* Efferent nerves reach the salivary glands via the glossopharyngeal and facial nerves. Acinar secretion is stimulated by the release of acetylcholine, which acts via the muscarinic receptors. The only hormonal effect on saliva secretion is from aldosterone, which increases ductal Na^+ absorption and K^+ secretion.

SWALLOWING

Swallowing (deglutition) carries food from the pharynx into the esophagus. There is a **voluntary stage** when food is shaped into a bolus, collected on the tongue, and pushed into the pharynx. The tongue is then raised against the hard palate to create a pressure gradient that forces the bolus into the pharynx and beyond. When food enters the pharynx, the following involuntary events of the **swallowing reflex** occur:

- The nasopharynx is closed by the **soft palate.**

- Food is prevented from entering the airway by elevation and forward displacement of the larynx and deflection of the food bolus by the **epiglottis.**

- The **upper esophageal sphincter** relaxes to allow the bolus to enter the esophagus. *The upper esophageal sphincter tone prevents the aspiration of the esophageal contents into the airway.* It also prevents the entry of air into the esophagus, since the esophageal body exists at below atmospheric pressure in the thorax.

The above events are coordinated by a center in the reticular formation, which also inhibits breathing until food is in the esophagus. *The oral and pharyngeal component of swallowing is controlled solely by extrinsic nerves.* Neurologic damage (e.g., the result of a **stroke**) can adversely affect this phase of swallowing.

ESOPHAGUS

The function of the esophagus is to move food and liquid to the stomach and to keep it there. The esophagus has **three functional zones:**

1. The **upper zone,** which is 6–8 cm long, is closely related to the pharyngeal musculature and consists of striated muscle.

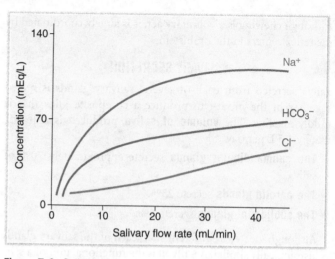

Figure 7-6: Salivary flow rate curves. The salivary ducts reabsorb NaCl without water, causing saliva to become hypotonic. Saliva is more hypotonic at slow flow rates because ducts have more time to reabsorb NaCl.

2. The **middle zone** (main body), which is 12–14 cm long, consists of smooth muscle.

3. The **lower zone,** which is 3–4 cm long, consists of smooth muscle and corresponds with the **lower esophageal sphincter.**

The area of the esophagus between the upper and lower esophageal sphincters remains quiescent until called upon to transport gas, fluids, or solids. Swallowing induces a wave of peristalsis in the esophagus known as **primary peristalsis.** If this wave is insufficient to move a bolus all the way to the stomach, distension of the esophageal wall by a remaining bolus induces **secondary peristalsis,** which is repeated until the bolus enters the stomach.

The technique of **esophageal manometry,** in which pressures are simultaneously measured at several locations along the esophagus, is used to assess swallowing and esophageal function (Figure 7-7). The **resting esophagus** has several notable features, including:

- Resting pressures are high at the **upper and lower esophageal sphincters** because both sphincters exhibit continuous resting smooth muscle tone.

- In the lumen of the **body of the esophagus** above the diaphragm, pressure is subatmospheric because the esophagus is passing through the intrathoracic space.

A different pattern of esophageal pressures is observed **upon swallowing:**

- The **upper esophageal sphincter briefly relaxes,** allowing the food bolus to pass into the esophagus.

- A **contractile (peristaltic) wave** sweeps down the esophagus.

- The **lower esophageal sphincter and the proximal stomach relax** to allow the bolus to enter the stomach.

 Gastroesophageal reflux disease (GERD) occurs when the lower esophageal sphincter is incompetent, allowing

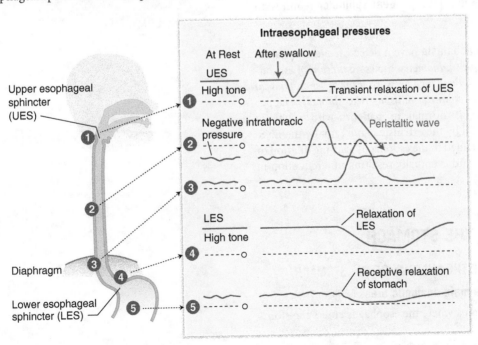

Figure 7-7: Esophageal manometry. Pressure sensors are located at each numbered location. Intraesophageal pressures are shown by solid lines; dashed lines indicate atmospheric (zero) pressure. The arrow indicates the moment at which a solid bolus was swallowed.

the flow of gastric juices and contents back into the esophagus. Factors that reduce the lower esophageal sphincter tone and predispose to GERD include smoking, obesity, pregnancy, hiatal hernia, and smooth muscle relaxants (e.g. nitroglycerin, blockers, and calcium channel blockers). Systemic diseases such as scleroderma can also affect the lower esophageal sphincter. GERD presents clinically as "**heartburn**" (substernal chest pain) and a sour taste in the mouth. However, reflux of acid is a common trigger for cough and asthma-like symptoms or more rarely a cause of aspiration pneumonitis.

Recurrent reflux of gastric acids damages the esophageal mucosa causing esophagitis, esophageal ulcers, and strictures. *Chronic esophagitis can induce a metaplastic change in the esophageal mucosa.* **Barrett's esophagus** *is a gastrointestinal metaplasia of the lower esophagus that results from chronic GERD-induced esophagitis.* This is the body's attempt to protect the esophagus from further damage. However, the transformation from squamous epithelium to intestinal epithelium (metaplasia) predisposes the cells to undergo dysplasia and eventual development of adenocarcinoma. As such, *Barrett's esophagus is the main risk factor for adenocarcinoma of the lower esophagus. (Note: carcinoma of the upper esophagus is typically squamous cell carcinoma and is related to smoking and alcohol consumption.)* ▼

The **control of swallowing** and esophageal peristalsis involves interaction between the extrinsic nerves and the ENS.

- The **upper esophageal sphincter** is part of the pharyngeal musculature and is controlled by the extrinsic cranial nerves.

- The **peristaltic wave** is coordinated by the ENS and involves a wave of relaxation preceding a wave of contraction. Relaxation is mediated by the neurotransmitter nitric oxide, and contraction is mediated by the release of acetylcholine.

- Relaxation of the **lower esophageal sphincter** requires an intact ENS.

▼ Patients with **achalasia** have a defect in the esophageal ENS. *Esophageal manometry shows disruption of esophageal peristalsis and sustained high pressure at the lower esophageal sphincter because the sphincter fails to relax properly.* Upper esophageal function is normal in patients with achalasia because it is controlled by the extrinsic nerves, not by the ENS. Swallowed food is retained in the esophagus, causing dilation of the esophageal body and eventually resulting in a reduction in peristalsis. ▼

THE STOMACH

OVERVIEW OF THE ANATOMY OF THE STOMACH

The stomach has **five main anatomic areas** (Figure 7-8):

1. **The cardia** is the area where the esophagus enters the stomach.
2. The **fundus** is the rounded area above the cardiac area.
3. The **body of the stomach** is below the cardiac region.

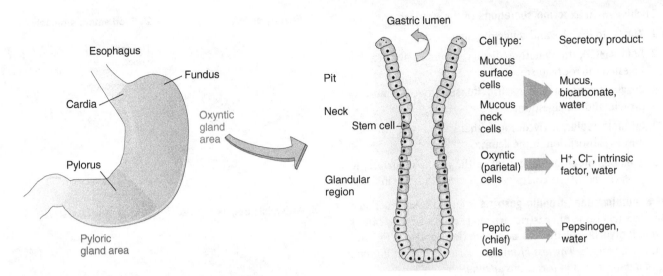

Figure 7-8: Cell types and secretory products of gastric glands.

4. The **gastric antrum** is the distal part of the stomach.

5. The **pyloric sphincter** guards the exit of the stomach into the small intestine.

From a functional perspective, the cardia, the fundus, and the body of the stomach comprise the **oxyntic (parietal) gland area,** which occupies roughly the proximal 80% of the stomach. The major exocrine secretions are all derived from this area. The **pyloric gland area** is the major source of gastric hormones, and comprises the distal 20% of the stomach.

The stomach mucosa consists of **gastric pits** and **gastric glands** (Figure 7-8). The surface mucosa and pits are lined by mucous cells. The oxyntic glands project downward and are composed of the **oxyntic (parietal) cells,** which secrete **hydrochloric acid (HCl)** and **intrinsic factor,** and the **peptic (chief) cells,** which secrete **pepsinogen.** Gastric glands in the antrum and pyloric area consist of endocrine cells, which secrete **gastrin** and **somatostatin.**

▽ **Gastritis** (inflammation of the gastric mucosa) has many causes, but it is most commonly caused by an infection by the bacteria *Helicobacter pylori.* Other common causes include smoking, use of alcohol and nonsteroidal anti-inflammatory drugs (NSAIDs), and chronic stress. *Regardless of the cause, if the surface epithelium of the stomach is acutely damaged, it rapidly regenerates in a process called* **restitution.** This repair results from rapid division of **stem cells,** which are located in the neck of gastric glands. ▽

OVERVIEW OF GASTRIC FUNCTIONS

The stomach is an important control point in the gastrointestinal tract because it must regulate the delivery of ingested food to the small intestine and present it at an appropriate rate and in a form that can be digested. This is achieved by integration of the following gastric **motor and exocrine functions:**

The **motor (motility) functions** of the stomach include acting as a reservoir for ingested food, followed by mixing and grinding of food prior to its regulated delivery into the small intestine.

The five main **exocrine secretions** of the stomach are:

1. **Water,** to dissolve and dilute ingested food.

2. **Acid** (HCl), to denature dietary proteins and to kill ingested microorganisms.

3. **Enzymes (pepsin and gastric lipase),** to contribute to protein and fat digestion.

4. **Intrinsic factor,** a glycoprotein that is necessary for vitamin B_{12} absorption in the ileum.

5. A **mucus-bicarbonate barrier** at the mucosal surface, to protect against the corrosive properties of gastric juice.

▽   **Autoimmune atrophic gastritis** is an antibody-mediated destruction of gastric parietal cells, which causes **hypochlorhydria** (insufficient acid secretion) and a deficiency of intrinsic factor. *The loss of intrinsic factor results in vitamin B_{12} malabsorption and pernicious anemia.* ▽

Endocrine functions of the stomach include the secretion of the hormones gastrin, somatostatin, and ghrelin. Gastrin and somatostatin are produced in the gastric antrum and regulate gastric acid secretion. Ghrelin is produced in the body of the stomach and is a factor involved in the regulation of hunger and satiety (see Chapter 2).

GASTRIC MOTILITY

Patterns of stomach motility that occur in the fed state differ from those that occur in the fasting state (Figure 7-9).

During **fasting,** the stomach is almost always in a quiescent state. It is interrupted at approximately 90-minute intervals by a series of peristaltic waves called the **migrating motor complex.** During these intervals, the larger indigestible components of food remaining in the stomach after a meal are flushed out into the small intestine.

Ingestion of a meal requires transient relaxation of the proximal stomach with the arrival of each bolus of food, which is known as **receptive relaxation.** As a large amount of food accumulates in the stomach, there is gradual relaxation and dilation of the entire stomach, called **accommodation,** which allows storage of the food without an increase in intragastric pressure. *Vagovagal reflexes are important in mediating both receptive relaxation and accommodation.*

Once food is ingested, the proximal stomach exhibits slow, sustained **tonic contractions** that gradually press food into the distal stomach. *Tonic contraction of the proximal stomach determines intragastric pressure, which is the main determinant of gastric emptying of liquids.*

The distal stomach contracts rhythmically in a phase called **antral systole,** when food is mixed with gastric juice to reduce the particle size. Food is broken down by **retropulsion,** when food is forcefully reflected back from the pyloric sphincter into the stomach. The meal then becomes a suspension of partially dissolved particles called **chyme.** Peristaltic waves occur at a rate of 3–4 per minute in the distal stomach during antral systole. Each peristaltic wave pushes about 1 mL of chyme through the pyloric sphincter, which, at this stage of digestion, only allows small particles (about 0.5–2 mm) to pass through.

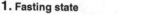
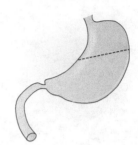
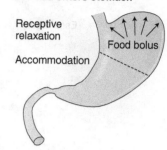
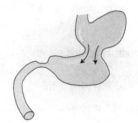
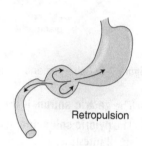

1. Fasting state

2. Food enters stomach

Receptive relaxation

Accommodation

Food bolus

3. Peristalsis begins

4. Antral systole

Retropulsion

Figure 7-9: Gastric motility. **1.** The stomach is quiescent most of the time between meals. **2.** Receptive relaxation of the proximal stomach facilitates the entry of food from the esophagus after swallowing. Accommodation is progressive relaxation of the entire stomach as it fills to prevent increased intragastric pressure during a meal. **3.** Peristalsis begins in the midstomach. **4.** Antral systole is the vigorous peristaltic rhythm in the distal stomach. Retropulsion is forceful reflection of food off the closed pyloric sphincter.

MECHANISM OF GASTRIC ACID SECRETION

Inhibitors of gastric acid secretion are among the most commonly used drugs, including both prescription and over-the-counter drugs. To understand the action of antacids, it is necessary to have a knowledge of the cellular mechanism of acid secretion and of the neuroendocrine control processes that stimulate acid secretion. The **oxyntic cells produce and secrete acid,** described as follows (Figure 7-10):

- H^+ is produced through the action of **carbonic anhydrase,** which produces carbonic acid from CO_2 and H_2O.

- The **H^+/K^+-ATPase** is used to pump H^+ from the cytoplasm into the stomach lumen in exchange for K^+. K^+ used in this exchange process is available from food or saliva, but it is also secreted via a luminal membrane K^+ channel.

- Cl^- must be secreted to yield HCl. Cl^- uptake into oxyntic cells from the extracellular fluid occurs via the **Cl^-/HCO_3^- exchange** at the basolateral cell membrane. *HCO_3^- exits the cell in such a large quantity that the gastric venous blood becomes alkaline; this is known as the **postprandial alkaline tide.***

- Cl^- is secreted into the lumen via a **Cl^- channel** in the luminal membrane, which results in the generation of a large lumen-negative transepithelial potential difference across the stomach mucosa. H^+ is transported against a large electrochemical gradient, which is reduced by a lumen-negative voltage.

▽ **Proton pump inhibitors** (e.g., omeprazole) are very potent inhibitors of the H^+/K^+-ATPase pump on the luminal surface of oxyntic (parietal) cells. *Omeprazole binds irreversibly to the H^+/K^+-ATPase pump, thereby inhibiting H^+ secretion until new H^+/K^+-ATPase protein is synthesized.* ▽

TWO-COMPONENT MODEL OF ACID SECRETION Approximately 1–2 L of gastric juice composed of mixed secretions from several cell types is produced per day. The composition of gastric juice changes with the overall secretion rate; at low secretion rates, it resembles interstitial fluid, but at high secretion rates, gastric juice becomes a solution composed primarily of HCl. The change in composition with the secretion rate is explained, as follows, by the **two-component model:**

1. The **oxyntic component** is the exocrine fluid secreted by the oxyntic cells and contains approximately 140 mM H^+, 20 mM K^+, 5 mM Na^+, and 165 mM Cl^-.

2. The **nonoxyntic component** is the collective secretions from all the other cell types present. Nonoxyntic secretion is a mildly alkaline fluid of constant composition and low volume.

When the stomach is stimulated, gastric juice is dominated by oxyntic cell secretion.

STIMULATION OF GASTRIC ACID PRODUCTION

There are several pathways that function together to stimulate gastric acid secretion. There is neural stimulation by the **vagus nerve** (which releases the neurotransmitter acetylcholine), endocrine stimulation from **gastrin,** and paracrine stimulation from **histamine.** Oxyntic cells express receptors for acetylcholine,

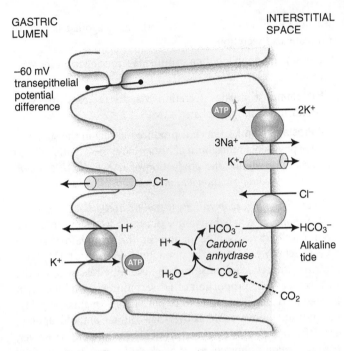

Figure 7-10: The mechanism of gastric acid secretion by the oxyntic (parietal) cells. H^+ and HCO_3^- are generated inside the cell by the action of carbonic anhydrase. H^+ is pumped across the luminal membrane by H^+/K^+-ATPase. HCO_3^- exits the basolateral membrane; the alkaline tide is the resulting alkalinity of gastric venous blood that is created during gastric stimulation. ATP, adenosine triphosphate.

gastrin, and histamine, and each individual agonist is able to stimulate acid secretion.

- **Gastrin** and **acetylcholine** stimulate secretion via an increase in intracellular Ca^{2+}.

- **Histamine** stimulates secretion via an increase in cyclic adenosine monophosphate (cAMP).

  - **Prostaglandin E_2,** which is produced locally in the stomach, is a physiologic antagonist of histamine at the oxyntic cell and acts by inhibiting the production of cAMP. ***NSAIDs** inhibit prostaglandin formation and increase gastric acid secretion.*

There is strong cooperativity between acetylcholine, gastrin, and histamine. When histamine occupies its receptor at the oxyntic cell, there is potentiation of the stimulatory action of acetylcholine and gastrin upon the secretion of H^+. Both gastrin and acetylcholine stimulate histamine release from the ECL cells; a large proportion of H^+ secretion caused by gastrin is mediated via histamine secretion. This explains why H_2-receptor antagonists, sold as over-the-counter **antacid agents,** are effective at reducing gastric acid production. However, *because proton pump inhibitors block acid secretion at the final common pathway of all agonists (the H^+/K^+-ATPase pump), these drugs are much more effective at blocking acid secretion than are the H_2-receptor antagonists.*

PHASES OF THE GASTROINTESTINAL RESPONSE The terms cephalic, gastric, and intestinal are used when describing the phases that control the gastrointestinal responses to a meal. The **cephalic phase** is characterized by the anticipation and the sight, smell, and taste of food. The **gastric and intestinal phases** overlap and refer to the period when food is present in the stomach and intestines, respectively. Significant stimulation of gastric secretion occurs during the cephalic and gastric phases, whereas there is inhibition of secretion in the stomach during the intestinal phase.

During the **cephalic phase,** several stimuli result in vagal stimulation, including the thought of a food and the smell and taste of food during chewing and swallowing. There are two ways in which **vagal innervation** stimulates H^+ secretion (Figure 7-11):

1. Direct release of **acetylcholine** by the postganglionic nerve terminals at the oxyntic cells.

2. Release of the neurotransmitter **gastrin-releasing peptide (GRP)** from the postganglionic nerves ending on the antral G cells. However, the response of gastrin secretion at this stage is relatively small because it is inhibited by low pH in the gastric lumen.

*At least 50% of the acid secretion in response to a meal occurs during the **gastric phase.*** Food entering the stomach neutralizes the acidity, which can cause the pH to increase to as high as six. At this point, the tonic suppression of gastrin secretion by low gastric pH is removed. The following two stimuli actively promote gastrin secretion:

1. **Distension of the stomach** triggers vagovagal and ENS reflexes, which stimulate G cells.

2. **Breakdown products of protein digestion** directly stimulate the G cells.

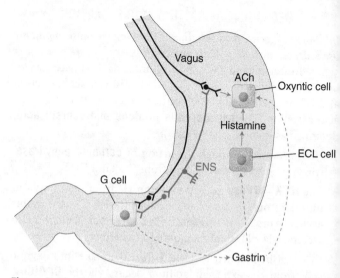

Figure 7-11: Regulation of gastric acid secretion. Efferent vagal nerve fibers and local enteric nervous system (ENS) stretch reflexes stimulate oxyntic (parietal) cells directly and stimulate antral G cells to secrete gastrin. Gastrin stimulates the oxyntic cells directly and stimulates histamine release from the enterochromaffin-like (ECL) cells. Histamine stimulates acid secretion by the oxyntic cells. ACh, acetylcholine.

▽ In **Zollinger-Ellison syndrome,** there is hypersecretion of gastric acid and peptic ulceration. Zollinger-Ellison syndrome is caused by a **gastrin-producing tumor (gastrinoma)** that is usually located in the pancreas. The *sine quo non* of gastrinoma is ulceration located distal to the duodenal bulb. About half of all patients with a gastrinoma have **multiple endocrine neoplasia syndrome.** ▽

The period between meals is referred to as the **interdigestive phase.** During the interdigestive phase, the stomach contains a small volume of very acidic gastric juice due to a continued oxyntic cell secretion at about 10% of the maximal rate.

INHIBITION OF STOMACH SECRETION AND MOTILITY

The mechanisms that inhibit gastric secretion are an important counterbalance to stimulatory mechanisms and are necessary because of the corrosive nature of gastric juices. The level of acidity in the stomach and negative feedback from the small intestinal hormones are the main ways in which gastric activity is inhibited. Gastric acid secretion is maximal about 1–2 hours after the ingestion of a balanced meal. The buffering capacity of the meal eventually becomes saturated, and the gastric pH begins to decrease; at this stage, a significant proportion of the meal has entered the small intestine. There are two ways in which a **decreasing gastric pH inhibits gastrin secretion:**

1. **Direct inhibition** of G cells by H^+ when the pH is reduced below 3.

2. **Paracrine inhibition** of G cells by **somatostatin;** the secretion of somatostatin from D cells is stimulated by low gastric pH.

Feedback inhibition of gastric H^+ secretion by the small intestine occurs due to hormones that are collectively known as **enterogastrones.** The luminal factors that trigger the release of enterogastrones include H^+, fatty acids, and hypertonicity. *Secretin is the primary enterogastrone and is released in response to the low pH in the duodenum.* Figure 7-12 illustrates the enterogastrone concept and some mechanisms that are thought to be involved in this process.

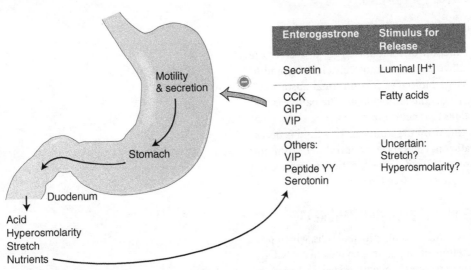

Enterogastrone	Stimulus for Release
Secretin	Luminal $[H^+]$
CCK GIP VIP	Fatty acids
Others: VIP Peptide YY Serotonin	Uncertain: Stretch? Hyperosmolarity?

Figure 7-12: Negative feedback inhibition of gastric emptying by enterogastrones. The duodenum senses acidity, osmolarity, distension, and nutrient composition of the luminal contents to gauge the rate of gastric emptying. An increase in these variables stimulates the release of the hormones shown, resulting in feedback inhibition of gastric motility and secretion. This mechanism ensures that the rate of gastric emptying is not excessive. CCK, cholecystokinin; GIP, glucose-dependent insulinotropic polypeptide; VIP, vasoactive intestinal polypeptide.

PEPSINS

Pepsins are proteolytic enzymes that attack the internal peptide bonds in proteins. They are secreted as two types of inactive **pepsinogens** in the stomach:

Type I pepsinogen is secreted in the oxyntic gland area.

Type II pepsinogen is secreted in the pyloric gland area.

The conversion of pepsinogen to pepsin occurs spontaneously when the pH is below 5; once active pepsin is present, it autocatalyses the conversion of pepsinogen to pepsin in a **positive feedback** manner. *Pepsinogen secretion is stimulated by acetylcholine from the vagal and ENS efferent neurons.* Stimuli include a local **acid-sensitive reflex** that ensures that pepsinogen is released when H⁺ is available for its conversion to pepsin.

GASTRIC MUCOSAL PROTECTION

A layer of **mucus** located at the mucosal surface serves as a barrier mechanism that prevents acid erosion of the mucosa. *This layer is effective in neutralizing acid because HCO_3^- secreted from the surface cells is trapped in the mucus* (Figure 7-13). There is no mucus layer inside the gastric glands to protect cells in this area from high levels of luminal acidity. The oxyntic cells have a thick plasma membrane for protection, and the tight junctions between oxyntic cells have a very high resistance to prevent H⁺ back-diffusion into the submucosa.

▽ **Erosive gastritis** can occur as a result of chronic use of NSAIDs. The mechanism by which NSAIDS cause gastritis involves the inhibition of prostaglandin synthesis in the stomach. *Prostaglandins normally maintain the physicochemical barrier on the gastroduodenal mucosal surface by stimulating the secretion of mucus and bicarbonate.* Loss of the protective mucus and bicarbonate barrier renders the gastric mucosa susceptible to damage by the acidic environment. ▼

THE PANCREAS

PANCREATIC FUNCTION

The main digestive function of the pancreas is to secrete the **enzymes** that break down the macromolecules in food and to produce smaller nutrient molecules for intestinal absorption. *Pancreatic enzymes are essential for digestion.* The pancreas also secretes an **alkaline fluid** that neutralizes the acidic chyme that enters the small intestine from the stomach. This fluid is necessary because pancreatic enzymes have a neutral pH optimum. The pancreas has a separate endocrine function to secrete the hormones insulin and glucagon (see Chapter 8).

STRUCTURE OF THE EXOCRINE PANCREAS

Most of the pancreas is comprised of epithelial cells, which produce an exocrine secretion of digestive enzymes in a HCO_3^--rich solution. Digestive enzymes are synthesized and secreted by grape-like acini, which consist of 20–50 pyramidal cells that surround a small luminal space. Pancreatic acini produce a low-volume, enzyme-rich fluid that drains via a series of ducts

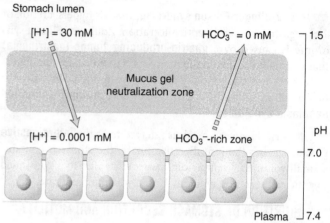

Figure 7-13: The mucus-bicarbonate barrier for gastric mucosal protection. Surface epithelial cells secrete HCO_3^-, which become trapped in a layer of mucus at the mucosal surface. H⁺ is neutralized by HCO_3^- as it diffuses through the surface mucus.

into the main pancreatic duct. **Pancreatic duct** epithelial cells produce a copious amount of **HCO₃⁻- rich fluid,** which is added to the acinar secretion. The main pancreatic duct joins the common bile duct to form a common excretory duct, which is guarded by the **Sphincter of Oddi.** Exocrine pancreatic secretions and bile enter the duodenum when the Sphincter of Oddi is relaxed. About 1–2 L of pancreatic juice, consisting of a mixture of secretions from the acini and ducts, is secreted per day (Figure 7-14).

ACINAR CELL SECRETION

Acinar cells produce hydrolytic enzymes to aid in the digestion of fats, proteins, carbohydrates, and nucleic acids. The apical region of acinar cells is packed with secretory granules awaiting a stimulus to bring about their release by exocytosis (Figure 7-15). Several hormones and neurotransmitters, called **secretagogues,** stimulate pancreatic enzyme secretion. *The two most important secretagogues are* **acetylcholine,** *secreted from vagal efferents, and the hormone* **cholecystokinin**; both of these agonists act by causing an increase in cytosolic Ca^{2+} concentration.

PREVENTION OF PANCREATIC AUTODIGESTION

Several features of **enzyme synthesis and activation** help to prevent autodigestion of the pancreas, including:

- Most enzymes are produced as inactive precursors called **zymogens.**

- Enzymes are sequestered in **membrane-limited vesicles** throughout synthesis to the point of exocytosis, avoiding contact with the acinar cell cytoplasm.

- Activation of zymogens occurs in the small intestine. The process depends on the conversion of the proenzyme trypsinogen to the active proteolytic enzyme trypsin. Trypsinogen is cleaved by the enzyme **enterokinase,** which is bound to the apical cell membranes of enterocytes lining the small intestine. *Once trypsin is activated, it cleaves and activates all other zymogens.*

- The pancreas produces a **trypsin inhibitor** to prevent activation of zymogens within the pancreas if trypsin is inappropriately activated inside the gland.

▽ **Pancreatitis** occurs when pancreatic enzymes are activated within the pancreas (and surrounding tissues), resulting in autodigestion of the tissues. *The most common causes of pancreatitis are gender specific and include gallstones in women and alcohol use in men.* Pancreatitis is a painful condition, and is classically described as an epigastric pain radiating from the epigastrium to the back and is often relieved by leaning forward. ▼

PANCREATIC DUCT

The mechanism of Na^+ and HCO_3^- secretion by the pancreatic duct cells occurs via the following steps (Figure 7-16):

- HCO_3^- secretion from the cell cytoplasm into the lumen occurs via the **Cl⁻/ HCO₃⁻ exchange** in the luminal cell membrane.

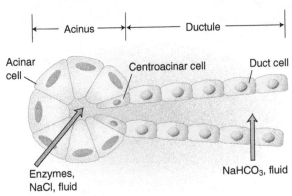

Figure 7-14: Schematic of the pancreatic structure. Pancreatic juice is a composite of two secretions; acinar cells produce enzymes in an isotonic NaCl solution, and pancreatic ducts secrete an isotonic NaHCO₃⁻ solution.

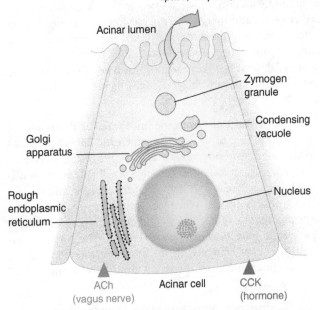

Figure 7-15: Enzyme synthesis and secretion by the pancreatic acinar cells. Enzymes are synthesized and stored in zymogen granules in the apical region of the cell. Acetylcholine (ACh) and cholecystokinin (CCK) are secretagogues that stimulate exocytosis of zymogens into the acinar lumen.

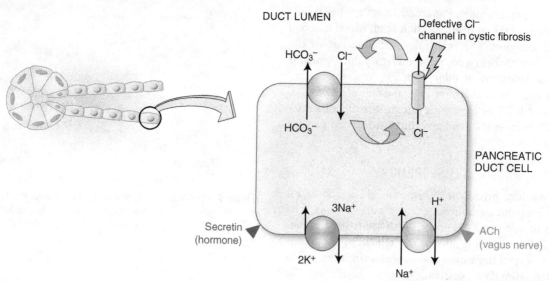

Figure 7-16: Cellular model of pancreatic duct cell secretion. HCO_3^- secretion requires Cl^- recycling via a Cl^- channel in the apical cell membrane. The channel is missing or defective in patients with cystic fibrosis, causing failure of $NaHCO_3^-$ and fluid secretion by the pancreatic ducts. ACh, acetylcholine.

- To supply enough intracellular Cl^- to sustain the rate of Cl^-/HCO_3^- exchange, Cl^- is recycled from the lumen into the cell via the **cystic fibrosis transmembrane conductance regulator (CFTR)** Cl^- channel.

- **Na^+** is secreted into the duct lumen following HCO_3^- secretion; **water** follows by osmosis to produce fluid secretion.

*Pancreatic duct cells are stimulated to secrete HCO_3^- in response to the hormone **secretin**, which acts via cAMP and opens the CFTR channels.*

▽ Patients with **cystic fibrosis** lack a functional Cl^- channel in the luminal membrane, which results in defective ductal fluid secretion. The ducts become blocked with precipitated enzymes and mucus and the pancreas undergoes fibrosis (hence the name of the disease). Blocked ducts impair secretion of needed pancreatic enzymes for digestion of nutrients, resulting in malabsorption. Treatment of this type of malabsorption includes oral pancreatic enzyme supplements taken with each meal. ▼

The composition of pancreatic juice varies with the rate of fluid secretion (Figure 7-17). The pancreatic **flow-rate curves** reflect changing proportions of acinar and ductal secretions in the pancreatic juice. Acini secrete a small volume of NaCl-rich solution, whereas duct cells produce a larger volume of a $NaHCO_3^-$-rich solution. *When the pancreas is stimulated, there is a predomination of duct cell fluid and the overall composition of pancreatic juice becomes rich in HCO_3^-. The Na^+ concentration does not change with the secretory rate because the primary acinar and duct secretions both have a similar Na^+ concentration.*

CONTROL OF PANCREATIC SECRETION

During the interdigestive state, there is only minimal secretion of pancreatic juice. Stimulation of pancreatic secretion begins during the cephalic phase of gastric acid production with the anticipation and sight, smell, and taste of food. Stimulation of

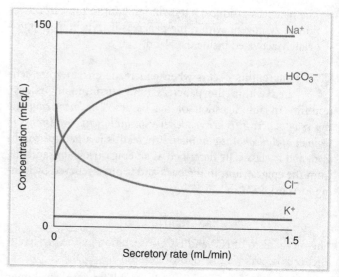

Figure 7-17: Pancreatic flow rate curves. At high flow rates, pancreatic juice becomes bicarbonate-rich due to stimulation of the pancreatic duct secretion by the hormone secretin.

the **cephalic phase** is mediated via the **vagus nerve** and the release of acetylcholine. There is minimal additional stimulation of the pancreas during the gastric phase. *Most pancreatic stimulation occurs in the* **intestinal phase** *so that secretion is coordinated when chyme enters the small intestine.*

- **CCK** stimulates acinar enzyme secretion; the secretion of CCK is stimulated by long-chain fatty acids and protein digestive products in the small intestine.

- **Secretin** stimulates ductal HCO_3^- secretion; acid entering the duodenum from the stomach stimulates the secretion of secretin.

- *Acetylcholine and CCK both potentiate the effect of secretin on ductal HCO_3^- and fluid secretion.* This potentiation is necessary because food buffers gastric acidity so that the pH of the duodenum may not be low enough to produce high secretin levels.

As food moves beyond the duodenum, the stimuli for pancreatic secretion gradually diminish and the pancreas returns to its resting condition, with a low secretory rate.

THE LIVER

LIVER FUNCTION

The digestive and excretory functions of the liver are associated with the secretion of **bile** via the biliary tract. Bile is a complex fluid that contains organic and inorganic secretions from the liver, which are important in the digestion of fats. The liver also serves many other **functions,** some of which are:

- **Carbohydrate metabolism.** *The liver is both a source and a "sink" for glucose, and is a key effector in control of the blood glucose concentration.* Glycogenolysis and gluconeogenesis add glucose to the blood. Glycogen synthesis, glycolysis, oxidative metabolism, and fat synthesis all consume blood glucose.

▽ One of the key pathogenic mechanisms in patients with **diabetes mellitus** is an inappropriately high output of hepatic glucose. The antidiabetic drug **metformin** has many mechanisms of action, one of which is to reduce hepatic glucose output, thereby decreasing plasma glucose levels. ▽

- **Fat metabolism.** Dietary lipids circulating in the form of chylomicrons (see fat absorption) are partially broken down during passage through the microcirculation by the enzyme **endothelial lipoprotein lipase.** The glycerol and fatty acids that are produced then enter the adipose and muscle cells. Remnant chylomicrons containing cholesterol, as well as long-chain fatty acids, are taken up by the liver. *The liver uses fatty acids for energy metabolism via beta oxidation or for the synthesis of ketones.*

- **Cholesterol metabolism.** The major sources of cholesterol are found in the diet plus *de novo* synthesis of cholesterol by the liver. *The major elimination pathway for cholesterol is in bile,* as native cholesterol, and via hepatic synthesis of bile acids. Bile acids are subsequently excreted in feces.

Amino acid and protein synthesis. The liver expresses a wide range of amino acid uptake carriers. A large amount of amino acid is consumed for synthesis of serum proteins (e.g., albumin, clotting factors, and hormone-binding proteins). Amino acids can also be used for oxidative metabolism. *Urea is formed as the final amino acid breakdown product.*

▽ The **assessment of liver function** in a patient with suspected liver disease includes determination of hepatocyte damage and synthetic function.

- **Hepatocyte damage** is indicated by elevated serum levels of the marker enzymes **alanine aminotransferase (ALT)** and **aspartate aminotransferase (AST)**.

- **Synthetic function** can be determined by measuring the **serum albumin concentration.** The adequacy of hepatic blood clotting factor production can also be assessed using the **prothrombin time** (see Chapter 3). ▼

Storage functions. *The liver is the main storage site for the fat-soluble vitamins A, D, E, and K, and vitamin B_{12}, iron, and copper.* Pathologic iron overload, a condition known as **hemochromatosis,** can cause liver damage due to excessive iron deposition in the liver.

Detoxification and biotransformation. *Removal of the bioactivity of many organic molecules, including steroids and hydrophobic drugs, occurs in the liver,* generally in two phases:

- **Phase I biotransformation** involves the cytochrome P450 enzymes.

- **Phase II biotransformation** involves conjugation to generate products that are more soluble for excretion. Conjugation reactions involve the addition of glucuronate, sulfate, or glutathione to the parent molecule.

▽ In the setting of **liver failure,** accumulating toxins can cause a myriad of clinical signs and symptoms. For example, **accumulation of estrogen** is thought to be responsible for gynecomastia, testicular atrophy, spider hemangiomas, and palmar erythema. ▼

Immune function. *Kupffer cells in the liver are the largest group of fixed macrophages in the body.* These cells are responsible for ingesting foreign bodies entering the blood via the gastrointestinal tract.

FUNCTIONAL ANATOMY OF THE LIVER

The liver is composed of histologically defined **lobules** (Figure 7-18). Chains of hepatocytes, usually composed of a single cell layer, separate the large blood-filled **sinusoids,** which are lined by very permeable fenestrated endothelia. The sinusoids of a single lobule drain into a central vein. The central veins of neighboring lobules unite to form the hepatic veins, which drain into the inferior vena cava. *The portal vein provides 75% of hepatic blood flow, and the hepatic artery contributes to the other 25%.* Blood from both the portal vein and the hepatic artery is mixed in the sinusoids. Because a large proportion of the blood supply is portal venous blood, hepatocytes are forced to function under low oxygen conditions.

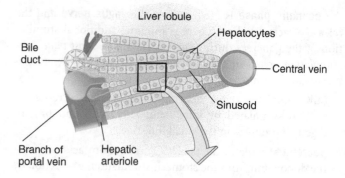

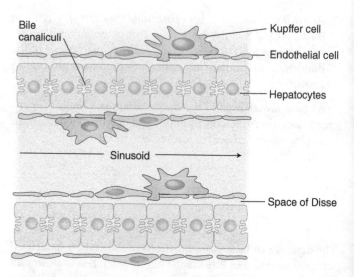

Figure 7-18: Anatomy of liver lobules. Sinusoids are wide, permeable capillaries containing a mixture of blood from the hepatic artery and the portal vein. Sinusoidal blood flows toward the central vein. Bile secreted by the hepatocytes flows in the opposite direction toward bile ductules at the periphery of the lobule.

Although the liver lobule is a convenient structure to visualize on histologic sections, it is not regarded as the functional unit of the liver. The function of hepatocytes is strongly influenced by the cellular microenvironment, which is mainly a function of the blood supply. The **liver acinus** is the smallest functional unit of the liver and consists of those hepatocytes that all receive a blood supply from the same hepatic arteriole and portal venule. An acinus is a three-dimensional ball of cells spanning more than one lobule. The vascular anatomy of the liver results in a "zonal" relationship between hepatocytes in an acinus and their arteriole. Different **cellular microenvironments** give rise to differences in cellular function.

- **Zone I** is closest to the arteriole, where cells receive the greatest delivery of oxygen and nutrients. *Cells in zone I preferentially undertake oxidative metabolism, ureagenesis, and bile acid production.*

- **Zone II** is a transitional zone between zones I and III.

- **Zone III** is furthest away from the arteriole, where the concentration of oxygen and nutrients is the lowest. *Zone III cells undertake glycolysis, ketogenesis, and detoxification reactions.*

▽ Chronic **passive congestion of the liver** secondary to congestive heart failure results in centrilobular edema (edema around the central hepatic veins), a condition known as "**nutmeg liver.**" ▽

BILIARY SYSTEM

Bile is a complex fluid secreted by the liver and consists of organic molecules in an alkaline solution. The biliary tract consists of a series of ducts that convey bile from the liver to the duodenum. **Bile has three functions:**

1. It facilitates the **assimilation of dietary lipid;** approximately 50% of dietary lipid appears in feces if bile is excluded from the small intestine. Bile facilitates fat digestion by promoting its emulsification and solubilization. This is achieved through the formation of **mixed micelles,** which enhance lipase action and then assist in the delivery of the digestive products to be absorbed by the enterocytes.

2. It provides a pathway to **excrete hydrophobic molecules** that may not be readily excreted by the kidney.

3. It assists in **neutralizing gastric acid** because it is an alkaline solution.

Hepatocytes secrete bile into the **canaliculi,** which are small 1-μm spaces bounded by neighboring hepatocytes. Canaliculi join together and convey hepatic bile toward small terminal ductules at the periphery of the liver lobules. Bile moves through a sequence of progressively larger ducts in each lobe of the liver and emerges in a hepatic duct. The hepatic ducts from each lobe join outside the liver to form the common hepatic duct. The cystic duct from the gallbladder joins the common hepatic duct to form the common bile duct. This network of ducts is known as the **biliary tree** (Figure 7-19).

Bile is stored between meals in the **gallbladder,** where it is concentrated. The integrated response to a meal includes contraction of the gallbladder during the intestinal phase. Bile,

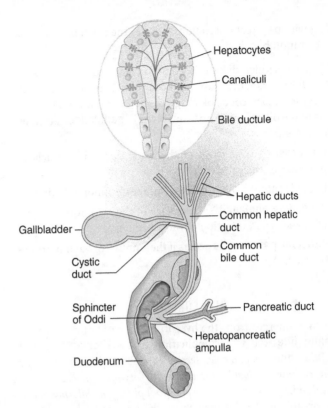

Figure 7-19: The biliary tract.

along with pancreatic secretions, reaches the small intestine via the common bile duct.

▽ Gallbladder disease is common and occurs in several forms, ranging from asymptomatic cholelithiasis (gall-stones) to biliary colic (blockage of the cystic duct). Different areas of the biliary tract can be involved in **gallbladder disease.** For example:

- **Cholecystitis** is blockage of the cystic duct with associated infection of the gallbladder.
- **Choledocholithiasis** is blockage of the common bile duct.
- **Ascending cholangitis** is blockage of the common bile duct with associated infection of the bile ducts.
- **Gallstone pancreatitis** occurs if the ampulla of Vater becomes blocked. ▼

BILE FORMATION

Bile that emerges from the liver in the hepatic ducts is called **hepatic bile** and is a combination of **canalicular bile** and **ductular bile.** *Hepatocytes secrete canalicular bile, an isotonic fluid containing NaCl, together with organic molecules that include bile salts, cholesterol, phospholipids, and bile pigments.* The organic molecules may be synthesized by hepatocytes or taken up by hepatocytes from the sinusoidal blood. Canalicular bile flows into the biliary tree, where ductular bile is added by epithelial cells called **cholangiocytes,** which line the biliary ducts. *Cholangiocytes resemble pancreatic duct cells and produce a HCO_3^--rich fluid in response to the hormone secretin.*

ORGANIC MOLECULES IN BILE **Bile acids** are the most abundant organic molecules in bile and comprise approximately 70% of the organic constituents of bile. Bile acids are **amphipathic** molecules with a hydrophobic nucleus on one side and several polar groups on the other. Hepatocytes synthesize and secrete the **primary bile acids** cholic acid and chenodeoxycholic acid, which are mostly conjugated with either glycine or tau-rine to produce, for example, glycocholate and taurocholate. **Conjugation** causes bile acids to ionize more readily into **bile salts,** which are more soluble in water (Figure 7-20). When bile acids are exposed to the small intestinal lumen, some of the pri-mary bile salts undergo bacterial modification. About 10–20% of bile salts undergo **deconjugation,** returning them to native bile acids. Native bile acids are reabsorbed in the small intestine and reconjugated in the liver prior to being secreted again. Dehydroxylation may also occur to create **secondary bile acids** (cholic → deoxycholic acid; chenodeoxycholic acid → lithocho-lic acid). Because of the loss of a polar –OH group, secondary bile acids become less soluble than the parent molecule.

When the bile acid concentration exceeds a "critical micellar concentration," bile salts interact to form aggregates known as **micelles.** The micelle provides a polar outer shell, which inter-acts with water, and a hydrophobic inner region. *Long-chain fatty acids, cholesterol, and other hydrophobic molecules readily dissolve inside the micelles.* The primary bile produced in the liver includes phospholipids, which are secreted by hepatocytes and constitute about 20% of the organic molecules in bile. Phospholipid molecules readily align with bile salts to form

Cholic acid

	Group at Position			% in Bile
	3	7	12	
Cholic acid	OH	OH	OH	50
Chenodeoxycholic acid	OH	OH	H	30
Deoxycholic acid	OH	H	OH	15
Lithocholic acid	OH	H	H	5

Figure 7-20: Bile acids and bile salts. Cholic acid and chenode-oxycholic acid are the primary bile acids produced by the liver. Conjugation with glycine and taurine favors ionization of bile acids to form more soluble bile salts. Dehydroxylation of the primary bile acids by intestinal bacteria produces the secondary bile acids deoxycholic acid and lithocholic acid.

mixed micelles, which have a greater capacity to dissolve other hydrophobic molecules than do bile salts alone.

Cholesterol, which is secreted by hepatocytes into canalicular bile, normally constitutes about 4% of the biliary solids. *Cholesterol is very hydrophobic and must be at the center of a micelle to be dissolved in aqueous solutions.* Other organic components of bile include bile pigments and a range of proteins.

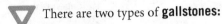 There are two types of **gallstones:**

1. **Cholesterol gallstones** are the most common type of gallstone. The main risk factor for cholesterol gallstone formation is excessive excretion of cholesterol, which is *common in obese patients.*

2. **Pigment gallstones** are mainly composed of calcium bilirubinate. *Patients with chronic hemolytic diseases are most at risk of developing this type of gallstone* due to the high levels of bilirubin excretion (bilirubin is a breakdown product of hemoglobin). The presence of calcium causes the radiopacity of pigment gallstones. ▼

ENTEROHEPATIC CIRCULATION OF BILE ACIDS The **enterohepatic circulation** is a circuit in which solutes are secreted by the liver only to be returned to the liver via intestinal reabsorption. **Molecules in the enterohepatic circulation** are:

░ Secreted into bile by hepatocytes.

░ Delivered to the small intestine via the biliary tract.

░ Reabsorbed from the small intestine.

░ Returned to the liver via the portal venous system to become available again for uptake and secretion by hepatocytes.

Many hydrophobic drugs (e.g., acetaminophen) are deactivated by the liver and excreted into bile; enterohepatic recycling frequently occurs, slowing the rate of drug elimination.

Enterohepatic recycling is physiologically important for bile salts and bile acids because the **bile acid pool** *is not large enough to assimilate the lipid content of a typical meal* (Figure 7-21). Bile salts and bile acids are recycled approximately two times during each meal, and about six to eight times each day via the enterohepatic circulation. About 95% of the bile salts that arrive in the intestine are reabsorbed. Bile salts that become deconjugated revert to bile acids, which are mostly undissociated and are reabsorbed by simple diffusion in the jejunum. Most primary and secondary bile salts are reabsorbed via **Na⁺-bile salt cotransport** when they reach the **distal ileum.** A small amount of bile acid (mostly as lithocholic acid) is lost in fecal excretion each day. The rate of bile acid loss in feces is matched by the rate of hepatic bile acid synthesis, thereby maintaining the bile acid pool.

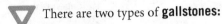 The enterohepatic circulation of bile acids can be intentionally disrupted as a treatment for high blood cholesterol levels (**hypercholesterolemia**). Disruption can be achieved by ingestion of **bile-binding resins** (e.g., cholestyramine), which prevent bile acid reabsorption in the distal ileum, thereby causing fecal bile acid excretion. When bile acids fail to return to the liver, the hepatic synthesis of new primary bile acids is stimulated, which requires an increased supply of cholesterol. The increased demand for cholesterol is met in two ways:

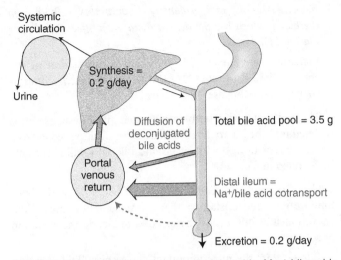

Figure 7-21: Enterohepatic circulation of bile acids. Most bile acids are reabsorbed in the distal ileum and are returned to the liver, via the portal vein, for recycling.

1. *Increased uptake of **low-density lipoproteins (LDLs)** from the blood, which has the desired therapeutic effect of reducing plasma LDL levels.*

2. Increased new cholesterol synthesis via stimulation of the enzyme **HMG-CoA reductase** (3-hydroxy-3-methyl-glutaryl-coenzymeA reductase) in the liver.

The additional cholesterol is converted into bile acids and is secreted into the biliary tract. In the setting of impaired enterohepatic circulation, the bile acids and bile salts will eventually be excreted in feces. ▼

CHOLERESIS Choleresis is the secretion of bile fluid by the liver. **Choleretics** are substances that stimulate choleresis. **Fluid secretion into bile** occurs by osmosis following the secretion of solutes:

- Bile salts are the most important choleretics. Fluid secretion into the canaliculi is **bile salt-dependent,** demonstrated by the increase in bile fluid flow as bile salt secretion increases (Figure 7-22). This occurs physiologically when bile salts return to the liver in the enterohepatic circulation and are taken up again by hepatocytes. *Choleresis can also be stimulated pharmacologically by administering bile salts (e.g., ursodiol).*

- Canalicular bile contains several other solutes, which are secreted by hepatocytes and grouped together as "nonbile acids." These solutes entrain a fairly constant background of bile fluid secretion, described as the **non–bile salt-dependent fraction** (Figure 7-22).

- Hepatic bile includes additional fluid secreted as **ductular bile.** Secretion of fluid by the cholangiocytes is driven by active $NaHCO_3$ secretion.

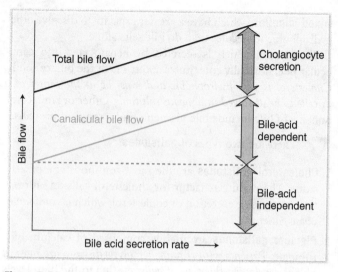

Figure 7-22: Determinants of biliary fluid secretion. Total bile flow is the sum of canalicular and ductular bile secretion. Canalicular bile flow is driven by secretion of bile acids and other solutes, which are grouped together as nonbile acids.

GALLBLADDER

The gallbladder is a blind **outpouching of the biliary tree.** It is a distensible muscular organ with a capacity of only 20–50 mL. The function of the gallbladder is to store and concentrate bile between meals and to eject bile into the duodenum during the digestion of a meal. During the interdigestive phase, the gallbladder is relaxed and the sphincter of Oddi is contracted, promoting storage of hepatic bile in the gallbladder. Contraction of the gallbladder during the intestinal phase of a meal delivers the maximum amount of bile into the small intestine at the time when nutrients are present. Therefore, **the control of the gallbladder** has several components (Figure 7-23A):

- During the cephalic phase, there is gradual rhythmic contraction of the gallbladder, mediated by the **cholinergic vagal neurons.**

- The entry of a meal into the small intestine stimulates **CCK** secretion. *CCK is the most powerful signal for gallbladder contraction and also mediates the relaxation of the sphincter of Oddi, allowing biliary and pancreatic secretions to enter the duodenum.*

- During the intestinal phase, increasing levels of **secretin** stimulate cholangiocyte secretion, providing additional HCO_3^- to neutralize acidic chyme.

- Once enterohepatic recycling of the bile acids begins, **choleresis** occurs and hepatic bile secretion accelerates.

Bile is secreted at a fairly constant rate between meals, with more than 50% of the daily hepatic bile produced entering the gallbladder during this interdigestive period. This volume of hepatic bile far exceeds the volume of bile in the gallbladder, and the excess fluid volume must be absorbed by epithelial cells lining the gallbladder. *Concentrated bile is more effective for promoting fat digestion.* The mechanism of salt and fluid absorption is shown in Figure 7-23B. The surface epithelium of the gallbladder secretes mucins and H⁺ for protection against the alkaline bile in the gallbladder lumen.

BILE PIGMENTS

The major bile pigment is **bilirubin,** which is a breakdown product of hemoglobin. The **pathway from the formation of bile pigments to their final excretion** is complex, and is responsible for the normal coloration of both feces and urine (Figure 7-24).

- *The process begins with ingestion of senescent red blood cells by macrophages.* **Heme oxygenase** is the key enzyme in macrophages that is required to break down the heme moiety from hemoglobin; **bilirubin** is the end product of this pathway.

- *Bilirubin is released from macrophages and bound to albumin in the plasma because of its low solubility in water.* This protein-bound form of bilirubin is referred to as **unconjugated (or indirect) bilirubin.**

- *Hepatocytes take up free bilirubin from plasma and convert it to bilirubin diglucuronide* via the enzyme **glucuronyl transferase;** this form of bilirubin is called **conjugated (or direct) bilirubin** and is water soluble.

- *Hepatocytes secrete conjugated bilirubin into bile canaliculi.*

- About half the conjugated bilirubin delivered to the intestine is excreted unaltered in feces. The action of intestinal bacteria metabolizes the remaining conjugated bilirubin to the colorless molecule **urobilinogen.**

- About 80% of urobilinogen passes to the colon, where it is metabolized by bacteria and colors feces with the brown pigment **stercobilin.**

- The remaining 20% of intestinal urobilinogen enters the enterohepatic recycling pathway; however, some urobilinogen escapes hepatic reuptake and enters the systemic circulation. Urobilinogen in blood is filtered at the kidney and colors the urine yellow when it is oxidized to the pigment **urobilin.**

▽ **Jaundice** is a disease that manifests with yellowing of the sclera, the mucous membranes, and the skin, and occurs when plasma bilirubin concentration (unconjugated or conjugated) exceeds about 2 mg/dL. **Excess production of bilirubin,** or a failure of the hepatocytes to take up or conjugate bilirubin, results in an accumulation of the unconjugated form in blood. If the hepatocytes fail to adequately secrete bilirubin, or if the bile duct is obstructed, then there is an accumulation of the conjugated form of bilirubin. The different types of hyperbilirubinemias that can lead to jaundice are outlined in Table 7-1 and classified as follows:

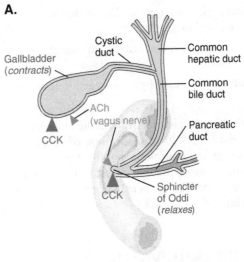

A.

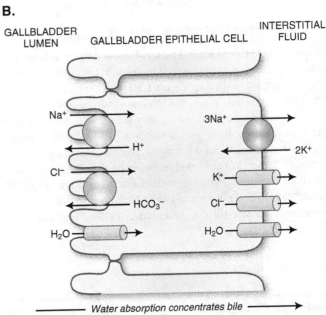

B.

Figure 7-23: A. Coordination of gallbladder motility. Cholecystokinin (CCK) is the main agent causing contraction of the gallbladder and simultaneous relaxation of the sphincter of Oddi. **B.** Mechanism of isotonic NaCl and fluid reabsorption by the gallbladder epithelium. ACh, acetylcholine.

1. **Prehepatic** jaundice is caused by conditions that present an excessive bilirubin load to the liver.
2. **Hepatic** jaundice results from an inability to take up, metabolize, or excrete bilirubin.
3. **Posthepatic jaundice** is caused by an obstruction to the biliary tract.

Obstructive jaundice, such as occurs with a malignant tumor of the head of the pancreas, results in suppression of hepatic bile flow and reabsorption of conjugated bile into the circulation. Suppressed bile flow results in **acholic (light or clay-colored) stool,** whereas reabsorbed bile is excreted in urine, causing **dark urine (bilirubinuria).** ▼

THE SMALL INTESTINE

STRUCTURE OF THE SMALL INTESTINE

The small intestine is several meters long and extends from the pyloric sphincter of the stomach to the junction with the large intestine at the ileocecal sphincter. It has three regions: the short **duodenum** proximally and the **jejunum** and the **ileum** distally. Exocrine secretions from the salivary glands, the stomach, and the pancreas and liver, plus secretions of the small intestine itself, are mixed with food for digestion and absorption. Several anatomic features of the small intestine amplify the surface area for absorption, including transverse folds in the mucosa (**plicae circulares**), the arrangement of the mucosa into **villi,** and the presence of **microvilli** on the enterocytes that line the small intestine (Figure 7-25).

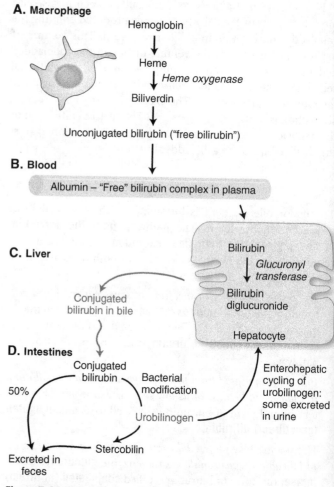

Figure 7-24: Bile pigments. **A.** Breakdown of hemoglobin in macrophages produces bilirubin. **B.** Carriage of free bilirubin in plasma. **C.** Conjugation of bilirubin by hepatocytes. **D.** Excretion of bilirubin.

TABLE 7-1. Causes of Unconjugated (Indirect) Versus Conjugated (Direct) Hyperbilirubinemias

Type of Hyperbilirubinemia	Unconjugated (Indirect) Bilirubinemia	Conjugated (Direct) Bilirubinemia
Prehepatic	**Hemolytic anemias** • Sickle cell disease • Hereditary spherocytosis **Ineffective hematopoiesis** • Thalassemia **Physiologic jaundice** • Neonates	
Hepatic	**Hereditary** • Crigler-Najjar syndrome (types 1 and 2) • Gilbert's syndrome	**Hereditary** • Dubin-Johnson syndrome • Rotor's syndrome **Liver disease** • Hepatitis (viral, toxin) • Cirrhosis
Posthepatic		**Biliary tract disease** • Gallstones • Tumors (bile duct, gallbladder, or pancreas) • Primary biliary cirrhosis • Primary sclerosing cholangitis

The ***villus*** *is the functional unit of the intestine.* The villus epithelium consists of **enterocytes,** mucous-secreting goblet cells, and endocrine cells. **Three regions of a villus** form a functional continuum: the crypt, the maturation zone, and the villus tip.

1. The **crypt** contains rapidly dividing **stem cells** that force migration of cells up the side of a villus. The cells initially produced in the intestinal crypts are immature and do not express enzymes or membrane transporters for nutrient absorption. *Crypt cells are the source of intestinal fluid secretion.*

2. The **maturation zone** is an intermediate zone where cells are moving toward the tip of the villus and are beginning to expresses enzymes and absorptive membrane transport proteins.

3. At the **villus tip,** enterocytes are fully differentiated and undertake the **absorption** of nutrients, electrolytes, and fluid. *After 3–4 days, the cells are sloughed off the villus tip as a defense mechanism against insults from the luminal contents.*

▽   **Celiac sprue** is a malabsorption syndrome caused by hypersensitivity to wheat **gluten** and **gliadin,** resulting in immune-mediated destruction and denudation of the small intestinal villi. *The denuded small intestine results in malabsorption of nutrients,* causing diarrhea (excess fecal fluid) and steatorrhea (excess fecal fat), with associated abdominal bloating and flatulence. *Removal of gluten from the diet will resolve the condition.* However, resolution of the malabsorption will not occur immediately upon dietary change because the crypt cells require a few days to mature and rebuild the absorptive intestinal villi. ▼

MOTILITY

During the fed state, there is a great deal of motor activity in the small intestine. The **three functions of small intestinal motility** during the fed state are:

1. **Mixing** of foodstuffs with digestive secretions and enzymes.

2. **Distribution** of the luminal contents around the mucosa for absorption.

3. **Propulsion** of the luminal contents in the aboral direction (away from the mouth).

When nutrients enter the small intestine, transit is initially fast and chyme is spread along the small bowel; transit then slows to promote absorption. There are two major **types of motility** that occur in the small intestine during the fed state (Figure 7-26):

1. **Segmentation** contractions produce a string of segments that constantly form and reform. *The main function of segmentation contractions is mixing of the luminal contents.*

2. **Peristalsis** consists of a wave of contractions that moves a bolus aborally. *The function of peristalsis is propulsion of luminal material.* Peristalsis is a reflex, and the main stimulus is moderate distension of the gut wall. The circular muscle contracts in the upstream contracting segment, forcing the bolus forward; **receptive relaxation** of the circular muscle in the downstream segment reduces the force needed to move the bolus aborally.

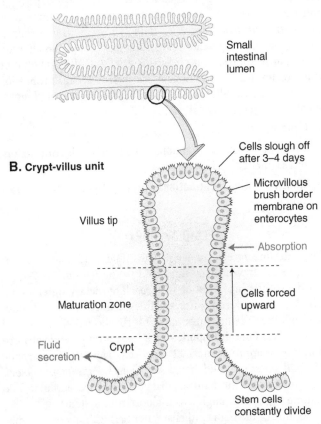

A. Plicae circulares

Small intestinal lumen

B. Crypt-villus unit

Cells slough off after 3–4 days

Microvillous brush border membrane on enterocytes

Villus tip

Absorption

Cells forced upward

Maturation zone

Fluid secretion

Crypt

Stem cells constantly divide

Figure 7-25: A. Amplification of the absorptive area of the small intestine. Plicae circulares are transverse folds of intestinal mucosa. **B.** The crypt-villus unit. The surface area is greatly increased by villi and microvilli on the apical membrane of the enterocytes. The crypt-villus unit is the functional unit of the small intestine. Stem cell division produces immature cells in crypts, which secrete fluid; mature cells at the villus tip absorb nutrients, electrolytes, and fluid.

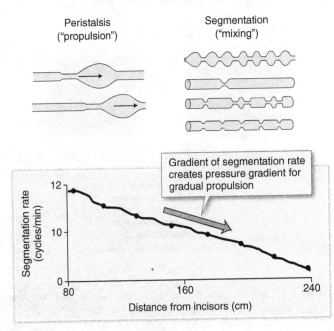

Peristalsis ("propulsion")

Segmentation ("mixing")

Gradient of segmentation rate creates pressure gradient for gradual propulsion

Segmentation rate (cycles/min)

12

10

0

80   160   240

Distance from incisors (cm)

Figure 7-26: Patterns of small intestinal motility.

The numerous contractions of the small intestine in the presence of food appear chaotic, and there is overlap in the function between peristaltic and segmenting contractions. *Most peristaltic contractions travel less than 2 cm and thus contribute to mixing.* Segmenting patterns are faster in the upper small intestine than in more distal areas; this **gradient of segmentation rate** creates a pressure gradient that assists aboral propulsion (Figure 7-26). An **alternative classification of intestinal movements** defines three variations:

1. **Tonic contraction** of sphincters.
2. **Rhythmic phasic contractions** (small peristaltic contractions and segmentation).
3. **Giant migrating contractions** (powerful peristaltic contractions).

FLUID ABSORPTION

The intestine receives a large daily fluid load that must be absorbed. A typical daily fluid load to the jejunum is 7–10 L per day, consisting of about 1–2 L each of dietary water, saliva, gastric juice, pancreatic juice, and intestinal secretion, and about 0.5 L of bile. The small intestine reabsorbs about 6–8 L per day of fluid by **isosmotic transport,** with a maximum possible absorption rate of approximately 12 L per day. *The rate of absorption of small intestinal fluid is not subject to significant physiologic regulation* by the mechanisms that govern the extracellular fluid volume (e.g., renin-angiotensin-aldosterone system).

Because of the high epithelial water permeability of the small intestine, there is rapid **osmotic equilibration** between the duodenal chyme and plasma. If food has a high water content and is hypotonic to plasma, there is rapid water uptake. *More frequently, a meal is hypertonic and water initially enters the small intestine from the extracellular fluid by osmosis.* Subsequent absorption of fluid depends on the active transport of nutrients and electrolytes (Figure 7-27). Na^+ uptake at the luminal membrane is driven by low intracellular Na^+ concentration. The driving force for Na^+ uptake is maintained by active Na^+ extrusion at the basolateral membrane by the Na^+/K^+-ATPase.

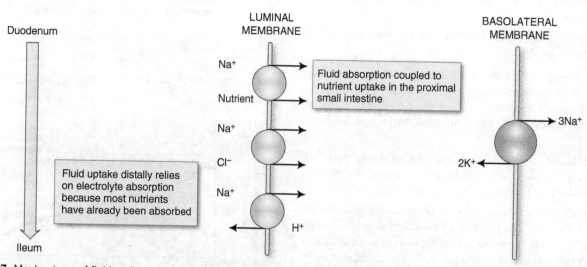

Figure 7-27: Mechanisms of fluid reabsorption along the small intestine. Different luminal entry mechanisms of Na^+ exist at different locations along the gastrointestinal tract. The gradient for passive Na^+ uptake into the enterocytes is maintained by active Na^+ extrusion across the basolateral cell membranes. Water reabsorption occurs by osmosis, secondary to Na^+ absorption.

Fluid absorption in the upper small intestine is mainly coupled to **Na⁺/nutrient uptake,** although Na⁺/H⁺ exchange is also present in this area of the gut. *By the time the food reaches the ileum, most sugars have been absorbed and fluid absorption is more dependent on NaCl reabsorption.*

Approximately 2 L per day of fluid is delivered to the **large intestine,** which is roughly the initial dietary fluid load. The colon absorbs approximately 1.9 L, leaving about 0.1 L per day in feces. The maximum reabsorptive capacity of the colon is approximately 5 L per day; *diarrhea results if the total fluid delivery to the colon exceeds 5 L per day.*

FLUID SECRETION

Both the small intestine and the large intestine secrete fluid from the crypt cells. Secretion is necessary for lubrication, as evidenced by the high incidence of obstruction of the gut when secretion is impaired in diseases such as **cystic fibrosis.** Fluid secretion also provides a source of Na⁺ for *coupling to nutrient absorption,* which is needed when a meal contains insufficient Na⁺ for sugar and amino acid uptake. Antibodies secreted in the area of the intestinal crypts also require fluid secretions to reach the lumen in the gut.

The mechanism of intestinal fluid secretion is clinically important because it is activated by a number of **bacterial enterotoxins** that cause **secretory diarrhea.** The key step in the mechanism of fluid secretion from the crypt enterocytes is opening of the Cl⁻ channels in the luminal cell membrane (Figure 7-28). There are **two types of Cl⁻ channels** present:

1. **cAMP-activated** Cl⁻ channels, for which the ENS neurotransmitter **VIP** is an important secretagogue.

2. **Ca²⁺-activated** Cl⁻ channels, for which **acetylcholine** from ENS neurons and **serotonin** from the EC cells are both secretagogues.

▽ Enterotoxic ***Escherichia coli*** (traveler's diarrhea due to *E coli*) and ***Vibrio cholera*** (cholera *due to V cholera*) both produce enterotoxins that utilize cAMP to induce **secretory diarrhea.** Cholera, for example, irreversibly activates **adenylyl cyclase,** causing continuous production of cAMP and a severe Cl⁻-rich watery diarrhea. There can be a significant fluid loss, and death can occur if there is a delay in rehydration and electrolyte replacement. ▼

INTESTINAL Ca²⁺ ABSORPTION

Ca²⁺ is reabsorbed in the **duodenum** and upper jejunum; about 30–80% of dietary Ca²⁺ typically is absorbed. About one third of the net Ca²⁺ uptake occurs passively via the paracellular route across the tight junctions. The remaining fraction occurs actively through **regulated Ca²⁺ transport pathways** in the enterocytes (Figure 7-29):

- Ca²⁺ enters the enterocytes down a steep electrochemical gradient via the **Ca²⁺ channels.**

- To prevent an increase in intracellular free Ca²⁺ concentration, Ca²⁺ binds to the protein **calbindin** within the cytoplasm.

- Extrusion of Ca²⁺ from the cells occurs by primary active transport (**Ca²⁺-ATPase**) and secondary active transport (**3Na⁺/Ca²⁺ exchange**), against a large electrochemical gradient.

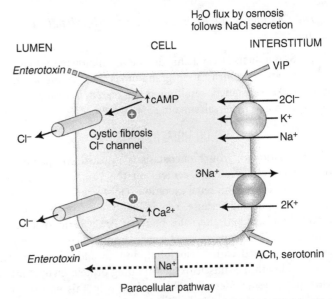

Figure 7-28: Mechanism of intestinal fluid secretion. Opening the luminal membrane Cl⁻ channels initiates secretion. Na⁺ secretion follows passively via the paracellular pathway, and water secretion occurs by osmosis. Secretagogues, including bacterial enterotoxins, can activate fluid secretion via cyclic adenosine monophosphate (cAMP) or increased intracellular Ca²⁺ concentration. VIP, vasoactive intestinal polypeptide; ACh, acetylcholine.

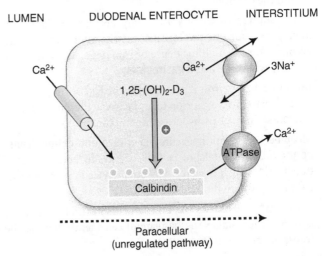

Figure 7-29: Mechanism of intestinal calcium absorption. Vitamin D₃ stimulates intestinal Ca²⁺ uptake by stimulating calbindin expression, as well as activating Ca²⁺ transport proteins.

The Ca^{2+} uptake mechanism is stimulated by **vitamin D** *(see Chapter 8).*

▼ **Sarcoidosis** is a systemic disease of unknown etiology. It produces noncaseating granulomas that secrete a vitamin D-like substance, resulting in increased intestinal Ca^{2+} absorption and hypercalcemia in some patients. ▼

IRON HOMEOSTASIS

The regulation of iron homeostasis is unusual compared to other minerals because it centers on the control of dietary uptake rather than on renal excretion. Tight regulation of iron levels is important because iron is highly reactive due to its redox chemistry and alternates between Fe^{3+} (ferric, oxidized iron) and Fe^{2+} (ferrous, reduced iron). About 70% of total body iron is associated with **hemoglobin,** and an additional 3% is associated with the muscle oxygen-binding protein **myoglobin.** Most of the remainder of total body iron is in a tissue storage form bound to the protein **ferritin.**

Iron is transported in blood plasma using a binding protein called **transferrin.** The iron bound to transferrin is in equilibrium with the very small amounts of free Fe^{2+} in the extracellular fluid and with iron that is bound to ferritin in the tissues. The total amount of iron in the body is subject to negative feedback regulation (Figure 7-30A). When the iron ferritin store in the liver is full, the liver releases an iron regulatory factor called **hepcidin.** Increased hepcidin inhibits Fe^{2+} uptake by the intestinal enterocytes, preventing iron overload.

Normal daily losses of iron are small, with only 0.6 mg per day in men and about double this amount in women (due to variable menstrual loss). Iron intake generally exceeds 20 mg per day in the typical Western diet, so only a small fraction of ingested iron needs to be absorbed. However, *in the developing world, dietary iron deficiency is the most common cause of anemia.* **Intestinal iron absorption** occurs through several mechanisms (see Figure 7-30B):

- In a typical nonvegetarian diet, most dietary iron arrives associated with **heme,** which has its own intestinal transport protein; iron is released by the action of **heme oxygenase** within the enterocyte.

- Other sources of **dietary iron** only become available following exposure to the low pH gastric environment. This accounts for the high incidence of iron deficiency anemia in patients who have had a **gastrectomy.**

- Most free dietary iron is presented in the Fe^{3+} form and must be converted to Fe^{2+} prior to uptake via the enzyme Fe^{3+} **reductase** in the brush-border membrane.

- Most Fe^{2+} absorption occurs via a **divalent cation transporter (DCT1).** Uptake of Fe^{2+} also occurs by endocytosis of **transferrin,** which is secreted by enterocytes into the intestinal lumen, where it binds free Fe^{2+}.

- Once inside the enterocyte, iron can either bind to ferritin or is transported across the basolateral cell membrane via the transport protein **ferroportin.**

▼ **Hemochromatosis** is an autosomal recessive disease caused by mutations in a gene referred to as **HFE.** *The abnormal HFE gene is unable to regulate iron absorption, resulting*

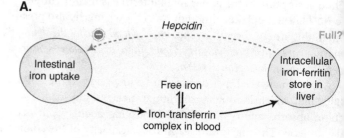

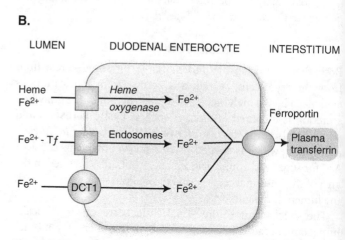

Figure 7-30: A. Overview of iron homeostasis. **B.** Mechanisms of intestinal iron uptake. DCT, Divalent cation transporter-1.

in toxic iron overload. Although the pathogenesis is not completely understood, the hepcidin system becomes less effective, which results in loss of negative feedback to stop excess iron absorption. The most common tissues (and toxic manifestations) affected by the **iron toxicity** are the liver (cirrhosis), the skin (bronze discoloration), and the pancreas (diabetes). Changes in the skin and pancreas illustrate why hemochromatosis is said to cause "**bronze diabetes.**" ▼

NUTRIENT DIGESTION AND ABSORPTION

The major classes of nutrients are carbohydrates, proteins, and fats. Most nutrients are large molecules that must be broken down into smaller molecules that can be absorbed. Digestion is the chemical **breakdown of food by enzymes** and can occur at three sites (Figure 7-31A):

1. **Luminal digestion** occurs within the lumen of the gastrointestinal tract and is mediated by enzymes from the salivary glands, the stomach, and the pancreas.

2. **Membrane digestion** is the action of enzymes fixed to the brush-border membrane of enterocytes. Such enzymes are synthesized by enterocytes and inserted into the membrane.

3. **Intracellular digestion** is mediated by cytoplasmic enzymes within enterocytes.

Nutrient absorption occurs in the small intestine (see Figure 7-31B). The proximal small intestine absorbs almost all of the **iron** and **Ca^{2+}** that is assimilated from food.

Carbohydrates can be absorbed along all parts of the small intestine, but their absorption is usually completed in the proximal small intestine. Absorption of other nutrients (including **protein, fat, salts, and water**) is spread more uniformly along the small intestine. *Bile acids and vitamin B_{12} are absorbed specifically in the distal ileum.*

CARBOHYDRATE DIGESTION Carbohydrates are the major source of calories in the Western diet, with about 400 g per day consumed. Approximately 60% is starch, about 30% is sucrose, and about 10% is lactose. *Digestion reduces carbohydrates to their component **monosaccharides:** glucose, galactose, and fructose.* Figure 7-32A summarizes the main dietary carbohydrates, the specific enzymes that break down the carbohydrates, and the final products of digestion.

Starch is a polymer of glucose; its luminal digestion begins with **salivary amylase** and is completed by **pancreatic amylase.** Although salivary amylase has a neutral pH optimum, it remains active for a long time in the stomach within a food bolus, where it is buffered from gastric acidity. Amylase breaks the α-1,4 glucose linkages to produce oligosaccharides of various lengths, known as **dextrins.** Much of the oligosaccharide and disaccharide digestion occurs by membrane digestion. The enzymes **glucoamylase** and **isomaltase** break down oligosaccharides; the disaccharides sucrose, lactose, and maltose are broken down by sucrase, lactase, and maltase, respectively.

▽ **Lactase deficiency** is common in adults from nonwhite populations and results in milk intolerance, with

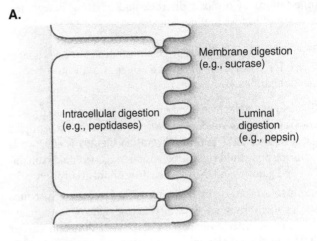

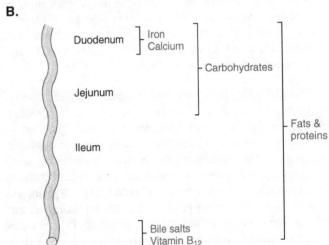

Figure 7-31: A. Sites of digestive enzyme action. **B.** Overview of nutrient absorption in the small intestine.

manifestations of osmotic diarrhea and bloating due to fermentation of lactose in the colon. ▼

CARBOHYDRATE ABSORPTION The small intestine has a very large capacity for absorption of sugars, which are all absorbed as **monosaccharides** (see Figure 7-32B).

▪ **Glucose and galactose** uptake from the gut lumen occur, with equal affinity, by secondary active transport via the Na⁺-coupled cotransporter **SGLT-1. Oral rehydration therapy** is effective at restoring body fluid volume because the ingested fluid contains Na^+ and glucose, and their uptake drives fluid absorption.

▪ **Fructose** is taken up by facilitated diffusion across the brush border membrane via **GLUT5**. Fructose, glucose, and galactose all exit enterocytes via the facilitated diffusion carrier **GLUT2** in the basolateral cell membranes. A small number of patients do not express functional SGLT-1 and are unable to reabsorb glucose; these patients can survive with adequate dietary fructose because it can be absorbed via GLUT5 and converted into glucose by the liver.

PROTEIN DIGESTION Dietary protein is assimilated either as amino acids or small peptides. A combination of luminal digestion, membrane digestion, and intracellular digestion is used to break down proteins. Luminal digestion begins with **pepsin** in the stomach. The partially digested proteins that enter the small intestine are hydrolyzed by three pancreatic **endopeptidases** (acting on internal peptide bonds): **elastase, chymotrypsin,** and **trypsin.** The oligopeptides produced by endopeptidases are further broken down by **ectopeptidases,** which act from the carboxy terminus of a peptide to remove one amino acid at a time. *Carboxypeptidase A digests the products produced by the actions of chymotrypsin and elastase, and **carboxypeptidase B** acts on the products of trypsin digestion.* The enzyme **aminooligopeptidase** is anchored to the enterocyte brush-border membrane and acts at the amino terminus of short peptides to release amino acids.

AMINO ACID AND PEPTIDE ABSORPTION Amino acids are a chemically diverse group of molecules, and several transport systems are needed for their absorption. Most of the systems are cotransporters that couple amino acid entry to that of Na⁺; others are facilitated diffusion carriers, which are Na⁺ independent. The normal mixture of amino acids and small peptides produced by enzyme digestion are absorbed faster than the same quantity of only amino acids. This phenomenon is called **kinetic advantage** and is explained by the mechanism of **H⁺-linked cotransport** systems for dipeptides and tripeptides, which operate independent of amino acid carriers (Figure 7-33). Short peptides that are absorbed by enterocytes are quickly broken down inside the cell to amino acids and are transported across the basolateral membrane into the blood. Each transport cycle of a dipeptide or a tripeptide carrier transports the equivalent of two or three amino acids into the enterocyte, accounting for rapid net uptake of protein products from the lumen through this pathway.

FAT DIGESTION *Triglycerides are the most abundant dietary form of lipid.* Other lipids include phospholipids, sphingolipids, sterols, and the fat-soluble vitamins A, D, E, and K. Nondietary sources of fats include lecithins and cholesterol from bile,

A.

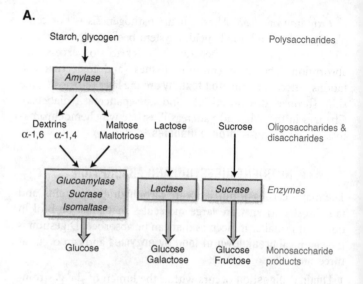

B.

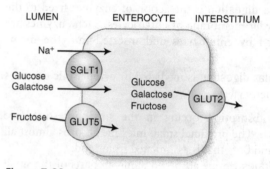

Figure 7-32: A. Major dietary forms of carbohydrates and their digestion. **B.** Absorption mechanisms for glucose, galactose, and fructose. SGLT-1 is a Na⁺/glucose cotransporter; GLUT2 and GLUT5 are uniporters for facilitated diffusion.

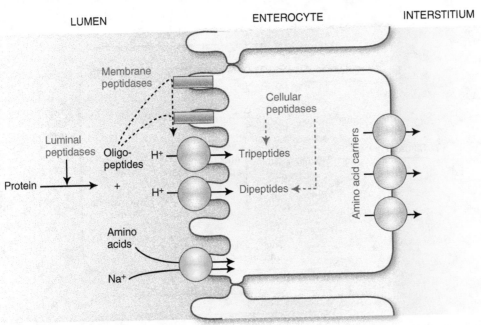

Figure 7-33: Protein digestion and absorption. Protein digestion includes the luminal, membrane, and intracellular digestion sites. Products of enzyme digestion include amino acids and small peptides, which are absorbed by a range of facilitated or Na^+-linked amino acid carriers as well as by H^+-linked dipeptide and tripeptide carriers.

sloughed enterocytes, and microbes. Lipid digestion involves a mechanical phase and a chemical phase.

The **mechanical phase** includes chewing and grinding peristalsis in the stomach, which together create an **emulsion** with large fat droplets being sheared into smaller droplets. When chyme enters the small intestine, bile is added. Bile salts reduce surface tension at the fat droplet and water interface and further aid the formation of a fine emulsion.

The **chemical phase** of fat digestion occurs when **lipases** remove fatty acids from the triglyceride molecules. Lipases are termed as acid or alkaline lipases, based on their pH optimum. **Lingual lipase** from the salivary glands and **gastric lipase** from the fundus of the stomach are **acid lipases** with a pH optimum between 3.5 and 5.5. *In adults, acid lipases account for about 20% of total lipolysis, but in neonates this can be over 50% of the total lipolytic activity.* **Alkaline lipase** is secreted by the pancreas and has a pH optimum between 6 and 8. The action of pancreatic lipase on triglycerides produces a monoglyceride and two free fatty acids. Pancreatic lipase requires **colipase** to effectively hydrolyze fats. Colipase is secreted by the pancreas and acts at the surface of a micelle by displacing a bile salt molecule, thereby providing a binding site for pancreatic lipase. Long-chain fatty acids produced by the action of pancreatic lipase are insoluble in water and must enter the core of a micelle to be dissolved. Other lipases include **phospholipase A₂**, which degrades lecithins and other phospholipids, and **carboxyl ester lipase (nonspecific lipase),** which is able to hydrolyze cholesterol esters.

▽   *Because the pancreas normally oversecretes lipase, ingested fats can be hydrolyzed with only 10% of the lipase secreted.* A patient with **chronic pancreatic insufficiency** is likely to have experienced very extensive destruction of the gland by the time the clinical signs of **maldigestion** become apparent (e.g., steatorrhea, bloating, colonic distension, gas, and nutrient excretion in feces). ▽

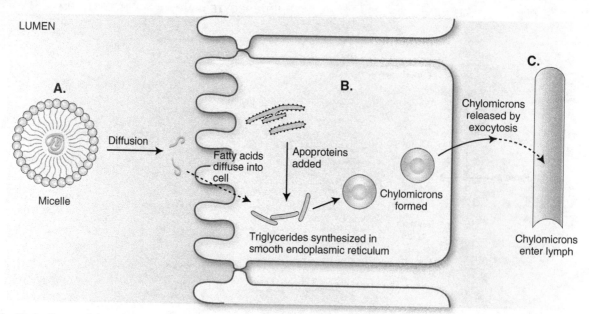

Figure 7-34: Absorption and intracellular processing of fatty acids. **A.** Diffusion of micelles through the unstirred surface fluid layer. **B.** Intracellular synthesis of triglyceride and formation of chylomicrons. **C.** Exocytosis of chylomicrons to lymphatic vessels.

FAT ABSORPTION *Medium-chain fatty acids* *are able to freely* *diffuse from the intestinal lumen into the blood without modi-* *fication*; however, most triglyceride digestion produces **long-chain fatty acids.** Absorption occurs via the following steps (Figure 7-34):

- Long-chain fatty acids dissolve in micelles, which provide a means for hydrophobic molecules to diffuse through an **unstirred fluid layer** at the intestinal surface (Figure 7-34A).

- The unstirred fluid layer has a lower pH than the neutralized chyme, which destabilizes micelles as they approach surface cells; long-chain fatty acids escape the micelle and **enter the enterocyte by diffusion** through the plasma membrane.

- *Enterocytes convert long-chain fatty acids back into triglycerides within the smooth endoplasmic reticulum.*

- Triglycerides are complexed with **apoproteins** within the smooth endoplasmic reticulum.

- The Golgi apparatus delivers the lipoprotein complexes in large vesicles called **chylomicrons,** which are transported across the basolateral membrane by exocytosis. *Chylomicrons are too large to pass across the capillary endothelia and instead enter the* **lymphatic** *vessels.*

- Chylomicrons enter the systemic blood when lymph drains into the venous system.

- The action of the enzyme **endothelial lipoprotein lipase** liberates fatty acids from chylomicrons, primarily for uptake by adipose tissue and muscle cells; the remnant chylomicrons are processed by the liver.

▼   **Fat malabsorption** results in increased levels of fecal fat excretion. **Steatorrhea** is the presence of more than 7 g per day of fatty acids in the stool. There are many potential **causes of fat malabsorption,** including:

Fat emulsification is poor in patients who have had a **gastrectomy** and who experience rapid dumping of ingested food into the small intestine.

Patients with **hypersecretion of gastric acid** (e.g., Zollinger-Ellison syndrome) may have an acidic duodenal environment that inhibits pancreatic lipase.

Biliary obstruction or **cholecystectomy** (removal of the gallbladder) reduces the availability of bile.

Patients with **pancreatic insufficiency** (e.g., cystic fibrosis) have inadequate pancreatic lipase secretion.

Abetalipoproteinemia is a rare condition in which the assembly of triglyceride and apoproteins is defective. ▼

VITAMIN ABSORPTION

Vitamins are organic molecules that are required for metabolism but cannot be synthesized in the body; therefore vitamins must be present in the diet. Table 7-2 lists recognized vitamins, summarizes their major functions, and describes the main

TABLE 7-2. Functions of Vitamins and the Effects of Deficiencies

Vitamin	Function	Deficiency
A (β-carotene)	Pigment in retina	Night blindness Hyperkeratosis
B$_1$ (thiamine)	Coenzyme in pyruvate and α-ketoacid metabolism	Beriberi
B$_2$ (riboflavin)	Coenzyme in mitochondrial oxidative metabolism	Normocytic anemia
B$_3$ (niacin)	Coenzyme in mitochondrial oxidative metabolism	Pellagra
B$_6$ (pyridoxine)	Coenzyme in amino acid synthesis	Normocytic anemia
B$_{12}$ (cobalamin)	Facilitates formation of erythrocytes and neuronal myelin sheath	Pernicious anemia
C (ascorbic acid)	Coenzyme in hydroxyproline formation, used in collagen	Scurvy
D (cholecalciferol)	Increased Ca^{2+} absorption	Rickets (childhood deficiency)
E (α-tocopherol)	Antioxidant	Peripheral neuropathy
K$_1$ (phylloquinone)	Blood clotting: needed for synthesis of factors VII, IX, X, and prothrombin	Hemorrhage
Folate	Purine synthesis	Megaloblastic anemia
Biotin	Coenzyme for carboxylation reactions	Neurologic signs
Pantothenic acid	Coenzyme A: needed for metabolism of carbohydrate and fat via acetyl-coenzyme A and amino acid synthesis	Neurologic and gastrointestinal signs

features of vitamin deficiencies. **Vitamins A, D, E, and K are fat-soluble;** a meal must contain fat if these vitamins are to be assimilated from food. Fat-soluble vitamins enter micelles and are absorbed into enterocytes by simple diffusion; they appear in chylomicrons unaltered by metabolic processes in the enterocyte. *Fat malabsorption is associated with a deficiency of fat-soluble vitamins because the vitamins are excreted along with excess fecal fat.*

The **water-soluble group** of vitamins includes the **B vitamins, vitamin C, folate, biotin, and pantothenic acid.** Intestinal absorption of these water-soluble molecules by simple diffusion is slow. Although not yet fully understood, separate carrier-mediated transport mechanisms have recently been identified for each of the water-soluble vitamins.

VITAMIN B$_{12}$ UPTAKE Vitamin B$_{12}$ deficiency may take months to manifest clinically because the liver stores a significant amount of the vitamin. *Untreated vitamin B$_{12}$ deficiency results in anemia.*

The following steps are involved in **vitamin B$_{12}$ uptake** (Figure 7-35):

- When vitamin B$_{12}$ is **ingested,** it is bound to the proteins in food and must be released in the stomach by the action of pepsin.

- Vitamin B$_{12}$ forms a complex with a glycoprotein called **haptocorrin,** which is secreted into the saliva and gastric juice.

- Pancreatic proteases hydrolyze haptocorrin to liberate vitamin B$_{12}$, which is then available to bind to **intrinsic factor** within the small intestine.

- The vitamin B$_{12}$-intrinsic factor complex is required for vitamin B$_{12}$ absorption via a specific **receptor-mediated mechanism in the distal ileum.**

- Vitamin B$_{12}$ encounters the binding protein **transcobalamin** in blood, which carries it to the liver for storage.

▽ The mechanism for assimilation of vitamin B$_{12}$ requires normal function in several gastrointestinal organs. As a result, there are multiple etiologies that lead to **vitamin B$_{12}$ deficiency,** including:

- **Dietary deficiency.**
- **Lack of intrinsic factor** (known as **pernicious anemia**), which may be caused, for example, by autoimmune destruction of the parietal cells or by gastric atrophy.
- **Pancreatic insufficiency** (e.g., cystic fibrosis).
- **Surgical resection of the ileum.**
- **Terminal ileum disease** (e.g., Crohn's ileitis); the ileum is the most common location of **Crohn's disease.**
- **Intestinal organisms** (e.g., *Diphyllobothrium latum,* a fish tapeworm).

Regardless of its cause, vitamin B$_{12}$ deficiency manifests as **megaloblastic anemia** and neurologic degeneration caused by **demyelination** of the peripheral nerves, the spinal cord, and the cerebrum. *Treatment of vitamin B$_{12}$ deficiency with only supplemental folic acid should never be attempted; the folic acid will resolve the anemia but without vitamin B$_{12}$ replacement, the patient will have irreversible neurologic dysfunction.* ▽

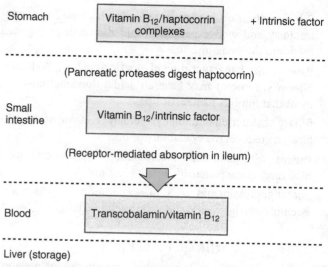

Figure 7-35: Vitamin B$_{12}$ assimilation. Haptocorrin binds vitamin B$_{12}$ in the stomach. Intrinsic factor secreted by the stomach is required for intestinal uptake of vitamin B$_{12}$. Binding of vitamin B$_{12}$ to intrinsic factor occurs in the small intestine.

THE LARGE INTESTINE

The large intestine is wider than the small intestine and begins beyond the ileocecal sphincter and ends at the anus. The large intestine consists of the **cecum;** the **ascending colon, transverse colon, descending colon,** and **sigmoid colon;** the **rectum;** and the **anal canal.** The longitudinal layer of smooth muscle is arranged in three discrete strips called **teniae coli.** Contractions of this discontinuous muscle layer cause the wall of the large intestine to form bulges known as **haustra.** The colon is lined with transporting epithelial cells called **colonocytes,** which absorb fluid and transport electrolytes but do not express digestive enzymes.

Nutrient absorption should be completed by the time the luminal contents reach the large intestine. The main functions of the large intestine are completion of **fluid absorption** and the storage and elimination of **fecal waste.** Most water absorption occurs in the **right colon** (the cecum, the ascending colon, and the first half of the transverse colon). Prior to defecation, fecal waste is stored in the **left colon** (i.e., the distal half of the transverse colon, the descending colon, and the sigmoid colon) (Figure 7-36). By the time fecal material reaches the rectum, it consists of a small volume of **K⁺-rich fluid** containing **undigested plant fibers,** bacteria, and inorganic material.

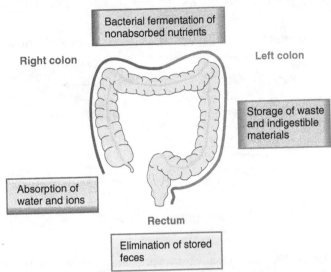

Figure 7-36: Areas and functions of the large intestine. The right colon includes the cecum, the ascending colon, and the proximal half of the transverse colon; the left colon includes the distal half of the transverse colon, the descending colon, the sigmoid colon, and the rectum.

COLONIC MOTILITY

Both **segmentation** and **peristalsis** in the colon produce motility patterns that facilitate fluid and electrolyte absorption and allow the storage and orderly evacuation of feces (Figure 7-37A). The segmenting contractions ("**haustral shuttling**") occur most often in the large intestine and function to gradually turn over the fecal contents. *Segmenting contractions are more rapid in the left colon than in the right colon, which tends to slow the movement of feces toward the rectum, allowing more time to complete fluid absorption* (see Figure 7-37B). Peristaltic contractions occur infrequently and act to forcefully propel feces into the rectum prior to defecation. Peristaltic contractions are giant migrating-type contractions called **mass movements.** These peristaltic waves typically occur 3–5 times per day, and each wave moves the fecal contents aborally 20 cm or more.

COLONIC FLUID TRANSPORT

Colonic fluid absorption reduces the 2 L per day of fluid that enters from the small intestine to about 0.1 L of fluid excretion in feces. The **mechanisms for Na⁺ absorption** that function in the right and left colon are as follows (Figure 7-38):

▪ In the **right (proximal) colon,** most Na⁺ uptake occurs via the Na⁺/H⁺ exchange, via a mechanism that resembles Na⁺ uptake in the ileum.

▪ In the **left (distal) colon,** Na⁺ absorption occurs via a Na⁺ channel, and K⁺ secretion occurs at the same time via K⁺ channels. *The transport model in the distal colon resembles that of the cortical collecting duct in the kidney* (see Chapter 6). In both locations, the hormone aldosterone stimulates Na⁺ absorption and K⁺ secretion.

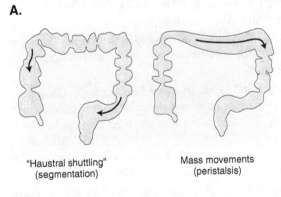

A.

"Haustral shuttling" (segmentation)   Mass movements (peristalsis)

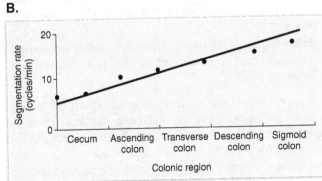

B.

Figure 7-37: A. Colonic motility patterns. **B.** The gradient of segmentation rates along the colon. A more rapid segmentation distally slows the aboral movement of the feces. Propulsion is achieved by giant migrating peristaltic contractions (mass movements).

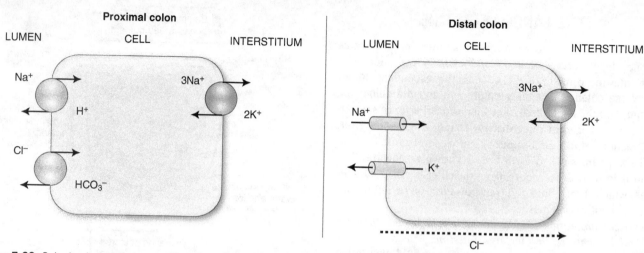

Figure 7-38: Colonic electrolyte transport in the proximal (right) colon **(A)** and in the distal (left) colon **(B)**.

The colon is also capable of fluid secretion, which is produced from the colonic crypts by the same mechanism as described above for the small intestine.

▽ Although rare, **villous adenomas** of the rectosigmoid colon can cause a **secretory diarrhea syndrome,** which results in hypokalemia and hypovolemia. ▼

▽ **DIARRHEA** Diarrhea is defined as an increase in stool fluid volume of more than 200 mL within 24 hours. In general terms, diarrhea may result from the delivery of more fluid to the colon than the colon can absorb, or it may result if feces move too rapidly through the colon to allow the colon to adequately absorb fluid. The **general causes of diarrhea** are:

- **Osmotic diarrhea** occurs when there is an agent in the intestine that causes water to be retained in the lumen. The agent may be a malabsorbed nutrient or an exogenous agent such as saline laxatives.

- **Secretory diarrhea** occurs when there is excess endogenous fluid secretion by enterocytes and colonocytes. Bacterial **food poisoning** is a common cause of secretory diarrhea (e.g., traveler's diarrhea caused by enterotoxic *E coli*). Rare causes of secretory diarrhea include hormone-secreting tumors that release secretagogues such as VIP or serotonin.

- **Rapid intestinal motility** may cause diarrhea due to transit times that are too brief to complete fluid and electrolyte absorption.

- **Inflammation** of the bowel may cause diarrhea as a result of increased fluid secretion and motility (e.g., inflammatory bowel disease).

Diarrhea may cause excessive loss of K^+ and HCO_3^- in feces, resulting in **hypokalemia** *and* **metabolic acidosis.** The principles underlying K^+ loss in diarrhea are the same as those that explain urinary K^+ loss from diuretic use (see Chapter 6). In this case, diarrhea causes large amounts of fluid and Na^+ delivery to the distal colon, which drives more Na^+ uptake via the Na^+ channels (Figure 7-38). This depolarizes the colonocyte apical membrane potential and increases the driving force for K^+ secretion. The diarrheal fluid entering the distal colon also has a low K^+ concentration and presents a more favorable diffusion gradient for K^+ secretion into the colon. Increased loss of HCO_3^- in feces occurs because of the Cl^-/HCO_3^- exchange in the apical cell membranes along the ileum and the colon. Luminal fluid contains NaCl; as more fluid flows past surface epithelial cells, there is more Cl^- available to drive HCO_3^- secretion. ▼

DIETARY FIBER

The main undigested material in feces is **nonstarch polysaccharides,** including cellulose, hemicellulose, lignin, pectin, gums, and algal polysaccharides, which are collectively called **dietary fiber.**

▽ A **high-fiber diet** improves colonic motility and reduces the incidence of constipation. Health benefits in other body systems are also associated with high-fiber diets, including reduced incidence of **coronary heart disease** and improved control of blood glucose concentration in type 2 diabetes mellitus, also called **non–insulin-dependent diabetes mellitus,** or NIDDM. ▼

Dietary fiber undergoes fermentation by bacteria in the colon, which produces the **short-chain fatty acids** acetate, propionate, and butyrate. Short-chain fatty acids create a more acidic colonic fluid, which prevents bacterial overgrowth. Fermentation reactions also produce gases (e.g., hydrogen, methane, carbon dioxide, and hydrogen sulfide), which are excreted as **flatus.**

ENTERIC MOTILITY

The functions of different motility patterns include **propulsion** (i.e., aboral movement of luminal material), **mixing** of luminal contents, or the creation of reservoirs for temporary **storage** of material (e.g., distal colon). The gastrointestinal tract is involved in a great deal of rhythmic contraction, which is facilitated by spontaneous electrical activity in gastrointestinal smooth muscle, known as the **basic electrical rhythm.** The sphincters along the gastrointestinal tract separate the gut into functional segments (Table 7-3). Sphincters are characterized as zones of high resting pressure that relax in response to an appropriate stimulus. Distention of the gut segment immediately distal to a sphincter causes it to contract, preventing retrograde flow. The actions of enteric nerves and hormones integrate motility behavior in each region of the gastrointestinal tract to promote digestion and absorption of nutrients.

SLOW WAVES

The phasic contractions that underlie mixing and propulsion of the intestinal contents are facilitated by the presence of a **basic electrical rhythm** (slow waves) in the gastrointestinal smooth muscle (Figure 7-39).

Slow waves in the gastrointestinal smooth muscle are spontaneous oscillations in the membrane potential. The distal stomach is the first location in the smooth muscle to exhibit slow waves.

TABLE 7-3. Sphincters in the Gastrointestinal Tract

Sphincter	Segments Separated
Upper esophageal sphincter	Mouth and pharynx
Lower esophageal sphincter	Esophagus and stomach
Sphincter of Oddi	Common bile duct and duodenum
Pyloric sphincter	Stomach and duodenum
Ileocecal sphincter	Ileum and cecum
Anal sphincter	Rectum and external environment

Spike potentials are triggered if the peak of a slow wave depolarizes the membrane to a threshold potential. Spike potentials are slow action potentials caused by the opening of Ca^{2+} channels.

Ca^{2+} entry into smooth muscle cells occurs during spike potentials and triggers **muscle contraction;** *this explains why the amount of force developed by muscle contraction correlates with the appearance of spike potentials.*

If spike potentials occur with every slow wave, a rhythmic contraction occurs with the same frequency as the slow wave. *The maximum frequency of rhythmic contraction in a given region of the gut, therefore, is set by the local rate of slow wave generation.* The observed pattern of gut motility (e.g., segmentation) is programmed by the ENS, which determines when slow waves will produce spike potentials and give rise to a contraction. **Excitatory transmitters** often cause nonselective cation channels in the smooth muscle cells to open; the resting membrane potential is depolarized and more slow waves cross the threshold for the generation of a spike potential. **Inhibitory transmitters** often act by opening the K^+ channels in smooth muscle cells, hyperpolarizing the membrane potential and preventing the slow waves from reaching threshold.

INTERSTITIAL CELLS OF CAJAL *The origin of the basic electrical rhythm is a network of fibroblast-like cells called the interstitial cells of Cajal,* which are positioned between the longitudinal and the circular smooth muscle layers. The interstitial cells of Cajal have multiple processes, many of which are electrically coupled to the smooth muscle cells via gap junctions and conduct the **pacemaker currents** to smooth muscle cells. Slow waves propagate down the gastrointestinal tract for variable distances via the extensive network of cell-to-cell contacts between the interstitial cells of Cajal.

MOTILITY PATTERNS ALONG THE GASTROINTESTINAL TRACT

Each of the areas of the gastrointestinal tract, as defined by the presence of sphincters (Table 7-3), shows patterns of motility that are distinct from other areas. In most cases, the observed motility patterns are strongly influenced by the characteristics of the locally generated slow waves.

ESOPHAGUS AND STOMACH There are no slow waves in the esophagus, which remains quiescent unless stimulated by swallowing or by the presence of a bolus in the lumen.

The proximal stomach does not exhibit rhythmic contraction nor does it produce slow waves. A steady tone in the proximal stomach presses on the gastric contents, pushing the contents toward the pylorus. *Slow waves are first encountered in the distal stomach,* and are driven by a pacemaker of the interstitial cells of Cajal in the **greater curvature** of the stomach. Slow waves occur at about 3–4 per minute and underlie the rhythmic contractions of **antral systole** that are observed when food is present.

SMALL INTESTINAL MOTILITY A pacemaker in the duodenum produces about 12 slow waves per minute. The rate of pacemaker activity declines progressively along the small bowel to about six to eight cycles per minute in the ileum. This pattern of slow

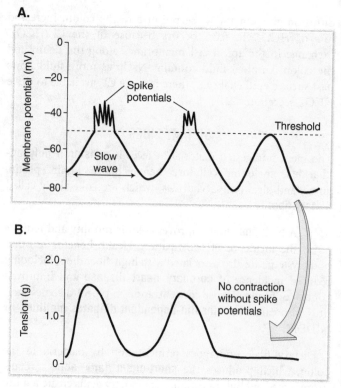

Figure 7-39: A. Basic electrical rhythm (slow waves) in gastrointestinal smooth muscle. **B.** Correlation of muscle contraction to the spike potentials. Spike potentials are Ca^{2+}-mediated action potentials triggered when slow waves cross a threshold potential.

waves produces a **gradient of segmenting contraction rates,** which is more rapid proximally than distally and promotes gradual aboral movement of food along the intestine.

The **terminal ileum** participates in reflexes that regulate intestinal motility and emptying of the stomach. If nutrients reach the terminal ileum, this reflects inadequate absorption at more proximal sites. The **ileal brake** is a mechanism that reduces stomach emptying and intestinal motility, and is mediated by the release of the hormones **glucagon-like peptide-1 and peptide YY.** A neuronal pathway operating through the ENS and the extrinsic nerves, known as the **ileogastric reflex,** augments the ileal brake when there is distension of the terminal ileum. The distal ileum is also able to sense inappropriate retrograde flow of colonic material into the small intestine. The distal ileum reacts to **short-chain fatty acids** derived from the colon by increasing peristalsis and quickly returning material to the colon. *If the distal ileum is surgically removed, a common effect is disrupted small intestinal motility.*

LARGE INTESTINAL MOTILITY *Most contractions of the large intestine are segmenting contractions that continually mix the fecal contents.* Occasional giant peristaltic contractions (mass movements) propel fecal material into the rectum. Mass movements are increased in frequency and intensity by the **gastrocolic reflex,** which is triggered by the entry of food into the stomach and duodenum. The neuronal pathway includes both the ENS and the autonomic nerves. **Fecal continence** is maintained by the action of several anal sphincters.

- The **internal anal sphincter** is a thickening of smooth muscle around the anal canal and is controlled by the autonomic nerves.

- The **external anal sphincter** is distal to the internal sphincter and is composed of skeletal muscle around the anal canal.

- The **pelvic diaphragm** is also important in the maintenance of fecal continence and is a sling of skeletal muscle, originating from the bony pelvis that forms the **acute anorectal angle.**

Rectal distension initiates the **rectosphincteric reflex,** in which the internal anal sphincter initially relaxes and the intraluminal pressure recorded in the anal canal decreases (Figure 7-40). As fecal material moves down into the upper part of the anal canal, it initiates the urge to defecate. Voluntary contraction of the external anal sphincter can override the rectosphincteric reflex. Voluntary contraction of the external sphincter causes the internal sphincter to regain tone; the rectal wall relaxes to reduce rectal pressure, and feces are temporarily **accommodated** in the rectum. If the defecation reflex is allowed to continue, the internal and external anal sphincters both relax. Coordinated voluntary acts of straining occur in conjunction with propulsive involuntary contractions of the left colon and rectum to expel feces.

MIGRATING MOTOR COMPLEX

The migrating motor complex is a pattern of motility that occurs about every 90 minutes between meals. It involves an interval of strong propulsive contractions, which pass down

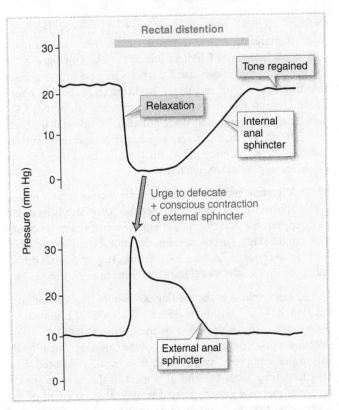

Figure 7-40: Rectosphincteric reflex. Pressure recordings within the internal and the external anal sphincters are shown during sustained rectal distension. Pressure at the internal sphincter decreases, indicating relaxation of the sphincter muscle. Increased pressure in the external anal sphincter reflects conscious contraction and causes the internal sphincter to regain its tone. The rectum relaxes to accommodate and store feces until an appropriate time for defecation.

the distal stomach and small intestine (Figure 7-41). The function of migrating motor complexes is to sweep the stomach and small intestine of indigestible materials. During a meal, the stomach only allows small particles to pass into the small intestine, leaving behind larger particles (e.g., dietary fiber). The migrating motor complex is an intrinsic property of the gastrointestinal tract that does not require external innervation. The appearance of migrating motor complexes in infants indicates the developmental maturity of the intestines and can be absent in **premature neonates.**

▽ **Migrating motor complexes** rarely disappear as a person ages or in pathologic states; however, they have been found to disappear, for example, in patients after treatment of cancer with **radiotherapy.** Loss of the migrating motor complex can cause bacterial overgrowth in the small intestine, suggesting that it normally prevents **bacterial colonization** of the upper intestine. ▽

The clock that sets the regular 90-minute intervals of contraction is found within the ENS. The motor program that is initiated includes secretion of the hormone **motilin,** which stimulates propulsive contractions of the intestine. The migrating motor complexes continue until a meal is ingested. The length of time from the end of a meal to the next migrating motor complex is linearly related to the caloric content of the meal rather than to ingestion of a specific nutrient. The start of an **interdigestive period** is defined by the first migrating motor complex that occurs after a meal.

▽ **Gastrointestinal distress** (i.e., nausea, vomiting, and diarrhea) is the most common adverse effect of **erythromycin,** a macrolide antibiotic. Erythromycin binds to motilin receptors, causing increased gastrointestinal motility, which is responsible for the unfavorable adverse effects of this drug. ▽

▽ **VOMITING** Vomiting removes noxious or harmful irritants from the gastrointestinal tract and can be initiated by several mechanisms, including:

▪ Noxious stimuli in the **gut lumen** (e.g., infected food) stimulate sensory receptors in the gut wall, resulting in the subjective sensation of nausea carried by autonomic nerves to the CNS.

▪ **Higher brain centers** can induce nausea and vomiting in the absence of noxious stimuli in the gut (e.g., as a result of seeing a disturbing image, smelling a nauseating odor, or by motion sickness).

▪ Chemicals in the circulation can induce vomiting by acting on a region of the area postrema on the lateral wall of the fourth ventricle, called the **chemoreceptor trigger zone.** The dopamine agonist **apomorphine** is an example of a stimulant of the chemoreceptor trigger zone that may be used in patients who have Parkinson's disease. Antiemetics must be given prophylactically to prevent vomiting when apomorphine is used. ▽

▽ The CNS **vomiting center** integrates stimuli and coordinates the act of vomiting, which involves reverse peristalsis in the small intestine and stomach, together with sequential relaxation of the pyloric, the lower esophageal, and the upper esophageal sphincters. Serotonin (5-HT) and dopamine (D) are

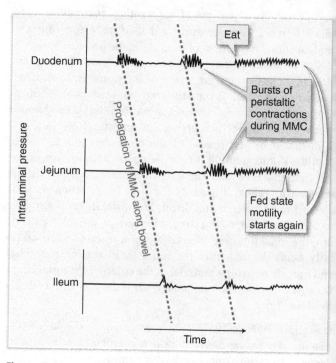

Figure 7-41: The migrating motor complex (MMC). Intraluminal pressure is measured at several sites along the small intestine. Isolated clusters of pressure spikes indicate the presence of the MMC at a given location. Dashed lines follow propagation of the MMC along the small intestine.

important transmitters in the central vomiting pathway; antagonists at the 5-HT$_3$ (e.g., ondansetron) and the D$_2$ receptors (e.g., prochlorperazine) are effective **antiemetics.** ▼

SPLANCHNIC CIRCULATION

The splanchnic circulation is the largest regional circulation at rest and receives about 30% of the cardiac output. The splanchnic circulation is also the largest reservoir of blood that can be redirected to other vascular beds (e.g., during exercise). Most of the blood in the splanchnic circulation is distributed to the gastrointestinal organs via the celiac and superior mesenteric arteries. Most of the venous drainage from the digestive system passes to the liver via the hepatic portal vein.

*The **sympathetic nervous system** is a dominant effector that controls splanchnic vascular resistance.* The release of norepinephrine by the postganglionic nerves causes **vasoconstriction** and **venoconstriction.** Norepinephrine is responsible for the decrease in splanchnic blood flow associated with the general cardiovascular stressors that activate the sympathetic nervous system, including reduced blood pressure, reduced blood volume, and fear and pain. *The gastrointestinal system is vulnerable to low blood flow and ischemia in states of **shock,** which can result in the release of toxins or the entry of pathogens.*

▽ **Mesenteric ischemia** results from low blood flow to the bowel. The most common cause of this disorder is due to the rupture of an **atheroma** (plaque in the arterial wall) with associated blockage of blood vessels. Clinically, this condition is most common in elderly people and presents as unremitting abdominal pain that is out of proportion to physical findings and is associated with bloody diarrhea. Bacterial migration across the injured bowel wall quickly results in **potentially fatal peritonitis.** The mortality rate in patients with mesenteric ischemia is over 50%. ▼

The period of increased splanchnic blood flow after a meal is called **postprandial hyperemia.** Splanchnic vasodilation results from several factors, including the hormonal environment (e.g., high levels of CCK) and the action of enteric nerves (e.g., VIPergic neurons). In addition, the generalized increase in parasympathetic nerve activity after a meal stimulates gastrointestinal secretion and motility, which indirectly increases splanchnic blood flow as a result of increased local metabolism (see Chapter 4).

STUDY QUESTIONS

Directions: Each numbered item is followed by lettered options. Some options may be partially correct, but there is only *ONE BEST* answer.

1. A healthy 28-year-old woman participated in a study of gastrointestinal function. She ingested a single nutritionally balanced meal containing small inert plastic beads, which could be visualized using medical imaging techniques. What is the most likely location of the beads 8 hours after ingestion of the meal?

   A. Arrested at lower esophageal sphincter
   B. Arrested at the pyloric sphincter
   C. Duodenum
   D. Ileum
   E. Sigmoid colon
   F. Excreted in feces

2. A 9-year-old boy awoke in the night complaining of abdominal pain that was dull and poorly localized. Which of the following pathways conveys these sensations of pain to consciousness?

   A. Myenteric plexus
   B. Sacral parasympathetic nerves
   C. Splanchnic sympathetic nerves
   D. Submucosal plexus
   E. Vagus nerve

3. A 49-year-old university professor volunteered to be the subject in a clinical demonstration in which a pressure sensor was passed an unknown distance into his esophagus via the nasopharynx. At one moment, the sensor was located in a region of tonically high resting pressure. When he was asked to swallow, there was an immediate decrease in pressure, followed by a rapid increase in the pressure at this location. Where was the pressure sensor located?

   A. Upper esophageal sphincter
   B. Thoracic esophageal body
   C. Abdominal esophageal body
   D. Lower esophageal sphincter
   E. Fundus of stomach

4. A 61-year-old man saw his physician with a complaint of progressive difficulty swallowing solid food. He reported a weight loss of about 18 kg (40 lb) despite trying to eat. He was frequently aspirating his food. The results of a radiology series and esophageal manometry suggested a diagnosis of achalasia. Which element of esophageal function would be LEAST affected in this patient?

   A. Relaxation of the upper esophageal sphincter
   B. Peristalsis in the upper esophageal body
   C. Peristalsis in the lower esophageal body
   D. Relaxation of the lower esophageal sphincter

5. Experiments were conducted using an in vitro stomach preparation to determine individual dose-response relationships for the stimulation of gastric acid production by histamine, gastrin, and acetylcholine. The dose corresponding to 50% stimulation was selected for each agonist. Which combination of agonists at this dose would produce the greatest stimulation of acid production?

   A. Histamine alone
   B. Gastrin alone
   C. Acetylcholine alone
   D. Gastrin + acetylcholine
   E. Histamine + gastrin
   F. Histamine + acetylcholine
   G. Histamine + gastrin + acetylcholine

6. A 17-year-old girl with cystic fibrosis has a history of recurrent lung infections. Until recently, she has reported few gastrointestinal symptoms. Due to recent weight loss and problems with bloating and discomfort, her pancreatic function is now being assessed using a secretin stimulation test. Which of the following abnormal responses to intravenous injection of secretin would be observed in this patient when compared with a normal subject?

   A. Increased secretion of pancreatic enzymes
   B. Increased pancreatic bicarbonate secretion
   C. Reduced gastric acid secretion
   D. Reduced volume of pancreatic juice

7. A 41-year-old woman with a history of biliary colic and gallstone disease was taken to the emergency department because of severe acute pain in the epigastric region. The patient also reports pain in the right shoulder area. Physical examination revealed generalized yellowing of skin and scleral membranes. Which profile of bile pigments would be expected in this patient?

	Free Plasma Bilirubin	Conjugated Plasma Bilirubin	Plasma Urobilinogen
A.	High	High	Normal
B.	High	Normal	High
C.	High	High	Low
D.	Normal	Normal	High
E.	Normal	High	Normal

8. A 22-year-old woman who has Crohn's disease underwent surgical removal of the distal ileum. Without supportive therapy, this patient is most likely to develop which of the following conditions within 1 year?

   A. Anemia

   B. Calcium deficiency

   C. Caloric malnutrition

   D. Iron deficiency

   E. Lactase deficiency

9. A 52-year-old man visited his physician because of persistent epigastric pain. The patient reported defecating at least five times a day and had lost weight despite trying to eat more. A 24-hour fecal sample revealed high rates of fat excretion. Which of the following differential diagnoses should be considered?

   A. Hypersecretion of gastric acid

   B. Inflammatory bowel disease

   C. Obstructive gallstone disease

   D. Pancreatic insufficiency

   E. All of the above

10. A 4-week-old boy was brought to the emergency department in a semiconscious state. He was severely dehydrated and an electrocardiogram showed abnormal waveforms. The boy's parents reported that he had severe acute diarrhea that had worsened over the past 24 hours. No vomiting had occurred. They had tried to treat the child with fluids orally. Serum analysis revealed a potassium concentration of 1.9 mM. Which mechanism accounts for severe hypokalemia in this case?

   A. Excess secretion of potassium in the small intestine

   B. Excess secretion of potassium in the large intestine

   C. Failure to absorb potassium in the small intestine

   D. Failure to absorb potassium in the large intestine

ANSWERS

1—D. The microspheres travel with the meal and reflect the transit time of the meal. After 8 hours, the meal would typically progress to the distal small intestine. The beads are small enough not to be arrested by sphincters.

2—C. Most afferent nerves conveying pain in the gastrointestinal tract travel in the sympathetic division of the autonomic nervous system.

3—A. High resting pressure indicates the sensor was located in a sphincter. The pattern of pressure changes upon swallowing describes the action of upper esophageal sphincter.

4—A. Achalasia is a condition that affects the intrinsic nerves of the ENS in the esophagus. Relaxation of the lower sphincter and the organization of peristalsis are particularly affected. The upper esophageal sphincter is controlled by extrinsic nerves and is minimally affected by achalasia.

5—G. There is potentiation between histamine, gastrin, and acetylcholine so that the combined response is greater than the sum of individual responses.

6—D. Cystic fibrosis Cl^- channels are required for fluid secretion by pancreatic ducts, which secrete most of the volume of pancreatic juice. Cl^- channels supply Cl^- from the cell to drive HCO_3^- secretion into the duct lumen. The secretion of HCO_3^- drives Na^+ secretion and fluid secretion. Without a functional Cl^- channel, fluid secretion is reduced very significantly.

7—C. The clinical signs and symptoms suggest blockage of the lower biliary tract with a gallstone. Obstructive jaundice develops, in which the liver conjugates bilirubin, which leaks into the systemic circulation. The capacity of hepatocytes to continue conjugating bilirubin decreases when the outflow pathway into the biliary tract is blocked. Therefore, serum free bilirubin levels increase. The lack of conjugated bilirubin entering the intestines prevents formation of urobilinogen; therefore the levels of urobilinogen are low.

8—A. The distal ileum is a specific site for absorption of vitamin B_{12}. Deficiency of this vitamin leads to pernicious anemia.

9—E. The patient has fat malabsorption. Hyperacidity can denature pancreatic lipase. Pancreatic insufficiency results in inadequate pancreatic lipase secretion. Obstructive gallstone disease limits bile delivery and reduces fat assimilation. Inflammatory bowel disease may prevent adequate absorption of dietary fat even when digestion is normal.

10—B. Potassium secretion in the distal large intestine occurs through luminal membrane potassium channels. The delivery of increased amounts of sodium and fluid to the large intestine in diarrhea drives excess potassium secretion.

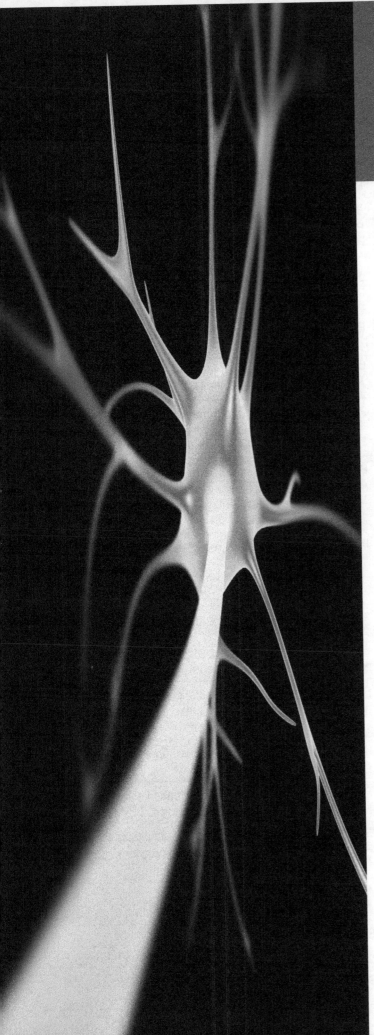

CHAPTER 8

ENDOCRINE PHYSIOLOGY

THE ENDOCRINE SYSTEM

OVERVIEW

A **hormone** is a chemical that is produced by the body and has a specific regulatory effect on a target cell or organ. Classic endocrinology was concerned with the functions of anatomically defined glands such as the thyroid gland or the pituitary gland. It is now recognized that almost every organ secretes hormones and that endocrine cells may be dispersed throughout the body (e.g., in the gut mucosa). The more recent study of endocrinology encompasses all processes concerned with the physiology of hormones. Certain diseases commonly encountered in general medical practice, such as diabetes mellitus or thyroid disorders, are caused by a **deficiency** or an **excess** of specific hormones. Many other common diseases not directly caused by endocrine dysfunction have prominent endocrine components, including cancer and atherosclerosis. Table 8-1 summarizes the hormones produced by the major endocrine organs.

INTERCELLULAR COMMUNICATION SYSTEMS

The maintenance of homeostasis requires the coordination of cells, tissues, and organs. Most communication between cells is achieved by the release of chemical messengers. The **modes of intercellular communication** are described as follows (Figure 8-1):

TABLE 8-1. Summary of Hormones Produced by the Major Endocrine Organs

Endocrine Gland	Hormone(s) Produced	Chemical Structure	Overview: Major Function(s)
Hypothalamus	Corticotropin-releasing hormone (CRH)	Peptide	• Stimulates adrenocorticotropic hormone (ACTH)
	Growth hormone-releasing hormone (GHRH)	Peptide	• Stimulates growth hormone (GH) release
	Growth hormone inhibitory hormone (GHIH; also known as somatostatin)	Peptide	• Inhibits GH release
	Gonadotropin-releasing hormone (GnRH)	Peptide	• Stimulates luteinizing hormone (LH) and follicle-stimulating hormone (FSH) release
	Prolactin-inhibiting factor (PIF; also known as dopamine)	Peptide	• Inhibits prolactin release
	Thyrotropin-releasing hormone (TRH)	Peptide	• Stimulates thyroid-stimulating hormone (TSH) and prolactin release
Anterior pituitary	ACTH	Peptide	• Trophic to adrenal cortex • Stimulates synthesis and secretion of cortisol, aldosterone, and androgens
	FSH	Peptide	• Promotes sperm maturation via Sertoli cells in testes • Stimulates ovarian follicle development
	GH	Peptide	• Acute metabolic effects oppose insulin • Chronic growth-promoting effect via insulin-like growth factor 1 (IGF-1)
	LH	Peptide	• Stimulates Leydig cells of testes to secrete testosterone • LH surge important for ovulation & formation of corpus luteum
	Prolactin	Peptide	• Required in lactation for mammary growth, initiation of milk secretion, and maintenance of milk production
	TSH	Peptide	• Stimulates synthesis and secretion of thyroid hormones
Posterior pituitary	Antidiuretic hormone (ADH) (also called arginine vasopressin, or AVP)	Peptide	• Increases water retention at kidney • Vasoconstricts arterioles
	Oxytocin	Peptide	• Stimulates uterine contractions during labor • Milk ejection in lactation
Thyroid	Triiodothyronine (T_3) & thyroxine (T_4)	Amine	• Increase metabolic rate • Required for normal growth and development
Adrenal cortex	Aldosterone	Steroid	• Decreases urinary Na^+ excretion • Increases urinary K^+ and H^+ excretion
	Cortisol	Steroid	• Released in response to stress • Multiple metabolic actions

Endocrine Gland	Hormone(s) Produced	Chemical Structure	Overview: Major Function(s)
Adrenal medulla	Epinephrine & norepinephrine	Amine	• Produces effects similar to actions of the sympathetic nervous system
Pancreas	Insulin (β cell)	Peptide	• Promotes storage of glucose as glycogen in liver and muscle • Promotes uptake of glucose and storage as triglyceride in adipose tissue and liver
	Glucagon (α cell)	Peptide	• Increases blood glucose by promoting glycogenolysis, gluconeogenesis, and ketogenesis in liver
Parathyroid	Parathyroid hormone (PTH)	Peptide	• Regulates serum $[Ca^{2+}]$ • Increases Ca^{2+} resorption from bone • Increases renal and intestinal Ca^{2+} absorption • Increases renal phosphate excretion
Testes	Testosterone	Steroid	• Required for male puberty; development and maintenance of male reproductive organs and secondary sex characteristics
Ovaries	Estrogens	Steroid	• Required for female puberty; development and maintenance of female reproductive organs and secondary sex characteristics
	Progesterone	Steroid	• Supports secretory phase of endometrial cycle • Important in maintenance of pregnancy
Other Endocrine Organs			
Placenta	Human chorionic gonadotropin (hCG)	Peptide	• Maintains corpus luteum early in pregnancy
	Human chorionic somatomammotropin (hCS) (also called human placental lactogen, or hPL)	Peptide	• Supports breast development in pregnancy • Regulates fuel metabolism of fetoplacental unit
Stomach	Gastrin	Peptide	• Stimulates HCl secretion by parietal cells of gastric mucosa
Small intestine	Cholecystokinin (CCK)	Peptide	• Stimulates release of pancreatic enzymes • Contracts gallbladder • Relaxes sphincter of Oddi • Inhibits stomach motility • Acts as satiety signal
	Secretin	Peptide	• Increases fluid and HCO_3^- secretion by pancreatic duct • Feedback inhibition of gastric H^+ secretion
Kidney	Renin	Peptide	• Cleaves circulating angiotensinogen to angiotensin I • Rate-limiting step in renin-angiotensin II-aldosterone axis
	1-25-Dihydroxycholecalciferol $(1,25\text{-}(OH)_2D_3)$	Steroid	• Stimulates gastrointestinal Ca^{2+} and phosphate absorption
	Erythropoietin (EPO)	Peptide	• Stimulates red blood cell production
Heart	Atrial natriuretic peptide (ANP)	Peptide	• Increases renal Na^+ excretion

■ **Neural** communication occurs by rapid information transfer using electrical signals; the release of neurotransmitters at synapses between neurons or at a target cell such as a muscle produces a response.

■ **Endocrine** communication occurs by the release of a chemical transmitter (hormone) by specialized endocrine cells and is carried to a distant site of action via the blood.

■ **Neuroendocrine** control is a hybrid of neural and endocrine communication in which neurons release a chemical transmitter (**neurohormone**) that is carried to a distant site of action via the blood; for example, the release of an antidiuretic hormone from the axon terminals in the posterior pituitary gland.

■ **Paracrine** communication involves cells that secrete chemical transmitters locally into the surrounding interstitial fluid; the target cells are near "neighbors" and are reached by diffusion of the hormone rather than by its transport in the blood.

■ **Autocrine** signaling occurs when a cell regulates itself by the release of a chemical messenger.

CLASSES OF HORMONES

Most hormones can be grouped into one of **three major chemical classes:** peptides, amines, and steroids.

1. **Peptides** are the largest group of hormones. Peptide hormones are synthesized in the rough endoplasmic reticulum of endocrine cells, typically as inactive preprohormones. A series of cleavage steps occurs in the endoplasmic reticulum and during passage of the prohormones through the Golgi apparatus into the secretory vesicles. Peptide-secreting endocrine cells store active hormones in intracellular vesicles until a stimulus triggers hormone secretion by exocytosis. Peptide hormones are generally water soluble and do not require carrier molecules in the blood.

2. **Amines** are a small group of hormones that includes the catecholamines (dopamine, epinephrine, and norepinephrine) and the thyroid hormones. Catecholamines are synthesized from tyrosine and stored in preformed vesicles, awaiting release by exocytosis. Catecholamines are water-soluble hormones that do not require carrier proteins in the plasma. Thyroid hormones are also derived from the amino acid tyrosine but are poorly soluble in water and do require carrier proteins in the blood.

3. **Steroid hormones** are synthesized from **cholesterol** and include cortisol, aldosterone, testosterone, estrogen, and progesterone. Steroid hormones are not stored in vesicles and rapidly diffuse out of the cell once synthesized due to their high lipid solubility. Steroids generally require carrier proteins in the blood due to their low water solubility. The properties of steroid hormones are compared to peptide hormones in Table 8-2.

There are several other types of hormones that have been discovered that are not included in the major chemical classes, including the **purines** (e.g., adenosine and adenosine triphosphate [ATP]) and some **gases** (e.g., nitric oxide and carbon monoxide).

PLASMA HORMONE CONCENTRATION

The magnitude of a response to a hormone depends on how many receptors are occupied at the target cell, which in turn depends

Neural

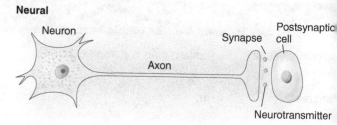

Endocrine

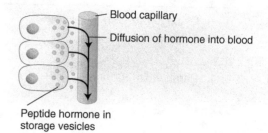

Neuroendocrine

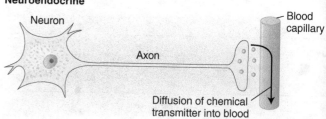

Paracrine

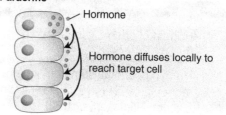

Autocrine

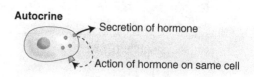

Figure 8-1: Modes of intercellular communication.

TABLE 8-2. Properties of Different Chemical Classes of Hormones

Hormone Characteristic	Peptide Hormone*	Steroid Hormone
Water soluble	Yes	No
Uses carrier protein in plasma	No	Yes
Is stored in vesicles prior to secretion	Yes	No
Receptor location at target cell	Plasma membrane	Intracellular
Mechanism of action	Mainly second messengers	Mainly altered gene expression
Speed and duration of action	Usually fast onset but short-acting responses	Usually slow onset but long-lasting responses

*The amine class has variable characteristics; catecholamines have properties more like peptides, whereas thyroid hormones share many of the characteristics of steroids.

on the free hormone concentration in the extracellular fluid. The plasma **free hormone concentration** is affected by:

1. The rate of hormone **secretion.**

2. The rate of hormone **elimination.**

3. The extent of hormone **binding to plasma proteins.**

FEEDBACK CONTROL OF HORMONE SECRETION In most cases, the rate of hormone secretion is under negative feedback control (Figure 8-2A). *Simple negative feedback occurs when a hormone, or a response to a hormone, directly inhibits further secretion of that hormone.* For example, insulin secretion by the β cells in the pancreas causes a decrease in the blood glucose concentration, which directly inhibits further insulin release.

In some cases, hormone secretion is under **hierarchical control** (complex negative feedback); for example, hormone secretion from a primary target gland that is controlled by the anterior pituitary hormones, which in turn are controlled by hypothalamic factors (see Figure 8-2B). Negative feedback can operate at the level of the primary gland, the anterior pituitary, or the hypothalamus. **Endocrine disorders** can be classified as primary, secondary, or tertiary.

- **Primary** disorder is an excess or deficiency of secretion by the target gland.

- **Secondary** disorder is an excess or deficiency of secretion by the pituitary gland.

- **Tertiary** disorder is an excess or deficiency of secretion by the hypothalamus.

In a few cases, the rate of hormone secretion may be controlled by **positive feedback,** in which the effects of the hormone result in further hormone secretion. For example, the surge in the plasma luteinizing hormone concentration, which occurs just prior to ovulation, is due to positive feedback stimulation by estrogen (see Chapter 9, Female Reproductive Physiology).

For some hormones, the plasma hormone concentration is strongly influenced by a rhythmic pattern of secretion. For example, the steroid hormone cortisol has a distinctive **circadian** (day/night) pattern of secretion, with the highest hormone concentration in the early morning hours and less concentration during late afternoon and evening. A **pulsatile** pattern of hormone

A. Simple negative feedback

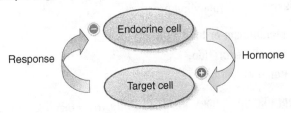

B. Complex negative feedback

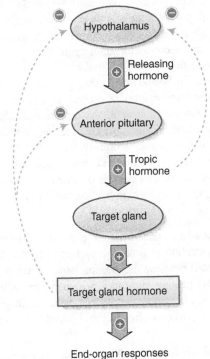

End-organ responses

Figure 8-2: Negative feedback control secretion. **A.** Simple negative feedback in which a hormone, or a response to the hormone, inhibits further hormone secretion. **B.** Complex (hierarchical) negative feedback in which a hormone secreted from a primary target gland exerts negative feedback on the hypothalamus and pituitary gland.

release is often superimposed on such rhythms (e.g., secretion of hypothalamic hormones). The existence of cyclic and pulsatile patterns of hormone secretion suggests that a single blood sample may not provide useful information about the adequacy of the plasma hormone concentration. For example, when hypercortisolism is suspected in a patient, it is important to collect a urine sample over a 24-hour period and measure the levels of free cortisol. *Dynamic tests to measure changes in hormone levels upon stimulation are often more meaningful than single blood samples* that are taken to determine the adequacy of hormone secretion (e.g., the adrenocorticotropic hormone [ACTH] stimulation test used to assess adrenocortical insufficiency).

HORMONE ELIMINATION Plasma hormone concentration is strongly influenced by the rate of hormone elimination. The **half-life** of a hormone is the time it takes to reduce the plasma hormone concentration by one half, and is used as an indicator of the rate of hormone elimination. The **metabolic clearance rate** of a hormone is the volume of plasma cleared of a hormone per minute. The metabolic clearance rate is calculated by dividing the rate of hormone removal from plasma by the plasma hormone concentration. **Hormones can be removed from plasma** by the following processes:

- **Metabolism or binding** in the tissues.
- **Hepatic excretion.**
- **Renal excretion.**

HORMONE TRANSPORT IN BLOOD Only free hormone molecules can diffuse out of capillaries and bind to their receptors at the target cell. Binding of a hormone to plasma proteins reduces the free concentration available. For example, steroids and thyroid hormones are poorly soluble in water and must bind to plasma proteins to be carried in plasma; typically, more than 90% of the total hormone concentration is protein bound. *The protein-bound hormone fraction remains in the plasma and is inactive.* The half-life of protein-bound hormones is generally long because the protein-bound fraction acts as a reservoir of the hormone. Water-soluble hormones such as peptides and catecholamines dissolve easily in the blood plasma and are able to freely diffuse from the plasma to their site of action. Water-soluble hormones that are not extensively protein bound tend to have a faster onset of action and act for shorter periods of time (e.g., catecholamines) than do hormones with a high fraction bound to carrier proteins in plasma (e.g., thyroid hormones).

▼ Alterations in serum protein concentration can affect the **concentration of protein-bound compounds.** This principle is illustrated by using the example of Ca^{2+}, which is approximately 50% protein bound (primarily to albumin). In hypoalbuminemic states, such as liver failure or nephrotic syndrome, the proportion of free (active) ionized Ca^{2+} increases. ▼

MEASUREMENT OF HORMONE CONCENTRATION *Hormones are effective at very low concentrations, in the 10^{-9} to 10^{-12} molar range.* **Radioimmunoassay** is the prototype technique used for determining the hormone concentration. This technique is based on the principle of competitive binding, and requires an antibody that specifically binds to the hormone plus radioactively labeled hormone. Radioactive hormone is incubated with limiting amounts of antibody, and a standard curve is prepared by adding known amounts of unlabeled hormone to displace radioactive hormone (Figure 8-3). The standard curve provides the relationship between the radioactivity remaining and the unlabeled hormone concentration; as more unlabeled hormone is added, less radioactivity remains. The standard curve is used to determine the hormone concentrations in plasma samples; there is less radioactivity remaining when a sample contains a large hormone concentration.

HORMONE RECEPTORS AND INTRACELLULAR SIGNALING

A response to a particular hormone is seen only in cells with specific receptors for that hormone. Receptors are proteins that may be in the surface membrane (e.g., peptide hormones and catecholamines), in the cell cytoplasm (e.g., steroid hormones), or in the nucleus (e.g., thyroid hormones). The response to a hormone is affected by the number of available receptors; downregulation or upregulation of the receptor number determines the **sensitivity** of a target cell to a hormone. In most cases, activation of a receptor by hormone binding changes the target cell activity either through the generation of **intracellular second messengers** or via changes in **gene transcription and translation.**

▽ **Schizophrenia** is a disease that is associated with an excess of dopamine in the brain. Pharmacologic management of the patient focuses on blocking specific dopamine receptors. However, long-term blockage of the dopamine receptors causes upregulation of the receptor, which is thought to be responsible for some of the adverse effects associated with antipsychotic medications (e.g., tardive dyskinesia). ▽

SECOND MESSENGER SYSTEMS FOR PEPTIDES AND CATECHOLAMINES
There are many examples in which the binding of a hormone (first messenger) to its receptor causes the generation of intracellular signaling molecules (second messengers). *Second messengers amplify the hormonal signal within the target cell.* A common means that second messengers use to bring about changes in cellular activity is through the stimulation of **kinases,** which are enzymes that phosphorylate target proteins. In the case of peptide hormones and catecholamines, the process of second messenger generation usually begins when the hormone-receptor complex associates with intracellular **heterotrimeric G proteins** (Figure 8-4A). G proteins have three subunits: α, β, and γ. Interaction with the hormone-receptor complex causes the **Gα subunit** to dissociate from the βγ subunit. The Gα subunit can interact with one of several effector proteins to regulate second messenger production. The G protein family is large, and different G proteins activate different **second messenger pathways,** including the ubiquitous cyclic adenosine monophosphate (cAMP) pathway and the diacylglycerol (DAG) and the inositol 1,4,5-triphosphate (IP_3) pathways.

▪ **cAMP** is formed from ATP by the membrane-bound enzyme **adenylyl cyclase.** The activity of adenylyl cyclase depends on the relative activation of the **stimulatory ($G_{\alpha s}$)** or **inhibitory ($G_{\alpha i}$)** G proteins. *The presence of stimulatory and inhibitory G proteins, coupled to different hormone-receptor*

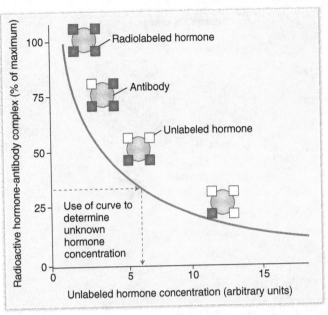

Figure 8-3: Radioimmunoassay standard curve used to measure hormone concentrations. A specific antibody to the hormone is incubated with radiolabeled hormone. A standard curve is created by introducing known concentrations of unlabeled hormone to displace radiolabeled hormone. The amount of radioactivity remaining is a function of unlabeled hormone concentration. When unknown samples are used, the measurement of the radioactivity remaining allows the hormone concentration to be read from the standard curve.

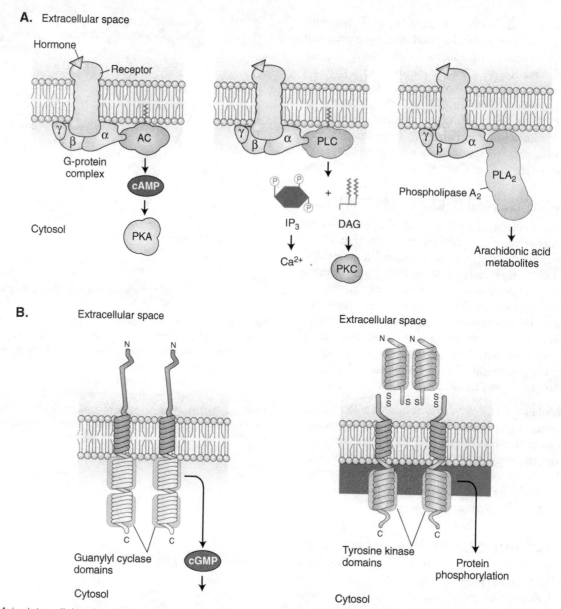

Figure 8-4: Major intracellular signaling systems used by peptide hormones and catecholamines. **A.** Coupling of the hormone-receptor complex to generation of intracellular second messengers by heterotrimeric G proteins. **B.** Hormone receptors that do not interact with G proteins. For example, some hormone receptors express enzyme activity when the hormone binds, including receptor guanylyl cyclases and receptor tyrosine kinases. AC, adenylyl cyclase; cAMP, cyclic adenosine monophosphate; PKA, protein kinase A; PLC, phospholipase C; IP₃, inositol 1,4,5-triphosphate; DAG, diacylglycerol; PKC, protein kinase C; cGMP, cyclic guanosine monophosphate.

complexes, demonstrates the principle that hormones can have antagonistic actions. For example, in the gastric parietal cells, histamine stimulates acid secretion through cAMP signaling via $G_{\alpha s}$, whereas prostaglandin E_2 inhibits cAMP formation via $G_{\alpha i}$ (see Chapter 7). When cAMP is produced inside a cell, it activates **protein kinase A,** which affects cellular activity through phosphorylation of the effector proteins. The cAMP signal is terminated when cAMP is broken down by the action of a **phosphodiesterase enzyme.**

▽ **Phosphodiesterase type III** is responsible for the breakdown of cAMP in cardiac muscle and blood vessels. **Milrinone** is a cardiovascular drug used in the acute management of patients with decompensated heart failure; it belongs to a unique class of drugs known as **inotropic vasodilators.**

Milrinone inhibits phosphodiesterase type III, thereby potentiating the effects of cAMP in cardiac muscle (increased contractility) and blood vessels (vasodilation). ▼

- **DAG and IP$_3$** are produced by the action of the membrane-bound enzyme **phospholipase C.** Phospholipase C is activated via the **G protein G$_{\alpha q}$,** and cleaves the membrane lipid phosphatidylinositol 4,5-bisphosphate (PIP$_2$) to generate DAG and IP$_3$. In the presence of Ca^{2+}, DAG activates **protein kinase C,** which in turn phosphorylates target proteins to bring about changes in cellular behavior. IP$_3$ causes the release of Ca^{2+} from the endoplasmic reticulum Ca^{2+} store. An increase in the intracellular [Ca^{2+}] alters the activity of many cellular proteins.

There are several **intracellular signaling systems** that are not dependent on the G proteins to couple the hormone-receptor complex to the generation of a second messenger (see Figure 8-4B):

- **Receptor tyrosine kinases** (e.g., the insulin receptor) directly initiate cascades of phosphorylation reactions within the cell when occupied by their hormone. Cytoplasmic tyrosine kinases such as **Janus kinase (JAK)** are activated when a hormone binds to tyrosine kinase-associated receptors (e.g., the growth hormone receptor).

▽ *Upregulation of tyrosine kinase receptors is linked to various endocrine neoplasms.* For example, the **RET protooncogene** encodes for a receptor tyrosine kinase that is used in cell signaling. Mutations in the RET protooncogene that lead to an increase in function are associated with **medullary thyroid cancer** and **multiple endocrine neoplasia (MEN) types 2 and 3.** ▼

- **Cyclic guanosine monophosphate (cGMP)** is generated from guanosine triphosphate (GTP) via the enzyme **guanylyl cyclase.** In some cases, the hormone receptor acquires guanylyl cyclase activity when the hormone occupies the receptor (e.g., the atrial natriuretic peptide receptor). Soluble guanylyl cyclase also exists in the cell cytoplasm of some cells and can be activated, for example, by **nitric oxide.** Like cAMP, the cGMP signal is terminated when cGMP is broken down by the action of a phosphodiesterase enzyme.

▽ **Phosphodiesterase type V** is responsible for the breakdown of cGMP in pulmonary vascular smooth muscle and in erectile tissue. **Sildenafil** (Viagra) inhibits phosphodiesterase type V and increases the vasodilatory effects of cGMP in both the pulmonary vascular bed and in the penis, making it an appropriate treatment for either pulmonary hypertension or erectile dysfunction. ▼

EICOSANOIDS The eicosanoids are a group of second messengers that are derived from **arachidonic acid;** the group includes **prostaglandins, prostacyclins, thromboxanes, and leukotrienes.** Eicosanoids differ from other second messengers because they themselves are hormones rather than intracellular signals. Arachidonic acid is produced from membrane lipids when the enzyme **phospholipase A$_2$** is activated via **G$_{\alpha q}$ or G$_{\alpha 11}$.** Therefore, the binding of a first hormonal messenger to its receptor can result

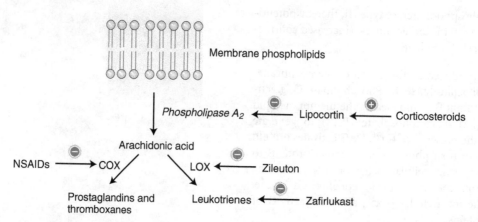

Figure 8-5: Pharmacologic interventions affecting the synthesis or actions of eicosanoids. Arachidonic acid is the precursor of eicosanoids, including prostaglandins, thromboxanes, and leukotrienes. Corticosteroids inhibit arachidonic acid production by inducing lipocortins, which block phospholipase A₂. Nonsteroidal anti-inflammatory drugs (NSAIDs) reversibly inhibit cyclooxygenase (COX), which decreases the formation of prostaglandins and thromboxanes *(note: acetylsalicylic acid [aspirin] irreversibly inhibits COX)*. Zileuton inhibits lipoxygenase (LOX), which decreases leukotriene production. Zafirlukast (and other "lukast" drugs) block leukotriene receptors and are used in the treatment of asthma.

in the generation of a second hormonal messenger. Different eicosanoids can be produced from arachidonic acid, depending on the enzymes expressed in the target cell (e.g., cyclooxygenase or lipoxygenase). Figure 8-5 illustrates the eicosanoid pathway and the key sites of pharmacologic inhibition.

STEROID AND THYROID HORMONE SIGNALING The effects of steroids and thyroid hormones occur slowly when compared with the effects of the peptide hormones. *The effects of the classic steroid hormone are slow because they occur due to changes in gene transcription and translation.* (Some fast steroid responses have recently been identified and may be attributed to surface membrane receptors.)

Most steroid hormone receptors are present in the cytoplasm and are accessed when steroids diffuse through lipid membranes to enter target cells (Figure 8-6). *Once a steroid receptor binds to its hormone, it enters the nucleus to interact with DNA.* An activated steroid receptor partners with another steroid receptor to form a **receptor dimer** as it binds to DNA. Binding to DNA occurs at a specific sequence of DNA known as a **steroid response element,** which is located at the 5′ region of a gene, upstream from the starting point for gene transcription. The nucleotide sequences of steroid response elements are highly conserved and are recognized by several steroid receptors. The specificity of steroid response in a given target cell is mainly determined by the type of steroid receptor present in the cell. Thyroid hormone receptors are widely expressed among the body tissues and function in the same manner as steroid receptors.

THE HYPOTHALAMUS AND THE PITUITARY GLAND

The pituitary gland (**hypophysis**) can be viewed as a master gland because it controls the secretion of several target endocrine glands. The secretion of pituitary hormones is controlled by release factors from the hypothalamus, giving rise to the

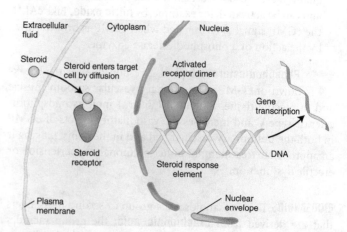

Figure 8-6: Mechanism of steroid hormone action. Steroids bind to intracellular receptors, usually located in the cytoplasm (as shown). Steroids enter target cells by diffusion. Receptors with a bound steroid molecule are chaperoned to the nucleus. Steroid-bound receptors form dimers and bind to steroid response elements in DNA to direct gene transcription.

concept of the **hypothalamic-pituitary axis.** Negative feedback from the primary target gland modulates the secretion of both pituitary and hypothalamic hormones. The pituitary gland lies in a bony cavity, known as the sella turcica, located at the base of the brain. It is connected to the **median eminence** of the hypothalamus via the **pituitary stalk.** The pituitary gland has two major lobes, the anterior pituitary and the posterior pituitary.

ANTERIOR PITUITARY GLAND

With the exception of prolactin, the anterior pituitary hormones are all **tropins,** *which control the release of another hormone from a target gland.* The anterior pituitary gland secretes the following **six major peptide hormones:**

1. **Growth hormone** (GH)
2. **Thyroid-stimulating hormone** (TSH)
3. **Adrenocorticotropic hormone** (ACTH)
4. **Follicle-stimulating hormone** (FSH)
5. **Luteinizing hormone** (LH)
6. **Prolactin**

The following **five major cell types** are **present in the anterior pituitary gland:**

1. **Somatotropes** secrete GH.
2. **Thyrotropes** secrete TSH.
3. **Corticotropes** secrete ACTH.
4. **Gonadotropes** secrete both LH and FSH.
5. **Lactotropes** secrete prolactin.

The anterior pituitary has a rich blood supply that arrives via the **hypothalamic-hypophysial portal venous system** (Figure 8-7). Blood arriving in the anterior pituitary first passes through capillaries in the inferior hypothalamus. The hypothalamic neurons secrete neurohormones into the pituitary portal blood supply, which control the release of the anterior pituitary hormones. In most cases, the anterior pituitary hormones are influenced by the following **stimulatory hypothalamic release factors:**

- Secretion of TSH is stimulated by **thyrotropin-releasing hormone** (TRH).
- Secretion of ACTH is stimulated by **corticotropin-releasing hormone** (CRH).
- Secretion of FSH and LH is stimulated by **gonadotropin-releasing hormone** (GnRH).
- Secretion of GH is controlled by a balance between the stimulatory factor **growth hormone-releasing hormone** (GHRH) and the inhibitory factor **somatostatin.** *GHRH control is dominant, because severing the pituitary stalk decreases GH secretion.*

Prolactin is the only anterior pituitary hormone that is not secreted in response to a stimulatory hypothalamic hormone. The secretion of prolactin is only under negative control by the **prolactin inhibitory factor (PIF)** (now known to be dopamine). *Without tonic inhibition by dopamine, the secretion rates of prolactin are greatly increased.*

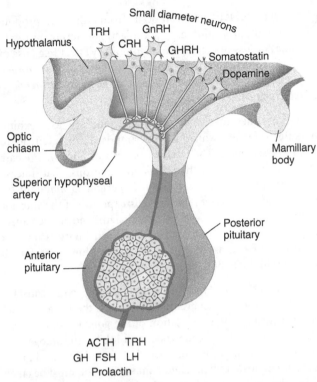

Figure 8-7: Anterior pituitary gland. Hypothalamic neurohormones reach the anterior pituitary gland via the hypothalamic-hypophysial portal venous system. TRH, thyrotropin-releasing hormone; CRH, corticotropin-releasing hormone; GnRH, gonadotropin-releasing hormone; GHRH, growth hormone-releasing hormone; ACTH, adrenocorticotropic hormone; TRH, thyrotropin; GH, growth hormone; FSH, follicle-stimulating hormone; LH, luteinizing hormone.

▽ **Hyperprolactinemia** can occur from either overproduction of prolactin (e.g., a prolactin-secreting pituitary adenoma) or loss of the dopamine inhibitory effect (e.g., use of antipsychotic drugs or damage to the pituitary stalk). *Regardless of the cause, the key clinical indicator of hyperprolactinemia is* **galactorrhea** *(milky nipple discharge).* ▽

All hormones in the hypothalamic-pituitary axis exhibit **pulsatile release,** which is superimposed on a circadian rhythm of secretion. The bursting pattern of hormone release reflects activity of the hypothalamic neurons that release neurohormones. *Pulsatile release is important to maintain the sensitivity of the anterior pituitary cells;* exposure of the anterior pituitary to a constant level of hypothalamic hormone causes receptor downregulation and loss of sensitivity. Complex negative feedback, as shown in Figure 8-2, functions for all hormones in the hypothalamic-pituitary axis.

▽ When the GnRH agonist **leuprolide** is given in constant high doses, it will eventually suppress the release of LH and FSH through downregulation of the gonadotropin receptors. The suppressed gonadotropes will inhibit steroidogenesis and cause a chemical form of castration, a modality used in the treatment of **advanced prostate cancer.** Caution must be taken during the initiation of leuprolide therapy because the initial injection can induce a surge of LH and FSH, causing a rapid increase in testosterone and a "flair" of the prostate cancer. Therefore, simultaneous use of an androgen receptor blocker such as flutamide must be used during the initial phase of leuprolide therapy. ▽

GROWTH HORMONE

There are **two general effects of GH:**

1. *It is the most important endocrine regulator of final* **body size.** Stimulation of linear growth occurs indirectly through stimulation of **insulin-like growth factor (IGF)-1** secretion. IGF-1 is also known as **somatomedin C.**

2. GH causes the following **acute metabolic effects** that oppose the effects of insulin:

   ▫ Lipolysis in adipose tissue.

   ▫ Reduced glucose uptake in muscle.

   ▫ Gluconeogenesis in the liver.

The control of GH secretion reflects both of the broad functions mentioned above. Figure 8-8A shows that there is marked variation in the serum GH levels throughout a 24-hour period. *There is typically intense pulsatile secretion during the first 2 hours of deep sleep, which accounts for about 70% of daily GH secretion.* **Acute stress** (e.g., exercise or trauma) stimulates GH secretion, utilizing the antiinsulin actions of GH to increase the blood glucose concentration.

Both the short-term and the long-term nutritional status of a patient can strongly influence GH secretion. In the short term, **hypoglycemia** stimulates GH release through a mechanism that involves the release of the gastrointestinal peptide hormone and the potent GH secretagogue **ghrelin.** In the longer term, **starvation** is a potent stimulus for GH secretion, especially when it is associated with cellular protein deficiency.

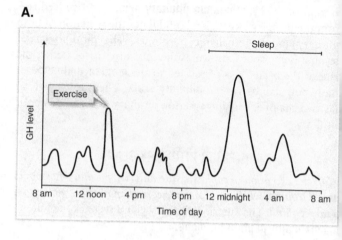

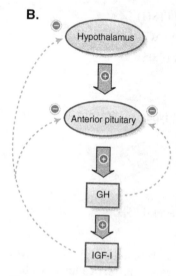

Figure 8-8: Growth hormone (GH) secretion. **A.** Circadian rhythm of GH secretion, with the greatest secretion in the early hours of sleep. GH secretion in response to acute stress is superimposed on the circadian rhythm. **B.** Hierarchical (complex) negative feedback of GH secretion. Insulin-like growth factor-I (IGF-1) secretion is stimulated by GH, and both hormones contribute to negative feedback control. GHRH, growth hormone-releasing hormone.

IGF-1 Control of GH secretion is influenced by negative feedback from IGF-1. GH stimulates the secretion of IGF-1 in many tissues, although the liver is the largest source of plasma IGF-1. IGF-1 is unusual as a peptide hormone because it has binding proteins in the blood, and more than 90% of IGF-1 is protein bound. *Protein binding extends the half-life and provides a relatively constant level of IGF-1 in the plasma despite wide minute-to-minute fluctuations in GH levels.* In addition to IGF-1 being present in the circulation, IGF-1 is produced locally in many tissues, where it can act in a paracrine manner to promote growth. The **negative feedback pathways that regulate GH secretion** are illustrated in Figure 8-8B.

- GH inhibits its own secretion at somatotropes.
- IGF-1 inhibits GH secretion directly at somatotropes.
- IGF-1 inhibits hypothalamic GHRH.
- IGF-1 stimulates hypothalamic somatostatin.

GROWTH AND GROWTH DEFECTS There are many different factors involved in normal human growth, including adequate emotional well-being during infancy and normal functioning of several endocrine systems. *The GHRH-GH-IGF-1 axis is particularly important for the growth of cartilage, bone, and muscle during linear growth.* Other endocrine systems, including the thyroid hormones, sex steroids, insulin, adrenal steroids, and growth factors, all contribute to final size as well as to the integration of growth among organs and tissues.

Defects in GH secretion in childhood can dramatically affect height because the epiphyseal growth plates in the long bones are open. A GH-secreting pituitary tumor is a cause of **gigantism** (Figure 8-9). Growth retardation and **dwarfism** result from a deficiency in GH.

▽ **Panhypopituitarism** is a cause of GH deficiency and refers to the absence or destruction of the entire anterior pituitary gland. When panhypopituitarism occurs in children, dwarfism occurs due to the lack of GH, and there is a lack of development of secondary sex characteristics due to the loss of gonadotropins. The gonadotropins and GH are typically the first hormones to be affected in patients with panhypopituitarism, whereas ACTH function is relatively preserved and usually the last hormone to be affected. ▼

▽ In adults, linear height is fixed due to closure of the growth plates in the long bones. Excess secretion of GH after puberty results in **acromegaly.** The hands, feet, jaw, forehead, and nose continue to grow, giving patients a characteristic appearance (Figure 8-10). GH excess is frequently associated with hyperglycemia and likely to cause **diabetes mellitus** due to the antiinsulin actions of GH. The major cause of mortality in patients with acromegaly relates to the continued growth of the internal organs, in particular the heart (resulting in cardiomegaly). *Congestive heart failure is the most common cause of death in acromegaly.* ▼

The other anterior pituitary hormones are discussed in more depth later in this chapter, together with their primary target gland (e.g., TRH and TSH are discussed in the section on Thyroid Hormones).

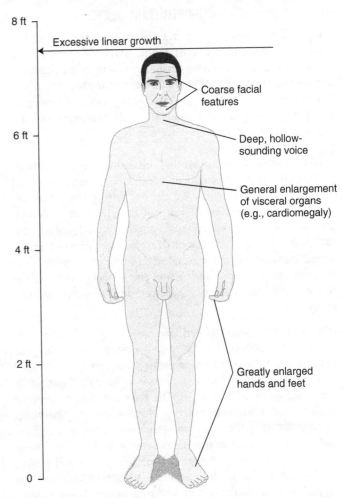

Figure 8-9: Characteristic features of gigantism caused by a pituitary tumor. The patient is a 14-year-old boy; his linear height is 226 cm (7 ft 5 in).

Excessive linear growth

Coarse facial features

Deep, hollow-sounding voice

General enlargement of visceral organs (e.g., cardiomegaly)

Greatly enlarged hands and feet

POSTERIOR PITUITARY GLAND

The posterior pituitary secretes the neurohormones **antidiuretic hormone (ADH)** and **oxytocin.** ADH and oxytocin are peptides produced in neurons that originate in the **paraventricular nucleus** and the **supraoptic nucleus** of the hypothalamus. The nerve tracts run through the pituitary stalk and terminate in the posterior pituitary (Figure 8-11). *ADH is mainly formed in the supraoptic nucleus and oxytocin is mainly formed in the paraventricular nucleus.*

ADH and oxytocin are synthesized in the neuron cell bodies from the larger precursor molecules preprooxyphysin and preprepressophysin, which are cleaved during the formation of the secretory vesicles. Cleavage of the precursor molecules produces the active hormone plus another peptide called **neurophysin.** Neurophysins are carrier proteins that assist in the axonal transport of oxytocin and ADH to the axon terminals in the posterior pituitary gland. Action potentials in these neurons result in the cosecretion of a hormone and its neurophysin by exocytosis.

ADH *ADH is the principal hormone controlling water balance in the body,* and acts at the kidney to concentrate the urine and to cause free water retention in the body (see Chapter 6). *ADH secretion is mainly controlled by changes in body fluid osmolarity and blood volume.* The rate of ADH secretion is most sensitive to altered extracellular osmolarity, which is sensed by neuronal **osmoreceptors** in the organum vasculosum laminae terminalis and the subfornical organ. Osmoreceptors alter their firing pattern in response to changes in their cell volume and project to the supraoptic nucleus and the paraventricular nucleus to regulate the synthesis and secretion of ADH. *An increase in plasma osmolarity of just 1% is sufficient to increase ADH secretion and to induce the sensation of thirst.* Water retention by the kidney, together with water ingestion, should reduce the plasma osmolarity to normal. Conversely, a decrease in the plasma osmolarity suppresses ADH secretion, resulting in greater urinary excretion of water.

ADH secretion is also affected by changes in blood volume. A change in blood volume is sensed by venous (low pressure) baroreceptors in the atria and to a lesser extent by arterial baroreceptors. Neuronal afferents project from baroreceptors to the paraventricular nucleus and the supraoptic nucleus in the hypothalamus to alter ADH secretion. *A decrease in blood volume of more than 15% is a highly potent stimulus for ADH secretion* and results in renal water conservation. Increased blood volume stretches the atria, which suppresses ADH secretion and results in increased urinary water excretion.

The effects of ADH on the kidney are mediated through the **V$_2$ receptors.** ADH is also known as **vasopressin** because it causes generalized arteriolar vasoconstriction when acting through the **V$_1$ receptors** in vascular smooth muscle. *ADH produces an integrated response to a decrease in both blood volume and blood pressure by increasing fluid retention at the kidney and by increasing blood pressure through vasoconstriction.*

▽   Failure of ADH secretion results in the formation of copious amounts of dilute urine in which the urine osmolarity will be less than that of plasma. This condition is called **central diabetes insipidus** (see Chapter 6). ▼

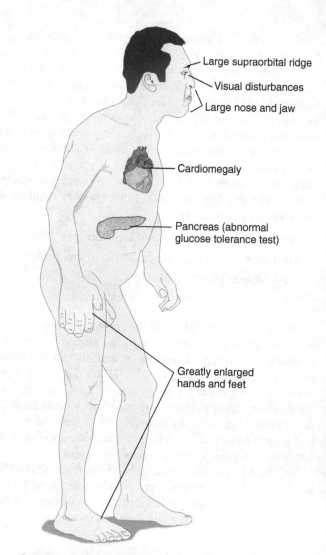

Figure 8-10: Characteristic features of acromegaly.

- Large supraorbital ridge
- Visual disturbances
- Large nose and jaw
- Cardiomegaly
- Pancreas (abnormal glucose tolerance test)
- Greatly enlarged hands and feet

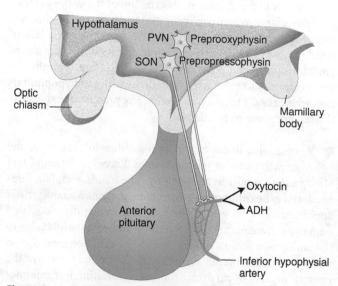

Hypothalamus
PVN — Preprooxyphysin
SON — Preprepressophysin
Optic chiasm
Mamillary body
Anterior pituitary
Oxytocin
ADH
Inferior hypophysial artery

Figure 8-11: Posterior pituitary gland. The neurohormones antidiuretic hormone (ADH) and oxytocin are synthesized in neurons located in the hypothalamic paraventricular and supraoptic nuclei from the precursor peptides preprepressophysin and preprooxyphysin, respectively. ADH and oxytocin are secreted into the systemic blood from axon terminals in the posterior pituitary gland. PVN, paraventricular nucleus; SON, supraoptic nucleus.

OXYTOCIN The **three major functions of oxytocin** are stimulating uterine contractions, stimulating milk ejection from the lactating breast, and promoting maternal behavior.

1. **Uterine contraction.** Oxytocin is important for **parturition.** Uterine sensitivity to oxytocin increases late in pregnancy, causing a powerful uterine response to oxytocin during **labor.** Distention of the uterine cervix stimulates the release of oxytocin via the neuronal pathways. The uterine contractions that result cause further cervical distension. A cycle of **positive feedback** develops during the later stages of labor in which progressive cervical distention stimulates more oxytocin release. The cycle terminates with the birth of the infant.

2. **Milk let-down** and **milk ejection** in the lactating breast. A suckling stimulus when an infant is breast-feeding provokes the secretion of oxytocin. Emotional stimuli such as the mother hearing a crying infant can also stimulate oxytocin secretion. Contraction of the myoepithelial cells in the mammary gland results in milk let-down and milk ejection.

3. Promotion of **maternal behavior** toward the neonate. In nonhuman mammals, injection of oxytocin into the brain induces maternal behavior. In humans, there is increased neuronal activity in the brain regions that are rich in oxytocin receptors during maternal bonding.

▽ **Pharmacologic use of oxytocin** in the peripartum period may be indicated for:

1. **Induction of labor.** Allowing a fetus to mature beyond 42 weeks' gestation results in a large fetus that poses an increased risk for both the mother and the infant during labor. Therefore, using oxytocin to induce labor prior to 42 weeks can alleviate this risk.

2. **Treatment of postpartum hemorrhage.** The most common cause of postpartum hemorrhage is uterine atony. Injection of oxytocin can stimulate the atonic uterus to contract, which will stop the hemorrhage. ▽

THE THYROID GLAND

*The thyroid hormones **thyroxine (T₄)** and **triiodothyronine (T₃)** play a major role in the overall control of the metabolic rate.* The thyroid gland is palpable in the anterior neck in front of the trachea, and consists of the main right and left lobes and a connecting branch, the isthmus. The thyroid gland has a characteristic histologic appearance due to the presence of the **thyroid follicles,** which contain **thyroid colloid.** Colloid is a protein-rich extracellular material that is produced by the endocrine cells surrounding each follicle, called **follicular cells** (Figure 8-12). The major protein in colloid is **thyroglobulin,** which contains T_4 and T_3 as part of its primary structure.

The thyroid gland secretes the hormone **calcitonin** from the **parafollicular cells (thyroid C cells),** which are not part of the follicular unit. Calcitonin is a minor hormone involved in Ca^{2+} and phosphate homeostasis (see Parathyroid Hormone and Vitamin D).

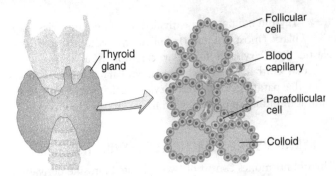

Figure 8-12: The location and histologic features of the thyroid gland.

▽ **Thyroid cancer** can be divided into four categories: papillary (most common), follicular, medullary, and anaplastic. Papillary and follicular carcinomas arise from the follicular epithelial cells, whereas medullary carcinoma arises from the parafollicular cells. Elevated calcitonin levels are a common finding in patients with medullary carcinoma. ▼

SYNTHESIS AND SECRETION OF THYROID HORMONES

Thyroid hormones consist of two iodinated tyrosine derivatives coupled together. Each tyrosine derivative can be iodinated at two locations, providing a total of four possible iodination sites. The following **patterns of iodination** occur naturally (Figure 8-13):

▪ Complete iodination at all four sites produces T_4.

▪ Iodination at three sites produces either T_3 or **reverse T_3 (rT_3)** depending on which sites are iodinated. *T_3 is the most biologically active thyroid hormone, whereas rT_3 is inactive.*

Thyroid hormones are synthesized within thyroid colloid and attached to the protein thyroglobulin. Before thyroid hormones can be secreted into the blood, there must first be uptake and hydrolysis of T_4- and T_3-linked thyroglobulin by the follicular cells. Thyroid hormones are then available for secretion by exocytosis into the extracellular fluid. The following five steps can be identified in **thyroid hormone synthesis** (Figure 8-14):

1. **Iodine trapping** by the follicular cells is the rate-limiting step. Iodide (I^-) is an essential dietary nutrient and is rapidly absorbed by the small intestine. Iodide is taken up by the follicular cells from the extracellular fluid via **Na^+/I^- cotransport** to fill an intracellular **iodide pool** and is secreted into the colloid via anion channels.

2. **Thyroglobulin** is synthesized in the follicular cells and secreted into the colloid by exocytosis. This large protein contains tyrosyl groups, which will be iodinated. The enzyme **thyroid peroxidase** is secreted into the colloid together with thyroglobulin. Thyroid peroxidase oxidizes iodide ions into iodine atoms, which can react with tyrosyl residues on thyroglobulin.

3. **Conjugation** (joining together) of two iodinated tyrosyl groups on thyroglobulin produces T_4 and T_3, continuing to be linked to thyroglobulin.

4. **Endocytosis** of thyroid colloid into the follicular cells. Hydrolysis of thyroglobulin occurs when endocytic vesicles enter the lysosomal pathway and produces a mixture of free T_4 and T_3, as well as the incompletely iodinated residues **diiodothyronine (DIT)** and **monoiodothyronine (MIT).** DIT and MIT are inactive and are deiodinated in a recycling pathway that returns iodide to the intracellular iodide pool within the follicular cells.

5. Thyroid hormones are secreted by **exocytosis** into the extracellular fluid. *Ninety percent of secreted hormone is T_4, and the remaining 10% is T_3.*

▽ **Iodine deficiency** is the most common cause of **goiter** worldwide. Lack of iodine in the diet reduces thyroid hormone synthesis, which results in increased TSH. The trophic effects of TSH cause enlargement of the thyroid gland (goiter). ▼

PERIPHERAL ACTIVATION OF T_4 After secretion into the blood, T_4 and T_3 must be bound to plasma proteins because they are

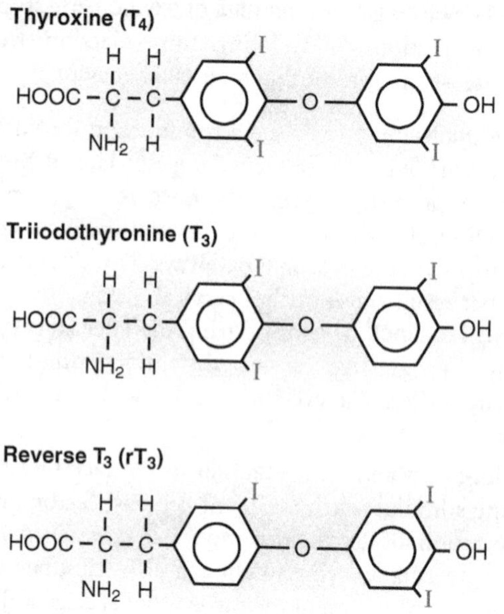

Thyroxine (T_4)

Triiodothyronine (T_3)

Reverse T_3 (rT_3)

Figure 8-13: Iodination sites for thyroid hormones. Thyroid hormones are tyrosine derivatives, with four potential iodination sites. Iodination of all four sites produces thyroxine (T_4), the major hormone secreted by the thyroid gland. The enzyme 5'-deiodinase converts T_4 to the more active hormone triiodothyronine (T_3) in the peripheral tissues. The enzyme 5-deiodinase converts T_4 to the inactive hormone reverse triiodothyronine (rT_3).

poorly soluble in water. More than 99% of T_4 and T_3 are bound in plasma to either **thyroid-binding globulin, transthyretin,** or albumin. *Protein binding provides a large reservoir of thyroid hormones in the plasma and produces a long half-life.*

Although most secreted thyroid hormone is in the T_4 form, *T_3 has much greater biologic activity than T_4. About 75% of circulating T_3 is derived from deiodination of T_4 in the peripheral tissues.* The enzyme **5′-deiodinase** converts T_4 to T_3. There are **two major forms** of 5′-deiodinase:

▨ **Type 1 5′-deiodinase** produces T_3 in most target tissues.

▨ **Type 2 5′-deiodinase** is expressed in the pituitary gland, where locally produced T_3 augments the negative feedback inhibition of TSH secretion.

During starvation, a different expression of type 1 and type 2 5′-deiodinase occurs, which allows a low rate of thyroid hormone secretion to be maintained. *The basal metabolic rate is therefore reduced during starvation, which conserves the body's energy stores.* Type 1 5′-deiodinase expression is reduced, causing a decrease in the concentration of circulating T_3. In contrast, type 2 5′-deiodinase activity is unaffected in starvation, ensuring that the local pituitary levels of T_3 are high enough to maintain suppression of TSH secretion.

THYROID HORMONE ACTIONS

Thyroid hormones exert long-lasting effects by changing gene transcription and translation. The thyroid hormone receptor is contained in the cell nuclei and is widely expressed throughout the body in different cell types. Thyroid hormone receptors act via **thyroid response elements** in many different genes to induce changes in gene expression. Only free (unbound) T_4 and T_3 can enter cells, which occurs either by diffusion or by carrier-mediated transport. Once in the cell nucleus, T_3 has a higher affinity for binding to the receptor than does T_4. The **primary effects of thyroid hormones** are to increase the basal metabolic rate, induce gluconeogenesis, and coordinate normal growth and development.

1. Thyroid hormones **increase the basal metabolic rate** by the following mechanisms:

   ▨ The primary mechanism through which thyroid hormones increase the metabolic rate is **stimulation of "futile cycles."** The **catabolism** (breakdown) and **anabolism** (synthesis) of triglycerides and proteins occurs simultaneously during the futile cycles. This seems to be a wasteful process, but it is important for the generation of body heat.

   ▨ Thyroid hormones increase heat production in **brown adipose tissue.** *This form of heat generation is normally only available in neonates.* Brown adipose tissue uncouples oxidative metabolism in the mitochondria, producing heat instead of ATP.

   ▨ Increased expression of **β-adrenergic receptors** in response to thyroid hormones is an indirect mechanism for increased metabolic rate. Increased sympathoadrenal activity stimulates metabolic activity in several tissues.

▽ In **hyperthyroidism,** the balance of anabolism and catabolism is skewed so that catabolism predominates. As a result, patients experience muscle wasting and loss of fat stores. ▽

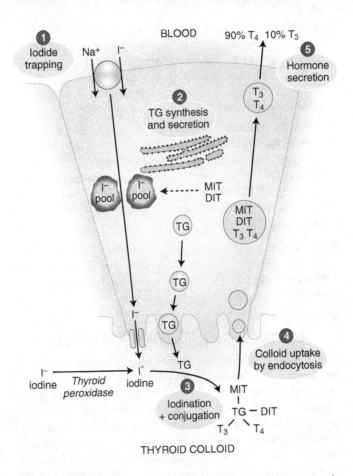

Figure 8-14: Synthesis and secretion of thyroid hormones by thyroid follicles. Steps 1–5 are fully described in the text. ❶ Iodine trapping; ❷ thyroglobulin secretion into the thyroid colloid; ❸ iodination and conjugation of thyroglobulin; ❹ endocytosis of colloid; ❺ secretion of thyroid hormones into extracellular fluid by exocytosis. DIT, diiodothyronine; MIT, monoiodothyronine; T_3, triiodothyronine; T_4, thyroxine; TG, thyroglobulin.

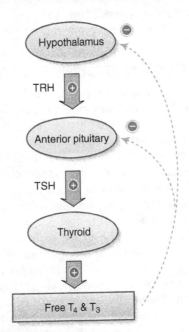

Figure 8-15: Hierarchical negative feedback control of thyroid hormone secretion. TRH, thyrotropin-releasing hormone; TSH, thyroid-stimulating hormone; T_4, thyroxine; T_3, triiodothyronine.

2. In addition to the effects on fat and protein metabolism, thyroid hormones increase hepatic glucose production by **gluconeogenesis.** However, *patients with excess secretion of thyroid hormone usually do not have elevated blood glucose concentrations if their insulin production is normal* (see Endocrine Pancreas).

3. Thyroid hormones contribute to the coordination of **normal growth and development** in addition to the GH-IGF-1 axis. Adequate thyroid hormone levels are required for normal growth and development in children. The goal of neonatal screening for **hypothyroidism** is to evaluate thyroid function 2–4 days after birth and implement therapy within 2 weeks of birth.

▽ *The most serious effect of thyroid hormone deficiency during childhood is irreversible mental retardation, called* **cretinism.** *Dwarfism also results from thyroid deficiency but is reversible with thyroid hormone treatment.* ▽

CONTROL OF THYROID HORMONE PRODUCTION

Hierarchical control of the synthesis and secretion of thyroid hormones occurs via the hypothalamic-pituitary-thyroid axis. Hypothalamic neurons secrete TRH into the pituitary portal blood. TRH acts on anterior pituitary thyrotropes to increase the secretion of TSH. *TSH in turn stimulates all the steps in thyroid hormone synthesis and secretion by the thyroid follicular cells.* TSH has a trophic effect on the thyroid gland; a sustained excess of TSH in plasma causes growth (**hyperplasia**) of the thyroid gland. Negative feedback control of thyroid hormone production is exerted by T_4 and T_3 through the inhibition of both TRH and TSH secretion (Figure 8-15).

▽ **Biochemical assessment of thyroid function** typically begins with TSH. *TSH measurement is the most sensitive means of determining actual thyroid hormone activity, assuming pituitary function is normal.* Low TSH indicates hyperthyroidism; high TSH indicates hypothyroidism. ▽

DISORDERS OF THYROID FUNCTION

Hypothyroidism is a common endocrine disorder that affects about 1% of the adult population at some time. Inadequate thyroid hormone production can result from failure at the level of thyroid gland itself (**primary hypothyroidism**), or it can be due to a lack of stimulation from TSH. Low TSH levels can result from pituitary dysfunction (**secondary hypothyroidism**) or from lack of pituitary stimulation by hypothalamic TRH (**tertiary hypothyroidism**). Primary hypothyroidism is characterized by low plasma concentrations of thyroid hormones but high levels of TSH due to a lack of negative feedback (Figure 8-16A). Secondary hypothyroidism is characterized by low levels of TSH, resulting in low levels of thyroid hormones (see Figure 8-16B). The symptoms of hypothyroidism (from all causes) include **chronic fatigue** and **weight gain** due to the reduction in the metabolic rate. Patients often develop **myxedema,** a syndrome with clinical manifestations of thick coarse skin and peripheral edema. **Depression** is another common finding in patients with hypothyroidism.

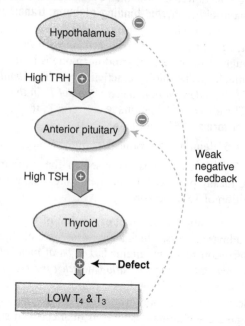

A. Primary hypothyroidism

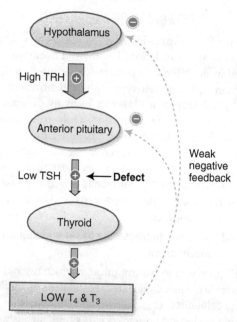

B. Secondary hypothyroidism

Figure 8-16: Hypothyroidism. **A.** Primary hypothyroidism results from failure of the thyroid gland and causes low plasma thyroid hormone levels. There is loss of negative feedback on thyrotropin-releasing hormone (TRH) and thyroid-stimulating hormone (TSH) secretion. **B.** Secondary hypothyroidism results from the failure of the anterior pituitary to secrete TSH and causes a lack of stimulation of thyroid hormone secretion. High TRH levels result from loss of negative feedback on the hypothalamus. T_3, triiodothyronine; T_4, thyroxine.

▽ **Primary hypothyroidism** is the most common cause of inadequate plasma thyroid hormone concentration. Sustained high plasma concentrations of TSH in primary hypothyroidism often cause the development of a painless **goiter** (swelling in the anterior neck due to enlargement of the thyroid gland), reflecting the trophic effect of TSH on the thyroid gland. There are **two major causes of primary hypothyroidism:**

1. The most common cause of primary hypothyroidism worldwide is **dietary iodide deficiency.**

2. **Hashimoto's thyroiditis** is an autoimmune condition that causes destruction of the thyroid cells, and is the most common cause of primary hypothyroidism in the United States. Autoantibodies against **thyroid peroxidase** (anti-TPO antibodies) and **antithyroglobulin antibodies** are commonly found in the serum of patients with Hashimoto's thyroiditis. ▽

Hyperthyroidism (excess secretion of thyroid hormones) can result from primary or secondary causes. In primary hyperthyroidism, high levels of plasma thyroid hormones and low levels of TSH are due to negative feedback inhibition of TSH secretion (Figure 8-17A). In secondary hyperthyroidism, there are high levels of both TSH and thyroid hormones (see Figure 8-17B). *The symptoms of thyroid hormone excess include high metabolic rate, weight loss, heat intolerance, sweating, and muscle weakness. A hypersympathetic state frequently occurs, with tachycardia and tremor due to over expression of β-adrenergic receptors.*

▽ The most common cause of thyroid hormone excess is **primary hyperthyroidism.** In most cases, primary thyroidism results either from a secretory tumor of the thyroid gland or from an autoimmune condition called **Graves' disease.** In Graves' disease, **thyroid-stimulating immunoglobulins** are produced by the immune system. *Thyroid-stimulating immunoglobulins are agonists at the TSH receptor, causing both hypersecretion of thyroid hormones and growth of the gland to produce a goiter.* Some patients with Graves' disease have wide bulging eyes, a condition known as **exophthalmos** (Figure 8-18). Secondary hyperthyroidism occurs more rarely and is caused, for example, by a TSH-secreting tumor of the pituitary gland. ▽

THE ADRENAL GLANDS

The adrenal glands consist of two functionally distinct parts: the **adrenal cortex,** which secretes steroids, and the **adrenal medulla,** which secretes catecholamines.

STRUCTURE OF THE ADRENAL GLANDS

Each kidney has an adrenal gland located above its upper pole. An adrenal gland consists of two distinct parts: an outer cortex and an inner medulla. The adrenal cortex secretes steroid hormones from **three distinct zones** (Figure 8-19):

1. The **glomerulosa layer** is the outermost zone and secretes **aldosterone.**

2. The **fasciculata layer** is the middle zone and secretes **cortisol** and **androgens.**

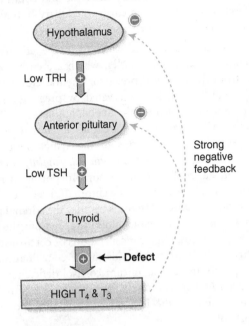

A. Primary hyperthyroidism

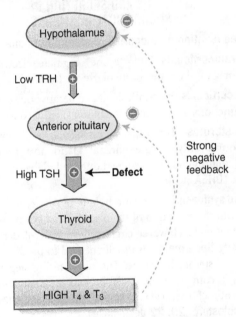

B. Secondary hyperthyroidism

Figure 8-17: Hyperthyroidism. **A.** Primary hyperthyroidism results from the uncontrolled secretion of thyroid hormones by the thyroid gland, which exerts strong negative feedback on thyrotropin-releasing hormone (TRH) and thyroid-stimulating hormone (TSH) secretion. **B.** Secondary hyperthyroidism results from the uncontrolled secretion of TSH from the anterior pituitary, which drives thyroid hormone secretion. TRH levels are strongly suppressed. T_3, triiodothyronine; T_4, thyroxine.

3. The **reticularis layer** is the inner zone and continues from the fasciculata layer to the corticomedullary boundary. The reticularis layer secretes cortisol and androgens.

The adrenal medulla is distinct from the adrenal cortex and consists of **chromaffin cells,** which are embryologically derived from the neuronal precursor (neural crest) cells. The adrenal medulla is richly innervated by preganglionic sympathetic neurons, which release **acetylcholine** as their neurotransmitter. Chromaffin cells are the functional equivalent of the postganglionic neurons of the sympathetic nervous system (see Chapter 2). *Chromaffin cells mainly secrete epinephrine* plus a small amount of norepinephrine in response to preganglionic stimulation. The chromaffin cells receive high concentrations of adrenal steroids because the adrenal medulla receives a direct portal venous blood supply from the adrenal cortex (Figure 8-20). High concentrations of cortisol stimulate epinephrine synthesis, which aids in the coordination of the stress response. In fact, significant cortisol deficiency, such as occurs in an **Addisonian crisis,** can result in potentially fatal hypotension due to the loss of catecholamine potentiation from cortisol.

SYNTHESIS AND SECRETION OF ADRENOCORTICAL HORMONES

The **three functional categories of steroid hormone** are:

1. **Mineralocorticoids** (aldosterone) regulate electrolyte balance in several organs, particularly the kidney.

2. **Glucocorticoids** (cortisol), so named because one of their several functions is to increase the blood glucose concentration.

3. **Sex steroids** (androgens, estrogens, and progestins) are found only in the adrenal gland and produce the **weak androgens** androstenedione and dehydroepiandrosterone (**DHEA**).

Steroid synthesis begins with cholesterol. All steroid-producing tissues, with the exception of the placenta, can synthesize cholesterol from acetate. However, circulating cholesterol, derived from **low-density lipoproteins,** is usually needed to produce adequate amounts of steroid hormone. The rate-limiting step in steroid synthesis is conversion of cholesterol to **pregnenolone,** which occurs in mitochondria via the **side-chain cleavage enzyme** (also called **cholesterol 20, 22 desmolase**).

The identity of the final steroid hormone that is synthesized depends on which other enzymes are expressed in a given steroid-producing cell (see Figure 8-20). In the adrenal cortex, the following primary steroid products are produced:

■ **Aldosterone** is only produced in the *glomerulosa* cells because these cells are the only ones that express the enzyme **aldosterone synthase.**

■ **Cortisol** is produced by the *fasciculata* and *reticularis* cells because these cells are the primary source of the required enzyme **17α-hydroxylase.**

■ **Weak androgens** are the sex steroids produced by the adrenal glands because the cells lack the enzymes needed to produce testosterone and estrogens. Progesterone is produced as an intermediate but is used in the synthesis of cortisol and aldosterone rather than being secreted by the adrenal gland.

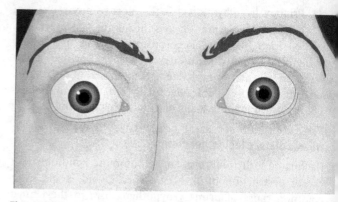

Figure 8-18: Characteristic wide-eyed appearance of exophthalmos in a woman with Graves' disease.

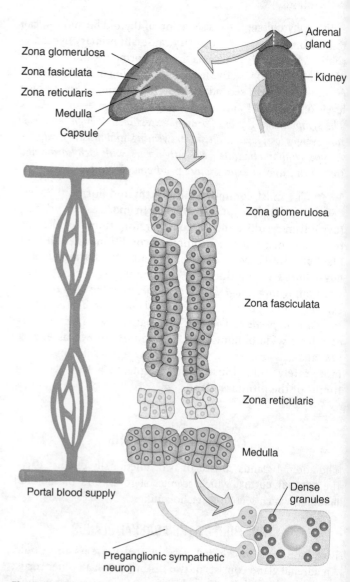

Figure 8-19: The adrenal gland. The adrenal cortex and the adrenal medulla are distinct structures visible in a cross-section of the adrenal gland. The adrenal cortex has three cellular layers, the *zona glomerulosa,* the *zona fasciculata,* and the *zona reticularis.* The adrenal medulla is composed of chromaffin cells, which receive a rich preganglionic sympathetic innervation and a portal blood supply from the adrenal cortex.

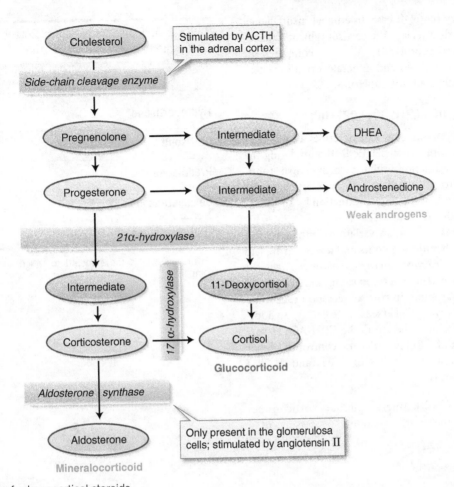

Figure 8-20: Synthesis of adrenocortical steroids.

ACTIONS OF CORTISOL

Cortisol affects many cell types due to the wide expression of glucocorticoid receptors. Free cortisol molecules diffuse into the target cells and bind to the cytoplasmic glucocorticoid receptors. The activated receptors enter the nucleus and alter gene expression via interactions with the **glucocorticoid response elements** found on DNA. Less than 5% of plasma cortisol is free to diffuse into the target cells, with about 90% bound to the **corticosteroid-binding protein (transcortin)** and a further 5% bound to albumin.

Cortisol is secreted in response to virtually all forms of stress, including trauma, infection, illness, temperature change, and mental stress; in the absence of cortisol, even minor illnesses can be fatal. Cortisol mobilizes glucose, amino acids, and fatty acids, and resists inflammatory and immune responses. The "glucocorticoid" action of cortisol (to increase blood glucose) occurs by several mechanisms, including stimulation of hepatic gluconeogenesis, mobilization of amino acids from muscle cells, reduced cellular metabolism of glucose, and reduced sensitivity to insulin (see Endocrine Pancreas).

▼ **Synthetic corticosteroids** (e.g., prednisone and dexamethasone) exhibit different levels of glucocorticoid and mineralocorticoid activity. Corticosteroids with stronger anti-inflammatory and immunosuppressant (glucocorticoid) effects are widely used in an attempt to control chronic inflammatory conditions such as arthritis, chronic obstructive pulmonary disease, and inflammatory bowel disease. In adrenal insufficiency, corticosteroids are used to replace the cortisol (glucocorticoid) and aldosterone (mineralocorticoid). Table 8-3 compares the estimated relative glucocorticoid and mineralocorticoid potencies of several commonly used corticosteroids. ▼

CONTROL OF CORTISOL SECRETION

The **hypothalamic-pituitary-adrenal axis** describes a cascade of hormones that begins with hypothalamic **CRH** stimulating the release of **ACTH** from the anterior pituitary, which in turn stimulates cortisol release from the adrenal cortex. Cortisol exerts negative feedback control over its own production by suppressing the secretion of both CRH and ACTH (Figure 8-21A).

Cortisol secretion has a circadian variation, with hormone levels highest in the early morning hours and lower during late afternoon and evening. *The circadian rhythm of cortisol helps the body in becoming active and alert in the morning and in reducing activity prior to sleep.* Variations in cortisol secretion reflect the pulsatile release of CRH and ACTH (see Figure 8-21B). In addition to the circadian rhythm inherent in the CRH-ACTH-cortisol axis, the secretion of CRH is under the control of higher brain centers, demonstrated by peaks of CRH (and ACTH) release in response to stress.

SYNTHESIS AND ACTIONS OF ACTH Anterior pituitary corticotropes synthesize ACTH by the posttranslational processing of a

TABLE 8-3. Estimated Relative Potencies of Common Corticosteroids

Drug	Glucocorticoid Activity	Mineralocorticoid Activity
Hydrocortisone*	1.0	1.0
Cortisone	0.8	0.8
Prednisone	4.0	0.25
Dexamethasone	30.0	0.0
Fludrocortisone	10.0	400.0

*Hydrocortisone is the standard to which all other corticosteroids are compared.

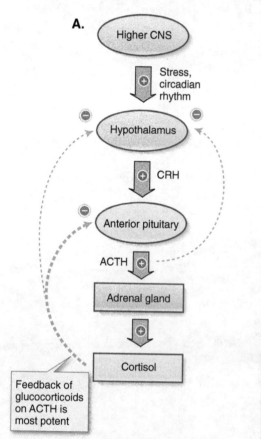

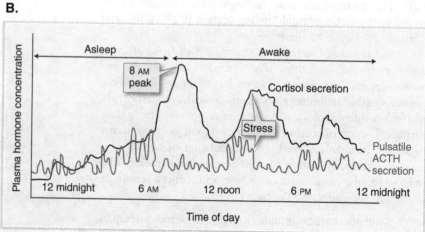

Figure 8-21: Cortisol secretion. **A.** Hierarchical negative feedback control operates via the hypothalamic-pituitary-adrenal axis. **B.** Cortisol secretion is driven by pulsatile adrenocorticotropic hormone (ACTH) secretion and has a circadian rhythm, with the greatest secretion in the early morning. ACTH secretion is driven by corticotropin-releasing hormone (CRH) from the hypothalamus. Other peaks of cortisol concentration occur in response to stress, when higher parts of the central nervous system drive greater CRH secretion.

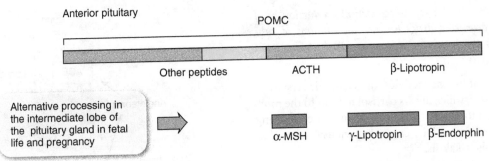

Figure 8-22: Processing of pro-opiomelanocortin (POMC) to produce various peptide hormones. ACTH, adrenocorticotropic hormone; MSH, melanocyte-stimulating hormone.

large precursor protein called **pro-opiomelanocortin (POMC).** Several other peptide hormones of uncertain physiologic importance are generated from POMC, including **β-lipotropin, β-endorphin,** and **melanocyte-stimulating hormone (MSH)** (Figure 8-22). The administration of large doses of MSH stimulates the production of the dark skin pigment melanin, by melanocytes in skin; thus the name MSH.

The primary action of ACTH is stimulation of cortisol secretion from the adrenal cortex, although receptors for ACTH are present in all three cortical cell layers. Cortisol secretion is only stimulated in the fasciculata and reticularis layers because these are the sites of **17α-hydroxylase** expression. *Aldosterone secretion is primarily controlled by angiotensin II* (see Renin-angiotensin System) and is only weakly stimulated by ACTH.

▽ **Excess ACTH** can occur in many conditions, including as a result of an ACTH-secreting pituitary adenoma; as a paraneoplastic syndrome associated with small cell lung carcinoma; or from the lack of negative feedback inhibition in the setting of primary adrenocortical insufficiency. ACTH is a trophic hormone; an excess causes growth of the adrenal glands. *Increased skin pigmentation is a characteristic of ACTH hypersecretion* and is thought to be either due to higher levels of MSH secretion or due to ACTH acting as an agonist at the MSH receptor.

ACTH deficiency causes secondary failure of cortisol secretion and atrophy of the fasciculata and reticularis layers of the adrenal cortex. The glomerulosa cells are spared because they are also supported by a trophic effect from angiotensin II. ▼

ACTIONS OF ALDOSTERONE

Aldosterone is required for the maintenance of normal extracellular fluid volume through the conservation of Na⁺. The main action of aldosterone is stimulation of Na⁺ reabsorption and K⁺ secretion at the distal renal tubule, although similar actions occur in other epithelia (e.g., distal colon, sweat glands, and salivary glands). The effect is to conserve Na⁺ in the extracellular fluid and promote K⁺ excretion. *In the total absence of aldosterone, there is severe Na⁺ depletion and K⁺ retention; without treatment, the condition is fatal.*

The effects of aldosterone are mediated via the **mineralocorticoid receptor.** Cells that express mineralocorticoid receptors also express the enzyme **11β-hydroxysteroid dehydrogenase,** which deactivates cortisol through its conversion to cortisone. This is necessary to prevent cortisol from acting as an agonist at the mineralocorticoid receptor (Figure 8-23).

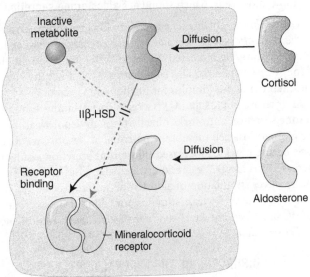

Figure 8-23: Metabolism of glucocorticoids by the enzyme 11β-hydroxysteroid dehydrogenase (HSD) in the mineralocorticoid target cells.

Fluid retention is a side effect of excess cortisol production or of therapy with glucocorticoid drugs because the amount of substrate overwhelms the level of endogenous 11β-hydroxysteroid dehydrogenase activity.

▽ **Licorice** inhibits the activity of 11β-hydroxysteroid dehydrogenase, which allows cortisol to bind to the mineralocorticoid receptors and to activate them. The resulting excess mineralocorticoid activity causes hypertension, hypokalemia, and metabolic alkalosis. ▽

CONTROL OF ALDOSTERONE SECRETION

The renin-angiotensin system is the most important stimulus for aldosterone secretion. Renin is secreted from the granular **juxtaglomerular cells** of the renal **juxtaglomerular apparatus** in response to low effective circulating blood volume. The **stimulus for renin release** is provided by three mechanisms acting together:

1. **Reduced distension of the renal afferent arteriole.**

2. **Tubuloglomerular feedback** signaling due to the low glomerular filtration rate and the low renal tubular fluid flow (see Chapter 6).

3. **Stimulation of the renal sympathetic nerves** due to activation of the baroreceptor reflex by decreased blood pressure (see Chapter 4).

The **secretion** of renin results in an increase in plasma angiotensin II and aldosterone concentrations as follows (Figure 8-24):

1. Renin acts on the circulating precursor protein **angiotensinogen,** which is produced by the liver. Angiotensinogen is cleaved by renin to the inactive decapeptide **angiotensin I.**

2. Angiotensin I is cleaved to produce the octapeptide **angiotensin II** by the action of **angiotensin-converting enzyme (ACE).** ACE is present on the vascular endothelial cells, with about 50% of ACE activity localized in the lung.

3. Angiotensin II binds to its AT_1 receptor in the adrenal cortical glomerulosa cells, which stimulates **aldosterone secretion.**

The combined responses of angiotensin II and aldosterone result in the restoration of the normal effective circulating volume; for example, through increased Na^+ and water retention in the kidney (see Chapter 6). This completes a cycle of negative feedback, removing the stimulus for further renin secretion.

An increase in **plasma [K^+]** is a secondary stimulus for aldosterone secretion and works directly through depolarization of the glomerulosa cell membrane potential. A negative feedback cycle occurs in which increased aldosterone secretion results in increased urinary K^+ excretion, which decreases plasma [K^+] and removes stimulation of aldosterone secretion.

ACTH is a very weak stimulus for aldosterone secretion; *aldosterone does not exert any negative feedback control over ACTH secretion.*

DISORDERS OF THE ADRENAL CORTEX

ADRENOCORTICAL INSUFFICIENCY *Most cases of adrenocortical insufficiency (**Addison's disease**) are due to primary failure of the entire adrenal cortex rather than to secondary or tertiary*

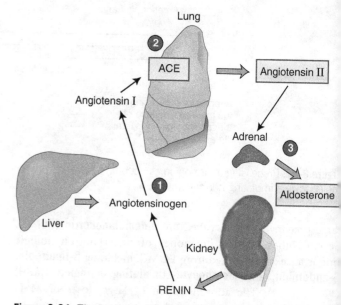

Figure 8-24: The renin-angiotensin-aldosterone system. Steps 1–3 are fully described in the text. ❶ Renin cleaves circulating angiotensinogen to produce angiotensin I; ❷ angiotensin-converting enzyme (ACE) converts angiotensin I to angiotensin II; ❸ angiotensin II stimulates aldosterone secretion from the adrenal cortex.

causes. One of the most common causes of primary failure is autoimmune adrenalitis.

The following **major signs and symptoms of adrenocortical insufficiency** result from the loss of cortisol and aldosterone:

- Cortisol deficiency causes **hypoglycemia** between meals, due to low rates of hepatic gluconeogenesis, and **hypotension,** as a result of the lack of potentiation of catecholamines. Patients typically experience weakness and fatigue. They may become severely debilitated by the inability to produce cortisol in response to stress, and are then described as being in **Addisonian crisis.**

- Aldosterone deficiency results in **hypovolemia** and **hyponatremia** as a result of urinary losses of NaCl and water. **Hyperkalemia** and **metabolic acidosis** result from reduced urinary excretion of K^+ and H^+.

- *In primary adrenal insufficiency, lack of negative feedback results in high levels of ACTH and a characteristic increase in skin pigmentation* (Figure 8-25).

- Deficiency of adrenal androgens in females is likely to result in **reduced libido** and thinning of the pubic hair. These effects do not occur in males due to secretion of the gonadal androgens (see Chapter 9, Male Reproductive Physiology).

▽ **Chronic systemic glucocorticoid therapy,** such as that used in the treatment of rheumatologic conditions (e.g., rheumatoid arthritis) or chronic inflammation, can suppress the hypothalamic-pituitary-adrenal axis through feedback inhibition. *Adrenal insufficiency may occur if treatment is abruptly stopped.* To avoid adrenal insufficiency, the steroid dose can be slowly tapered down, allowing time for the hypothalamic-pituitary-adrenal axis to become active again. When concerned about adrenal insufficiency in the acutely ill patient, the hypothalamic-pituitary-adrenal axis can be quickly tested using the **ACTH stimulation test.** After administration of an ACTH analogue (e.g., cosyntropin), the serum cortisol levels should increase appropriately; failure to do so indicates adrenocortical insufficiency. ▽

HYPERCORTISOLISM Hypercortisolism, or **Cushing's syndrome,** is characterized by the following signs and symptoms, which result from an **excess of glucocorticoids** (Figure 8-26):

- **Hyperglycemia** is due to enhanced gluconeogenesis.

- **Muscle wasting** and weakness are due to protein catabolism.

- **Truncal obesity** and a characteristic rounding of the face called **moon face** are caused by redistribution of body fat.

- **Hypertension** is common due to the mineralocorticoid effects of excess glucocorticoids.

Cushing's syndrome is caused by endogenous or exogenous sources such as use of glucocorticoid therapy. Cushing's syndrome is classified as primary, secondary, and tertiary. The different patterns of plasma cortisol and ACTH concentration in these disorders are summarized in Table 8-4 and as follows:

- **Primary hypercortisolism** may be due to an adenoma of the adrenal cortex.

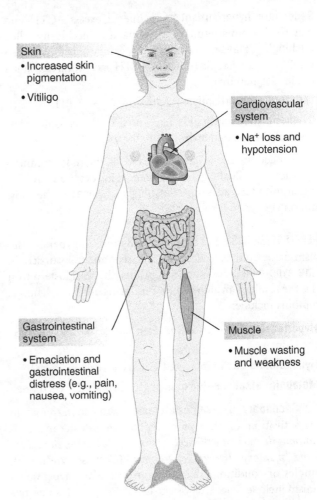

Figure 8-25: Characteristic features of a patient with chronic primary adrenocortical insufficiency (Addison's disease).

- **Secondary hypercortisolism** is due to excess ACTH and may result from a pituitary adenoma; it is specifically called **Cushing's disease.** Secondary hypercortisolism can also result from an ectopic source of ACTH secretion (e.g., small cell lung carcinoma).

- **Tertiary hypercortisolism** results from excess CRH.

- **Synthetic glucocorticoids** (e.g., used in the chronic treatment of rheumatoid arthritis).

▼ Exogenous use of glucocorticoids is the most common cause of **Cushing's syndrome.** However, an ACTH-secreting pituitary adenoma (**Cushing's disease**) is the most common endogenous cause. ▼

HYPERALDOSTERONISM The signs and symptoms of hyperaldosteronism arise from the effects of excessive mineralocorticoids. **Conn's syndrome** is also known as primary hyperaldosteronism and is the result of an aldosterone-producing adrenal adenoma. Symptoms include:

- **Hypertension** due to excessive retention of Na$^+$ and fluids by the kidney.

- **Hypokalemia** due to increased urinary K$^+$ excretion.

- **Metabolic alkalosis** due to increased urinary H$^+$ excretion.

▼ **Secondary hyperaldosteronism** occurs in response to activation of the renin-angiotensin-aldosterone axis. *Conditions that activate this axis are far more common than those causing primary hyperaldosteronism* (Conn's syndrome). Examples of conditions that result in secondary hyperaldosteronism include renal artery stenosis, cirrhosis, and congestive heart failure. ▼

ADRENOGENITAL SYNDROME In most disorders of the adrenal cortex, the clinical picture is dominated by the consequences of inappropriate levels of glucocorticoids and mineralocorticoids. The adrenal androgens have weak effects compared to the effects of testosterone produced by the male gonads. Therefore, an excess or a deficiency of the adrenal androgens has little impact on adult males. *The effects of the adrenal androgens are more apparent in children and women since they do not secrete gonadal androgens.* Tumors of the adrenal cortex can secrete an excess of adrenal androgens; children and adult females develop male secondary sex characteristics, and there is marked growth of the clitoris or the penis, called the **adrenogenital syndrome.**

21α-HYDROXYLASE DEFICIENCY Mutations of enzymes in the steroid biosynthetic pathway can occur, resulting in failure to manufacture a given hormone. In this event, there is an accumulation of the precursor steroids proximal to the enzyme defect in the synthetic pathway. *The most common congenital error in adrenal steroid metabolism is 21α-hydroxylase deficiency.* Loss of 21α-hydroxylase function causes the following complications (Figure 8-27):

- Symptoms of **primary adrenal insufficiency** due to the inability to synthesize cortisol or aldosterone.

- Massive **accumulation of adrenal androgens,** as steroid precursors are shunted along the androgen synthesis pathway.

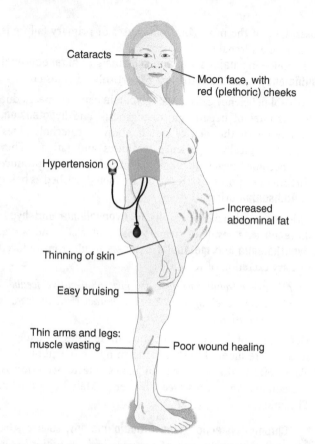

Figure 8-26: Characteristic features of a patient with Cushing's syndrome.

TABLE 8-4. Levels of Cortisol and Adrenocorticotropic Hormone (ACTH) in Cushing's Syndrome

Disorder	Endogenous Cortisol Levels	ACTH Levels
Primary hypercortisolism (e.g., adrenal adenoma)	↑	↓
Secondary hypercortisolism (e.g., Cushing's disease)	↑	↑
Tertiary hypercortisolism	↑	↑
Exogenous glucocorticoid treatment	↓	↓

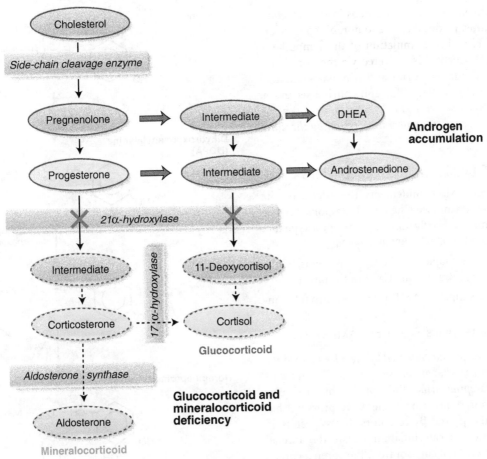

Figure 8-27: Shunting of adrenal steroid synthesis toward androgen production in 21α-hydroxylase deficiency.

■ **Adrenal hyperplasia,** due to high levels of ACTH caused by loss of negative feedback inhibition from cortisol.

▽ The clinical syndrome caused by 21α-hydroxylase deficiency is called **virilizing congenital adrenal hyperplasia.** *This congenital defect is most readily apparent in female infants because the influence of androgens in utero produces ambiguous genitalia.* ▼

SYNTHESIS AND SECRETION OF CATECHOLAMINES

As a part of the stress response, the adrenal medulla secretes catecholamines in concert with activation of the sympathetic nervous system. The adrenal medulla synthesizes epinephrine and norepinephrine, which are derived from the amino acid tyrosine via a series of enzymatically controlled reactions (Figure 8-28). The rate limiting step is the production of **L-dopa** from tyrosine via the enzyme **tyrosine hydroxylase.** The final conversion from norepinephrine to epinephrine is catalyzed by **phenylethanolamine-*N*-methyltransferase** and only occurs in the chromaffin cells; in the sympathetic postganglionic neurons, the pathway ends with the production of norepinephrine. Epinephrine and norepinephrine are stored within the **dense granules** of the chromaffin cells in association with the binding protein chromogranin.

The release of catecholamines by the adrenal medulla is controlled by the central nervous system (CNS) via the preganglionic sympathetic neurons. The neurotransmitter acetylcholine is released and acts at the **nicotinic cholinergic**

receptors on the chromaffin cells. The steps in the catecholamine synthetic pathway from tyrosine to norepinephrine are stimulated by ACTH and by stimulation of the sympathetic nerves (Figure 8-28). Cortisol is delivered via the portal vessels directly from the adrenal cortex and stimulates the final enzyme in the pathway necessary for epinephrine secretion. *Thus, the stress response sensed in the hypothalamic-pituitary-adrenocortical axis sustains epinephrine secretion by the adrenal medulla.*

ACTIONS OF CIRCULATING CATECHOLAMINES

The CNS-epinephrine axis complements the effects of the sympathetic nervous system (see Chapter 2). Responses in the target cells depend on the specific adrenergic receptor type that is expressed. There are **five major receptor types:**

- The α_1 **receptors** are coupled to the $G_{\alpha q}$ G proteins, which give rise to increased intracellular $[Ca^{2+}]$ in the target cells.

- The α_2 **receptors** suppress cAMP responses through coupling to $G_{\alpha i}$.

- The β_1, β_2, **and** β_3 **receptors** all increase cAMP via $G_{\alpha s}$.

The major endocrine product released by the adrenal medulla is epinephrine, whereas the major sympathetic neurotransmitter released is norepinephrine. Epinephrine has a similar binding affinity to norepinephrine at the α receptors but has greater affinity at the β_1 and β_2 receptors. Stress results in the enhanced secretion of catecholamines from the adrenal medulla and the secretion of cortisol from the adrenal cortex. Catecholamines coordinate a short-term response, which includes increased cardiac output, bronchodilation, and elevated blood glucose concentration (Table 8-5). Cortisol initiates a longer response, which includes the mobilization of glucose, fatty acids, and amino acids, and suppression of the immune system.

▽ Understanding the pharmacologic effects of **adrenergic agonists and antagonists** requires knowledge of the different adrenergic receptor types and their locations. For example, administering a β_2 agonist, such as **albuterol,** a drug that is often used in the treatment of asthmatic episodes, will result in relaxation of the smooth muscle in the lung. A knowledge of adrenergic receptor types can also be helpful in predicting the potential side effects of a drug. For example, using a selective α_1 antagonist such as **prazosin** in the setting of benign prostatic hyperplasia allows more complete bladder emptying by relaxing the urinary sphincter; however, as a result of blocking the α_1 receptors on the blood vessels, prazosin can also cause postural hypotension or reflex tachycardia. ▼

INACTIVATION OF CIRCULATING CATECHOLAMINES Circulating catecholamines are rapidly broken down by a series of enzymatic reactions, as illustrated in Figure 8-29. Endothelial cells in the heart, liver, and kidney express the enzyme **catecholamine-O-methyltransferase (COMT),** which converts epinephrine to **metanephrine** and norepinephrine to **normetanephrine.** A second enzyme, **monoamine oxidase (MAO),** converts both of these metabolites to **vanillylmandelic acid (VMA),** which is excreted in the urine. *Catecholamine production by the adrenal*

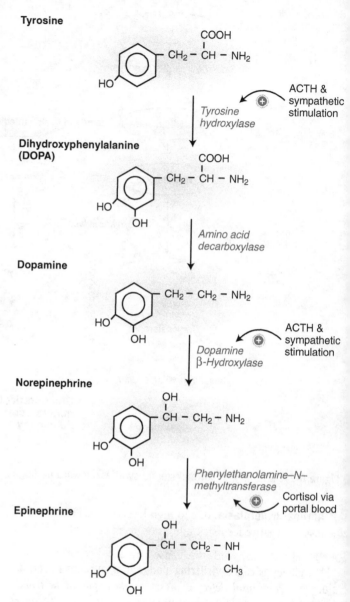

Figure 8-28: Catecholamine synthesis in the adrenal medulla. ACTH, adrenocorticotropic hormone.

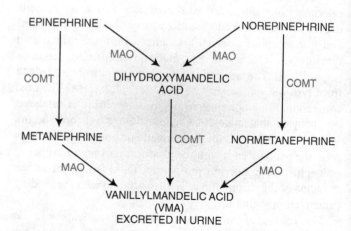

Figure 8-29: Degradation of circulating catecholamines. MAO, monoamine oxidase; COMT, catechol-O-methyltransferase.

medulla is assessed by measuring the levels of catecholamines, metanephrines, and VMA in the urine.

▽ Patients with **pheochromocytoma,** a secretory tumor of the adrenal medulla, hypersecrete catecholamines. Episodes of dramatic surges in the release of catecholamines result in transient hypertension, palpitations, sweating, increased body temperature, and increased blood glucose concentration. Diagnosis is aided by measuring the increased concentrations of catecholamines and their breakdown products in the urine. ▽

THE ENDOCRINE PANCREAS

The pancreatic hormones insulin and glucagon are the most important hormones that control the blood glucose concentration. **Diabetes mellitus** is a disorder of insulin secretion, or of tissue insulin insensitivity, that is characterized by metabolic abnormalities of the body's fuels (e.g., glucose, lipids, and amino acids) and results in hyperglycemia. The incidence of diabetes mellitus has reached epidemic proportions, and the disease is now a major cause of morbidity and mortality globally.

PANCREATIC ENDOCRINE CELLS

Endocrine cells in the pancreas form small aggregates called the **islets of Langerhans,** which are scattered among the exocrine pancreas. Islets of Langerhans have **three major endocrine cell types** (Figure 8-30):

▨ α **Cells** are mainly located at the periphery of the islets and secrete **glucagon.**

▨ β **Cells** are mainly located toward the center of the islets and secrete **insulin, proinsulin,** and **C peptide.**

▨ δ **Cells** secrete **somatostatin;** there are fewer δ cells than there are α and β cells.

▽ Serum levels of **C peptide** can be used to differentiate between endogenous hyperinsulinemia (e.g., insulinoma) and exogenous hyperinsulinemia (e.g., surreptitious insulin use). Both C peptide and insulin concentrations are elevated in a patient with an insulinoma, whereas C peptide will be absent if the hyperinsulinemia results from exogenous insulin injection. ▽

Blood flows through the islets of Langerhans from the center toward the periphery. Insulin is secreted by cells at the core of the islet so that the α cells toward the periphery receive a high concentration of insulin. This anatomic arrangement is significant because insulin and glucagon are antagonistic hormones in the regulation of blood glucose; *insulin suppresses glucagon secretion.*

INSULIN SYNTHESIS AND SECRETION

Transcription and translation of the insulin gene produces the precursor protein **preproinsulin** (Figure 8-31). Cleavage of a leader sequence produces proinsulin, which enters the rough endoplasmic reticulum. **Processing of proinsulin** occurs during transit through the Golgi apparatus and the

TABLE 8-5. Selected Effector Organ Responses to Adrenal Medullary Hormones and Sympathetic Nerve Stimulation

Organ	Receptor Type	Response
Heart		
Sinoatrial node	β_1	Increased heart rate
Atrioventricular node and the His-Purkinje system	β_1	Increased conduction speed
Myocardium	β_1	Increased contractility
Vascular smooth muscle	α_1	Constriction in skin, abdominal viscera, and kidney
	β_2	Dilation in skeletal muscle
Bronchiolar smooth muscle	β_2	Relaxation
Gastrointestinal tract		
Circular smooth muscle	α_2, β_2	Reduced motility
Sphincters	α_1	Constriction
Secretion	α_2	Inhibition
Liver	β_2	Glycogenolysis and gluconeogenesis
Adipose tissue	β_1, β_3	Lipolysis
Kidney	β_1	Renin secretion
Urinary bladder		
Detrusor wall	β_2	Relaxation of bladder
Sphincter	α_1	Constriction
Male sex organs	α_1	Ejaculation

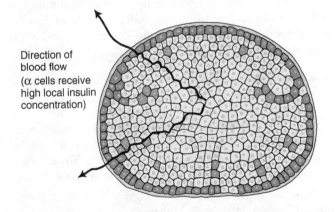

Direction of blood flow (α cells receive high local insulin concentration)

⬤ α Cells (glucagon)   ⬤ β Cells (insulin)   ⬤ δ Cells (somatostatin)

Figure 8-30: Endocrine cells in a pancreatic islet of Langerhans.

formation of secretory granules, and involves the following three steps:

1. **Proinsulin** is synthesized with three domains: A, B, and C. The C domain lies between the A domain and the B domain.

2. The C domain is cleaved from proinsulin to yield a free **C peptide.** *Urinary excretion of C peptide is a useful marker of insulin production* because it is produced in a 1 to 1 ratio with insulin and is not degraded after secretion.

3. The A and B chains of proinsulin are joined by disulphide bridges to form **insulin.**

ACTIONS OF INSULIN

The maintenance of a normal blood glucose concentration is particularly important for CNS function. Insulin is a key integrator of fuel metabolism as the body shifts between fed and fasted states; insulin secretion increases after a meal and returns to a low baseline level between meals. Insulin directs fuel metabolism toward the use of carbohydrates to prevent sustained increases in blood glucose concentration following a meal. As carbohydrate metabolism increases, protein and fat stores are conserved. *The net effect of insulin on the plasma metabolite levels is a reduction in glucose, amino acids, fatty acids, and ketoacids.* The **three major effector organs for insulin** are the liver, skeletal muscle, and adipose tissue.

1. **Liver.** Insulin regulates the activity of several metabolic enzymes in the liver, resulting in increased metabolism of glucose as a fuel, increased storage of glucose as glycogen, and the conversion of glucose to triglycerides. Insulin stimulates hepatic protein synthesis and inhibits protein breakdown.

2. **Skeletal muscle.** Insulin increases glucose uptake in muscle cells by stimulating the facilitated diffusion carrier GLUT4. It also directs the increased use of glucose as a fuel in muscle cells and increases glycogen synthesis. Finally, insulin reduces the use of circulating triglyceride as fuel in muscle, allowing more to be stored in adipose tissue.

▽ **Glycemic control** is improved in patients with diabetes mellitus who exercise because the GLUT4 uptake carrier is directly stimulated by increased muscle work. GLUT4 activity is increased by **adenosine monophosphate kinase,** which couples increased cellular metabolism in the muscle cell to increased glucose uptake independently of insulin. Therefore, diabetics who are insulin dependent require less insulin during exercise. ▼

3. **Adipose tissue.** Insulin stimulates glucose uptake in adipose tissue, via **GLUT4,** and increases glucose storage as a triglyceride within the adipocytes. Insulin increases the expression of the enzyme **endothelial lipoprotein lipase,** which releases fatty acids and glycerol from the circulating triglycerides in chylomicrons and very low-density lipoproteins. Free fatty acids and glycerol are taken up by adipocytes and stored as triglyceride.

An action of insulin that is unrelated to fuel metabolism is increased cellular uptake of K^+. Most meals contain a significant K^+ load, which must be sequestered into cells to prevent a potentially dangerous increase in the plasma $[K^+]$. The increase in insulin

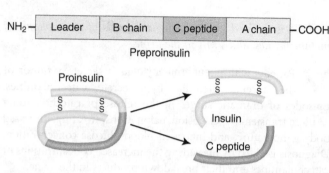

Figure 8-31: Processing of preproinsulin in the pancreatic β cells. Cleavage of C peptide from a region between the A and B chains of insulin produces equal amounts of C peptide and insulin. C peptide is stored in vesicles together with insulin, and both are secreted simultaneously during exocytosis.

secretion after a meal is important because it quickly sequesters ingested K^+.

▽ **Insulin infusion** can be used therapeutically to quickly reduce the plasma $[K^+]$ in patients with **hyperkalemia.** In the setting of hyperkalemia, insulin can be infused concomitantly with glucose to prevent hypoglycemia. ▽

The tissue effects of insulin are mediated via a **receptor tyrosine kinase.** The number of available insulin receptors is an important determinant of the cellular response to insulin. *In obesity, the expression of insulin receptors is reduced, which is an important cause of insulin insensitivity that can lead to diabetes mellitus.*

CONTROL OF INSULIN SECRETION

Blood glucose concentration is the primary regulator of insulin secretion. An increase in blood glucose concentration stimulates insulin secretion. The actions of insulin reduce the blood glucose concentration back to normal, thereby inhibiting further insulin secretion. **Stimulation of insulin secretion** by glucose requires the metabolism of glucose by the β cells and occurs by the following four steps (Figure 8-32):

1. Glucose is taken up via **GLUT2** and oxidized to produce ATP.

2. An increase in the cellular ATP and adenosine diphosphate (ADP) concentration ratio inhibits **ATP-sensitive K^+ channels,** resulting in depolarization of the β cell membrane potential.

3. Depolarization activates the **voltage-sensitive Ca^{2+} channels,** causing influx of Ca^{2+}.

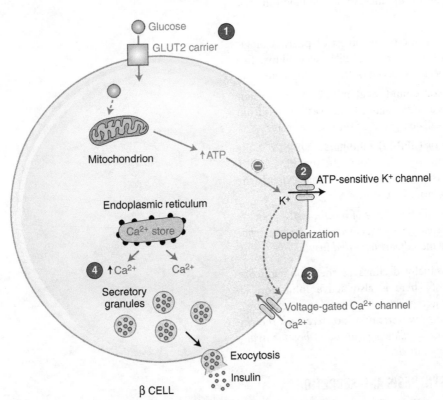

Figure 8-32: Cellular mechanism coupling increased plasma glucose concentration to insulin secretion from the pancreatic β cells. Steps 1–4 are fully described in the text. ❶ Uptake and oxidative metabolism of glucose; ❷ closure of adenosine triphosphate-sensitive K^+ channels; ❸ Ca^{2+} influx through voltage-operated Ca^{2+} channels following membrane depolarization; ❹ Ca^{2+}-induced Ca^{2+} release resulting in exocytosis of insulin and C peptide.

4. **Ca²⁺-induced Ca²⁺ release** augments an increase in intracellular [Ca²⁺], which triggers **exocytosis** of secretory granules containing insulin.

▽ Once formed, insulin is stored in the secretory granules, where it awaits the signal to be released. **Sulfonylureas** (e.g., glipizide and glyburide) are pharmacologic agents that bind to and inhibit the ATP-sensitive K⁺ channels. Sulfonylureas, therefore, stimulate the release of preformed insulin stored in vesicles, which results in reducing the blood glucose concentration. *(Note: sulfonylureas do not cause an increase in insulin synthesis.)* ▽

An increase in the plasma concentration of **arginine, leucine, or lysine** also stimulates insulin release. This is appropriate because insulin is an anabolic hormone that promotes protein synthesis. The terminal oxidation of these amino acids in the β cells results in increased cellular ATP and the same signaling cascade that was previously described for glucose.

Insulin is secreted as part of the integrated response to a meal even before glucose is absorbed by the intestine to increase plasma glucose concentration. The anticipation of a meal causes weak stimulation of the β cells via the **cholinergic vagal neurons.** When a meal enters the small intestine, the presence of nutrients in the lumen stimulates the secretion of **incretins,** the gastrointestinal peptide hormones that stimulate insulin secretion (see Chapter 7). The major incretins are **glucose-dependent insulinotropic peptide (GIP) and glucagon-like peptide-1 (GLP-1).** As glucose is being assimilated from a meal, the action of incretins allows an increase in the plasma insulin concentration and minimizes the increase in the blood glucose concentration.

▽ **Incretins** have been the recent object of pharmacologic development for the treatment of diabetes mellitus. Two **classes of drugs** have been borne out of this development:

1. **Incretin mimetics** (compounds that mimic incretins). For example, exenatide is a GLP-1 agonist that was isolated from the venom from the salivary gland of the Gila monster.

2. **Dipeptidylpeptidase IV (DPP-IV) inhibitors.** DPP-IV is the enzyme responsible for breaking down the incretins GLP-1 and GIP. Sitagliptin is a DPP-IV inhibitor that extends the half-life of the endogenous incretins.

Note: incretins only generate the release of insulin in the presence of elevated blood glucose concentrations, obviating the risk of hypoglycemia that is posed by the sulfonylureas and insulin. ▽

Insulin secretion gradually declines as the blood glucose concentration decreases. There is also active inhibition of insulin secretion during the stress response (e.g., exercise). *Catecholamines inhibit insulin secretion via α₂ receptors, thereby preventing hypoglycemia and allowing glucose to become available for uptake by working muscle.*

GLUCAGON SYNTHESIS AND SECRETION

Glucagon antagonizes the actions of insulin to increase the blood glucose concentration. Transcription and translation of the glucagon gene occurs in the pancreatic α cells and in the L cells of the intestinal mucosa. Several peptide hormones can

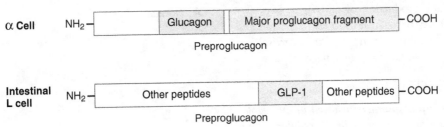

Figure 8-33: Processing of preproglucagon produces glucagon in pancreatic a cells and glucagon-like peptide in intestinal L cells. GLP-1, glucagon-like peptide-1.

be generated from preproglucagon; the α **cells** mainly produce glucagon, whereas the **L cells** mainly produce GLP-1 (Figure 8-33).

ACTIONS OF GLUCAGON

The main target organ for glucagon is the liver; the **primary effects of glucagon** are to increase the hepatic production of glucose and ketones.

▪ **Glucose production** is stimulated via glycogenolysis and gluconeogenesis.

▪ The major **ketones** are β hydroxybutyrate and acetoacetic acid, which are synthesized from fatty acids via acetyl coenzyme A. Ketones provide an alternative energy source to glucose in many tissues, including the brain. Use of ketones for fuel conserves glucose and the cellular protein stores as fasting progresses to starvation.

High concentrations of glucagon, such as those encountered during starvation, stimulate lipolysis in adipose tissue and proteolysis in muscle to maintain a supply of substrates required for cellular energy metabolism.

CONTROL OF GLUCAGON SECRETION

Glucagon secretion is stimulated by hypoglycemia and inhibited by hyperglycemia. This pattern of glucagon secretion is the inverse of insulin secretion and occurs because insulin directly inhibits glucagon secretion (i.e., high levels of insulin produce low levels of glucagon).

Ingestion of a protein-rich meal stimulates glucagon secretion. An increase in the plasma concentrations of the amino acids **arginine** and **alanine** in particular stimulate glucagon secretion. It is important to have increased glucagon secretion in response to protein ingestion because amino acids also stimulate insulin release. The increase in glucagon secretion minimizes a change in the ratio of plasma insulin to glucagon concentration and prevents the development of hypoglycemia due to an excess of insulin.

INTEGRATED CONTROL OF BLOOD GLUCOSE CONCENTRATION

Blood glucose concentration is determined by a balance between glucose input and output from the circulation (Figure 8-34). Glucose input to the circulation is dependent on the diet and on the production of glucose by the liver. Glucose output from the circulation is a function of tissue metabolism. Increased metabolic use and storage of glucose in response to hyperglycemia is due to insulin secretion. The decreased metabolic use of glucose

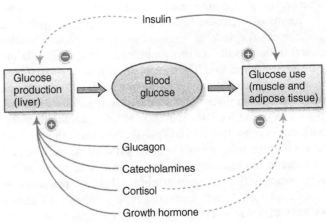

Figure 8-34: Integrated control of blood glucose concentration.

and the increased hepatic production of glucose in hypoglycemia result from interplay between hormones. *Glucagon and catecholamines act rapidly to counter hypoglycemia; cortisol and GH support a sustained counter response to hypoglycemia.*

DIABETES MELLITUS

Diabetes mellitus is a group of disorders involved in the regulation of insulin production or secretion or in the cellular actions of insulin; the result is hyperglycemia. Researchers recently have discovered that adipocytes are biologically active cells that produce chemicals that may contribute to the development of diabetes mellitus. The link between diabetes and obesity is quite clear as the prevalence of diabetes and **obesity** continues to increase in parallel. Obesity is associated with **insulin insensitivity,** which results in chronic hyperglycemia. *Hyperglycemia causes widespread organ damage; diabetes is currently the leading cause of blindness, nontraumatic lower extremity amputation, and end-stage renal disease.* Diabetes-related abnormalities associated with lipid metabolism also result in the accelerated development of atherosclerosis.

BLOOD GLUCOSE TESTING The normal blood glucose concentration following an overnight fast (>8 h) is in the range of 70–99 mg/dL. Patients with a fasting blood glucose concentration in the range of 100–125 mg/dL have **impaired fasting glucose,** which may reflect a prediabetic condition. *A reproducible fasting glucose concentration of ≥126 mg/dL is diagnostic for diabetes mellitus.*

A **glucose tolerance test** can be used to diagnose diabetes in a fasting patient given 75 g of an oral glucose solution (Figure 8-35A). Blood samples are drawn before glucose ingestion and at intervals of 30 minutes, 1 hour, 2 hours, and 3 hours after ingestion. *Diabetes is diagnosed if the plasma glucose concentration remains ≥200 mg/dL 2 hours after glucose ingestion.*

Obtaining a random (nonfasting) sample of a plasma glucose concentration of ≥200 mg/dL can also be diagnostic, but only if the patient is concomitantly experiencing the **classic symptoms of diabetes:** polyuria, polydipsia, and unintentional weight loss.

TYPE 1 DIABETES MELLITUS About 10% of patients with diabetes have **type 1 diabetes mellitus** (formerly known as insulin-dependent diabetes mellitus, or IDDM). Type 1 diabetes is usually **juvenile onset** and results from the autoimmune destruction of the pancreatic β cells. Figure 8-35B shows the results of a glucose tolerance test of a patient with type 1 diabetes. The lack of an increase in the plasma insulin concentration results in a very prolonged increase in the plasma glucose concentration. The loss of insulin in the continued presence of glucagon results in the overproduction of glucose and ketones by the liver and in a reduced ability of the peripheral tissues to utilize glucose. The body enters a **catabolic state,** with extensive proteolysis and lipolysis. Patients with untreated type 1 diabetes often present with **dehydration,** which is caused by **osmotic diuresis** when the rate of glucose filtration at the kidney exceeds the maximum rate of renal glucose reabsorption (see Chapter 6). A complication of type 1 diabetes is **diabetic ketoacidosis** due to ketone formation, which is a potentially fatal cause of metabolic acidosis (see Chapter 6).

A. Normal

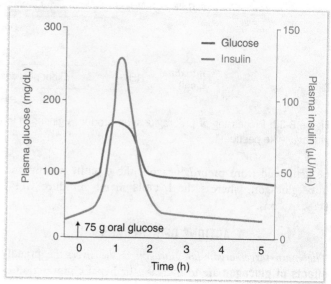

B. Type I diabetes mellitus

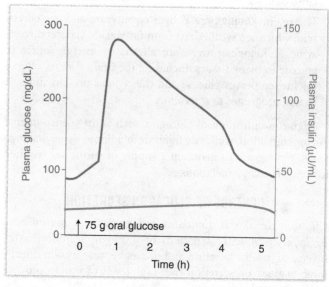

Figure 8-35: Glucose tolerance testing. **A.** In a normal fasting person, an oral glucose challenge of 75 g produces an increase in the blood glucose concentration and an insulin secretion response during the first 2 hours after glucose ingestion. The resting blood glucose concentration is reestablished within 2 hours. **B.** Patients with type 1 diabetes mellitus do not secrete insulin in response to a glucose challenge. A plasma glucose concentration of ≥200 mg/dL more than 2 hours after glucose ingestion is diagnostic of diabetes mellitus. U, international insulin units.

TYPE 2 DIABETES MELLITUS Approximately 90% of patients with diabetes have **type 2 diabetes mellitus** (formerly known as non–insulin-dependent diabetes mellitus, or NIDDM), which is characterized by some degree of reduced insulin secretion coupled with insulin resistance in the target cells. Unlike type 1 diabetes, the accumulation of ketones usually does not occur in patients with type 2 diabetes because there is a sufficient hepatic response to insulin to prevent glucagon from driving ketone formation.

Type 2 diabetes is strongly linked to **obesity** and, therefore, incidence of the disease has recently rapidly increased. Type 2 diabetes was formerly a disease that was associated with mature onset, but the dramatic increase in childhood obesity suggests that the term "mature onset diabetes" is no longer appropriate.

In many patients, the phenomenon of insulin resistance is part of a complex collection of disorders called the **metabolic syndrome**, which is associated with *increased risk of cardiovascular disease as well as with type 2 diabetes*. Patients with metabolic syndrome generally have coexisting measurements of truncal (visceral) obesity, hyperglycemia, dyslipidemia (including elevated triglycerides and low levels of high density lipoprotein), and hypertension.

PARATHYROID HORMONE, VITAMIN D, AND CALCITONIN

Parathyroid hormone (PTH) and vitamin D are the principal hormones that regulate Ca^{2+} and phosphate homeostasis. The homeostasis of Ca^{2+} and phosphate is linked because these hormones are both present in **hydroxyapatite** crystals, which form the major mineral component of bone. Ca^{2+} has many critical functions in addition to being a structural component of bone; for example, Ca^{2+} is critical for muscle contraction, exocytosis, intracellular signaling, and nerve conduction. Phosphate is required by all cells; for example, phosphate transfer reactions are the basis of cellular energy metabolism (e.g., ATP and ADP) and of the control of cellular function via phosphorylation and dephosphorylation reactions.

CA²⁺ AND PHOSPHATE BALANCE

The maintenance of normal plasma Ca^{2+} and phosphate concentrations requires a balance between inputs to the circulation and outputs from the circulation. Ca^{2+} and phosphate enter the circulation from the gastrointestinal system and from the resorption of bone. The processes of renal excretion and bone formation remove Ca^{2+} and phosphate from plasma. A typical Western diet contains more daily intake of Ca^{2+} and phosphate than is needed; net intestinal absorption is matched by urinary excretion. Bone is being continuously remodeled by the simultaneous formation of bone by **osteoblasts** and its resorption by **osteoclasts**. Depending on the balance between osteoblast and osteoclast activity, bone remodeling may either add Ca^{2+} and phosphate to plasma or it may remove these ions. After the completion of bone growth, daily rates of bone formation and resorption should be equal (Figure 8-36).

Ca^{2+} exists in three forms in plasma, in approximately the following proportions:

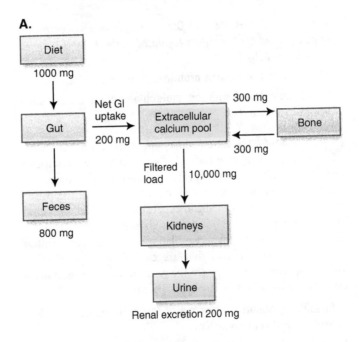

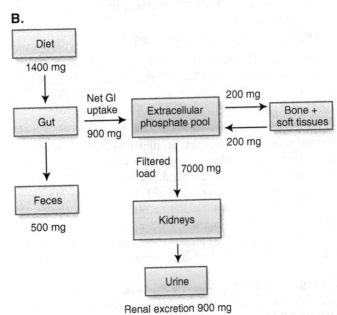

Figure 8-36: A. Normal daily Ca^{2+} balance. **B.** Normal daily phosphate balance. The normal Western diet includes a daily excess of Ca^{2+} and phosphate, which is only partially absorbed. Extracellular fluid contains a small proportion of total body Ca^{2+} and phosphate. In healthy adults, the net excretion of Ca^{2+} and phosphate by the renal system correlates with uptake from the diet. After growth has stopped, bone remodeling does not add or remove net Ca^{2+} or phosphate to or from the extracellular fluid. GI, gastrointestinal.

■ 45% exists as **free ionized Ca²⁺.** *The plasma concentration of free ionized Ca^{2+} is tightly regulated in the 1.0–1.3 mmol/L (4.0–5.2 mg/dL).*

■ 45% is **bound to plasma proteins,** particularly albumin.

■ 10% is **complexed with low-molecular-weight anions** such as citrate and oxalate.

▽ *The acid-base status of the patient affects the free [Ca²⁺] through changes in Ca^{2+} binding to protein.* H^+ competes with Ca^{2+} for binding sites on albumin (and on other proteins), resulting in increased free $[Ca^{2+}]$ in acidosis. In contrast, hypocalcemia may result from alkalosis because more Ca^{2+} will bind to albumin when the $[H^+]$ is decreased. In respiratory alkalosis, such as occurs during hyperventilation, patients may manifest with carpal-pedal spasms that are caused by hypocalcemia. Muscles spasms and tetany are the result of the increased muscle cell excitability caused by hypocalcemia. ▼

Phosphate occurs in two major forms in plasma, alkaline phosphate and acid phosphate:

1. **80%** exists as **alkaline phosphate (HPO₄²⁻)** at a normal plasma pH of 7.4.

2. **20%** exists as **acid phosphate (H₂PO₄⁻).**

The **plasma [phosphate]** is less strictly regulated than Ca^{2+}, and is within the range of 0.8–1.5 mmol/L (2.5–4.5 mg/dL).

PTH

PTH exerts dominant control of Ca^{2+} and phosphate homeostasis. Normally, there are four small parathyroid glands, with two on the back of each lobe of the thyroid gland. **Chief cells** are responsible for production of the peptide hormone PTH, which is formed from the cleavage of preproPTH. Like most peptide hormones, PTH is water soluble and circulates free in plasma. PTH is broken down by cleavage into smaller peptide fragments in the liver and by hydrolysis of the active N-terminal fragment in the kidney. PTH has a short half-life, of approximately 5 minutes.

ACTIONS OF PTH *PTH increases the free plasma Ca^{2+} concentration and decreases the plasma phosphate concentration.* The **direct effects of PTH** are:

■ **Stimulation of bone resorption,** which adds both Ca^{2+} and phosphate to plasma. The rate of resorption of the organic bone matrix can be assessed by measuring urinary excretion of **hydroxyproline.**

■ **Decrease in renal Ca²⁺ excretion,** due to PTH stimulation of Ca^{2+} reabsorption in the thick ascending limb and the distal tubule of the nephron.

■ **Increase in renal phosphate excretion,** due to the inhibition of phosphate reabsorption in the proximal renal tubule.

The direct actions of PTH on Ca^{2+} cause an increase in the plasma $[Ca^{2+}]$. The effect of PTH on phosphate is to cause movement of phosphate from bone to plasma and from plasma to urine, with the net effect of reducing the plasma phosphate concentration. PTH indirectly exerts more effects on Ca^{2+} and phosphate homeostasis by stimulating the final step in vitamin D synthesis in the kidney (see below).

CONTROL OF PTH SECRETION The **rate of PTH secretion** is regulated by the following three factors (Figure 8-37):

1. **Plasma free [Ca^{2+}].** *A decrease in the plasma [Ca^{2+}] is the most potent stimulus for PTH secretion.* Chief cells sense plasma Ca^{2+} concentration through expression of the **extracellular Ca^{2+}-sensing receptor (CaSR)**. The CaSR is a G-protein–coupled receptor, which is linked to the IP$_3$/DAG intracellular signaling pathway.

2. **Plasma [phosphate].** *A prolonged increase in phosphate concentration stimulates PTH secretion.*

3. **Vitamin D.** PTH stimulates vitamin D synthesis, which exerts negative feedback inhibition on PTH secretion.

VITAMIN D

Vitamin D is present in the body as **vitamin D$_2$ (ergocalciferol)** and **vitamin D$_3$ (cholecalciferol).** Vitamin D$_3$ is a precursor molecule that is modified to become the active hormone **1,25-dihydroxycholecalciferol,** which is sometimes referred to as **1,25-(OH)$_2$D$_3$,** or **calcitriol.** Calcitriol has multiple physiologic effects, of which the most clearly understood is the control of Ca^{2+} and phosphate homeostasis.

Cholecalciferol can be synthesized from **7-dehydrocholesterol** in the skin when the skin is exposed to an adequate amount of **ultraviolet light** (Figure 8-38). The reserve of cholecalciferol in adipose cells is released into the plasma if the circulating concentrations decrease. However, *people living in regions of the world where seasonal sunlight exposure is insufficient or people who do not expose their skin to sunlight rely on a dietary supplement of vitamin D.* Cholecalciferol is a fat-soluble vitamin that must be dissolved in bile acid micelles to be absorbed in the small intestine (see Chapter 7). Hydroxylation of cholecalciferol at the 25th position occurs in the liver and is not regulated. *Activation of vitamin D is completed by 1-hydroxylation in the kidney and is stimulated by PTH* and, to a lesser degree, by low plasma phosphate concentration.

▽ Patients with **chronic renal failure** are often deficient in vitamin D because the diseased kidneys are unable to sufficiently convert inactive vitamin D to its active form. ▼

ACTIONS OF VITAMIN D *The major effect of 1,25-(OH)$_2$D$_3$ is stimulation of dietary Ca^{2+} and phosphate absorption in the small intestine* (and to a lesser extent in the kidney). These actions of 1,25-(OH)$_2$D$_3$ cause the Ca^{2+} and phosphate ion product in plasma to increase, which provides the appropriate environment for bone mineralization. The actions of vitamin D are mediated through an intracellular receptor and by alterations in gene transcription. The integrated effects of vitamin D and PTH are discussed below.

CALCITONIN

Calcitonin is a peptide hormone produced by the thyroid C cells in response to hypercalcemia. In animals, studies have shown that calcitonin decreases bone resorption through inhibition of osteoclasts and that it increases urinary Ca^{2+} excretion to counter hypercalcemia. *However, in humans, calcitonin has weak effects of Ca^{2+} homeostasis,* and neither the absence nor the excess of calcitonin causes defects in Ca^{2+} or phosphate homeostasis.

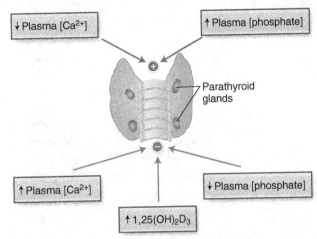

Figure 8-37: Regulation of parathyroid hormone secretion by plasma [Ca^{2+}], plasma [phosphate], and vitamin D. 1,25-(OH)$_2$D$_3$, 1,25 dihydroxycholecalciferol.

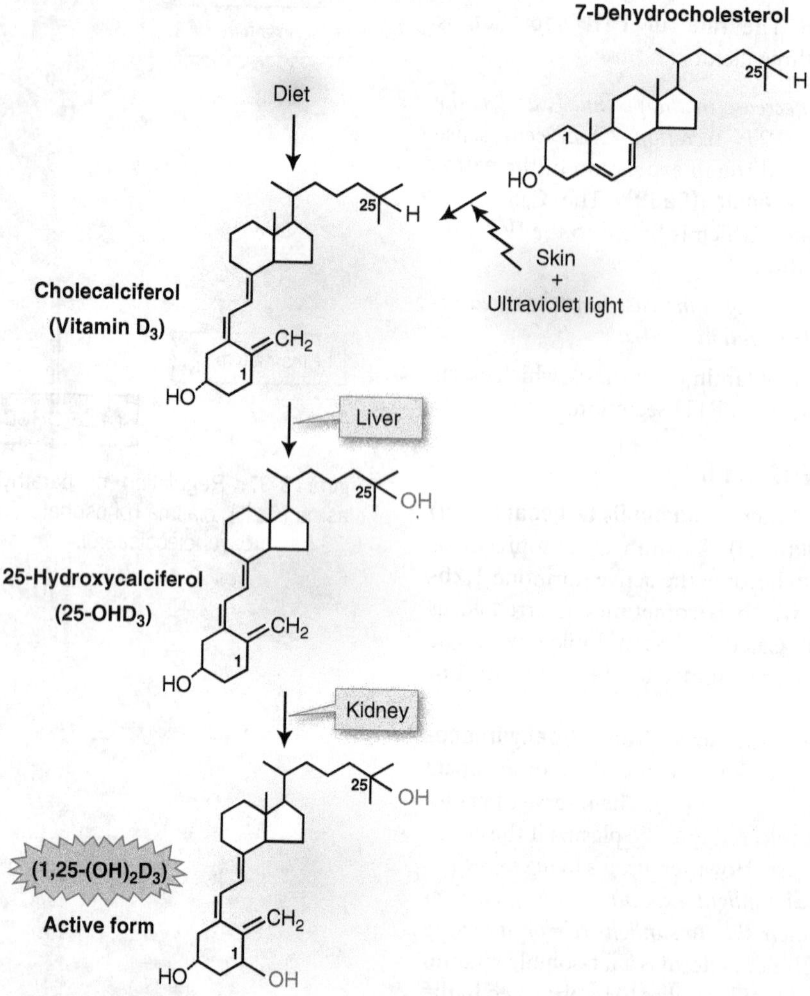

Figure 8-38: Synthesis and activation of vitamin D (cholecalciferol). Vitamin D is supplied from the diet and by synthesis from cholesterol-based precursors in the skin. Activation of vitamin D occurs in two stages: 25-hydroxylation in the liver (not regulated) and 1-hydroxylation in the kidney (stimulated by parathyroid hormone and hypophosphatemia).

▽ Despite its limited physiologic significance, calcitonin has a medical role as a tumor marker for medullary thyroid cancer and as an adjunctive therapy in hypercalcemia and in Paget's disease of the bone. Additionally, the use of calcitonin illustrates the important pharmacologic concept of **tachyphylaxis,** the development of rapid tolerance to drugs following repeated administration. Examples of drugs that undergo tachyphylaxis include calcitonin, nitroglycerin, and ephedrine. ▽

INTEGRATED CONTROL OF CA²⁺ AND PHOSPHATE BALANCE The control of Ca^{2+} and phosphate concentrations in plasma is complicated by the poor solubility of these ions when they are present together in solution. The opposing actions of PTH to mobilize Ca^{2+} and increase phosphate excretion are important to prevent an excessive Ca^{2+} and phosphate ion product and precipitation of calcium phosphate crystals, known as **metastatic calcification.** *In general, the control of plasma $[Ca^{2+}]$ is dominant over the control of plasma [phosphate].*

Both Ca^{2+} and phosphate are required in the context of increasing or maintaining **bone mineralization.** Both ions are available through the actions of vitamin D on the gut and kidney. Vitamin D suppresses PTH secretion, which is logical because PTH stimulates bone resorption and would otherwise oppose bone formation.

▽ A **deficiency of vitamin D** during childhood causes a bone deformity called **rickets,** which is due to the poor mineralization of bone (Figure 8-39). Because of the impaired calcification of cartilage at the growth plates in children with rickets, the clinical effects of the disease are most apparent at sites where bone growth is most rapid. Classic clinical findings include bowing of the lower legs, rachitic rosary (i.e., thickening of the costochondral margins), and Harrison's groove (i.e., lateral groove in the chest wall at the site of attachment of the diaphragm). ▽

Response to hypocalcemia Figure 8-40 shows the integrated response of the PTH-vitamin D axis to **hypocalcemia.** The plasma concentration of both hormones increases because hypocalcemia stimulates PTH secretion, which in turn stimulates the production of 1,25-$(OH)_2D_3$. To return the plasma Ca^{2+} concentration to normal, bone resorption and intestinal Ca^{2+} absorption increase and urinary Ca^{2+} excretion decreases. Bone resorption due to increased PTH concentration produces an unwanted phosphate input into the plasma; increased 1,25-$(OH)_2D_3$ causes further addition of phosphate to plasma through increased intestinal absorption. *An increase in plasma phosphate concentration is prevented because PTH strongly increases urinary phosphate excretion.*

▽ Hypocalcemia causes instability of membrane potentials, neuronal hyperexcitability, and muscle tetanus. **Hypocalcemic tetany** can be assessed clinically by attempting to elicit either **Chvostek's sign** or **Trousseau's sign.** Chvostek's sign is a facial spasm induced by tapping over the facial nerve just anterior to the ear. Trousseau's sign is attempting to induce carpal spasms by occluding the brachial artery for up to 3 minutes using a blood pressure cuff. ▽

Response to hypercalcemia To counter **hypercalcemia,** there is a decrease in PTH and vitamin D activity, shifting the balance of bone remodeling toward bone formation. Urinary Ca^{2+} excretion increases and intestinal Ca^{2+} absorption decreases, restoring normal plasma free $[Ca^{2+}]$.

▽ The phrase "bones, stones, moans, groans, and psychiatric overtones" indicates potential signs and symptoms of hypercalcemia:

- **Bones.** Bone pain.
- **Stones.** Kidney stones.
- **Moans.** Abdominal pains associated with constipation or pancreatitis.
- **Groans.** General malaise and weakness.
- **Psychiatric overtones.** Depression, delirium, and coma. ▽

Responses to hyperphosphatemia and hypophosphatemia Figure 8-41 shows the integrated response to correct sustained **hyperphosphatemia.** Increased plasma phosphate concentration stimulates PTH secretion, which increases urinary phosphate excretion. Normally, increased PTH concentration stimulates renal 1,25-$(OH)_2D_3$ production, but in the setting of hyperphosphatemia,

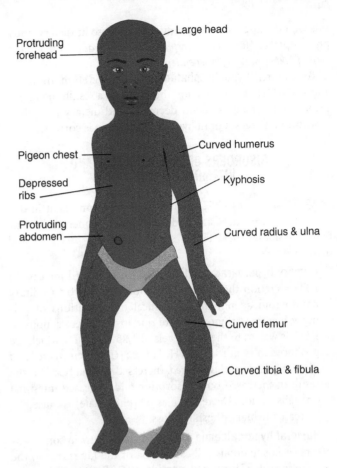

Figure 8-39: Bone deformities caused by vitamin D deficiency in childhood.

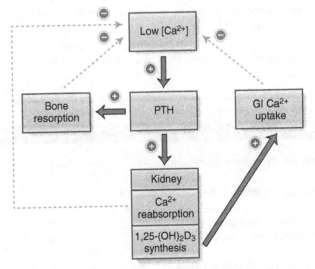

Figure 8-40: Integrated responses to hypocalcemia. PTH, parathyroid hormone; GI, gastrointestinal; 1,25-$(OH)_2D_3$, 1,25 dihydroxycholecalciferol.

this would cause a counterproductive increase in dietary phosphate uptake. *However, hyperphosphatemia reduces the production of 1,25-(OH)$_2$D$_3$ independently of PTH.*

To counter **hypophosphatemia,** PTH secretion decreases and 1,25-(OH)$_2$D$_3$ production increases. As a result, the rate of urinary phosphate excretion decreases and dietary phosphate absorption increases until hypophosphatemia is corrected.

DISORDERS OF PTH SECRETION AND VITAMIN D PRODUCTION

▽ Disorders of PTH or vitamin D secretion result in disturbances in Ca^{2+} and phosphate homeostasis. The pathophysiology of PTH is summarized in Table 8-6 and described below.

- **Primary hyperparathyroidism** is an uncontrolled increase in PTH secretion that is most commonly caused by a solitary parathyroid adenoma. The clinical manifestations of primary hyperparathyroidism are due to the direct actions of PTH as well as to the high levels of 1,25-(OH)$_2$D$_3$, which are produced in response to PTH. *Plasma [Ca^{2+}] is increased and plasma [phosphate] is reduced.* Increased plasma [Ca^{2+}] is the result of increased bone resorption and increased intestinal Ca^{2+} absorption. Decreased plasma [phosphate] is caused by increased urinary phosphate loss.

- **Humoral hypercalcemia of malignancy** occurs in some cancers (e.g., squamous cell carcinoma of the lung) due to the secretion of **PTH-related peptide (PTHrP)** by tumor cells. PTH-rP has the same actions as PTH; therefore patients develop increased plasma [Ca^{2+}] and decreased [phosphate]. *However, PTH concentration is low because secretion is suppressed by negative feedback from the high plasma [Ca^{2+}].* Primary hyperparathyroidism is the most common cause of hypercalcemia in the outpatient setting, whereas humoral hypercalcemia of malignancy is the most common cause of hypercalcemia in hospitalized patients.

- **Secondary hyperparathyroidism** often complicates end-stage renal disease. Chronic renal failure causes inadequate renal phosphate excretion, which results in increased plasma [phosphate]. PTH secretion is stimulated by increased plasma [phosphate], accounting for secondary hyperparathyroidism. High PTH levels often result in bone

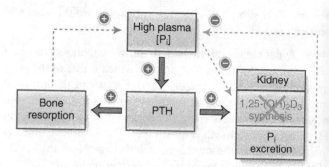

Figure 8-41: Integrated responses to hyperphosphatemia. PTH parathyroid hormone; 1,25-(OH)$_2$D$_3$, 1,25 dihydroxycholecalciferol.

TABLE 8-6 Pathophysiology of Parathyroid Hormone (PTH)

Endocrine Disorder	[PTH]	1, 25-(OH)$_2$D$_3$	Plasma [Ca^{2+}]	Plasma [Phosphate]
Primary hyperparathyroidism	↑	↑	↑	↓
Humoral hypercalcemia of malignancy	↓	↑	↑	↓
Secondary hyperparathyroidism of chronic renal failure	↑	↓	↓	↑
Primary hypoparathyroidism	↓	↓	↓	↑
Pseudohypoparathyroidism	↑	↓	↓	↑

demineralization in chronic renal disease, called **renal osteodystrophy.** Levels of $1,25\text{-}(OH)_2D_3$ are low because of reduced functional renal mass.

Surgical removal of the parathyroid glands is the most common cause of **primary hypoparathyroidism.** The effects are the opposite of those described above for primary hyperparathyroidism; plasma $[Ca^{2+}]$ is decreased and [phosphate] is increased.

Pseudohypoparathyroidism is caused by a defective G protein in the kidney and bone that produces tissue resistance to PTH. Patients present with low plasma $[Ca^{2+}]$ and high [phosphate] because the normal tissue responses to PTH do not occur. *Although PTH secretion is stimulated by hypocalcemia, tissue resistance to PTH prevents a response.* ▼

SEX STEROIDS AND BONE

The sex steroids estradiol (in females) and testosterone (in males) are required for maintenance of normal bone mass. *In postmenopausal women, there is a marked decline in estradiol levels, which is associated with a loss of bone mass, called* **osteoporosis,** *and a corresponding increase in bone fractures.* Osteoporosis is less common in males due to a smaller and more gradual decline in testosterone levels with age.

▽ **Fragility fractures** associated with osteoporosis are a major cause of morbidity and mortality. Characteristic fragility fractures occur in the vertebrae, hips, and distal radius (Colles' fracture). Hip fractures are associated with a 20% mortality rate, and about 50% of surviving patients have permanent disability. ▼

THE HYPOTHALAMIC-PITUITARY-GONADAL ENDOCRINE AXIS

Sex steroids are essential for the differentiation and maintenance of the gonads and other reproductive organs (see Chapter 9). Production of the **sex steroids** is under hierarchical control by pituitary and hypothalamic factors.

SEX STEROIDS

Steroid synthesis in the **ovary** and **testis** produces different products than those produced by the adrenal glands because the gonads do not express the enzymes 21α-hydroxylase or 11β-hydroxylase, which are necessary for corticosteroid synthesis (Figure 8-42). The **three classes of steroid produced by the gonads** are progestins, estrogens, and androgens.

1. **Progestins** are primarily female sex steroids. They prepare the uterine endometrium for implantation of a fertilized ovum and promote the development of the placenta and breasts during pregnancy. *The major progestin in the circulation is* **progesterone.**

2. **Estrogens** play a major role in puberty in girls and in the menstrual (ovarian) cycle. Natural estrogens include **estrone (E_1), estradiol (E_2),** and **estriol (E_3).** *Estradiol is the major estrogen that is secreted from the ovaries during the ovarian cycle.*

3. **Androgens** are the main sex steroids in males. *The major circulating androgen is testosterone, which is produced by*

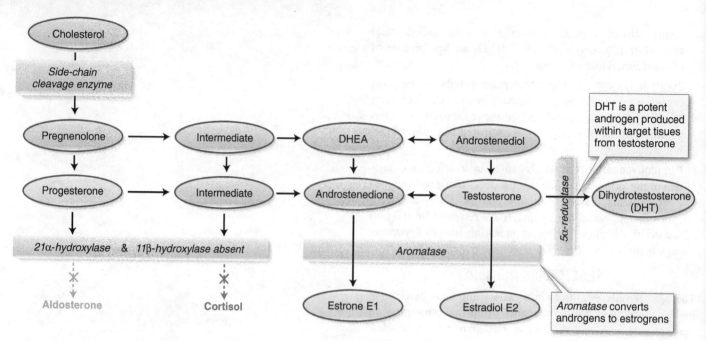

Figure 8-42: Gonadal synthesis of sex steroids. DHEA, dehydroepiandrosterone.

the Leydig cells in the testes. Testosterone is converted to **dihydrotestosterone** within target tissues, via the enzyme **5α-reductase.** Testosterone is a key factor for sexual differentiation of the male fetus and for the development and maintenance of male secondary sex characteristics. Adrenal androgens are produced as a byproduct of corticosteroid synthesis and produce weak effects in comparison to the effects produced by testosterone.

SECRETION OF GONADOTROPINS

Production of sex steroids from the gonads is controlled by the gonadotropins **luteinizing hormone (LH)** and **follicle-stimulating hormone (FSH).** Gonadotropes are stimulated by the hypothalamic neurohormone **gonadotropin-releasing hormone (GnRH).** *Secretion of GnRH occurs in a pulsatile pattern, which is necessary to maintain the stimulation of gonadotropes.* If the same amount of GnRH is continuously available, the gonadotropes become desensitized and do not secrete LH and FSH. **Human chorionic gonadotropin (hCG)** is a pregnancy-specific gonadotropin with a very high structural homology to LH. *hCG is secreted by the developing placenta and is necessary to maintain ovarian steroid production in early pregnancy* (see Chapter 9, Female Reproductive Physiology).

In the mature male reproductive system, the effects of FSH and LH result in the secretion of testosterone and the production of sperm cells. As with other hierarchical feedback control systems, the endocrine product of the primary target gland exerts negative feedback, which in this case is testosterone. Testosterone inhibits the secretion of FSH and LH by the gonadotropes and also inhibits GnRH secretion (Figure 8-43). Gonadotropin secretion can also be influenced by **inhibins** and **activins,** which are peptides hormones. As their names indicate, inhibins inhibit and activins activate gonadotrope function,

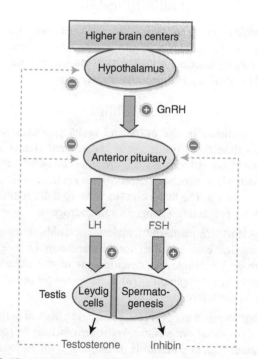

Figure 8-43: Hypothalamic-pituitary-gonadal axis in the male. LH, luteinizing hormone; FSH, follicle-stimulating hormone.

respectively. In males, FSH stimulates the testis to secrete inhibin, which exerts specific negative feedback on FSH secretion by the gonadotropes. The functions of the male gonads are discussed in more detail in Chapter 9.

The hypothalamic-pituitary-gonadal axis in females is more complex than in the male because of the cyclic changes in hormone secretion that occur during the ovarian cycle. There is also variable control of the gonadotropes by positive and negative feedback mechanisms (see Chapter 9).

STUDY QUESTIONS

Directions: Each numbered item is followed by lettered options. Some options may be partially correct, but there is only *ONE BEST* answer.

1. Analogues of guanosine triphosphate (GTP) such as GTP-γ-S can be used to activate G proteins in isolated cells. Which of the following signaling molecules would NOT be produced in response to GTP-γ-S?

    A. Arachidonic acid

    B. Cyclic adenosine monophosphate (cAMP)

    C. Diacylglycerol (DAG)

    D. Inositol 1,4,5-triphosphate (IP_3)

    E. Tyrosine kinase

2. A 28-year-old woman suffered severe trauma to the head in a horseback riding accident that resulted in the complete transection of the pituitary stalk. The plasma levels of which hormone would be expected to increase as a result of this accident?

    A. Adrenocorticotropic hormone

    B. Follicle-stimulating hormone

    C. Growth hormone

    D. Luteinizing hormone

    E. Oxytocin

    F. Prolactin

    G. Thyroid-stimulating hormone

    H. Vasopressin

3. A 4-year-old boy was diagnosed with visual disturbances due to a pituitary tumor secreting excess growth hormone. Which of the following conditions would this boy most likely develop without treatment?

    A. Acromegaly due directly to excess growth hormone

    B. Acromegaly due to excess insulin-like growth factor (IGF)-1 production

    C. Dwarfism due directly to excess growth hormone

    D. Dwarfism due to excess IGF-1 production

    E. Gigantism due directly to excess growth hormone

    F. Gigantism due to excess IGF-1 production

4. A 58-year-old woman complained of lethargy and weight gain over the past year. Further investigation revealed a painless goiter, thick coarse skin, peripheral edema, and low iodine levels. Which of the following most likely describes this patient's diagnosis and plasma thyroid-stimulating hormone (TSH) level?

    A. Primary hyperthyroidism, high TSH

    B. Primary hyperthyroidism, normal TSH

    C. Primary hyperthyroidism, low TSH

    D. Primary hypothyroidism, high TSH

    E. Primary hypothyroidism, normal TSH

    F. Primary hypothyroidism, low TSH

5. A 42-year-old man visited his physician with a complaint that he was always tired. He described craving salty foods and feeling lightheaded after missing lunch. Physical examination shows a blood pressure of 100/70 mm Hg. Laboratory studies show a decreased plasma [Na^+], increased plasma [K^+], and decreased fasting plasma [glucose]. Over the past several months, he said that his skin had become tanned despite avoiding sun exposure. The physician suspected that the patient's adrenal gland was not functioning properly. Which profile of cortisol and adrenocorticotropic hormone (ACTH) levels are consistent with the symptoms described?

    A. High cortisol, high ACTH

    B. High cortisol, low ACTH

    C. Low cortisol, high ACTH

    D. Low cortisol, low ACTH

6. A genetically female infant was born with ambiguous genitalia. She remained in the hospital because of continual urinary salt and water losses during the first week of life. The differential diagnosis of 21α–hydroxylase deficiency would be supported by determining which of the following hormonal plasma profiles?

	Cortisol	Aldosterone	Adrenal Androgens	ACTH
A.	Low	Low	Low	Low
B.	Low	Low	High	High
C.	High	High	Low	Low
D.	High	High	High	High
E.	Low	Low	Low	High
F.	High	High	High	Low

7. A 22-year-old man was treated with a selective $β_2$-adrenoceptor agonist. Which of the following effects is expected to occur?

    A. Generalized vasoconstriction

    B. Increased gut motility

    C. Increased heart rate

    D. Reduced airway resistance

    E. Penile erection

8. A 28-year-old man with type 1 diabetes mellitus self-administered his routine insulin injection. Which of the following effects on plasma concentrations of glucose, fatty acids, and ketones would be expected 1 hour after insulin treatment compared with 1 hour before insulin treatment?

A. ↑ glucose, ↑ fatty acids, ↑ ketones

B. ↑ glucose, ↓ fatty acids, ↑ ketones

C. ↑ glucose, ↓ fatty acids, ↓ ketones

D. ↓ glucose, ↑ fatty acids, ↑ ketones

E. ↓ glucose, ↓ fatty acids, ↑ increased ketones

F. ↓ glucose, ↓ fatty acids, ↓ ketones

9. A 58-year-old man presented to his physician feeling generally unwell and complaining of excessive urination and thirst. He was morbidly obese. The urinalysis showed glycosuria and proteinuria but no ketonuria. Which of the following conditions is most consistent with these findings?

A. Acromegaly

B. Central diabetes insipidus

C. Nephrogenic diabetes insipidus

D. Primary hypothyroidism

E. Type 1 diabetes mellitus

F. Type 2 diabetes mellitus

10. A patient is found to have a rare genetic defect in a G protein that causes tissue resistance to parathyroid hormone (PTH) in kidney and bone. Which of the following profiles for plasma Ca^{2+}, phosphate (P), and PTH concentration would be expected in this patient?

	Plasma [Ca^{2+}]	Plasma [P]	Plasma PTH
A.	Low	Low	Low
B.	Low	Low	High
C.	Low	High	High
D.	High	High	High
E.	High	High	Low
F.	High	Low	Low

ANSWERS

1—E. Tyrosine kinases do not couple to G proteins; all other choices are second messengers that are produced through activation of G-protein–coupled receptors.

2—F. Prolactin is the only hormone under primarily negative control from the hypothalamus, via dopamine release. Sectioning of the pituitary stalk therefore increases prolactin secretion, due to loss of dopamine action on lactotrope cells of the anterior pituitary.

3—F. Excess growth hormone produces gigantism in prepubertal children because the epiphyseal growth plates in long bones have not closed. The effects of growth hormone on linear growth are mediated via IGF-1.

4—D. Iodine deficiency prevents normal production of thyroid hormone by the thyroid gland, producing primary hypothyroidism. Lack of negative feedback inhibition by thyroid hormone on the hypothalamus and pituitary results in high TSH levels.

5—C. The symptoms describe adrenal insufficiency, with Na wasting, volume depletion, and K retention due to low aldosterone levels. Fasting hypoglycemia and fatigue are due to low cortisol levels. Increased pigmentation suggests high levels of ACTH. High ACTH would occur in primary adrenal insufficiency due to a lack of negative feedback from cortisol.

6—B. The enzyme 21-hydroxylase is required for cortisol and aldosterone synthesis (Figure 8-11). Low levels of cortisol result in high levels of ACTH due to loss of negative feedback. Build up of steroid precursors in adrenal cortex is shunted toward the formation of excess adrenal androgens, which causes virilization.

7—D. β_2 receptors mediate relaxation of bronchioles to reduce airway resistance. Vasodilation of skeletal muscle arterioles and mobilization of glucose and fatty acids in the liver also occur through activation of β_2 receptors.

8—F. Insulin directs increased uptake, use, and storage glucose, and increased storage of fatty acids as triglycerides. Ketone production in the liver is increased by glucagon and suppressed by insulin.

9—F. Glycosuria indicates diabetes mellitus. Mature onset and obesity are most likely to be associated with type 2 diabetes mellitus; the absence of ketonuria suggests type 2 rather than type 1 diabetes. Polyuria is due to osmotic diuresis from hyperglycemia. Proteinuria may indicate renal damage as a result of diabetes mellitus.

10—C. If PTH is ineffective due to tissue resistance, there is inadequate renal Ca^{2+} retention and failure to produce enough 1,25-(OH_2) D_3, in turn resulting in low dietary Ca^{2+} uptake. With ineffective PTH, there is low Ca^{2+} mobilization from bone. Urine phosphate excretion is inadequate. Low Ca^{2+} and high phosphate stimulate PTH secretion.

CHAPTER 9

REPRODUCTIVE PHYSIOLOGY

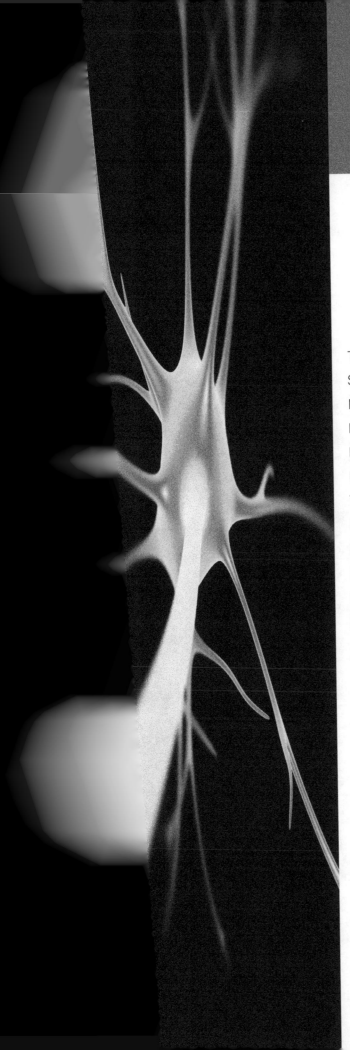

THE REPRODUCTIVE SYSTEM

OVERVIEW

The male and female gonads and the genitalia develop from common precursors in the first weeks of embryonic life, but the final stages of **sexual differentiation** are not completed until puberty. Human reproduction and sexuality are unique in that they are defined by recreation and pleasure in addition to procreation; physiological and psychological satisfaction are both of central importance. *In sexually mature males, millions of gametes (**spermatozoa**) are continually produced by the testes, whereas in females, fertility is cyclical and yields a single gamete (**oocyte**) approximately once per month.* If intercourse occurs at the appropriate time, **ejaculation** of sperm into the female reproductive tract enables the **fertilization** of the oocyte by a single sperm. **Implantation** of the developing embryo occurs in the uterus, and is rapidly followed by development of the **placenta.** The normal gestation period of 40 weeks ends with **labor** and **parturition** (childbirth). The final differentiation of the female breast occurs during pregnancy to allow **lactation** and breast-feeding. The complex events in male and female reproductive physiology are orchestrated by the pituitary, the gonadal, and (during pregnancy) the placental hormones.

SEXUAL DIFFERENTIATION

Sexual differentiation refers to the transformation of the undifferentiated gonads of the early embryo into functional male and female reproductive systems. Anatomic differentiation occurs in utero, but the final maturation that produces fully functional reproductive organs is not completed until puberty.

REPRODUCTIVE EMBRYOLOGY

The process that determines whether male or female reproductive organs develop depends on the complement of sex chromosomes present; female gametes (**oocytes**) all have the same 22X chromosomal makeup, whereas male gametes (**spermatozoa**) are either 22X or 22Y. The **chromosomal** sex of the fetus is determined at fertilization when the male and female gametes combine; XX is female and XY is male.

The default **phenotypic sex** *is female if the fetus does not have a Y chromosome.* The presence of a Y chromosome directs the undifferentiated gonad to become a testis rather than an ovary. A single gene (*SRY*), located in the **sex-determining region** of the Y chromosome, is required for male sexual differentiation.

Before sexual differentiation begins, the fetus has developed two parallel duct systems located near the undifferentiated gonads: the **mesonephric (wolffian) duct and the paramesonephric (müllerian) duct** (Figure 9-1). By week 10 of gestation, the fetal gonads can be distinguished as either **testes** or **ovaries.**

In **males,** the primordial germ cells have given rise to precursors of male gametes called **spermatogonia,** which, together with support cells called **Sertoli cells,** form the germinal epithelium that will later generate male gametes. The mesenchyme surrounding the germinal epithelium gives rise to interstitial cells called **Leydig cells,** which secrete testosterone.

In **females,** the primordial germ cells give rise to precursors of female gametes called **oogonia.** The epithelium surrounding the oogonia differentiates into **granulosa cells,** and the surrounding ovarian mesenchyme becomes **thecal cells.** In the sexually mature female, estrogens and progestins are secreted by the granulosa and theca cells.

Differentiation of the genitalia depends only on the presence or absence of hormones secreted by the testes. In the male fetus, the secretion of testosterone by Leydig cells directs each mesonephric duct to develop into an **epididymis,** a **vas deferens,** and a **seminal vesicle** (Figure 9-1). Leydig cells produce testosterone in response to the hormone human chorionic gonadotropin

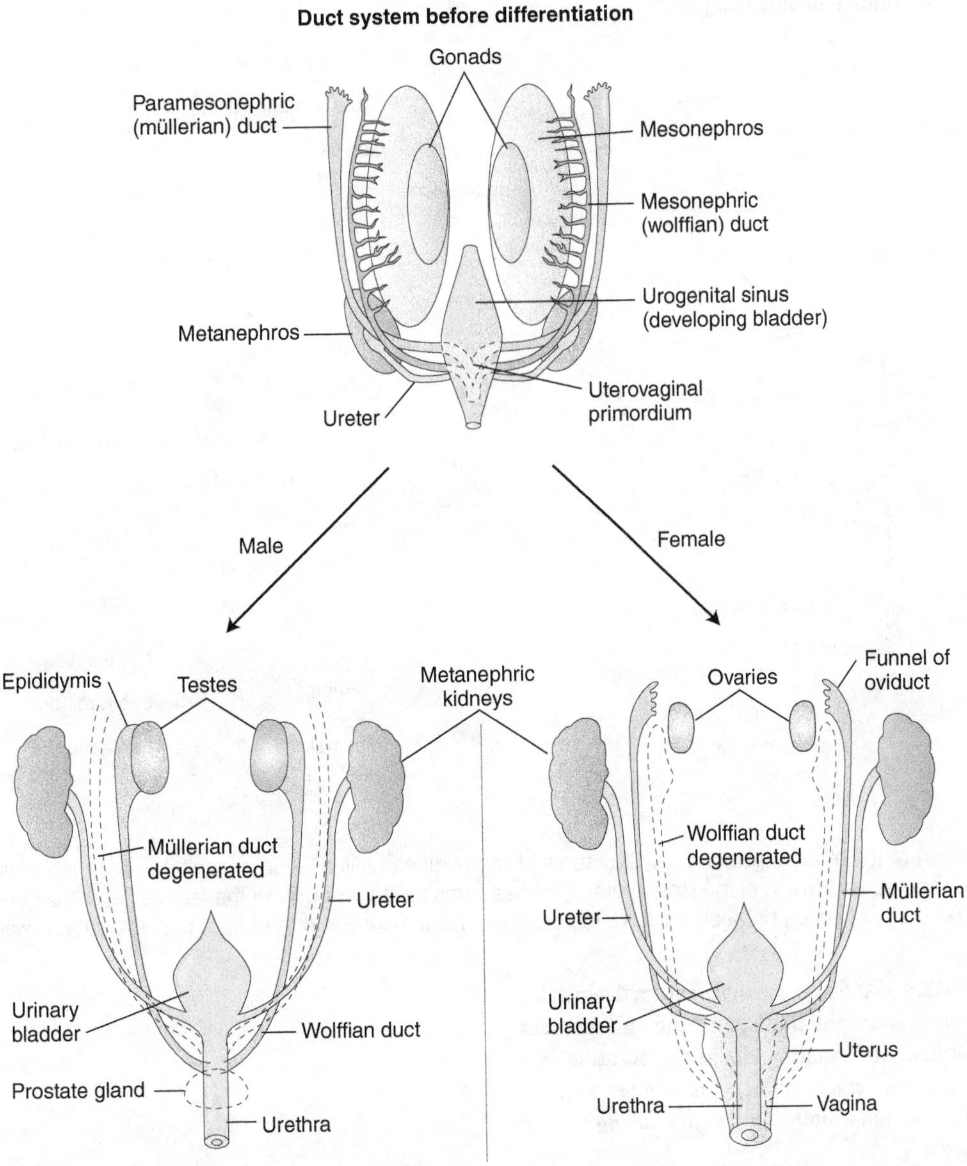

Duct system before differentiation

Figure 9-1: Differentiation of the internal reproductive organs. The mesonephric (wolffian) and paramesonephric (müllerian) duct systems of the early embryo run lateral to the undifferentiated fetal gonad. Secretion of testosterone in the male fetus results in the development of the mesonephric duct into the male reproductive organs; secretion of müllerian inhibiting substance by the Sertoli cells produces regression of the paramesonephric ducts. In the female fetus, the absence of testosterone allows the paramesonephric ducts to develop into the female reproductive organs and results in degeneration of the mesonephric ducts.

(hCG), which is secreted by the placenta. At the same time, the developing Sertoli cells are directed by *SRY* to secrete **müllerian-inhibiting substance,** causing regression of the müllerian duct system. Fetal ovaries are not necessary for the development of the female genitalia, which are able to continue to develop due to the high concentration of maternal estrogens that are present during pregnancy. The absence of the müllerian-inhibiting substance in the female fetus allows the müllerian duct system (instead of the wolffian duct) to develop, forming the **fallopian tubes,** the **uterus,** and the **upper vagina** (see Figure 9-1).

Undifferentiated external genitalia consist of a genital tubercle and a urogenital slit, bounded by two lateral genital folds and two labioscrotal swellings (Figure 9-2A). In males, the conversion of testosterone to **dihydrotestosterone,** via the enzyme **5α-reductase** within these target tissues, is necessary for

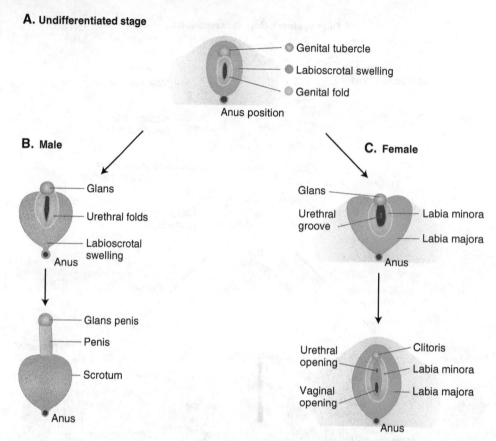

A. Undifferentiated stage

- Genital tubercle
- Labioscrotal swelling
- Genital fold

Anus position

B. Male

- Glans
- Urethral folds
- Labioscrotal swelling

Anus

- Glans penis
- Penis
- Scrotum

Anus

C. Female

- Glans
- Urethral groove
- Labia minora
- Labia majora

Anus

- Urethral opening
- Clitoris
- Labia minora
- Vaginal opening
- Labia majora

Anus

Figure 9-2: Differentiation of the external genitalia. **A.** Structures of the undifferentiated external genitalia. **B.** In the male fetus, fusion of the genital folds creates the penis, and fusion of the labioscrotal swellings forms the scrotum. **C.** In the female fetus, the genital folds do not fuse, allowing the vagina and urethra to open between the labia minora; the labia majora are formed from the labioscrotal swellings.

formation of the **prostate gland** and the male external genitalia. The genital folds fuse to form the **penis,** and the enlargement and fusion of the labioscrotal swellings form the **scrotum** (see Figure 9-2B). *Descent of the fetal testes into the scrotum requires the secretion of the fetal gonadotropins and occurs during the last trimester of pregnancy.*

▽ **Cryptorchidism** is the incomplete descent of the testis from the abdominal cavity to the scrotum, and is associated with testicular malignancy and infertility. In the setting of unilateral cryptorchidism, the fully descended testis may remain at risk of impaired sperm production or of becoming malignant. ▼

In females, the urogenital slit remains open to form the **introitus** (vaginal opening); the **labia minora** are formed from the genital folds, and the **clitoris** forms anterior to the urethral opening. The **labia majora** are formed from the labioscrotal swellings. *Exposure of the female fetus to androgens at this critical time of sexual differentiation can result in* **masculinization** *of the fetus, regardless of the genetic or gonadal sex.*

▽ **Virilization** of a fetus refers to a genetic female with normal ovaries and müllerian duct structures (e.g., fallopian tubes, uterus, and upper vagina), but with masculinization of the external genitalia (e.g., clitoromegaly, large phallus, and fusion of the labioscrotal folds to form a scrotum) due to excessive in utero exposure to androgens. ▼

MALE PSEUDOHERMAPHRODITISM

Sexual differentiation can be abnormal in genetically male or female infants. *Male pseudohermaphroditism occurs when the testes are present and the external and possibly internal genitalia have a female phenotype.*

▽ **Complete androgen insensitivity (testicular feminization)** results from the lack of functional **androgen receptors.** This condition illustrates the role of steroids in sexual differentiation.

- **Dihydrotestosterone** cannot direct the wolffian duct to develop into male genitalia; the testes remain undescended.
- **Müllerian-inhibiting substance** continues to be secreted from the Sertoli cells, resulting in the absence of the female internal genitalia. Patients have a short, blind-ended vagina without a cervix, uterus, or ovary.
- **Failure of masculinization during puberty** is due to the lack of androgen receptors. The low levels of estrogens present cause breast development at puberty, but there is only a small amount of pubic hair. *Diagnosis is often determined following failure of the onset of the menstrual cycle.* ▽

▽ A cause of male pseudohermaphroditism is **deficiency of the enzyme 5α-reductase,** which prevents the conversion of testosterone to dihydrotestosterone. The weaker androgenic effects of testosterone produce varying degrees of failure of the genital and labioscrotal folds to close. The presence of masculinization at puberty distinguishes this condition from complete androgen insensitivity. ▽

FEMALE PSEUDOHERMAPHRODITISM

▽ **Ambiguous genitalia** in a genetically female infant most commonly results from **congenital adrenal hyperplasia.** The most common example of congenital adrenal hyperplasia is deficiency of the enzyme **21α-hydroxylase** in the steroid synthesis pathway, which results in excessive production of adrenal androgens and virilization of a female fetus (see Chapter 8, Adrenal Glands). ▽

PUBERTY

Puberty is the final stage in the process of sexual differentiation and results in the mature individual, with the development of physical and behavioral attributes that allow reproduction. **Adrenarche,** which precedes puberty, is the stage of maturation when the contribution of the adrenal glands occurs before the visible onset of puberty, with increased secretion of adrenal androgens in both males and females. *Adrenarche occurs at about 6 to 8 years of age and is independent of adrenocorticotropic hormone (ACTH) or gonadotropins.* Increasing levels of the adrenal androgens initiate axillary and pubic hair growth during this time.

The first endocrine event of puberty is an increase in the pulsatile secretion of luteinizing hormone (LH) and follicle-stimulating hormone (FSH), which occurs during sleep. This increase is due to the loss of inhibition of the gonadotropin-releasing hormone **(GnRH) pulse generator** within the central nervous system. Toward the beginning of puberty, there is a marked diurnal cycle of LH and FSH secretion, which disappears after puberty. Figure 9-3 shows the typical time course of changes that occur in males and females between the ages of 6 and 21 years. Puberty visibly begins in males between *9 and 14 years of age,* with enlargement of the testes; in females, visible puberty begins between *8 and 10 years of age,* with breast enlargement (thelarche). Other **secondary sexual characteristics** appear over the next 2.5 years. In males, the first ejaculation (**thorarche**) occurs between the ages of 12 and 14 years; in females, the first menstrual cycle (**menarche**) occurs between the ages of 11 and 14 years.

Pubertal changes in males include:

- Increased size and maturation of the testes, involving secretion of testosterone by Leydig cells and **spermatogenesis** in the seminiferous tubules. *Enlargement of the testes in puberty results from FSH secretion and can be used as a clinical indicator of normal function in the developing hypothalamic-pituitary axis.*

- Enlargement of the **scrotum** and **penis.**

- **Male secondary sexual characteristics** develop as testosterone levels increase, and include increased and thickened hair on the axilla, face, trunk, and pubis. Bone mass and the mass and strength of skeletal muscle also increase. There is deepening of the voice and enlargement of the larynx.

▼ **Gynecomastia,** or enlargement of the male breast, can be a pathologic condition. However, normal physiologic gynecomastia occurs when estrogen levels are elevated, such as occurs during the neonatal period (due to high maternal estrogen levels) or during normal male puberty (due to increased testosterone secretion, which is converted to estrogen). Gynecomastia may also occur in elderly men due to increased conversion of testosterone to estrogen. ▼

Pubertal changes in females include:

- **Breast development,** which is mainly a response to the increasing levels of ovarian estrogen secretion. Breast development is characterized by growth of the lactiferous duct system and deposition of fat. *Final differentiation and development of the breast only occurs during pregnancy.*

- Establishment of the monthly **ovarian cycle** requires maturation of the hypothalamic-pituitary-ovarian axis (see Menstrual Cycle). First, there is an increase in FSH and LH secretion; next, ovarian steroid secretion occurs in response to gonadotropin; and finally, there is development of a mid-cycle positive feedback response to estrogen, causing an LH surge that initiates ovulation. *Initial menstrual cycles may be anovulatory and are often irregular as the hormonal axis matures.*

- **Secondary sexual characteristics** in females include enlargement of the uterus, the labia minora, and the labia majora, and keratinization of the vaginal mucosa. There is widening of the pelvis and deposition of fat on the hips and thighs.

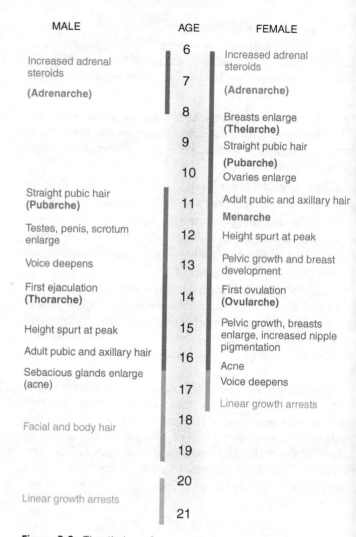

Figure 9-3: The timing of events during puberty in males and females.

PUBERTAL GROWTH SPURT A dramatic growth spurt occurs in both males and females during puberty. Somatic growth is primarily controlled by the **growth hormone (GH)–insulin-like growth factor (IGF)-1 axis** (see Chapter 8). Increased LH and FSH secretion at the beginning of puberty occurs together with increased GH secretion. *The increase in GH secretion is caused by increasing estrogen levels in both sexes*; in males, estrogen is produced from testosterone via the enzyme **aromatase.** The highest rates of GH secretion occur during puberty because the strength of negative feedback inhibition of GH secretion by IGF-1 is weak. After puberty, the rate of GH production declines with age.

Sex steroids are responsible for closure of the epiphyseal growth plates in long bones. *Early exposure to sex steroids is likely to result in short adult stature.* On average, men are 10–15 cm taller than women, which can be attributed to two phenomena:

1. Growth during **the pubertal growth spurt is more rapid in males** than in females.

2. **Puberty occurs later in males,** allowing about 2 additional years of prepubertal growth before closure of the epiphyseal plate is stimulated by sex steroids. Linear growth is completed in females by about age 17 and in males by about age 21.

▽ **Precocious puberty** refers to early pubertal development, often before 8 years of age in girls and before 9 years of age in boys. In addition to early sexual maturation, increased linear growth and skeletal maturation are also common features in both boys and girls. As a result, *children who experience precocious puberty are often tall for their age during childhood, but short for their age during adulthood.* ▼

MALE REPRODUCTIVE PHYSIOLOGY

The major components of the male reproductive system are shown in Figure 9-4. The reproductive function of the **penis** is vaginal penetration during **sexual intercourse,** allowing **ejaculation** of **semen** into the **vagina.** Semen contains **spermatozoa** (male gametes), which are produced in the **testis.** Most of the volume of semen is **seminal plasma,** which is composed of secretions from the **seminal vesicles** and the **prostate gland.** Spermatozoa contribute about 10% of semen volume, producing a final **sperm count** of approximately 20–50 million spermatozoa per mL of semen.

THE TESTIS

The paired **testes** are located outside the abdominal cavity, in the scrotum. The **two major functions of the testis** are:

1. **Spermatogenesis** (production of spermatozoa), which occurs in numerous coiled tubes called **seminiferous tubules** (see Figure 9-4B). The testes are located outside the abdominal cavity within the scrotum and are maintained at a temperature about 2°C below normal body temperature, which is necessary for spermatogenesis to occur. *Spermatogenesis is strongly inhibited by heat.*

2. **Testosterone secretion.** Steroid-producing Leydig cells are interstitial cells scattered between seminiferous tubules.

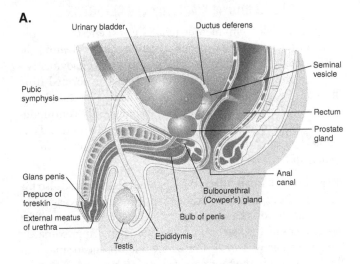

A.

Urinary bladder
Ductus deferens
Seminal vesicle
Pubic symphysis
Rectum
Prostate gland
Glans penis
Anal canal
Prepuce of foreskin
Bulbourethral (Cowper's) gland
External meatus of urethra
Bulb of penis
Testis
Epididymis

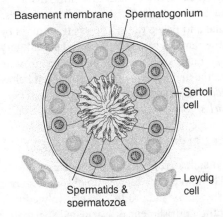

B.

Basement membrane   Spermatogonium
Sertoli cell
Leydig cell
Spermatids & spermatozoa

Figure 9-4: The anatomy of the male reproductive system. **A.** Midline vertical section showing the pathway taken by the vas deferens via the inguinal canal into the pelvis. Sperm from the testis and seminal plasma from the seminal vesicles and prostate gland are delivered into the prostatic part of the urethra during emission and are ejected from the penile urethra at ejaculation. **B.** Microscopic appearance of a single seminiferous tubule within the testis. Cells of the spermatogenic series, seen inside the tubule, are associated with the Sertoli cells. Steroid-secreting Leydig cells are located between the seminiferous tubules.

THE EPIDIDYMIS AND THE VAS DEFERENS

The ducts of the seminiferous tubules exit the testis and converge to form a comma-shaped structure that lies behind the testis, called the **epididymis.** The duct of the epididymis is a single, highly coiled tube, about 6-m long. It is formed from the convergence of the seminiferous tubules at the upper pole of the testis; the tail of the epididymis is continuous with the **vas deferens** at the lower pole of the testis. *Final maturation of spermatozoa occurs during their storage in the epididymis.*

▽ **Cystic fibrosis** affects the lungs and pancreas and also the genitourinary tract. More than 95% of males diagnosed with cystic fibrosis have azoospermia due to obliteration of the vas deferens by thick, tenacious fluid secretions. Approximately 20% of women with cystic fibrosis are infertile due to abnormal fluid transport in the cervix and fallopian tubes. ▼

The **vas deferens** is a muscular tube that expels spermatozoa to the urethra during **ejaculation.** It passes up behind the testis, enters the abdomen via the inguinal canal, and follows a course around the abdominal and pelvic walls. The vas terminates by joining the duct of the seminal vesicle to form the **ejaculatory duct.** The ejaculatory ducts on each side pierce the prostate gland and empty into the first portion of the urethra, just below the bladder. *At ejaculation, spermatozoa combine with secretions from the seminal vesicles.*

THE SEMINAL VESICLES AND THE PROSTATE GLAND

The paired **seminal vesicles** are glandular outpouchings of the vas deferens, located behind the bladder. *Seminal vesicles secrete about 70% of semen by volume* and produce an electrolyte fluid, rich in **fructose,** for the nourishment of ejaculated spermatozoa within the female reproductive tract.

The **prostate gland** surrounds the first portion of the urethra and consists of lobules that drain directly into the urethra through small ducts. Prostate secretion is an electrolyte fluid, rich is **acid phosphatase.** The prostate gland contains smooth muscle, which contracts to deliver secretions into the urethra during a phase called **emission,** just prior to ejaculation.

▽ **Benign prostatic hyperplasia (BPH)** causes enlargement of the prostate, typically in the periurethral zone. Impedance of urinary flow is a common finding in BPH. In contrast, **prostate cancer** most commonly arises in the peripheral (outer) zone of the prostate; urinary obstruction becomes a late complication. ▼

MALE EXTERNAL GENITALIA

The functions of the **penis** are urination and (after puberty) intercourse. The penis is composed of three columns of erectile tissue: two **corpora cavernosa** and the **corpus spongiosum.** The **penile urethra** traverses the corpus spongiosum, which ends as the expanded **glans penis;** urine and semen exit via the **external urethral meatus** of the glans. The prepuce, or **foreskin,** is a retractable fold of skin covering the glans penis, which is often surgically removed by **circumcision.**

Congenital anomalies of the penis include hypospadias and epispadias. **Hypospadias** is an abnormality in which the urethral opening is on the ventral surface of the penis and occurs when the urethral folds fail to fuse during development. **Epispadias** is a malformation in which the urethral opening is on the dorsal surface of the penis. ▼

SPERMATOGENESIS The **three phases** of spermatogenesis are:

1. **Proliferation of spermatogonia** to produce a large population of cells. Once a spermatogonium undergoes its final mitotic division, it becomes a **primary spermatocyte.**

2. **Generation of genetic diversity** by meiosis. After the first meiotic division, the developing gametes are called **secondary spermatocytes;** after the second (final) meiotic division, gametes are called **spermatids.**

3. **Maturation of sperm** with specializations that allow the journey to the oocyte within the female reproductive tract. Dramatic cellular remodeling of spermatids produces **spermatozoa** in a process called **spermiogenesis.**

The seminiferous epithelium consists of cells in the various stages of spermatogenesis. Moving from the periphery of a seminiferous tubule toward the lumen, germinal cells are progressing in their development from spermatogonia to spermatozoa (Figure 9-4B). Developing spermatocytes are embedded in cytoplasmic extensions from the large nongerminal **Sertoli cells,** which provide support and nutrition. The process of **spermiation** involves the release of spermatids from contact with Sertoli cells into the tubule lumen as spermatozoa.

Approximately 74 days are needed to produce mature spermatozoa from spermatogonia. Spermatozoa remain in the seminiferous tubule for about 60 days but have not yet acquired the motility needed to swim to the ovum within the female reproductive tract. Final maturation of spermatozoa in the **epididymis** takes approximately 2 weeks. Mature spermatozoa have a **head region** containing the nucleus, which is surrounded by a large secretory vesicle, the **acrosome;** there is a **middle connecting section,** which is rich in mitochondria, and a **tail region,** which provides a swimming action (Figure 9-5).

Endocrine control of spermatogenesis LH and FSH are secreted from the anterior pituitary under the control of GnRH from the hypothalamus. *LH stimulates Leydig cells to produce testosterone,* which enters the systemic circulation and also diffuses locally into the seminiferous tubules. *FSH stimulates the Sertoli cells,* resulting in the secretion of **androgen-binding protein** into the lumen of the seminiferous tubule. The function of androgen-binding protein is to increase the local concentration of testosterone at the site of spermatogenesis (Figure 9-6). FSH stimulates the secretion of **inhibin** from the Sertoli cells, which exerts negative feedback on FSH secretion by the anterior pituitary. Testosterone exerts negative feedback on the secretion of both FSH and LH.

ERECTION, EMISSION, AND EJACULATION *Penile erection is necessary for intercourse to occur and is controlled by the parasympathetic nervous system.* Erotic stimuli increase efferent parasympathetic activity, causing relaxation of vascular smooth muscle and vasodilation of penile blood vessels. **Nitric oxide (NO)** is the

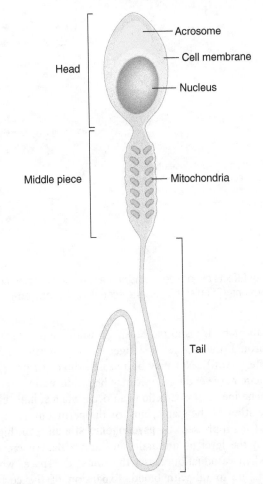

Figure 9-5: A spermatozoon. The head contains a large secretory vesicle, the acrosome, which releases hydrolytic enzymes on to the oocyte during fertilization. The middle section has many mitochondria, providing adenosine triphosphate (ATP) to power the swimming action of the tail.

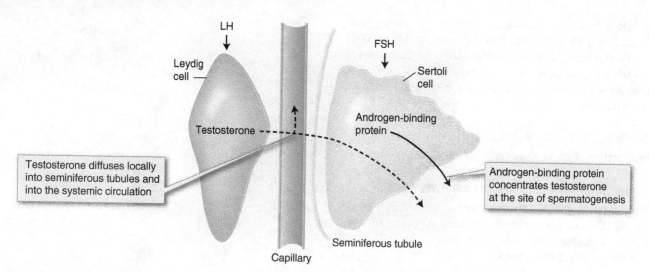

Figure 9-6: Effects of gonadotropins at the testis. Luteinizing hormone (LH) stimulates the Leydig cells to secrete testosterone. Follicle-stimulating hormone (FSH) stimulates the secretion of androgen-binding protein by the Sertoli cells into the lumen of the seminiferous tubules.

most important transmitter causing vasodilation in erectile tissue through the second messenger cyclic guanosine monophosphate (cGMP). NO may be released directly from parasympathetic nerve endings, or it may be produced in response to acetylcholine release. Erection can occur via a **spinal reflex,** by stimulation of the glans penis, or the perineum. It can be induced (or suppressed) by **psychogenic stimuli** from higher centers at the level of midbrain and amygdala. An erection results when vasodilation causes the sinusoidal spaces within erectile tissue to fill with blood. Expansion of the corpora cavernosa compresses venous outflow, further increasing rigidity of the penis. The corpus spongiosum does not contribute significantly to penile rigidity because the urethra must remain patent for passage of the ejaculate.

▽ **Impotence or erectile dysfunction** can be related to many conditions, including endocrine disorders (e.g., diabetes mellitus or low testosterone levels due to hypogonadism), drugs (e.g., antihypertensives or antidepressants), vascular disease, or psychogenic causes (e.g., stress). **Sildenafil** (Viagra) is a drug that is taken orally and can be used to treat some types of erectile dysfunction. Sildenafil inhibits phosphodiesterase type V, the enzyme responsible for breaking down cGMP. By inhibiting this key enzyme, *sildenafil potentiates the effects of cGMP, prolonging vasodilation of the erectile tissues.* ▼

As **ejaculation** approaches, there is sequential contraction of smooth muscle in the vas deferens, the prostate, and the seminal vesicles, which results in spermatozoa and seminal plasma moving into the urethra. This is called the **emission phase** and is coordinated by sympathetic nerves. At ejaculation, semen is ejected forcefully from the urethra; contraction of the internal bladder sphincter (by sympathetic neural stimulation) prevents retrograde ejaculation. Ejaculation is largely an involuntary spinal reflex that occurs after the entry of semen into the urethra during emission. Forceful contractions of the perineal musculature and pelvic floor are coordinated through somatic innervation via the **pudendal nerve. Orgasm** is the pleasurable sensation, which, in males, accompanies ejaculation.

If the internal bladder sphincter does not contract properly, the ejaculate can travel up the urethra and into the bladder, a condition known as **retrograde ejaculation.** Dysfunction of the internal bladder sphincter can result as a complication of diabetes mellitus, use of drugs (e.g., antidepressants), or prostate surgery (e.g., transurethral resection of the prostate, a surgical treatment for benign prostatic hyperplasia). ▼

FEMALE REPRODUCTIVE PHYSIOLOGY

The major components of the upper female reproductive tract are shown in Figure 9-7. The ovaries normally release a single **oocyte** (ovum or egg) into the reproductive tract, which occurs approximately once per month. The oocyte travels along a **fallopian tube** to a hollow muscular organ, the **uterus.** The fallopian tube is the normal site where **fertilization** of the ovum by a single sperm cell occurs; the uterus is the site of **implantation** and development of the embryo.

The lower reproductive tract consists of the **vagina** and the **vulva** (external genitalia). The functions of the vagina are to receive the penis during intercourse and to temporarily retain semen. The vagina and vulva also comprise the lowest part of the **birth canal.**

THE OVARIES AND THE FALLOPIAN TUBES

The paired **ovaries** are the female gonads. There is one ovary located laterally on each side of the pelvis. The ovary is the site of **gametogenesis (oogenesis)** and the major source of the sex steroids. The histologic appearance of the ovary varies throughout the ovarian cycle; oocytes in various stages of development within **follicles,** as well as a temporary endocrine gland, the **corpus luteum,** may be seen (Figure 9-8).

The **fallopian tubes** *transport the ovum and sperm to the site of* **fertilization,** *and transport the zygote to the site of* **implantation** *in the uterus.* There is one fallopian tube associated with each ovary and each one has **four areas** (Figure 9-7):

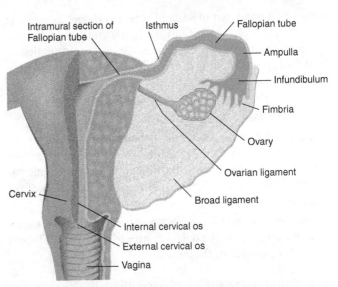

Figure 9-7: Female internal reproductive organs. The ovaries are placed laterally in the pelvis. Oocytes are released into the peritoneal cavity and caught by fimbria at the distal end of the fallopian tubes, which conduct the oocyte to the cavity of the uterus. The uterus communicates with the vagina via the cervix.

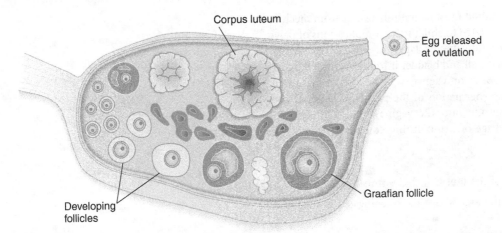

Figure 9-8: Microscopic appearance of the ovary. (Note: the structures shown are not all present at the same time). In the first half of the menstrual cycle, several oocytes begin to develop as a cohort of follicles. A single dominant follicle is visible about midcycle and has differentiated into a large graafian follicle. Ovulation occurs by forceful rupture of the graafian follicle. After ovulation, the graafian follicle transforms into the corpus luteum.

1. The most distal part of a fallopian tube is funnel-shaped and bears finger-like projections called **fimbria,** which receive the ovum when it is released from the ovary at **ovulation.** A ciliated epithelial lining propels the ovum along the fallopian tube toward the uterus.

2. *The usual site of fertilization of the oocyte is a dilated area called the* **ampulla.**

3. A narrow portion, called the **isthmus,** helps to retain the early embryo within the tube for 2–3 days after fertilization. During this time, there is final maturation of the **endometrium** (lining of the uterus) to facilitate implantation of the embryo.

4. Each fallopian tube has an **intramural** portion, where it joins the hollow uterus. The point of entry of the fallopian tube is called the **cornua** of the uterus.

▽ **Pelvic inflammatory disease (PID)** is caused by an ascending sexually transmitted disease. PID is most commonly due to **chlamydia** and **gonorrhea,** and ascends from the cervix to the endometrium, to the fallopian tubes, and to the pelvic cavity. As a complication, the fallopian tubes can become scarred, increasing the risk of an **ectopic tubal pregnancy,** which is a potentially fatal condition! *The most common site of implantation of an ectopic pregnancy is the ampulla of the fallopian tube.* ▽

THE UTERUS

The uterus is a pear-shaped muscular organ within the pelvis, located between the bladder and rectum. *The function of the uterus is to support the growing fetus during pregnancy.* There is dramatic growth of the uterus during pregnancy, occurring by a process of both muscle cell hyperplasia and production of new muscle cells from the resident stem cells. During **parturition** (childbirth), the uterine smooth muscle contracts powerfully to expel the fetus. The uterus is supported in position by several connective tissue **ligaments.** *Damage to the uterine ligaments (e.g., during childbirth) may result in* **prolapse** *of the uterus downward into the vagina.*

▽ **Pelvic relaxation** most commonly results from mechanical trauma related to childbirth. Complications of pelvic relaxation include uterine prolapse, cystocele (bulging of the anterior vaginal wall and bladder into the vagina), rectocele (bulging of the posterior vaginal wall and rectum into the vagina), enterocele (herniation of the pouch of Douglas containing small intestine into the vagina), and urinary stress incontinence (leakage of urine during coughing, sneezing, or laughing). ▽

The structure of the uterus includes three areas:

1. The **fundus** is the area above the openings of the fallopian tubes.

2. The **corpus** is the main body of the uterus. The lower third of the corpus is called the **lower uterine segment.** Contraction of this area draws the dilated cervix (lowest part of the uterus) upward during labor.

3. The **cervix** is about 4-cm long and is mainly composed of connective tissue; this contrasts with the corpus, which is mainly composed of smooth muscle. Approximately half of the cervix protrudes into the upper vagina. The **cervical canal** joins the vaginal lumen and uterine cavity, and is lined by a mucous-secreting epithelium. The properties of **cervical mucus** change significantly during the **menstrual cycle.** *About the time of ovulation at midcycle, under the influence of high estrogen and low progesterone, the mucus is thin and readily allows passage of sperm.* A sample of cervical mucus placed on a microscope slide at this time dries in a fern-like pattern, hence the term **ferning of cervical mucus.** *Later in the menstrual cycle, high concentrations of progesterone promote the secretion of thicker mucus, which resists the passage of sperm.*

▽ **Cervical cancer** most commonly occurs at the squamo-columnar junction, which is the transition zone between vaginal epithelium and cervical epithelium. The most effective screening tool for the detection of cervical cancer was developed by George Papanicolaou and is known as the **Pap smear.** Cells collected from the cervical squamocolumnar junction are stained with the multichromatic Papanicolaou's stain and examined under the microscope for signs of dysplasia. Infection with **human papillomavirus (HPV),** including **types 16 and 18,** plays an important etiologic role in the development of cervical cancer. HPV viral proteins have the capacity to inactivate tumor-suppressor genes, which may explain the carcinogenic effects of the virus. *The recent development of an HPV vaccine (Gardasil) protects women from persistent infection with the virus and may significantly alter the epidemiology of cervical cancer in the future.* ▽

ENDOMETRIUM The **endometrium** is the epithelial lining of the uterus and undergoes dramatic changes during the monthly cycle. There are **three phases of the monthly menstrual cycle:**

1. *The proliferative phase* occurs in the first half of the cycle prior to ovulation and is under the influence of high estrogen levels. During this time, there is marked thickening of the endometrium, growth of the **endometrial glands,** and the appearance of **spiral arteries.**

2. *The secretory phase occurs after ovulation, during the second half of the monthly cycle when there is progesterone dominance.* There is copious secretion of progesterone from the endometrial glands in preparation for implantation of an embryo at this time.

3. **The menstrual phase** occurs if implantation of an embryo does not occur; progesterone levels decrease toward the end of the cycle, causing the uterine spiral arteries to spasm. Tissue necrosis and bleeding (**menses**) occurs, usually over a period of 4–5 days, as the endometrial lining sloughs off.

THE VAGINA AND THE VULVA

The vagina is a tube that extends from the vaginal opening (**introitus**) to the cervix. Many mucus-secreting glands line the introitus and are stimulated during intercourse to provide lubrication. The largest and most important of these glands is **Bartholin's gland,** which is located posterolaterally. The vulva is the collective name for the female external genitalia and comprises the lower third of the vagina, the labia, and the clitoris (Figure 9-9). The clitoris is the female homologue of the penis and consists of erectile tissue of the paired corpora cavernosa, ending in the highly sensitive **glans clitoris.** The urethral opening lies between the clitoris and the introitus.

▽ **Condyloma acuminatum** (or genital warts) can occur in men or women. **HPV types 6 and 11** have been associated with this contagious venereal disease. ▼

OOGENESIS Oogenesis is the process through which the mature female gamete is formed. Oogenesis begins in fetal life but is not completed until the time of fertilization. The proliferation of oogonia by mitosis ends midway through fetal life, at which time oocytes are arrested in the first meiotic division. Thereafter, the number of oocytes gradually declines with age; there are about 1–2 million oocytes at birth and about 100,000 at puberty. Oocytes may be stimulated to develop for release at ovulation, or they will die through a process called **atresia.**

Oogenesis occurs in the ovary within structures called follicles. Each unstimulated follicle contains a single **primary oocyte** surrounded by a single layer of **granulosa cells,** which in turn are associated with **thecal cells.** *With each monthly menstrual cycle, several follicles are stimulated to develop, but only one will become the dominant follicle that continues to ovulation.*

▪ The **oocyte** and granulosa cells in developing follicles enlarge.

▪ A clear gelatinous ring of extracellular matrix appears around the oocyte, called the **zona pellucida.**

▪ The dominant follicle becomes a **graafian follicle** (Figure 9-10). After the LH surge, the oocyte within a graafian follicle completes the first meiotic division to become a **secondary oocyte.**

▪ Rupture of the graafian follicle at **ovulation** expels the oocyte into the peritoneal space near the fimbria of the fallopian tube.

▪ The ruptured follicle collapses and granulosa cells proliferate to fill the space. *Under the influence of LH, structural transformation to the* **corpus luteum** *occurs.*

▽ **Trisomy** (e.g., trisomy 21, also known as **Down syndrome**) is associated with increased maternal age. The mechanism that causes trisomy is thought to be related to **prolonged arrest of the first meiotic division** and age-dependent degradation of the meiotic proteins in the primary oocyte. The first meiotic division is arrested during fetal life and is not completed until that particular oocyte is "chosen" to become the dominant follicle for ovulation. ▼

THE MENSTRUAL (OVARIAN) CYCLE

The cyclic activity of the hypothalamic-pituitary-ovarian axis results in ovulation and the simultaneous development of a uterine environment that is capable of supporting pregnancy, should fertilization occur. The terms menstrual cycle and

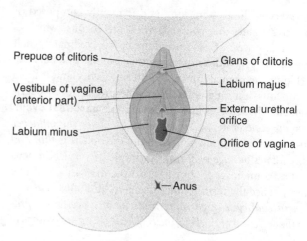

Figure 9-9: Female external genitalia.

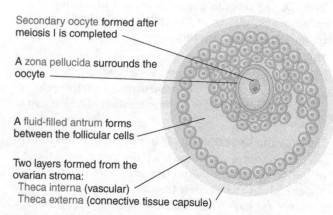

Figure 9-10: A graafian follicle. The oocyte is surrounded by a gelatinous ring (the zona pellucida) by the granulosa cells of the cumulus oophorus and by the follicular fluid (the antrum). Thinning of the outer follicular wall of thecal cells occurs just prior to ovulation. Rupture of the follicle at ovulation ejects the oocyte-cumulus complex.

ovarian cycle are both used to describe a sequence of events that recurs approximately every 28 days. *The first day of menstrual bleeding defines day 1 of a menstrual cycle.* From the perspective of events taking place in the ovary, the cycle is divided into **three phases** (Figure 9-11):

1. **The follicular phase (days 1–14).** The follicular phase is the first half of the menstrual cycle. Toward the end of the previous cycle, the corpus luteum dies, resulting in a sharp decrease in the blood levels of progesterone, estrogen, and inhibin. The loss of negative feedback inhibition of FSH

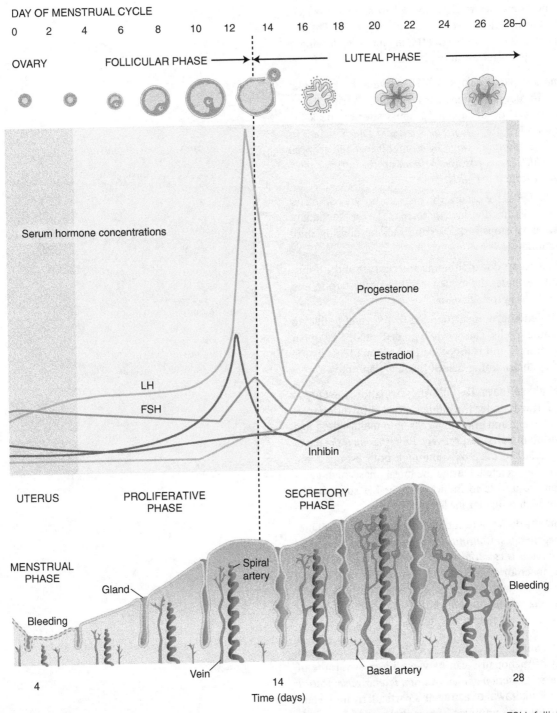

Figure 9-11: Ovarian, hormonal, and uterine events that occur during the menstrual cycle. LH, luteinizing hormone; FSH, follicle-stimulating hormone.

secretion allows plasma FSH concentration to increase. Under the influence of FSH, a cohort of primary follicles develops (a process that begins in the final 2–3 days of the previous cycle).

- **Granulosa cells** secrete estrogen and inhibin under the influence of FSH, accounting for the increase in plasma concentration of these hormones during the follicular phase (Figure 9-11). *Granulosa cells rely on a supply of androgens from thecal cells as a substrate for estrogen production.* By the midfollicular phase, FSH secretion is suppressed, preventing the recruitment of more follicles.

- A **dominant follicle** emerges, which has *high sensitivity to FSH,* and continues to develop and to secrete estrogen, despite the now low levels of circulating FSH. The less dominant follicles undergo **atresia** and die, leaving a single oocyte for release at ovulation.

2. **The ovulatory phase (days 13–15).** Ovulation occurs at the midpoint of a normal menstrual cycle. It is triggered by an LH surge and occurs about 12 hours after the peak LH concentration (Figure 9-11). *The dominant follicle signals its maturity to the pituitary gland by a rapid increase in estrogen secretion, which exerts positive feedback on the anterior pituitary by sensitizing it to GnRH.*

- When the LH surge occurs, the primary oocyte completes the first meiotic division to form a larger **secondary oocyte,** which stops in the second meiotic division until fertilization.

- **Ovulation** occurs due to thinning and rupture of the dominant follicle, under the influence of LH, progesterone, and locally released prostaglandins.

- The released oocyte is surrounded by the **zona pellucida** and granulosa cells. The oocyte is guided into the fallopian tube by fimbria and is propelled toward the uterus by the ciliated epithelial lining cells of the fallopian tube.

3. **The luteal phase (days 15–28).** After ovulation, the **corpus luteum** is formed, under the influence of LH by differentiation of both theca and granulosa cells, into **theca-lutein and granulosa-lutein cells,** respectively. *Progesterone is the major secretory product of these cells,* although both estrogen and inhibin are also secreted. During the luteal phase, high levels of estrogen are unable to induce another LH surge in the presence of high progesterone levels.

- If **pregnancy** does not occur, the corpus luteum spontaneously degenerates. *Continued progesterone secretion by the corpus luteum is essential to early pregnancy.* If implantation of an embryo occurs, the trophoblast cells of the developing placenta secrete the LH analogue *hCG, which supports the corpus luteum until the developing placenta assumes the production of progesterone.*

MENOPAUSE Menopause is a normal stage of life—the physiologic effects of menopause can be viewed as a syndrome of "ovarian failure." *Cessation of menstruation is a universal feature of menopause.* **Withdrawal of estrogen** is particularly important in accounting for the symptoms of menopause, which include insomnia, hot flushes, variable degrees of vaginal atrophy, and lecreased breast size. *Estrogen deficiency causes bone loss and increases the risk of* **osteoporosis.**

During menopause, there is marked reduction of estrogen and progesterone concentrations. The loss of ovarian function removes negative feedback on GnRH, producing high serum concentrations of FSH and LH. *FSH levels are particularly high in postmenopausal women* because inhibins, which exert selective negative feedback on FSH secretion, are no longer produced by the ovary.

▽ Despite the proposed cardioprotective effects of estrogen, the leading causes of death are similar in men and women: (1) cardiovascular disease, (2) cancer, and (3) stroke. The Women's Health Initiative studied the effects of **hormone replacement therapy** (combined use of estrogen and progestin, known as HRT) on postmenopausal women. The results showed that, compared to women in the placebo group, women on HRT had higher rates of breast cancer, coronary heart disease, stroke, and pulmonary embolism. The only benefits noted were reduced rates of hip fracture and colon cancer. These findings from the Women's Health Initiative have contributed to the controversy surrounding the use of combined estrogen and progestin. ▽

▽ **Endometrial cancer** is the most common malignant tumor of the female genital tract. It is primarily a disease of postmenopausal women and typically presents clinically as postmenopausal vaginal bleeding. Exposure to unopposed estrogen plays a critical etiologic role. Risk factors include obesity, nulliparity (no pregnancies), late menopause, chronic anovulation (e.g., polycystic ovarian syndrome), and use of estrogen replacement therapy. ▽

Andropause occurs in men; there is reduced testosterone secretion, but the effects of andropause are usually mild compared to the effects of menopause in most women.

HUMAN SEXUAL RESPONSES

The physiology of human sexual responses is categorized in four phases as **excitement, plateau, orgasm,** and **resolution.** Physiologic changes during the human sexual response include vascular congestion, generalized muscle tension, and increased cardiorespiratory activity.

THE MALE SEXUAL RESPONSE

The **four phases** of the male sexual response are as follows (Figure 9-12A):

1. Penile erection is the first response to effective sexual arousal in the **excitement phase,** and can occur through psychogenic or reflexogenic stimulation.

2. During the **plateau phase,** there is a small increase in penile erection, the testes enlarge due to vascular congestion, and the scrotum contracts to draw the testes upward toward the perineum. Emission occurs shortly before ejaculation, depositing spermatozoa and seminal plasma into the posterior urethra.

A. Male sexual response

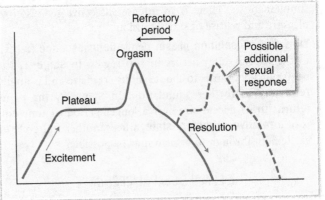

B. Female sexual responses

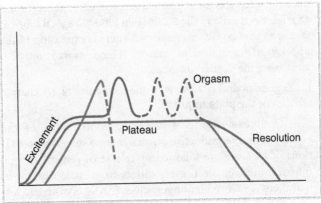

Figure 9-12: Phases of the human sexual response. **A.** The male sexual response involves penile erection in the excitement phase, emission of sperm and seminal plasma into the urethra in the plateau phase, a single orgasm associated with ejaculation, and a resolution phase with penile detumescence. **B.** The same phases are represented in the female sexual response, although the plateau and orgasm phases are more variable. There may be an extended plateau without orgasm, a short plateau with orgasm, or multiple orgasms due to the lack of a refractory period.

3. With adequate stimulation, **orgasm** and ejaculation occur simultaneously. There is an intense subjective sensation of pleasure and release of sexual tension.

4. During the **resolution phase,** penile **detumescence** (return to the flaccid state) occurs in two stages. In **stage 1,** the penis quickly returns to about half its erect size and is totally **refractory** to further stimulation. In **stage 2,** the penis returns to its flaccid size over a longer period of time and is in a **relative refractory state,** when another full cycle of excitement through to orgasm may be possible.

THE FEMALE SEXUAL RESPONSE

The **four phases** of the female sexual response are as follows (Figure 9-12B):

1. Psychogenic and reflexogenic pathways function similarly in males and females during sexual arousal. Clitoral erection is a variable response in the **excitement phase.** Vaginal lubrication is a more consistent response. There is expansion of the upper vagina, and the labia minora enlarge, moving outward away from the vaginal introitus.

2. Engorgement and reddening of the labia minora are characteristics of the **plateau phase.**

3. Female **orgasm** produces rhythmic contractions of the perineum and reproductive organs. Intense subjective sensations of pleasure are followed by release of general skeletal muscle tone. Female orgasm differs from male orgasm in that there is no ejaculation response; female orgasm can last longer and there is no refractory period before additional orgasms can occur.

4. The **resolution phase** involves relaxation of the vagina and vascular decongestion of the reproductive organs.

▽ **Dysfunction of the sexual response cycle** can occur at any stage; examples include desire disorders (more common in women), excitement disorders (e.g., inadequate vaginal lubrication), erectile dysfunction, anorgasmia (e.g., inadequate clitoral stimulation), dyspareunia (i.e., painful intercourse), and vaginismus (i.e., painful reflexive spasms of the paravaginal muscles inhibiting any vaginal penetration). ▽

FERTILIZATION AND THE ESTABLISHMENT OF PREGNANCY

At ejaculation, 100–600 million sperm are deposited into the vagina. After a few minutes, a small number of sperm have already reached the fallopian tube. **Sperm transport** results from the sperm's swimming motion and is assisted by contractions of the uterus and fallopian tubes during female orgasm (if it occurs). The oocyte is propelled along the fallopian tube by the action of cilia. The sperm and egg usually meet in the dilated ampulla of the fallopian tube. *Successful fertilization occurs within a short time window, several hours after ovulation.* The fertilized egg is usually retained in the fallopian tube for about 3 days, where it divides into a solid mass of 12 or more cells called a **morula.** The morula develops into a **blastocyst** during the proceeding 3 days as it floats freely in the uterine cavity. *Implantation of the blastocyst into the uterine endometrium occurs 6–7 days after ovulation.*

▽ **Infertility** is defined as the inability to conceive after 12 months of unprotected sexual intercourse. Approximately 17% of infertility is unexplainable, and 25% relates to male factors and about 58% relates to female factors. ▽

CAPACITATION OF SPERMATOZOA

Sperm must undergo a final maturation event to acquire the ability to penetrate the zona pellucida and fertilize the egg. This process is called **capacitation** and involves the removal of a protein coat that alters the membrane properties of the sperm. Capacitation occurs physiologically within the female reproductive tract, but it can also occur in vitro.

STAGES OF FERTILIZATION

There are **eight defined stages** during fertilization of the egg by a sperm (Figure 9-13):

1. The sperm head penetrates the layer of follicular cells surrounding the egg and **binds to specific proteins in the zona pellucida.**

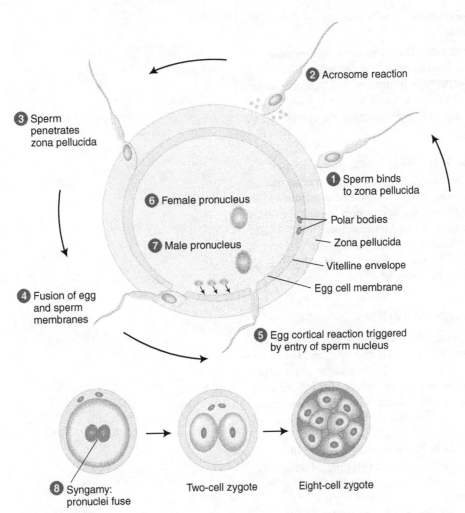

Figure 9-13: Fertilization. Refer to the text, Stages of Fertilization, for a more complete description of the numbered sequence of events shown in the figure.

2. The sperm undergoes **the acrosome reaction.** The acrosome is a large secretory vesicle containing hydrolytic enzymes, located in the head of the sperm. Binding of the sperm head to the zona pellucida produces an increase in intracellular $[Ca^{2+}]$ in the sperm, resulting in exocytosis of the contents of the acrosome on to the zona pellucida.

3. The sperm **penetrates the zona pellucida** to reach the oocyte membrane.

4. **The cell membranes of the sperm and egg fuse,** releasing the sperm nucleus and cytoplasm into the egg cytoplasm. This event causes depolarization of the egg cell membrane, which deters binding of other sperm heads to the egg.

5. The egg undergoes **the cortical reaction** in which enzymes are released by the egg, via exocytosis, and results in hardening of the zona pellucida. The cortical reaction is caused by entry of the sperm nucleus, triggering a large inositol triphosphate-dependent increase in intracellular $[Ca^{2+}]$ in the egg. *Together, with the egg cell membrane depolarization, hardening of the zona pellucida prevents entry of further sperm* (**polyspermy**).

6. The Ca^{2+} signal of the cortical reaction triggers **completion of the second meiotic division** by the secondary oocyte. Unfolding of chromosomes occurs to produce **the female pronucleus.**

7. Chromosomes in the sperm nucleus decondense, producing the **male pronucleus.**

8. **Male and female pronuclei fuse.** The union of chromosomes from the male and female, called **syngamy,** marks the end of fertilization. A **zygote** is formed with 23 chromosomes from each parent. *The chromosomal sex of the fetus has also been determined, depending on whether the sperm is 22X or 22Y.*

▽ **Hydatidiform mole** is a benign molar pregnancy that can be classified as either complete (most common) or incomplete. A complete hydatidiform mole results from fertilization of an empty egg with a single sperm, resulting in only paternally derived chromosomes. An incomplete hydatidiform mole results from fertilization of a normal egg with two sperm, resulting in triploidy (three sets of chromosomes). *Molar pregnancies are incompatible with life.* ▽

IMPLANTATION

The fertilized egg develops for 6–7 days before implantation. Synchronized development of the fertilized egg and the endometrium are required for successful implantation. The endometrium is in the secretory phase, under the influence of progesterone from the corpus luteum. Endometrial secretions nourish the developing embryo within the lumen of the uterus prior to implantation. Fluid within the uterine cavity is gradually absorbed via finger-like projections of the endometrium, called **pinopodes,** which appear only at this time. Fluid absorption brings the embryo closer to the endometrium to facilitate contact and implantation.

During the time when the developing embryo is floating in the uterine cavity, a process called "**hatching**" occurs, in

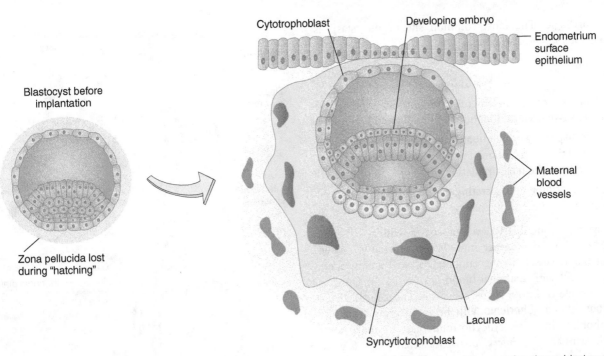

Blastocyst before
implantation

Zona pellucida lost
during "hatching"

Cytotrophoblast   Developing embryo   Endometrium
surface
epithelium

Maternal
blood
vessels

Lacunae

Syncytiotrophoblast

Figure 9-14: Embryo implantation. The embryo develops for approximately 1 week after fertilization of the egg, forming a blastocyst at the time of implantation. The endometrium is invaded by trophoblast cells that surround the blastocyst. Once implantation has occurred, the decidual reaction transforms the entire uterine endometrium into the decidual membranes of pregnancy.

which the zona pellucida and the follicular cells surrounding the blastocyst degenerate to expose the underlying embryonic cells. The blastocyst stage of a developing embryo is spherical; a fluid-filled cavity is surrounded by a layer of cells called the **trophoblast** (Figure 9-14). The **inner cell mass** is a collection of cells on one side of the cavity that will develop into the embryo. Once hatching is complete, the trophoblast cells are able to come into direct contact with the endometrium.

Implantation occurs in the following **three stages:**

1. **Apposition** is the formation of a loose connection between the trophoblast and the endometrium.

2. **Adhesion** occurs through specific ligand-receptor interactions when microvilli extend from the trophoblast cells. Adhesion is followed by rapid proliferation of trophoblast cells and differentiation into two layers: an inner **cytotrophoblast** cell layer and an outer multinucleated layer facing the endometrium, called the **syncytiotrophoblast.**

3. **Invasion** of the endometrial stroma by the syncytiotrophoblast causes the embryo to become completely embedded in the endometrium.

After invasion by the syncytiotrophoblast, the entire endometrium undergoes further biochemical and morphologic change, called **decidualization (decidual reaction),** and forms the "membranes of pregnancy" called the **decidua.** *Decidualization begins at the site of implantation and spreads in a concentric wave around the entire endometrium.*

▽ **Choriocarcinoma** is a malignant molar pregnancy that consists of both cytotrophoblasts and syncytiotrophoblasts. Due to the natural invasive nature of the syncytiotrophoblastic cells, it is of no surprise that this tumor is very invasive and hemorrhagic. The most common site of metastasis is hematogenous spread to the lung. ▼

THE PLACENTA

The placenta is formed by elements from both the mother and the fetus. The **two general functions of the placenta** are:

1. It is a **transporting epithelium.** Materials needed for fetal growth and development must pass across the placenta from the maternal to the fetal circulation.

2. It is an **endocrine gland,** secreting several hormones required for the maintenance of pregnancy.

The syncytiotrophoblast develops spaces within it called **lacunae,** as it invades deeper into the endometrium. When maternal blood vessels in the endometrial wall are invaded, these spaces fill with maternal blood (Figure 9-14). Lacunae eventually coalesce into a single blood-filled space, called the **intervillous space. Chorionic villi** begin to grow from the cytotrophoblast into the syncytiotrophoblast to make contact with lacunae. *The intervillous space behaves like a giant capillary, with fresh maternal arterial blood entering from the uterine spiral arteries and leaving via the placental veins.* Mature chorionic villi contain fetal blood capillaries at their core (Figure 9-15). Numerous chorionic villi project into the intervillous space, resembling a forest of trees "rooted" to a discrete area called the **chorionic plate.** Fetal blood flowing through the chorionic villi arrives via two **umbilical arteries,** which branch repeatedly as they enter the chorionic plate. Blood returns from the chorionic villi to the fetus via the **umbilical veins.** The **maternal-fetal exchange barrier** between fetal and maternal blood consists of the following three components:

1. The **fetal capillary endothelium.**

2. A layer of **cytotrophoblast** and **fetal mesenchymal cells.**

3. A layer of **syncytiotrophoblast** facing the maternal blood pool.

▽ The most common cause of bleeding during the third trimester is due to separation of the placenta from the uterine wall, a condition known as **placenta abruptio.** *This potentially fatal condition classically presents as painful vaginal bleeding in the third trimester.* ▼

PLACENTAL TRANSPORT Transport across the placenta occurs by a combination of active and passive mechanisms. Oxygen and carbon dioxide move by simple diffusion; glucose is transported to the fetus by facilitated diffusion; and amino acids are mostly transported by secondary active transport. Large molecules such as low-density lipoproteins (LDL), antibodies, and other peptides (e.g., transferrin) are taken up by the syncytiotrophoblast via receptor-mediated endocytosis. *Transport rates increase significantly in the final weeks of gestation, reflecting the accelerating growth rate of the fetus at this time.*

▽ Antibodies transported across the placenta augment the **fetal immune system.** The immune system of a newborn

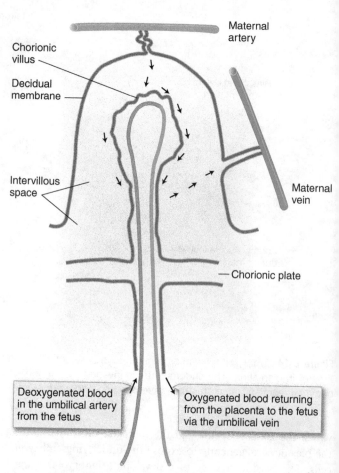

Figure 9-15: Schematic representation of the maternal-fetal exchange barrier.

predominately consists of maternal IgG. However, at approximately 6 months of age, the infant's immune system must begin to assume the major role in defense against infection due to the degradation of the maternal IgG over time. Thus, **immunodeficiency disorders** (e.g., *severe combined immunodeficiency [SCID]*) *do not begin to manifest until after 6 months of age.* ▼

Gas exchange across the placenta Umbilical arteries carry deoxygenated blood from the fetus to the placenta, and gas exchange with blood in the maternal intervillous space results in the *return of oxygenated blood to the fetus via the umbilical veins.* The average P_{O_2} of blood in the intervillous space is about 30–35 mm Hg, which, in adults, would only produce about 60% saturation of hemoglobin and would result in severely impaired arterial oxygen content (see Chapter 5). **Fetal hemoglobin** *has a higher oxygen affinity than adult hemoglobin,* allowing 80–90% saturation of hemoglobin with a P_{O_2} of only about 30 mm Hg in the umbilical venous blood (Figure 9-16).

The P_{CO_2} of umbilical arterial blood is about 50 mm Hg compared to the P_{CO_2} of about 42 mm Hg in the intervillous space. This diffusion gradient allows carbon dioxide excretion from the fetus to the mother; *the carbon dioxide produced by the fetus is excreted via the maternal lungs.*

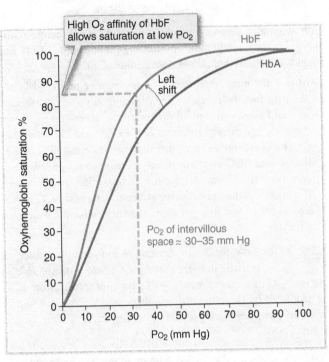

Figure 9-16: Oxyhemoglobin dissociation curves for fetal hemoglobin (HbF) and adult hemoglobin (HbA). The fetal curve shifts to the left, indicating the higher O_2 affinity of HbF that is necessary to ensure that O_2 is transferred in the direction from mother to fetus.

THE ENDOCRINOLOGY OF PREGNANCY

There are several hormones (e.g., peptides, amines, and steroids) that are essential to the maintenance of pregnancy. The placenta is a key endocrine organ, particularly after the first few weeks of gestation. The time course over which the plasma concentration of several hormones increases during pregnancy is shown in Figure 9-17.

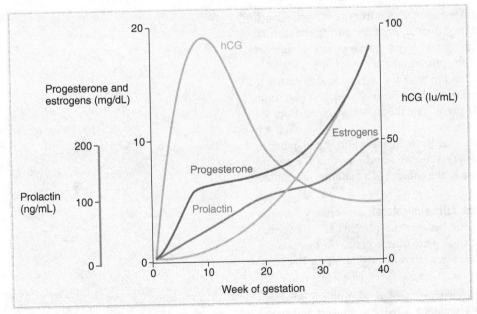

Figure 9-17: Changes in selected plasma hormone concentrations during pregnancy. The early peak of chorionic gonadotropin rescues the corpus luteum, which is responsible for the early rise in progesterone secretion. The placenta assumes production of progesterone by about gestation week 9. Estrogen secretion begins later because maturation of the fetal adrenal glands, which supplies androgen precursors to the placenta, is necessary for estrogen production.

PLACENTAL PEPTIDES

The two major placental peptides, which are only secreted during pregnancy, are **human chorionic gonadotropin** (hCG) and **human chorionic somatomammotropin** (hCS).

1. *hCG* is the most important peptide hormone produced by the placenta because it rescues the corpus luteum from degeneration and allows continued progesterone secretion to support the early pregnancy. At about 8–9 weeks' gestation, the placenta will assume the production of progesterone. Thereafter, the plasma hCG concentrations decrease to lower levels but continue to be important for maintaining progesterone secretion by the syncytiotrophoblast. Placental hCG secretion is controlled in a paracrine manner by locally produced GnRH.

▽ **Pregnancy tests** can detect the unique appearance of hCG in urine in early pregnancy. These tests are able to detect hCG in maternal urine 7–10 days after fertilization. hCG is produced by the syncytiotrophoblast and will be elevated in cases of twin pregnancy, hydatidiform mole, and choriocarcinoma. ▼

2. Levels of **hCS** (also called **human placental lactogen**) are high during pregnancy. *hCS is structurally similar to GH and prolactin.* Its metabolic effects are similar to those of GH, with suppression of maternal glucose use and reduced maternal insulin responsiveness, which may preserve glucose for fetal use. *Fatty acids and ketones are important energy sources in the fetus and placenta,* and hCS stimulates production of these substrates. Higher concentrations of hCS found later in pregnancy also promote mammary gland development.

STEROID HORMONE PRODUCTION BY THE MATERNAL-PLACENTAL-FETAL UNIT

Maternal levels of progesterone and estrogens are both much higher during pregnancy than at any time during the normal menstrual cycle. High steroid levels are necessary to support pregnancy. For example, *progesterone is needed in the uterus to maintain the decidua and to relax the uterine smooth muscle to prevent early expulsion of the fetus.* Beyond week 9 of gestation, most of the steroids present in the maternal circulation are secreted by the placenta.

The placenta is assisted by both the mother and fetus to provide all the necessary substrates and enzymes for steroid production, giving rise to the concept of a **maternal-placental-fetal unit** (Figure 9-18).

▌ **Maternally derived LDL cholesterol** is necessary for placental steroidogenesis because the placenta lacks enzymes needed to produce cholesterol from acetate. *The placenta can produce progesterone when provided with a supply of cholesterol.*

▌ The placenta lacks enzymes needed to produce estrogens but has very high **aromatase** activity to convert androgens to estrogens. *The **fetal adrenal glands** supply the placenta with weak androgens for conversion to estrogens.* These glands produce **dehydroepiandrosterone sulphate (DHEA-S),** most

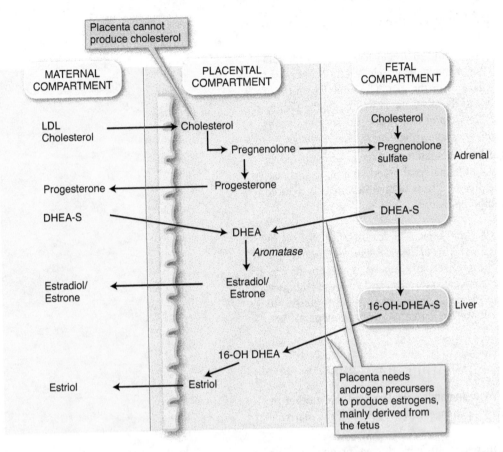

Figure 9-18: Steroid production by the maternal-placental-fetal unit. DHEA, dehydroepinandrosterone; DHEA-S, dehydroepiandrosterone sulfate; 16-OH-DHEA-S, 16-hydroxy-dehydroepiandrosterone sulfate; LDL, low-density lipoprotein.

of which is converted to 16-hydroxy-DHEA-S by the fetal liver.

■ **Estriol (E3)** is produced by the placenta from fetal 16-OH-DHEA-S. *Normally, estriol is not an important estrogen, but it is considered the major estrogen of pregnancy.* Estriol has weak estrogenic properties in most maternal organs, but increases uteroplacental blood flow.

■ The fetus does not produce progesterone or estrogens, thereby avoiding exposure to high concentrations of these steroids. Although the fetus produces large amounts of weak adrenal androgens, *masculinization of the female fetus does not occur because the placenta acts as a large sink for fetal androgens.*

MATERNAL HORMONES

The level of activity in several maternal endocrine axes is altered during pregnancy.

■ In pregnant women, *the total concentration of **thyroid hormones** (T_3 and T_4) is increased but the concentration of free T_3 and T_4 is normal.* Estrogens stimulate the maternal liver to increase the synthesis of many proteins, including thyroid hormone-binding globulin. Increased levels of thyroid-binding globulin cause an initial decrease in free thyroid hormone concentration, which produces feedback stimulation of the hypothalamic-pituitary-thyroid axis to restore free T_3 and T_4.

There is an increase in the maternal levels of **parathyroid hormone (PTH) and vitamin D,** which results in increased maternal Ca^{2+} uptake from the diet. The final activation of vitamin D_3 occurs in the placenta as well as in the kidney. *Changes in the PTH-vitamin D axis are necessary to support the very high demand of fetal growth on the Ca^{2+} supply.*

The **renin-angiotensin-aldosterone axis** is upregulated in pregnancy, allowing the maternal blood volume to increase. Sensitivity to the pressor effects of angiotensin II is reduced to prevent high blood pressure.

▽ *Preeclampsia* (also known as **toxemia**) is defined by pregnancy-induced onset of hypertension, proteinuria, and edema. Although the precise pathogenesis is unknown, preeclampsia results in systemic vasospasm and endothelial injury, causing multiorgan damage. If preeclampsia progresses to include seizure, the condition is referred to as **eclampsia.** ▽

MATERNAL ADAPTATION TO PREGNANCY

Numerous **physiologic demands** are placed on the mother by the fetus, which result in changes in virtually all of the maternal physiologic systems.

1. **Blood volume** increases 40–50% during pregnancy. The increase is necessary to provide a larger preload to meet the demands for increased cardiac output, to protect maternal venous return, and to provide a reserve against blood loss during childbirth. The increased maternal cardiac output supplies the increased demand from the pregnant uterus, the placenta, the kidney (for excretion), the skin (to liberate additional heat), the breast (developing in readiness for lactation), and the heart (to support increased cardiac work). The increase in maternal blood volume reflects an increase in both plasma volume and red cell mass. *Plasma volume increases due to upregulation of the renin-angiotensin-aldosterone axis in response to high levels of estrogen and progesterone.* The increase in plasma volume is greater than the increase in red cell mass, producing a **dilutional anemia** during pregnancy.

2. **Blood coagulability increases** to protect the mother from hemorrhage during childbirth.

▽ Pregnancy is a **hypercoagulable state** primarily because of increases in coagulation factors VII, VIII, and IX, and protein C. The hypercoagulable state of pregnancy predisposes the mother to the development of **deep vein thrombosis** and **pulmonary embolism.** ▽

3. **Alveolar ventilation** increases due to the action of progesterone on the medullary respiratory centers. Increased alveolar ventilation results from an increase in tidal volume rather than increased respiratory rate. *Maternal arterial P_{CO_2} decreases from about 40 mm Hg to about 30–34 mm Hg.* The kidney compensates for this mild respiratory alkalosis and returns the plasma pH to normal by reducing the plasma

bicarbonate concentration (see Chapter 6). When compared to the nonpregnant state, pulmonary function tests show a measurable decrease in residual volume and functional residual capacity because the diaphragm is displaced upward by the enlarged uterus.

4. The **glomerular filtration rate** increases by 40–50% by mid-pregnancy, with a consequent decrease in the concentrations of plasma creatinine and urea. *Glucose appears in the urine in 10–20% of pregnant women* because of increased filtered glucose load and relatively fixed tubular reabsorptive capacity for glucose.

5. **Nutritional demands** of pregnancy include notable increases in protein intake for growth of the fetus, placenta, uterus, and breasts. **Maternal iron deficiency** can develop due to the demands for production of fetal and maternal hemoglobin. *Folate supplementation is also needed for increased hemoglobin synthesis as well as to reduce the risk of fetal neural tube defects.*

6. **Suppression of cellular immunity** is important to avoid fetal rejection; however, this causes pregnant women to become more susceptible to viral infections.

▽ **Constipation** is a common problem during pregnancy because of the effects of progesterone on smooth muscle. Progesterone slows gastric and colonic motility, thereby increasing transit time and subsequent fluid absorption, which results in constipation. ▼

PARTURITION

The gestation period is approximately 40 weeks, and is measured from the first day of the last menstrual period. Expulsion of the fetus, its placenta, and other membranes from the uterus occurs during **labor.** This process is characterized by thinning and dilation of the cervix and by strong regular contractions of the uterus. The **four phases of uterine activity during pregnancy and labor** are:

▪ **Phase 0** is a long phase during which the uterus remains quiescent, under the influence of progesterone. The peptide **relaxin,** secreted by the corpus luteum, assists in maintaining the uterus in a relaxed state.

▪ **Phase 1** represents activation of the uterus when close to term. In the weeks preceding parturition (childbirth), there is weak, low-frequency myometrial activity called **contractures** (also known as **Braxton-Hicks** contractions or false labor). In phase 1, there is increased myometrial expression of receptors for **oxytocin** and excitatory **prostaglandins (PGE$_2$, PGF$_{2\alpha}$).** The appearance of many new **gap junctions** promotes coordinated contraction of the myometrial smooth muscle cells. These changes are associated with a transition from contractures to true contractions.

▪ **Phase 2** is the dramatic stage of labor when there is stimulation of the uterus, with increasing oxytocin and prostaglandin levels inducing true **uterine contractions** and **dilation of the cervix.** *The products of conception are delivered at parturition, ending phase 2.*

In **phase 3,** the uterus returns to its normal size with the assistance of sustained contraction of the myometrium, which also assists in **blood clotting.**

The **initiation of labor** is poorly understood because of considerable species differences that limit inferences from animal studies. In humans, there is evidence that prostaglandins and estrogens produced by the maternal-fetal-placental unit are important. Production of estrogens by the placenta requires fetal androgen precursors. An **increase in fetal androgen production** before labor may result from the placental secretion of corticotropin-releasing hormone, leading to the secretion of adrenocorticotropic hormone (ACTH) from the fetal pituitary gland. Fetal ACTH stimulates the fetal adrenal gland to produce androgen.

Once labor is initiated, the local release of **prostaglandins** is important for generating powerful uterine contractions. **Oxytocin** is secreted in large amounts from the posterior pituitary during the expulsive stage of labor. The positive feedback stimulation of oxytocin secretion due to increasing cervical distension is known as the **Ferguson reflex.**

▽ The powerful uterine contractions induced by **prostaglandins** can be utilized clinically to expel a fetus during abortion or ectopic tubal pregnancy or to stop postpartum hemorrhaging due to an atonic uterus. ▼

LACTATION

The gross anatomy of the lactating breast is illustrated in Figure 9-19A. The functional unit of milk production is the **mammary alveolus,** which consists of a lumen surrounded by alveolar epithelial cells (Figure 9-19B). Alveolar epithelial cells are capable of transcellular fluid and electrolyte secretion, receptor-mediated transport of maternal immunoglobulins, and the synthesis and transport of milk lipids and proteins. A cluster of alveoli comprise a **secretory lobule.** Each lobule delivers breast milk via a duct that widens at an **ampulla** and continues to the nipple via a **lactiferous duct.**

Initial breast development at puberty produces a rudimentary system of ducts. During the first weeks of pregnancy, under the influence of ovarian and placental steroids, there is rapid growth and development to produce mammary alveoli and a differentiated system of ducts. Other hormones, including insulin, cortisol, prolactin, and chorionic somatomammotropin, contribute to the final development of the breast during pregnancy.

BREAST MILK

Breast milk is a complex **emulsion of lipids in an isotonic solution,** which contains all the minerals founds in extracellular fluid.

▪ Fats, mostly in the form of **triglycerides,** constitute 3–5% of milk.

▪ Proteins make up about 1% of milk; the proteins **casein** and **lactalbumin** are only found in milk.

▪ The major sugar in milk is **lactose,** comprising about 7% of milk.

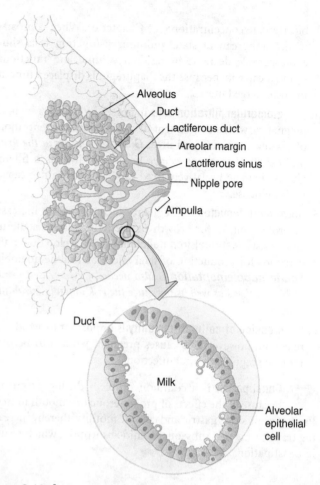

Figure 9-19: A. Gross anatomy of the lactating breast. **B.** The mammary alveolus.

Colostrum is the thin, yellowish fluid produced within the first few days after parturition, before the main milk production begins. It contains more protein than milk, including **antibodies** and immune cells, and provides the neonate with some immunologic protection.

▽ **Human breast milk** is the preferred food for full-term infants. Breast milk is rich in immunoglobulins (mainly IgA) and maternal macrophages, which are thought to protect the infant against upper respiratory tract and inner ear infections. In addition to reduced infections, breast-fed infants also have a lower incidence of allergic diseases (e.g., food allergies and intolerances to foods). Breast-feeding also promotes bonding between the mother and the infant and hastens the return to prepregnancy weight for the mother. ▼

ENDOCRINE CONTROL OF LACTATION

Prolactin and **oxytocin** are the two key hormones involved in the control of lactation; *prolactin is required for milk production, and oxytocin stimulates milk ejection from the breast* (see Chapter 8).

Prolactin is a peptide hormone secreted by the anterior pituitary lactotropes and is *essential for milk production by the lactating breast.* The control of prolactin secretion is unusual in that the dominant factor controlling prolactin secretion is inhibition by hypothalamic **dopamine.** Despite elevated prolactin levels during pregnancy, maternal milk production does not occur before the birth of the infant because high estrogen levels inhibit the effects of prolactin at the breast. There is a dramatic decline in estrogen levels after expulsion of the placenta at birth, which removes the inhibitory effects of estrogen on prolactin. *Milk production in response to prolactin begins approximately 2 days after birth.* During the first few days postpartum, the breast secretes colostrum, before lactation begins.

THE SUCKLING REFLEX The neuroendocrine responses that occur when an infant suckles are known as suckling reflexes. *The afferent limb of the reflex is neuronal, and the efferent responses are hormonal.* The **suckling reflexes have three major functions:**

1. Suckling is the most important stimulus for **prolactin secretion,** acting via neural pathways to inhibit hypothalamic dopamine release. Elevated prolactin levels are sustained for as long as an infant breast-feeds. Peaks of prolactin concentration occur with each feeding session so that *milk production meets the demands set by the infant.* The prolactin released during a feed serves to stimulate milk production in readiness for the next feed.

2. The suckling reflex stimulates **oxytocin secretion** from neurons in the posterior pituitary. Oxytocin causes contraction of myoepithelial cells and **milk ejection** (let-down) from the breast. The reflex can be conditioned, for example, by the sound of an infant crying.

3. The suckling reflex **inhibits the GnRH pulse generator,** which suppresses FSH and LH release and also *suppresses the menstrual cycle in most mothers who are breast-feeding.* The effectiveness of this suppression depends on feeding frequency and can result in the absence of menses for over

2 years. Mothers who do not breast-feed usually resume their menstrual cycles within 2–4 months after giving birth.

CONTRACEPTION

Many **methods of contraception** have been developed and apply strategies to intervene in the physiologic mechanisms of reproduction; for example:

- **Natural contraception** encourages the avoidance of coitus during the woman's midcycle fertile period, about the time of ovulation.

- **Barrier methods** such as condoms and the cap attempt to prevent the sperm from encountering the egg.

- **Intrauterine devices (IUDs)** disrupt implantation of the blastocyst.

- **Hormonal contraception** aims to disrupt the endocrinology of the menstrual cycle. **Combined oral contraceptives** contain both estrogen and progesterone and inhibit the increase of FSH that is needed to induce follicular development. **Progestin-only pills** produce thick cervical mucus that inhibits sperm passage, and they also disrupt normal endometrial development and inhibit gonadotropin production.

▽ Similar to pregnancy, **oral contraceptives** induce a hypercoagulable state and should be avoided in patients with a history of vascular disease (e.g., deep vein thrombosis or stroke). On the other hand, oral contraceptives have been associated with lower rates of ovarian and endometrial cancer. ▼

STUDY QUESTIONS

Directions: Each numbered item is followed by lettered options. Some options may be partially correct, but there is only *ONE BEST* answer.

1. A 34-year old-woman begins assisted fertility treatment to initiate ovulation. She is treated with an agent that acts via gonadotropin-releasing hormone (GnRH) receptors in the anterior pituitary. Which of the following treatments is most likely to be effective?

   A. GnRH agonist given in pulsatile doses

   B. GnRH agonist given continuously

   C. GnRH receptor blocker given in pulsatile doses

   D. GnRH receptor blocker given continuously

2. A 58-year-old man complained of loss of libido and reduced muscle strength. Serum analysis showed reduced levels of testosterone. Reduced activity in which of the following hormone-target cell axes could account for his symptoms?

   A. Luteinizing hormone (LH) – Leydig cell

   B. Follicle-stimulating hormone (FSH) – Leydig cell

   C. LH – Sertoli cell

   D. FSH – Sertoli cell

   E. LH – spermatogonium

   F. FSH – spermatogonium

3. A 17-year-old girl visited her physician because she had never had a menstrual period. Physical examination revealed a tall female with a short, blind-ended vagina and no palpable cervix. Ultrasound showed the absence of a uterus and no ovaries but the presence of undescended testes. Deficiency of which enzyme, hormone, or receptor is most likely to account for these findings?

   A. Androgen receptors

   B. Aromatase

   C. Estrogen receptors

   D. 21α-Hydroxylase

   E. Müllerian-inhibiting substance

   F. Progesterone

   G. 5α-Reductase

4. A 57-year-old man was prescribed the phosphodiesterase type 5 inhibitor sildenafil to enhance sexual function. Which of the following effects will most likely occur after he has taken sildenafil?

   A. Penile erection in the absence of erotic stimulation

   B. Enhanced penile erection following normal erotic stimulation

   C. Increased fluid release from seminal vesicles during emission

   D. Increased prostate secretion during emission

   E. Increased perineal muscle contractions during ejaculation

5. A blood sample is taken from a 27-year-old woman for hormone analysis. The sample contains low levels of follicle-stimulating hormone (FSH) and luteinizing hormone (LH) and high levels of estrogen, progesterone, and inhibin. Assuming a normal 28-day menstrual cycle, on which day of the woman's menstrual cycle was the blood sample taken?

   A. Day 1

   B. Day 7

   C. Day 14

   D. Day 21

   E. Day 28

6. A couple trying to conceive decided to use an ovulation predictor kit to indicate when intercourse should occur to maximize the probability of pregnancy. If ovulation occurs on day 15 of this woman's menstrual cycle, when would implantation of a successfully fertilized egg most likely occur in the uterus?

   A. Days 16–17

   B. Days 18–20

   C. Days 21–22

   D. Days 23–24

   E. Days 25–26

7. An experiment was performed in vitro in which motile sperm were placed in a dish with an egg that was released by natural ovulation. The sperm and egg were both loaded with fluorescent dyes that allowed intracellular $[Ca^{2+}]$ to be measured. A calcium signal was recorded in a single sperm, attached to the zona pellucida of the egg. This signal was most likely associated with which of the following events?

   A. Acrosome reaction

   B. Apoptosis

   C. Capacitation

   D. Cortical reaction

   E. Syngamy

8. Which of the following enzymes or substrates does the fetus provide for the placenta to produce estrogen?

A. Aromatase

B. Dehydroepiandrosterone sulfate (DHEA-S)

C. 21α-Hydroxylase

D. Pregnenolone

E. Progesterone

F. 5α-Reductase

G. Testosterone

9. A 23-year-old woman consulted her midwife 1 day after the uncomplicated delivery of her first child. She was concerned about her lack of milk production and that she was only producing "a thin yellow fluid" at the breast. The midwife reassured her that this was normal and that milk production would begin within 1–2 days. Which hormone was suppressing her milk production?

A. Estrogen

B. Inhibin

C. Oxytocin

D. Progesterone

E. Prolactin

10. A 65-year-old woman was taken to the emergency department after fracturing her hip when stepping off a high curb. X-rays show a fracture at the head of the femur and also reveal very low bone density in general. Which of the following hormonal profiles for the pituitary-gonadal axis is predicted in this patient?

	[FSH]	[LH]	[Estrogen]
A.	Low	Low	Low
B.	Low	Low	High
C.	Low	High	High
D.	High	High	High
E.	High	High	Low
F.	High	Low	Low

ANSWERS

1—A. Pulsatile GnRH mimics the physiologic release pattern. Continuous dosing is ineffective because it downregulates pituitary gonadotropes.

2—A. Leydig cells produce testosterone in response to LH.

3—A. The patient has complete androgen insensitivity (testicular feminization) in which androgen-induced development of the mesonephric duct fails. Sertoli cells continue to secrete müllerian-inhibiting substance, so female internal reproductive organs also fail to develop.

4—B. Sildenafil decreases the clearance of cyclic guanine monophosphate (cGMP), which mediates vasodilation in erectile tissues following NO release. NO is not produced or released unless parasympathetic nerves are activated by normal erotic stimulation. Emission and ejaculation are mediated via sympathetic nerves, independent of NO-cGMP.

5—D. A high concentration of estrogen, progesterone, and inhibin, all at the same time, indicates peak secretion from the corpus luteum about days 18–24. Negative feedback produces low LH and FSH.

6—C. Implantation normally occurs 6–7 days after ovulation.

7—A. Binding of the sperm head to specific proteins of the zona pellucida causes a calcium signal in the sperm, resulting in the acrosome reaction.

8—B. Human placenta has a very high aromatase enzyme activity that converts androgens to estrogens but lacks the ability to produce the androgen substrate. DHEA-S and its 16-hydroxylated derivative are produced by fetal adrenal for this purpose.

9—A. Estrogens suppress the milk-producing effects of prolactin during pregnancy to prevent milk production before birth. Expulsion of the placenta at birth removes the source of estrogen. At about day 2 postpartum, milk production in response to prolactin begins.

10—E. Ovarian failure after menopause causes estrogen, progesterone, and inhibin levels to decrease to very low levels. The loss of negative feedback results in high levels of gonadotropin secretion by the anterior pituitary. This patient has osteoporosis, a common complication of sustained low estrogen.

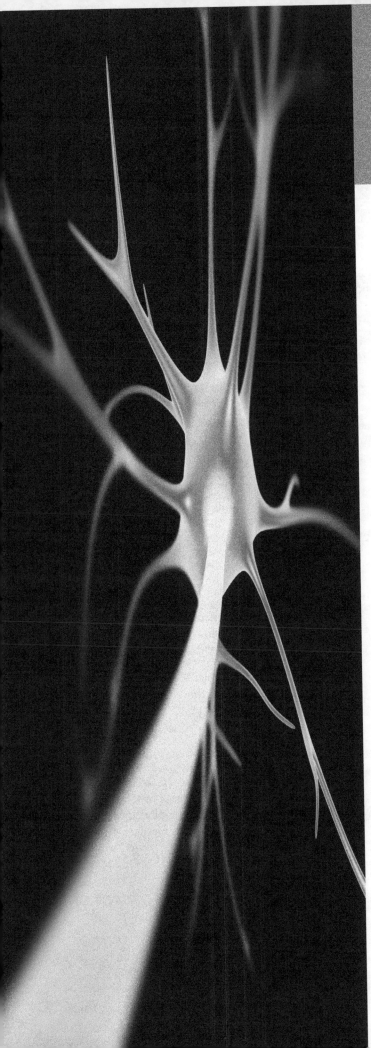

CHAPTER 10

FINAL EXAMINATION

Directions: Each numbered item is followed by lettered options. Select the best answer to each question. Some options may be partially correct, but there is only ONE BEST answer.

STUDY QUESTIONS

GENERAL PHYSIOLOGY AND NEUROPHYSIOLOGY

Questions 1–2

1. Nitrous oxide (N_2O) is a lipid soluble anesthetic gas. A 14-year-old girl was sedated with N_2O to relieve pain during an intra-articular injection. The N_2O concentration in her blood quickly equaled, but never exceeded, the alveolar N_2O concentration. What membrane transport mechanism is most likely to account for the uptake of N_2O from inspired air into her blood?

   A. Antiport with CO_2

   B. Cotransport with O_2

   C. Endocytosis

   D. Primary active transport

   E. Simple diffusion

2. The rate of N_2O uptake would increase if the:

   A. body temperature decreased

   B. diffusion distance from alveolus to blood increased

   C. inspired N_2O concentration increased

   D. rate of alveolar ventilation decreased

   E. rate of pulmonary blood flow decreased

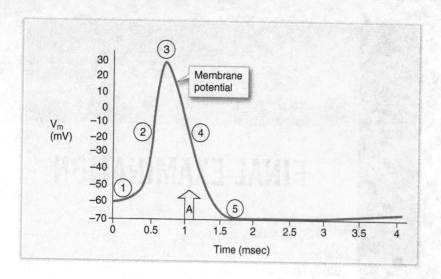

Questions 3–5

3. What change in ion channel activity is most responsible for the rapid depolarization of the neuronal membrane potential at position 2 (shown in the above figure)?

A. Opening of K^+ channels

B. Closure of K^+ channels

C. Inactivation of K^+ channels

D. Opening of Na^+ channels

E. Closure of Na^+ channels

F. Inactivation of Na^+ channels

4. During the repolarizing phase of the nerve action potential shown, which ionic currents are flowing when the membrane potential is 0 mV?

A. Net current is zero at 0 mV

B. Net inward K^+ current

C. Net inward Na^+ current

D. Net inward Cl^- current

5. If a second depolarizing stimulus of normal strength was applied at the arrow marked A on the figure, a second action potential

A. has a lower peak voltage than normal

B. has slower depolarization

C. is additive with the first action potential

D. is normal size but initiation is delayed

E. would not be triggered

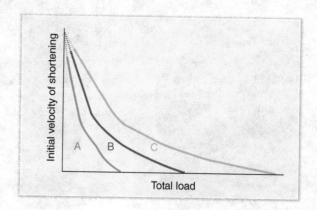

6. An isolated muscle was studied in the laboratory. The figure shows the relationship between shortening velocity and the total load placed on the skeletal muscle. A change in which of the following variables can explain the shift in this force-velocity relation from curve A to curve C?

A. Increased preload

B. Increased contractility

C. Increased afterload

D. Increased V_{max}

7. H^+ secretion was studied in selected cells taken from the human distal colon. H^+ secretion was found to be dependent on the presence of K^+ in the lumen of the colon, and was completely inhibited when the tissue was deprived of oxygen. Which mechanism of H^+ secretion is most consistent with the transport characteristics described?

A. Exocytosis

B. Facilitated diffusion

C. H^+/K^+ cotransport

D. H^+/Cl^- antiport

E. H^+ channels

F. H^+/K^+-ATPase

G. Simple diffusion through plasma membrane

8. A low serum K^+ concentration (hypokalemia) of 2.0 mM (normal range 3.5–5.5 mM) was measured in an 8-year-old boy after he experienced repeated episodes of diarrhea. K^+ was administered with intravenous fluids in an attempt to correct dehydration and hypokalemia. An excessive infusion of K^+ was given accidentally, which resulted in an acute increase in serum K^+ to 6.8 mM. What effect would this infusion have on the resting membrane potential (V_m) of most cells?

A. No change in V_m because V_m is independent of E_K

B. No change in V_m because E_K does not change

C. Depolarization due to E_K becoming less negative

D. Depolarization due to E_K becoming more negative

E. Hyperpolarization due to E_K becoming less negative

F. Hyperpolarization due to E_K becoming more negative

9. A skeletal muscle was stimulated with an increasing frequency of action potentials. The force of muscle contraction rose progressively to a plateau. The mechanism most likely to be responsible for this effect is

A. increased Ca^{2+} entry from interstitial fluid

B. increased amplitude of action potentials with increased stimulation frequency

C. phosphorylation of myosin light chain kinase

D. reduced sensitivity of troponin C to Ca^{2+}

E. reduced time for Ca^{2+} reuptake into sarcoplasmic reticulum

10. As part of a physiology laboratory class, a two-point discrimination test is conducted on the tip of the left index finger of a healthy student volunteer. The axons of the primary sensory neurons that mediate these sensations can be found at which of the following locations?

A. Left dorsal columns

B. Right lateral spinothalamic pathway

C. Left side of the thalamus

D. Left internal capsule

E. Left somatosensory cortex

11. A 52-year-old man developed a brain tumor that involved the suprachiasmatic nucleus. Which of the following functions or behaviors is likely to be abnormal as a result of this lesion?

A. Feeding behavior

B. Circadian rhythm generation

C. Sexual behavior

D. Short-term memory

E. Temperature regulation

F. Water balance

12. A 59-year-old woman was admitted to hospital with a 2-day history of altered mental status and headache. Her condition deteriorated, and she was transferred to the intensive care unit for airway protection. The woman was diagnosed with encephalitis due to herpes simplex virus infection. She remained hospitalized for 3 weeks and was treated with antiviral medication during this period. Upon recovery, she had aphasia, characterized by difficulty in comprehending written or spoken words. She mostly spoke in meaningless sentences and appeared to have memory loss. Which lobe of the brain was likely to have been most damaged as a result of the encephalitis?

A. Frontal

B. Insular

C. Parietal

D. Occipital

E. Temporal

13. A 29-year-old man was stabbed in the back during a fight. The knife caused severe damage to the right half of the spinal cord at T11. Which of the following neurologic deficits would result from this injury?

A. Loss of tactile sensation in the left leg

B. Loss of positional sense from the left leg

C. Paresis and spasticity of the left leg

D. Loss of pain sensation in the right leg

E. Loss of temperature sensation in the right leg

F. Paresis and spasticity of the right leg

14. An 81-year-old woman suffers compression of the right optic nerve by a large aneurysm of her internal carotid artery. Which of the following visual field defects may occur as a result?

A. Binasal hemianopia

B. Bitemporal hemianopia

C. Homonymous hemianopia

D. Macula degeneration

E. Monocular blindness

15. An 18-year-old man fails his driving test due to his inability to read the license plate on an automobile a few meters away. He visits an optometrist, who diagnoses nearsightedness. Which of the following lenses would correct this visual defect?

A. Concave

B. Convex

C. Cylindrical

D. Flat

16. A 17-year-old boy visited his physician because he had frequent headaches and because his academic performance at school was deteriorating despite his best efforts. He had also recently developed a slight tremor in his left hand. MRI scans revealed that both lateral ventricles and the third ventricle were enlarged; the fourth ventricle and subarachnoid space appeared normal. The physician determines that the boy has hydrocephalus. What is the most likely cause of hydrocephalus in this case?

A. Arachnoid granulation blockage

B. Cerebral aqueduct stenosis

C. Choroid plexus papilloma

D. Compression of the spinal canal

E. Ependymal cell dysfunction

17. Synaptic integration within a small neuronal network was studied in the laboratory. A recording electrode was placed in one output neuron, and stimulating electrodes were placed in several other input neurons. When weak stimulation was applied to any single input neuron, no action potentials were recorded in the output neuron. However, simultaneous stimulation of three or more input neurons consistently yielded action potentials in the output neuron. These results illustrate the phenomenon of

A. inhibitory postsynaptic potentials

B. quantal release

C. spatial summation

D. synaptic gating

E. temporal summation

18. A healthy 24-year-old woman runs 5 miles at a moderate pace. Her core body temperature increases to 40°C in the first 20 minutes of the run and remains stable at this value throughout the run (normal temperature = 36–38°C). Her sweating rate increases twofold during the run. Under these conditions, what is the most important mechanism through which sweating is stimulated?

A. Cholinergic parasympathetic neurons

B. Cholinergic sympathetic neurons

C. Circulating epinephrine

D. Norepinephrinergic parasympathetic neurons

E. Norepinephrinergic sympathetic neurons

19. A 68-year-old man was brought to the physician by his wife, who had noticed several changes in her husband over the past year. When greeting the patient, the physician noticed that the man had difficulty getting out of his

chair and took a long time to begin walking toward he office. The man walked with a slow shuffling gait and ha a characteristic tremor in both hands. He spoke slowl in a flat tone, without blinking. Physical examination revealed increased muscle tone in his arms and legs. Wha type of drug should this patient be prescribed to alleviat his symptoms?

A. Anticholinesterase

B. Barbiturate

C. Dopamine precursor

D. Sympathomimetic

E. Serotonin-reuptake inhibitor

20. A 59-year-old man is detained by police on suspicion of driving under the influence of alcohol after a minor automobile accident. The police officer assumed the man was severely impaired due to his very wide gait and inability to walk heel to toe in a straight line. However, a breath test revealed an alcohol level just below the legal limit. The man admitted being a heavy drinker for many years but insisted that he had not consumed any alcohol since the previous day. Neurologic examinations showed no sensory, cognitive, or memory deficits. Which of the following structures is most likely to be dysfunctional in this patient?

A. Amygdala

B. Basal ganglia

C. Cerebellum

D. Motor cortex

E. Vestibular labyrinth

21. A 35-year-old woman visited her physician because she had a severe throat infection for several days. She was prescribed an antibiotic but the infection was resistant to the drug and persisted for 5 weeks. After the inflammation had subsided, the woman complained of difficulty swallowing, loss of taste, and shooting pains in her throat. She had no speech problems. She also described frequent palpitations, which she had never felt before the throat infection. Which cranial nerve was most affected by this infection?

A. Abducens (CN VI)

B. Facial (CN VII)

C. Glossopharyngeal (CN IX)

D. Hypoglossal (CN XII)

E. Vagus (X)

22. A 44-year-old woman suffered a stroke that involved part of her midbrain. A hearing impairment resulted, which included a reduced ability to localize sound or to distinguish between sounds. Which structure in this area of the brain may have been damaged by the stroke and could account for these deficits?

A. Inferior colliculus

B. Medial lemniscus

C. Red nucleus

D. Reticular activating system

E. Substantia nigra

BLOOD AND CARDIOVASCULAR PHYSIOLOGY

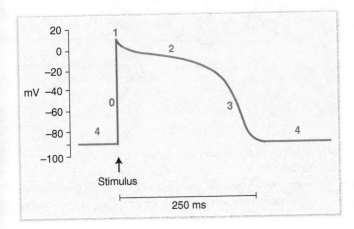

23. The above figure shows a single cardiac action potential measured in a normal ventricular myocyte. Which of the following stable ionic currents across the cell membrane is most responsible for phase 4?

A. Ca^{2+} current

B. Cl^- current

C. K^+ current

D. Na^+ current

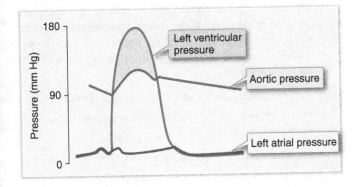

24. A 50-year-old man with a chronic heart valve abnormality is evaluated for valve replacement surgery. Cardiac catheterization produced the results shown in the figure above. Which of the following heart valve abnormalities does the patient have?

A. Aortic stenosis

B. Aortic insufficiency

C. Mitral stenosis

D. Mitral insufficiency

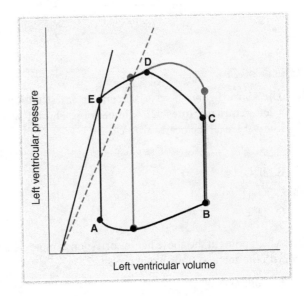

25. An 84-year-old woman visited her family physician complaining of severe shortness of breath at night and the need to urinate several times during the night. She said that she also became short of breath when lying down or during physical exertion. She was referred to a cardiologist for further investigation. Referring to the above figure, the patient's left ventricular pressure volume loop (*blue*) compared to the expected normal data (*black*). What changes would be expected in the left ventricular ejection fraction of this patient?

A. Decreased

B. Increased

C. No change

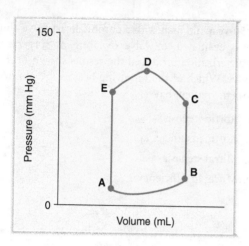

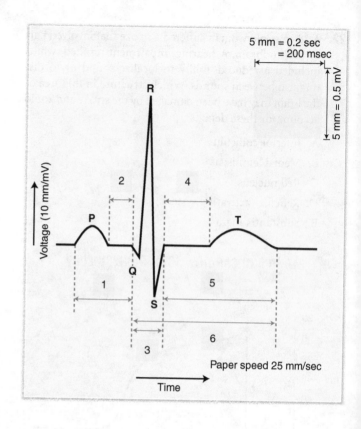

Questions 26–29

26. The above figure shows a schematic representation of a left ventricular pressure volume loop. During which interval are all the heart valves closed?

    A. A–B
    B. B–C
    C. C–D
    D. D–E

27. Which point in the above figure corresponds most closely with the aortic systolic blood pressure?

    A. Point A
    B. Point B
    C. Point C
    D. Point D
    E. Point E

28. At which point in the above figure does the mitral valve close?

    A. Point A
    B. Point B
    C. Point C
    D. Point D
    E. Point E

29. A heart murmur due to aortic stenosis would be heard throughout which of the following intervals?

    A. A–C
    B. B–D
    C. C–E
    D. D–A

30. The above figure shows a single cardiac cycle measured in lead II of a normal electrocardiogram (ECG); segments and intervals are indicated by the numbers 1–6. Ventricular myocytes are in which phase of the action potential during period 4?

    A. Phase 0
    B. Phase 1
    C. Phase 2
    D. Phase 3
    E. Phase 4

31. A 31-year-old woman fractured her pelvis in a skiing accident that resulted in a life-threatening hemorrhage. Because she was skiing in a remote area, 3 hours elapsed before the emergency services were able to administer a blood transfusion. When volume resuscitation was complete, her hematocrit was 40% but then decreased progressively to 24% after 10 days. Her plasma creatinine concentration increased from 1 mg/dL to 8 mg/dL over the same period. What is the most likely cause of this patient's anemia?

    A. Decrease in glomerular filtration rate (GFR)
    B. Decrease in erythropoietin (EPO) secretion
    C. Bone marrow failure at the fracture site
    D. Syndrome of inappropriate ADH secretion (SIADH)
    E. The destruction of transfused blood

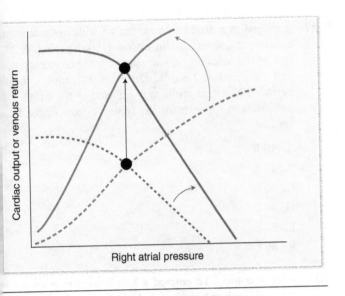

32. Solid lines in the figure show changes in cardiac output and systemic vascular function caused by an unknown stressor; dashed lines indicate the normal resting state. The cardiovascular response depicted on the figure would occur in response to which of the following stressors?

A. Digestion of food

B. Dynamic exercise

C. Hypothermia

D. Severe hemorrhage

RESPIRATORY, RENAL, AND ACID BASE PHYSIOLOGY

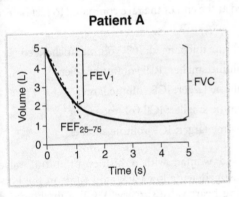

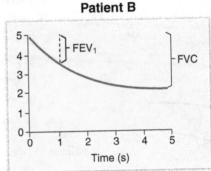

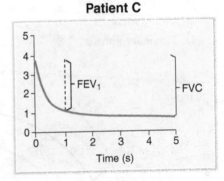

33. The above figure shows the results of a forced exhalation in three different male patients of similar age, height, and weight. Which one of the patients is most likely to have chronic bronchitis?

A. Patient A

B. Patient B

C. Patient C

D. No results are consistent with chronic bronchitis.

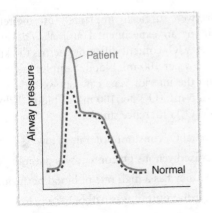

34. A 54-year-old woman with Guillain-Barré syndrome has received mechanical ventilation for the past 7 days. During the past 30 minutes, the amount of positive airway pressure required to deliver a tidal volume has increased. The above figure shows changes in airway pressure during a tidal breath in which a brief pause is applied just after the tidal volume is delivered. The red line shows the patient's current result; the dashed line shows the result of the same test applied 1 hour previously. What change in the patient's lung function can explain the present test result?

A. Decreased airway resistance

B. Increased airway resistance

C. Decreased static lung compliance

D. Increased static lung compliance

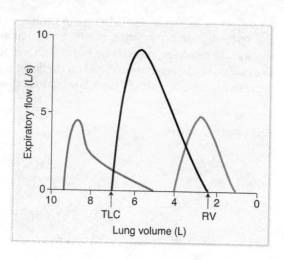

35. The above figure shows expiratory flow-volume curves for three female patients of similar age, height, and weight. Which diagnosis is consistent with the red curve?

A. Asthma

B. Chronic bronchitis

C. Emphysema

D. Plmonary fibrosis

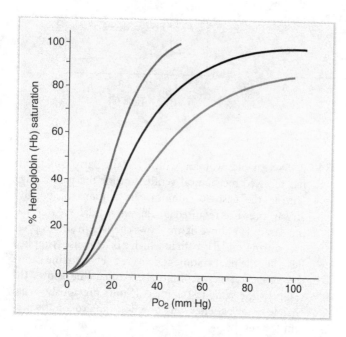

36. Which of the following changes in the properties of blood would result in a shift from the blue curve to the red curve shown in the above figure?

A. Decreased erythrocyte 2,3-bisphosphoglycerate (2,3-BPG) concentration

B. Decreased temperature

C. Decreased hematocrit

D. Increased partial pressure of CO_2

E. Increased pH

F. Increased plasma volume

37. A subject in a drug trial was infused with isotonic saline containing 200 mg inulin over a 1-hour period. At the end of the infusion period, plasma inulin concentration had stabilized at 1mg/dL. During the 1-hour infusion period, 100 mg of inulin was excreted in the urine. Use these data to approximate the subject's extracellular fluid volume.

A. 10 L

B. 20 L

C. 30 L

D. 40 L

E. 50 L

F. 60 L

38. A 24-year-old man entered a 5-mile road race on a hot day. Although in good health, he had not trained in preparation for the race, and he did not drink any replacement fluids during the race. What changes to his intracellular fluid (ICF) and extracellular fluid (ECF) volumes would be observed at the end of the race compared to just before the race?

A. ECF volume unchanged; ICF volume unchanged

B. ECF volume smaller; ICF volume smaller

C. ECF volume larger; ICF volume larger

D. ECF volume smaller; ICF volume larger

E. ECF volume larger; ICF volume smaller

39. A 52-year-old woman with a history of mitral valve disease developed acute low back pain while in the hospital awaiting heart valve surgery. A CT scan showed a single triangular area of infarction extending from the renal medulla to the outer cortex. Which feature of the renal blood supply accounts for this discrete pattern of infarction?

A. Countercurrent exchange in the vasa recta

B. Lack of anastomosis between the arcuate arteries

C. Low blood flow rate to the renal cortex

D. Low glomerular filtration of the cortical nephrons

E. Separate renal arteries to the upper and lower poles of the kidney

40. Cannulae were surgically implanted into the renal artery and vein of an experimental animal. The arterial-to-venous (A-V)O_2 content difference across the kidney was 1.5 mL (O_2) per 100 mL blood. Samples taken from the aorta and the inferior vena cava showed a systemic difference of 5 mL (O_2) per 100 mL of blood. Why was the renal A-V(O_2) difference smaller?

A. The renal O_2 consumption rate is low

B. The mixed venous O_2 content was pathologically low

C. The kidney has a high rate of blood perfusion

D. The cardiac output was pathologically low

41. A 56-year-old man visited his family physician for a routine health checkup. A urine test revealed significant excretion of albumin. Which cell type is most likely to be damaged or malfunctioning in this patient?

   A. Glomerular endothelial cell

   B. Juxtaglomerular cell

   C. Mesangial cell

   D. Podocyte

   E. Vascular smooth muscle in afferent arteriole

42. Infusion of the α_1-adrenoceptor agonist phenylephrine into an experimental animal caused an increase in renal vascular resistance; there was greater constriction of the afferent arteriole than the efferent arteriole. What effect on renal blood flow, glomerular filtration, and filtration fraction would result from treatment with phenylephrine?

	Renal Blood Flow (RBF)	Glomerular Filtration Rate (GFR)	Filtration Fraction (FF)
A.	Decrease	Decrease	Decrease
B.	Decrease	Decrease	Unchanged
C.	Decrease	Unchanged	Decrease
D.	Unchanged	Decrease	Decrease
E.	Unchanged	Unchanged	Decrease
F.	Unchanged	Unchanged	Unchanged

43. A 48-year-old man who is 178 cm (5 ft 10 in) tall and weighs 75 kg (165 lb) was in the hospital for minor elective surgery, but laboratory studies showed that his plasma creatinine concentration was five times higher than normal. Which of the following is the most likely cause of this finding?

   A. Acidosis

   B. Dehydration

   C. High plasma antidiuretic hormone (ADH) concentration

   D. Large muscle mass

   E. Low plasma Na^+ concentration

   F. Low glomerular filtration rate (GFR)

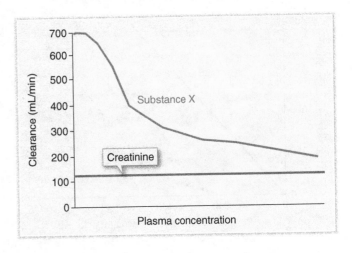

44. Based only on the information shown in the above figure, what can be deduced about the renal handling of substance X?

   A. There is net tubular reabsorption of substance X

   B. There is net tubular secretion of substance X

   C. Substance X is freely filtered at the glomerulus but is not reabsorbed or secreted

   D. Tubular transport of substance X occurs by simple diffusion

45. A 24-year-old man involved in an experiment is found to have a renal p-aminohippuric acid (PAH) clearance of 600 mL/min, a creatinine clearance of 100 mL/min, and a hematocrit of 50%. His rate of renal blood flow is calculated to be

   A. 50 mL/min

   B. 100 mL/min

   C. 300 mL/min

   D. 600 mL/min

   E. 800 mL/min

   F. 1000 mL/min

   G. 1200 mL/min

46. A 24-hour urine sample is collected from a patient who was admitted to the hospital because of severe renal colic. Results of the urinalysis show urine creatinine concentration = 20 mg/mL and average urine flow rate = 1 mL/min. Plasma creatinine concentration was 0.2 mg/mL. What is the filtered load of creatinine?

   A. 0.2 mg/min

   B. 1.0 mg/min

   C. 20 mg/min

   D. 100 mg/min

   E. 200 mg/min

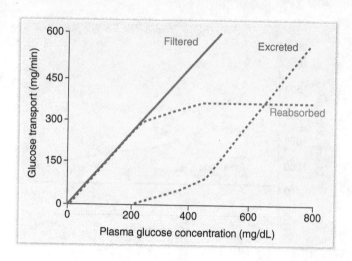

47. The above figure shows a renal titration curve for glucose. Use the figure to determine the renal threshold for glucose.

A. 0 mg/dL

B. 200 mg/dL

C. 600 mg/dL

D. 0 mg/min

E. 200 mg/min

F. 600 mg/min

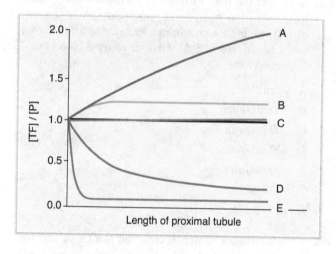

48. The figure shows tubular fluid-to-plasma (TF/P) concentration profiles for several solutes at increasing distance along the proximal tubule. Which solute would produce a profile similar to solute E?

A. Ca^{2+}

B. Creatinine

C. Glucose

D. K^+

E. Na^+

49. A 2-week-old infant was admitted to the hospital following a visit by the community nurse because he had not gained any weight since birth. On admission, he was found to be severely dehydrated and hypovolemic and was treated with intravenous fluids. Genetic tests were ordered because of the marked renal electrolyte wasting, which showed a mutation in the renal Na/2Cl/K cotransport system. Excessive renal loss of each of the following ions was measured EXCEPT

A. Ca^{2+}

B. Cl^-

C. K^+

D. Mg^{2+}

E. Na^+

F. phosphate

50. A 64-year-old woman with glaucoma is given the carbonic anhydrase inhibitor acetazolamide. Which ion would have the largest increase in its fractional excretion as a side effect of this drug?

A. Ca^{2+}

B. Cl^-

C. HCO_3^-

D. K^+

E. Na^+

51. A healthy 59-year-old woman ingested 1 L of water over a 20-minute period. Her urine flow rate increased after 30 minutes and remained elevated for 3 hours. Which of the following changes in her renal function can account for increased water excretion?

A. Aquaporin 2 expression in the collecting duct decreased

B. End proximal tubule fluid became dilute

C. Glomerular filtration rate (GFR) increased

D. Na^+ reabsorption in the thin descending limb increased

E. Renal urea production increased

52. A 15-year-old boy was busy with school activities and did not drink any liquids from 8 am to 5 pm. When he urinated late in the day, he noticed that his urine was dark yellow. All of the following events were occurring in his kidney during the day EXCEPT

A. reduced fractional Na^+ excretion

B. reduced fractional urea excretion

C. increased plasma antidiuretic hormone (ADH) concentration

D. increased Na^+ reabsorption in the thin descending limb

E. increased aquaporin 2 expression in the collecting duct

53. The urine concentrating ability is evaluated in a 90-year-old woman who complained of polydipsia and polyuria. During the test period, urine flow rate = 2 mL/min, urine osmolarity = 295 mOsM, and plasma osmolarity = 295 mOsM. Free water clearance was calculated to be

A. 0 mL/min

B. 0.5 mL/min

C. 1.0 mL/min

D. 2.0 mL/min

54. A 19-year-old man involved in an automobile accident suffered internal bleeding that resulted in a significant decrease in effective circulating blood volume. The plasma concentration of each of the following hormones would be elevated EXCEPT

A. aldosterone

B. angiotensin II

C. antidiuretic hormone (ADH)

D. atrial natriuretic peptide (ANP)

E. epinephrine

55. A healthy 22-year-old man ate 200 g of salted peanuts. As a result, he became extremely thirsty and drank 1 L of water. What changes would occur to the physical forces acting at renal peritubular capillaries in response to this ingestion of salt and water?

A. Increased hydrostatic pressure and reduced oncotic pressure

B. Increased hydrostatic pressure and increased oncotic pressure

C. Reduced hydrostatic pressure and reduced oncotic pressure

D. Reduced hydrostatic pressure and increased oncotic pressure

56. A 29-year-old man had complained to his wife about bone pain, frequent headaches, and fatigue for over 1 year but had not visited his physician. After an episode of acute renal colic, he was evaluated in the hospital and found to have kidney stones. He was diagnosed with primary hyperparathyroidism. Compared to individuals with normal parathyroid function, his fractional renal Ca^{2+} excretion is expected to be

A. increased

B. decreased

C. unchanged

57. A 32-year-old man fell from a ladder and fractured his skull. On admission to the hospital, he was unconscious because of a closed head injury. Arterial blood gas analysis showed:

PO_2 = 106 mm Hg

PCO_2 = 25 mm Hg

pH = 7.52

$[HCO_3^-]$ = 21 mEq/L

Base excess = −1 mEq/L

Which of the following primary acid-base disturbances is present?

A. Respiratory alkalosis

B. Respiratory acidosis

C. Metabolic alkalosis

D. Metabolic acidosis

58. A 14-year-old girl with a history of poorly controlled type 1 diabetes mellitus is found unresponsive in her bed. Her parents call 911, and she is taken by ambulance to the emergency department. The arterial blood gas analysis at this time showed:

PO_2 = 90 mm Hg

PCO_2 = 36 mm Hg

pH = 7.10

$[HCO_3^-]$ = 7 mEq/L

Base excess = -20 mEq/L

Which of the following primary acid-base disturbances is present in this patient?

A. Respiratory alkalosis

B. Respiratory acidosis

C. Metabolic alkalosis

D. Metabolic acidosis

59. A 27-year-old woman who weighs 60 kg was anesthetized using a drug that distributed equally throughout her total body water. Hepatic and renal function were both normal, and her body mass index was within the normal range. What is the approximate volume of distribution for the anesthetic in this patient?

A. 10 L

B. 20 L

C. 30 L

D. 40 L

E. 50 L

F. 60 L

60. A 64-year-old man was admitted to the hospital with evidence of low effective circulating blood volume. His past medical history includes a myocardial infarction 1 year ago but no previous kidney problems were noted. Clearance of PAH and creatinine are both reduced. Plasma creatinine is approximately three times higher than normal. Assuming normal diet and liver function, this patient's blood urea nitrogen (BUN) concentration would be expected to be

A. approximately the same as normal

B. approximately one third of normal

C. significantly less than one third of normal

D. approximately three times normal

E. significantly more than three times normal

61. A 21-year-old woman with a history of substance abuse was found unresponsive with a hypodermic needle in her arm. Arterial blood gas analysis showed:

$Po_2 = 68$ mm Hg

$Pco_2 = 84$ mm Hg

pH = 7.02

$[HCO_3^-] = 23$ mEq/L

Base excess = −2mEq/L

Which of the following primary acid-base disturbances is present?

A. Respiratory alkalosis

B. Respiratory acidosis

C. Metabolic alkalosis

D. Metabolic acidosis

62. A 56-year-old man with chronic renal insufficiency was evaluated in the hospital in preparation for hemodialysis. Arterial blood gas analysis showed:

$Po_2 = 90$ mm Hg

$Pco_2 = 28$ mm Hg

pH = 7.32

$[HCO_3^-] = 15$ mEq/L

Base excess = −10mEq/L

The patient was diagnosed with partially compensated

A. respiratory alkalosis

B. respiratory acidosis

C. metabolic alkalosis

D. metabolic acidosis

GASTROINTESTINAL PHYSIOLOGY

63. During surgery to remove a tumor, an area of normal small intestine was removed and placed in a tissue bath for study. A peptide with endocrine activity was added to the bathing solution. The peptide caused secretion of fluid from surface epithelium and simultaneous relaxation of smooth muscle. The peptide was most likely to be

A. cholecystokinin

B. gastrin

C. glucose-dependent insulinotropic polypeptide

D. motilin

E. vasoactive intestinal polypeptide

64. A novel antibiotic drug was tested in animals. Side-effects of the drug included increased intestinal motility, which was characterized by waves of peristaltic contractions approximately every 90 minutes. Which hormone is the antibiotic most likely to mimic?

A. Cholecystokinin

B. Gastrin

C. Glucagon-like peptide-1

D. Motilin

E. Secretin

65. A 62-year-old man was admitted to the hospital with low blood pressure and evidence of active bleeding from the upper gastrointestinal tract. He was administered fluid intravenously and a drug that vasoconstricts splanchnic blood vessels. The drug also reduces gastric acid production and pancreatic secretion. Which hormone does the drug mimic?

A. Acetylcholine

B. Cholecystokinin

C. Gastrin

D. Secretin

E. Somatostatin

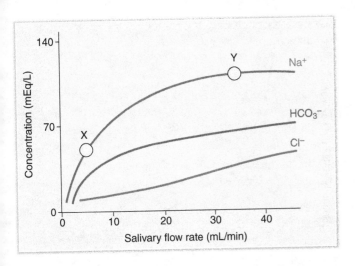

66. Which one of the following interventions would result in the sample taken at point Y in the figure compared to a control sample obtained at point X?

    A. Dehydration of the subject
    B. Exposure of the subject to low ambient temperature
    C. Induction of sleep by meditation
    D. Infusion of aldosterone
    E. Stimulation of parasympathetic nerves to the salivary gland

67. A 3-year-old boy swallowed a steel ball bearing 1 cm in diameter. An x-ray taken 6 hours later showed that the object was located in his distal ileum. Which pattern of gastric motility allowed the ball bearing to pass through the pyloric sphincter?

    A. Antral systole
    B. Migrating motor complex
    C. Phasic contractions of the fundus
    D. Tonic contraction of proximal stomach

68. A preparation of normal pancreatic acinar cells obtained from a surgical sample was studied in vitro. Fluorescent imaging was used to measure changes in intracellular Ca^{2+} concentration in response to a series of agonists. Which of the following hormones would produce the largest increase in intracellular $[Ca^{2+}]$?

    A. Cholecystokinin
    B. Gastrin
    C. Glucagon
    D. Secretin
    E. Vasoactive intestinal polypeptide

69. A 39-year-old woman is treated for pancreatic cancer by complete surgical removal of the pancreas and duodenum. Without supplemental treatment, which of the following mineral deficiencies would most likely develop in this patient in the following weeks and months?

    A. Iron and Ca^{2+}
    B. K^+ and Ca^{2+}
    C. K^+ and iron
    D. Na^+ and K^+
    E. Na^+ and Ca^{2+}

70. A 40-year-old man with hereditary hemochromatosis visited his physician because he was concerned about a recent darkening of his skin. A program of controlled blood removal by venipuncture was begun to reduce body iron levels. What process is responsible for iron overload in this patient?

    A. Excess production of transferrin
    B. Excess intestinal absorption of iron
    C. Excess hepatic secretion of hepcidin
    D. Failure of tissue ferritin production
    E. Inadequate renal iron excretion

71. Sugar absorption was studied in a segment of jejunum perfused in vitro. What is the most likely effect on glucose absorption of adding equimolar galactose to the luminal solution?

    A. Glucose absorption is abolished
    B. Glucose absorption continues at a reduced rate
    C. Glucose absorption is unaffected
    D. Glucose absorption continues at an increased rate

72. A 28-year-old man visited his physician because of diarrhea and bloating, which has been an increasing problem for the past 6 months. Fecal analysis showed that fecal osmolarity was not accounted for by the electrolytes present in the sample. Which condition could account for the presence of this "fecal osmolar gap"?

    A. Achalasia
    B. Diabetes mellitus
    C. Lactase deficiency
    D. Secretory diarrhea
    E. Xerostomia

73. A patient with chronic steatorrhea is most likely to develop deficiency of which of the following vitamins?

    A. Vitamins A and B_1
    B. Vitamins A and C
    C. Vitamins A and D
    D. Vitamins B_1 and C
    E. Vitamins B_1 and D
    F. Vitamins C and D

74. A 3-month-old infant was being breast-fed in the physician's reception room. Just before entering the physician's office for her examination, the child defecated into her diaper. Which of the following gastrointestinal reflexes is most likely to account for this untimely defecation?

   A. Enterogastrone reflex

   B. Gastroileal reflex

   C. Gastrocolic reflex

   D. Ileal brake

   E. Rectosphincteric reflex

75. A group of normal subjects was given a range of test meals, each of the same volume. The rate of gastric emptying was determined using noninvasive imaging procedures. Which of the following meals would take the longest time to empty from the stomach?

   A. Pure water, pH = 7.0

   B. 1% glucose solution, pH = 7.0

   C. 1% glucose + 0.1% oleic acid, pH = 7.2

   D. 1% glucose + 0.1% oleic acid + 0.9% saline, pH = 7.2

   E. 1% glucose + 0.1% oleic acid + 0.9% saline + HCl, pH = 6.2

ENDOCRINOLOGY AND REPRODUCTIVE PHYSIOLOGY

76. A stable derivative of cholesterol was synthesized as part of a drug discovery program. Which of the following properties is this new molecule most likely to have when injected into test subjects?

   A. Binds mostly to surface membrane receptors on target cells

   B. Circulates bound to plasma proteins

   C. Enters target cells by carrier-mediated transport

   D. Has effects lasting a few minutes

   E. Induces an increase in intracellular cAMP in target cells

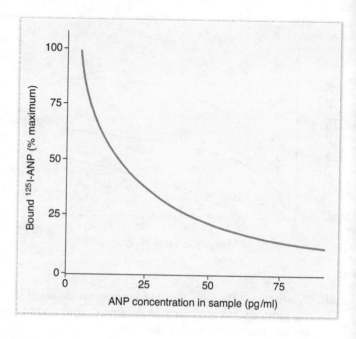

77. Plasma atrial natriuretic peptide (ANP) concentration was measured by radioimmunoassay in a healthy 31-year-old man. The standard curve shown in the figure above was obtained by displacing radioactive ^{125}I-ANP from anti-ANP antibodies with ANP standards. A sample of a patient's serum caused 50% of ^{125}I-ANP to remain bound to the antibody. What was the patient's approximate plasma ANP concentration?

   A. 0 pg/mL

   B. 20 pg/mL

   C. 40 pg/mL

   D. 60 pg/mL

   E. 80 pg/mL

78. A 54-year-old woman visited her physician because of persistent headaches and blurred vision. The physician noted that the woman has very large hands and feet, a wide jaw, a large tongue, and a prominent forehead. Which of the following metabolic abnormalities would most likely be present in this patient?

   A. Decreased blood fatty acid concentration

   B. Decreased hepatic gluconeogenesis

   C. Decreased protein synthesis

   D. Increased blood glucose concentration

   E. Increased uptake of glucose in skeletal muscle

79. A 19-year-old patient produced a copious amount of dilute urine following a head injury sustained in a motor vehicle accident. Damage to which of the following sites could account for these symptoms in this patient?

   A. Anterior pituitary

   B. Mamillary body

   C. Median eminence

   D. Superior hypophyseal artery

   E. Supraoptic nucleus

80. A healthy 29-year-old man was injected with thyroid-stimulating-hormone (TSH) as part of a clinical research study. Increased levels of serum thyroid hormones were detected within a few minutes. Which major form of thyroid hormone was detected in this subject?

A. Monoiodothyronine

B. Diiodothyronine

C. Triiodothyronine

D. Reverse triiodothyronine

E. Thyroxine

81. A 28-year-old woman visited her physician because of anxiety. She was perspiring heavily and complained about the high temperature of the waiting room. Physical examination showed a thin patient with notable tremor, muscle weakness, tachycardia. and an ophthalmopathy with a staring gaze. What is the most likely profile of serum thyroxine (T_4) and thyroid-stimulating hormone (TSH) concentrations in this patient?

A. Low T_4, high TSH

B. Low T_4, low TSH

C. High T_4, low TSH

D. High T_4, high TSH

82. A fine needle adrenal biopsy was performed in a 71-year-old man who had an unidentified adrenal mass. Tests performed on the sample included the expression of the enzyme aldosterone synthase. Which area of the adrenal gland would show positive staining for this enzyme?

A. Zona glomerulosa

B. Zona fasciculata

C. Zona reticularis

D. Medullary chromaffin cells.

83. A 2-year-old boy is brought to the pediatrician because he has acute viral laryngitis and has developed difficulty breathing. He was previously treated for 3 days with a large dose of oral glucocorticoids to reduce inflammation of his larynx. The effects of this treatment on the child's fasting plasma glucose and fatty acids levels would most likely be

A. increased glucose and increased fatty acids

B. increased glucose and decreased fatty acids

C. decreased glucose and increased fatty acids

D. decreased glucose and decreased fatty acids

84. Excessive licorice consumption may result in secondary hypertension due to inhibition of the enzyme 11β-hydroxysteroid dehydrogenase in renal epithelial cells. The Na^+ retention that follows is due to interaction between which agonist–receptor pair?

A. Glucocorticoids—glucocorticoid receptors

B. Mineralocorticoids—mineralocorticoid receptors

C. Mineralocorticoids—glucocorticoid receptors

D. Glucocorticoids—mineralocorticoid receptors

85. A 68-year-old woman became acutely ill while on holiday. She was confused and unable to give the attending physician her medical history. The physician noticed the patient had a moon face, truncal obesity, and bruising on large areas of skin on both legs. Laboratory studies showed fasting hyperglycemia and low levels of both cortisol and adrenocorticotropic hormone (ACTH). Which of the following conditions is consistent with the physical examination and laboratory data?

A. ACTH-secreting tumor

B. Chronic glucocorticoid medication

C. Cortisol-secreting tumor

D. Destructive tumor of the anterior pituitary

E. Primary adrenocortical insufficiency

86. A 45-year-old woman suffered episodes of headache, nausea, sweating, and palpitations that were becoming more frequent and severe. One such episode occurred while she was visiting a friend in the hospital. A nurse measured her heart rate and blood pressure during the episode, which were 142 beats/min and 180/145 mm Hg, respectively. A resident suggested the differential diagnosis of pheochromocytoma. Which of the following profiles of catecholamine excretion in the urine would support this diagnosis?

	Vanillylmandelic acid (VMA)	Metanephrine	Epinephrine
A.	Low	Low	Low
B.	Low	Low	High
C.	Low	High	High
D.	High	High	High
E.	High	High	Low
F.	High	Low	Low

87. A 28-year-old medical resident who was accustomed to eating regular meals was forced to skip breakfast and lunch one day because of a heavy work schedule. By midafternoon, he was feeling lightheaded and very hungry. Compared to his typical day, the plasma concentration of which of the following hormones would be decreased at this time?

A. Cortisol

B. Epinephrine

C. Glucagon

D. Growth hormone

E. Insulin

88. A healthy 21-year-old man was intravenously infused with a saline solution containing a mixture of amino acids, including arginine and leucine. Which pair of secretory responses in insulin and glucagon would occur in response to this challenge?

A. Increased insulin and increased glucagon

B. Increased insulin and decreased glucagon

C. Decreased insulin and decreased glucagon

D. Decreased insulin and increased glucagon

89. A healthy 12-year-old girl consumed a 100-g bar of chocolate. Her plasma insulin concentration increased significantly soon after eating, with only a modest increase in plasma glucose concentration. Which hormone is released by mucosal endocrine cells of the gastrointestinal tract that could help to account for these observations?

A. Enterogastrone

B. Gastrin

C. Glucagon

D. Glucagon-like peptide-1

E. Insulin

90. A 19-year-old woman visited her physician complaining of frequent urination and of being thirsty all the time. On physical examination, the woman appeared extremely malnourished. Plasma analysis showed high concentrations of both glucose and ketones. Which hormone is most responsible for the presence of high ketone concentrations in this patient?

A. Cortisol

B. Epinephrine

C. Glucagon

D. Growth hormone

E. Insulin

91. A healthy 34-year-old woman runs 5 miles at a fast pace resulting in a large increase in the rate of glucose oxidation in her muscles. Which pair of hormones is most important to minimize the decrease in plasma glucose concentration during her run?

A. Cortisol and growth hormone

B. Cortisol and insulin

C. Epinephrine and insulin

D. Glucagon and epinephrine

E. Glucagon and thyroxine

F. Growth hormone and thyroxine

92. A 23-year-old medical student ingests several liters of cola in an effort to stay awake over a 24-hour period of studying. This ingestion of cola represents a large intake of phosphate ions, which results in increased urinary phosphate excretion. Which hormone is most responsible for stimulating phosphate excretion in this case?

A. Calcitonin

B. Ergocalciferol

C. Parathyroid hormone

D. 1,25-$(OH)_2$ Vitamin D_3

93. A 46-year-old man with bone cancer is found to have high plasma levels of parathyroid hormone-related peptide (PTH-rp). Which of the following profiles for plasma Ca^{2+}, phosphate (P), and parathyroid hormone (PTH) concentration would be expected in this patient?

	Plasma [Ca^{2+}]	Plasma [P]	Plasma [PTH]
A.	Low	Low	Low
B.	Low	Low	High
C.	Low	High	High
D.	High	High	High
E.	High	High	Low
F.	High	Low	Low

94. A 17-year-old girl visited her physician because she had never had a menstrual period. Physical examination revealed a tall female with a short, blind-ended vagina and no palpable cervix. Ultrasound showed the absence of a uterus and no ovaries and the presence of undescended testes. Deficiency of which enzyme, hormone, or receptor is most likely to account for these findings?

A. Androgen receptors

B. Aromatase

C. Estrogen receptors

D. 21α-Hydroxylase

E. Müllerian-inhibiting substance

F. Progesterone

G. 5α-Reductase

95. A blood sample is taken from a 27-year-old woman for hormone analysis. The sample contains low levels of follicle-stimulating hormone (FSH) and luteinizing hormone (LH) and high levels of estrogen, progesterone, and inhibin. Assuming a normal 28-day menstrual cycle, on which day of this woman's menstrual cycle was the blood sample taken?

A. Day 1

B. Day 7

C. Day 14

D. Day 21

E. Day 28

96. An indicator dilution technique was used to estimate plasma volume in a pregnant woman at the beginning of her third trimester. Plasma volume was found to be about 30% higher than that expected for a nonpregnant woman of similar height and weight. Increased secretion of which hormone accounts directly for this large increase in plasma volume?

A. Aldosterone

B. Atrial natriuretic peptide

C. Chorionic gonadotropin

D. Cortisol

E. Estrogen

F. Oxytocin

G. Progesterone

97. An arterial blood sample was taken from a 28-year-old pregnant woman. Blood gas analysis showed:

$Po_2 = 91$ mm Hg

$So_2 = 97\%$

$Pco_2 = 31$ mm Hg

$pH = 7.42$

$HCO_3^- = 21$ mEq/L

Which primary physiologic adaptation to pregnancy is responsible for changes in acid-base status compared to normal nonpregnant women?

A. Increased alveolar ventilation

B. Decreased alveolar ventilation

C. Increased insulin responsiveness

D. Decreased insulin responsiveness

E. Increased glomerular filtration rate

F. Decreased glomerular filtration rate

98. A 37-year old-woman who is breast-feeding her 4-month-old son is taking the train to see her mother who lives several hours away. When the woman hears the cry of another infant, she notices that milk has been expressed from both her breasts. The release of which hormone can account for this response?

A. Estrogen

B. Inhibin

C. Oxytocin

D. Progesterone

E. Prolactin

99. A 36-year-old woman who is pregnant with her third child is in labor. Her serum oxytocin levels were measured at regular intervals over a 24-hour period. Measurements were taken at the onset when the woman began having low back pains 1 day before delivery and ended 3 hours after delivery of the infant, just before the woman was to begin breast-feeding the infant. A normal vaginal delivery was completed without medical intervention. At what time was the oxytocin concentration in maternal blood most likely to be highest?

A. Before labor

B. At the onset of back pain

C. Uterine contractions 20 minutes apart

D. During the expulsive stages of labor

E. Three hours after delivery

100. A 32-year-old woman and her partner were trying to conceive a child. The woman had regular menstrual cycles of about 30 days in length. Four days after missing her menstrual period, she bought a commercial pregnancy testing kit. The couple was excited to discover that her urine sample indicated a positive result for pregnancy. Which of the following hormones was detected in her urine?

A. Human chorionic gonadotropin

B. Estrogen

C. Follicle-stimulating hormone

D. Gonadotropin-releasing hormone

E. Inhibin

F. Luteinizing hormone

G. Progesterone

101. Fetal acquisition of glucose occurs by placental glucose transport. What is the first cell layer within the placenta that glucose must cross during transport from maternal to fetal blood?

A. Cytotrophoblast

B. Decidua

C. Inner cell mass

D. Mesenchyme

E. Syncytiotrophoblast

102. The luteinizing hormone surge measured during the ovulatory phase of the menstrual cycle results from positive feedback exerted by which of the following hormones?

    A. Estrogen

    B. Follicle-stimulating hormone

    C. Gonadotropin-releasing hormone

    D. Inhibin

    E. Progesterone

103. A 36-year-old woman visited her gynecologist to have a routine annual examination. A cervical Pap smear was performed to check for abnormal cells. The mucus sample was thin and produced a fern-like pattern when it dried on a microscope slide. Assuming a normal 28-day menstrual cycle, on which day of this woman's menstrual cycle was the smear taken?

    A. Day 1

    B. Day 7

    C. Day 14

    D. Day 21

    E. Day 28

104. A 37-year-old man with four children elected to have a vasectomy. This procedure prevents conception because

    A. no sperm are ejaculated

    B. secretion from seminal vesicles is not ejaculated

    C. secretion from the prostate gland is not ejaculated

    D. no semen is ejaculated

105. A child born with ambiguous genitalia was found to have a 46XY karyotype. Testes were present at birth, and there was a small phallus with a urethral opening at its midpoint. The child entered puberty late, but masculinization was evident. Which deficiency could account for these findings?

    A. Aromatase

    B. 21α-Hydroxylase

    C. Luteinizing hormone receptor

    D. 5α-Reductase

    E. Testosterone

106. Ovarian granulosa cells were grown in primary cell culture in vitro. The cells failed to secrete significant amounts of estrogen when exposed to follicle-stimulating hormone (FSH) and luteinizing hormone (LH) until they were cultured together with ovarian thecal cells. A likely explanation for the failure of granulosa cells to produce estrogens when cultured alone is

    A. inability of granulosa cells to synthesize cholesterol

    B. lack of androgen precursors from which to produce estrogens

    C. lack of aromatase activity

    D. lack of 5α-reductase activity

    E. lack of progesterone precursor from which to produce estrogens

107. When the gas composition of umbilical arterial blood is compared to umbilical venous blood, the arterial blood has

    A. lower P_{O_2} and higher P_{CO_2}

    B. lower P_{O_2} and lower P_{CO_2}

    C. higher P_{O_2} and lower P_{CO_2}

    D. higher P_{O_2} and higher P_{CO_2}

    E. the same P_{O_2} and P_{CO_2}

108. An 18-year-old man visited his physician because he was concerned about his height. He is 152 cm tall (5 ft). He described himself when he was in elementary school as being self-conscious because he was taller than his peers. He also recalled developing pubic and axillary hair at about age 7 or 8. Physical examination showed a healthy male of short stature with normal genitalia and male secondary sexual development. Which endocrine abnormality best explains the findings in this patient?

    A. Early maturation of the hypothalamic-pituitary-gonadal axis

    B. Failure of pulsatile gonadotrophin-releasing hormone secretion at puberty

    C. Growth hormone excess in early childhood

    D. Insulin-like growth factor-1 deficiency

    E. Panhypopituitarism

ANSWERS

1—E. Small lipid soluble gas molecules such as N_2O readily diffuse through biological membranes. The inability to increase blood N_2O concentration above that in the lung alveolus is consistent with simple diffusion and the absence of any primary or secondary active transport process.

2—C. According to Fick's law of diffusion, the rate of simple diffusion of N_2O is proportional to its membrane permeability and to its concentration gradient. The N_2O concentration gradient is increased if the inspired N_2O concentration is increased, but is decreased if alveolar ventilation or pulmonary blood flow are decreased. The rate of simple diffusion is slower at colder temperatures or if the diffusion distance is increased.

3—D. When a depolarizing stimulus causes the threshold membrane potential (of about −55 mV) to be exceeded, voltage sensitive Na^+ channels rapidly open, resulting in fast depolarization.

4—C. At 0 mV during repolarization, Na^+ channels are inactivating but many remain open. K^+ channels are opening rapidly at this time. The electrochemical driving force is inward for Na^+ and outward for K^+. Therefore, there is net outward K^+ flow and net inward Na^+ flow at this time. A significant Na^+ conductance must still be present to account for a membrane potential of 0 mV.

5—E. The stimulus is applied during the absolute refractory period. No second action potential is possible because too many Na^+ channels are now inactivated.

6—A. Curves intersect the x-axis when there is zero shortening ("isometric" contraction). The total force on the muscle at this point is indicative of preload; therefore curve C has the largest preload. If a total load is selected on the x-axis and a vertical line is drawn, the curves may be compared; increased preload results in faster muscle shortening.

7—F. Primary active transport has a direct dependence on adenosine triphosphate hydrolysis and would be inhibited under anaerobic conditions. Secretion moves H^+ out of the cell; dependence on external K^+ suggests an exchange with H^+.

8—C. In most cells, V_m is a function of $[K^+]_o$ because K^+ channels provide the dominant membrane conductance at rest. Acutely increasing $[K^+]_o$ results in a less negative value for E_K, according to the Nernst equation. V_m becomes less negative, or depolarize as a result.

9—E. The question describes temporal summation, in which the muscle is tetanized. The basis of this effect is accumulation of Ca^{2+} in the sarcoplasm with repeated stimulation due to insufficient time for Ca^{2+} reuptake by sarcoplasmic reticulum. A plateau is reached when maximal cross-bridge cycling has occurred.

10—A. The primary sensory neurons for touch, vibration, and proprioception are conveyed by the ipsilateral dorsal columns. Second-order neurons cross over in the medulla and ascend to the thalamus; third-order neurons are conveyed via the internal capsule to the somatosensory cortex.

11—B. The suprachiasmatic nucleus is a key site for the "body clock" and therefore the generation and maintenance of circadian rhythms.

12—E. The patient has aphasia consistent with damage to Wernicke's area, which is at the junction of the temporal and parietal lobes. The presence of memory loss is consistent with damage to the hippocampal formation, which is in the medial temporal lobe.

13—F. Transection of the right lateral corticospinal tracts (which have already crossed over) causes loss of upper motor neurons controlling movement of the right leg. Therefore, there is right leg paresis and spasticity. Transection of the right dorsal columns causes loss of touch, vibration, and proprioception from the right leg because these neurons cross over in the medulla. Transection of the anterolateral spinothalamic tracts results in loss of contralateral (left in this case) pain and temperature sensation; these modalities are absent two to three spinal segments below the lesion due to the path of sensory neurons via Lissauer's tract.

14—E. Loss of an optic nerve involves only the affected eye. Bitemporal hemianopia is caused by damage to fibers crossing at the optic chiasm; homonymous hemianopia (loss of one half of the visual field) is caused by lesions beyond the optic chiasm. Binasal hemianopia would require selective damage at the lateral aspect of the optic chiasm on both sides. Macular degeneration is loss of the central vision due to damage to the macula area of the retina.

15—A. Nearsightedness (myopia) is usually the result of eyeballs that are too long, causing light to be focused in front of the retina. A concave lens corrects this problem by causing light to diverge before it enters the eye. A convex lens would worsen the problem by converging light rays further; a cylindrical lens is used to correct for astigmatism.

16—B. Expansion of the ventricular system is isolated to areas upstream of the cerebral aqueduct, suggesting this is a site of obstruction that results in hydrocephalus.

17—C. Since only action potentials were being recorded in an output neuron, no synaptic events were measured directly. Simultaneous stimulation from several input neurons demonstrates spatial summation of inputs to reach threshold for action potential in the output neuron. If increased intensity of stimulation in a single input neuron produces action potentials in the output neuron, this would demonstrate temporal summation.

18—B. Physiologic sweating in response to increased body temperature is mediated by cholinergic sympathetic nerves, which are activated by the hypothalamic temperature controller. Adrenergic sweating can also occur to a lesser degree and may contribute, for example, to the presentation of sweating and vasoconstriction in patients with shock.

19—C. The patient has the classic clinical findings of Parkinson's disease. The paucity of movement reflects loss of dopaminergic input to the basal ganglia from the substantia nigra pars compacta. Exogenous administration of a dopamine precursor capable of entering the brain, such as levodopa, will alleviate symptoms.

20—C. The wide ataxic gait and inability to walk heel to toe without falling suggest a cerebellar problem; chronic alcohol abuse is a common cause of cerebellar damage. Loss of proprioception via the dorsal column pathways would also cause a similar pattern of symptoms.

21—C. The glossopharyngeal nerve is sensory to the pharynx and motor to several striated muscles involved in the pharyngeal component of swallowing. It conveys taste from the posterior third of the tongue. The sinus nerve joins the glossopharyngeal nerve; dysfunction in the baroreceptor reflex may, therefore, play a role in the appearance of palpitations. The facial nerve is secretomotor to salivary glands and serves taste to the anterior two thirds of the tongue; it may be affected, but it is not involved with swallowing or mediating sensations from the pharynx. The vagus nerve is important for modulation of gastrointestinal and cardiac function, but it is not necessary for swallowing or involved in oral sensations. The hypoglossal and abducens are only motor nerves to the tongue and extraocular muscles, respectively

22—A. The inferior colliculus is a key relay in the auditory pathway. The medial lemniscus is a sensory fiber tract; the red nucleus and substantia nigra are part of the motor system. The reticular activating system is part of the diffuse modulatory systems and is not directly related to the auditory system.

23—C. Phase 4 is the resting membrane potential, which is most dependent on the presence of open K^+ channels that mediate an outward K^+ current.

24—A. High left ventricular pressure is developed by the left ventricle to overcome the impedance to ejection of blood through a narrowed aortic valve. In severe valve disease such as this, the aortic systolic pressure is reduced due to low stroke volume.

25—A. The patient has a clinical history consistent with systolic heart failure. The pressure-volume relation confirms reduced ventricular contractility. The ejection fraction is reduced systolic heart failure. In contrast, ventricular contractility and ejection fraction would be preserved in diastolic heart failure, but cardiac filling would be reduced and diastolic heart pressures increased.

26—B. During isovolumic contraction, the atrioventricular valves close because of increasing ventricular pressure, but the semilunar valves are not yet open because ventricular pressure has not exceeded the pressure in the aorta (or the pulmonary artery).

27—D. The aortic valve opens at point C and ventricular ejection occurs from C–E; the peak left ventricular pressure is almost equal to the peak aortic (systolic) pressure.

28—B. Diastolic filling is completed from A–B; isovolumic contraction begins at B, causing the mitral valve to close.

29—C. Narrowing of the aortic valve causes turbulent blood flow during ventricular ejection. Therefore, the murmur is heard from the opening of the aortic valve at point C to its closure at point E.

30—C. Period 4 is the ST segment in which the ECG recording is on the isoelectric baseline, indicating that all ventricular cells are at the same potential (no electrical dipole is measured). In this period, ventricular cells are between depolarization (QRS complex) and repolarization (T wave) and are therefore in the plateau (phase 2) of the action potential.

31—B. Hematocrit is the percentage of whole blood contributed by red blood cells. Destruction of transfused blood is unlikely, assuming blood type is correctly matched. Dilution of red cells by water retention in SIADH is possible, but a decrease to 24% hematocrit represents massive water retention. GFR has decreased, as shown by the high plasma creatinine concentration, but GFR is not a direct determinant of the hematocrit. Low GFR indicates renal insufficiency, which will be accompanied by failure to secrete EPO, thereby causing anemia. There are many sites of active bone marrow away from the fracture site for erythrocyte production.

32—B. The stressor results in an increase in cardiac output and venous return associated with increased cardiac contractility (increased cardiac output for the same atrial pressure). Systemic vascular resistance is reduced, evidenced by the increased slope of the vascular function curve. During exercise, the activation of the sympathetic nervous system provides positive inotropic stimulation to the heart, thereby increasing cardiac output. Dilation of muscle blood vessels is responsible for reducing systemic vascular resistance. During digestion, blood would be redistributed to the gastrointestinal organs but without a change in cardiac output. In hypothermia, cardiac output would decrease because cooling inhibits heart rate and contractility. In severe hemorrhage, cardiac output would decrease due to decreased venous return.

33—B. Chronic bronchitis is an obstructive lung disorder, characterized by reduced FVC, FEV_1, and a reduced ratio of FVC to FEV_1.

34—B. The peak inspiratory pressure is increased, showing that dynamic compliance is reduced. However, the plateau pressure measured when no air is flowing is unchanged compared to the previous test, indicating that the increased peak airway pressure is associated with air flow. Increased airway resistance therefore accounts for the high airway pressure needed to ventilate the patient. If the plateau of pressure had increased, this would indicate that the lung and chest compliance were low.

35—D. The red curve depicts a patient breathing from a reduced resting lung volume. This occurs in pulmonary fibrosis due to low lung compliance. The blue curve depicts a patient with emphysema who breathes from an increased resting lung volume due to highly compliant lungs.

36—D. The red oxyhemoglobin dissociation curve is right-shifted, which may be caused by increased temperature, increased PCO_2, or increased erythrocyte 2,3-BPG concentration, or by decreased pH.

37—A. Inulin is a marker for ECF volume. Using Equation 1-1 (see Chapter 1), $V = (Q - q)/C$: $V = (200\,mg - 100\,mg)/1\,mg/dL = 100\,dL = 10\,L$.

38—B. Sweat is a hypotonic saline solution. Sweating reduces ECF volume and raises ECF osmolarity, causing water to flow from ICF to ECF. Both ICF and ECF have a reduced final volume and higher osmolarity (hyperosmotic volume contraction).

39—B. Lobar branching of a single renal artery reflects the embryologic development of the kidney in lobes. The arcuate arteries arising from the lobar arteries appear to meet and anastomose along the corticomedullary boundary, but there is little functional anastomosis.

40—C. The A-V(O_2) differences given in the question are normal, suggesting no pathologic problems. Renal A-V(O_2) is low because renal blood flow is normally very high, providing an excess of O_2 delivery despite high renal O_2 demand.

41—D. The glomerular barrier restricting protein filtration is located partly in the glomerular basement membrane and partly by filtration slits between foot processes of podocytes.

42—B. Constriction of afferent arteriole increases vascular resistance and reduces RBF. Blood flow into the glomerulus decreases, resulting in a decrease in P_{GC} and, therefore, a decrease in GFR. RBF and GFR both decrease, leaving the filtration fraction unchanged.

43—F. High plasma creatinine is most likely to indicate a decrease in GFR. Dehydration can also cause a decrease in GFR, but not so much as to cause a fivefold increase in P_{cr}. Creatinine levels are not affected by ADH or acid-base status. Increased creatinine is observed in body builders due to high muscle mass, but this patient has a low body weight that is not consistent with this explanation.

44—B. Clearance of substance X is larger than that of creatinine at all plasma concentrations. When clearance of a solute exceeds glomerular filtration, the solute must be secreted in addition to filtration. The decline in the clearance of substance X with increased plasma concentration indicates a saturable carrier-mediated transport process rather than simple diffusion.

45—G. C_{PAH} is the effective renal plasma flow rate. Applying Equation 6-6 (see Chapter 6), renal blood flow (RBF) = renal plasma flow (RPF)/(1-Hct): RBF = 600 mL/min/0.5 = 1200 mL/min.

46—C. In the case of creatinine, a marker for the glomerular filtration rate, the excretion rate equals the filtered load. Excretion rate is the product of urine concentration and urine flow rate: $FL_{cr} = 20\,mg/mL \times 1\,mL/min = 20\,mg/min$.

47—B. Renal threshold is defined as the plasma concentration at which a solute first appears in the urine. The blue curve indicates glucose excretion, which begins at a plasma glucose concentration of about 200 mg/mL.

48—C. The rapid decline in tubular solute concentration at the start of the proximal tubule indicates a preferentially absorbed solute. Nutrients and HCO_3^- have this pattern of proximal tubule absorption.

49—F. The infant has Bartter's syndrome. Loss of function in the thick ascending limb causes dramatic urinary electrolyte losses, reflecting what is normally reabsorbed in this segment. Phosphate is the only electrolyte listed that does not have a high rate of transport in the thick ascending limb; phosphate is mainly reabsorbed in the proximal tubule.

50—C. Carbonic anhydrase is required to recover filtered HCO_3^- in the proximal tubule. Inhibition by acetazolamide results in a large urinary loss of HCO_3^-. Note: in this case, acetazolamide was used for its effect on the eye to reduce the rate of aqueous humor secretion by the ciliary epithelium.

51—A. Ingestion of a large volume of water causes hypotonic plasma and suppresses antidiuretic hormone (ADH) secretion. Low ADH levels inactivate the countercurrent system. Water reabsorption is inhibited in the collecting duct because aquaporin 2 water channels are internalized by principal cells. Changes in free water excretion are not mediated by changes in GFR or proximal tubule absorption.

52—D. Dehydration increases plasma osmolarity and stimulates ADH secretion. ADH stimulates Na^+ and urea reabsorption as part of the countercurrent mechanism. Na^+ reabsorption is stimulated in the ascending limb, not the descending limb of the loop of Henle. Aquaporin 2 expression increases to allow water retention by the collecting duct.

53—A. Equations 6-7 and 6-8 (see Chapter 6) could be applied, but in this case urine is exactly isosmotic with respect to plasma, so no free water can have been added or removed in the formation of urine.

54—D. ANP causes excretion of more Na^+. This endocrine axis is suppressed in response to hemorrhage because blood volume and atrial stretch are reduced.

55—A. Increasing extracellular fluid (ECF) volume with salt and water ingestion dilutes plasma proteins and reduces plasma oncotic pressure generally. Increased ECF volume includes increased plasma volume, the largest fraction of which is in the systemic veins. Increased systemic venous pressure increases capillary pressures, including the peritubular capillary hydrostatic pressure. These changes to Starling's forces suppress tubular fluid reabsorption and therefore promote renal Na^+ and water excretion.

56—B. Parathyroid hormone stimulates renal Ca^{2+} reabsorption by the distal tubule, causing a decrease in fractional excretion.

57—A. Pco_2 is depressed. The patient is hyperventilating and has respiratory alkalosis. There is alkalemia with no metabolic compensation.

58—D. Plasma $[HCO_3^-]$ is very low and there is a large base deficit, defining metabolic acidosis. The pH is acidic, and there is no respiratory compensation present.

59—C. Total body water can be estimated as 50% of body weight in women of normal body mass index (and 60% of body weight in men). Therefore, a female patient weighing 60 kg would have approximately 30 L of body water.

60—E. The patient has low effective circulating volume and reduction in renal blood flow and filtration (C_{PAH} and C_{CR}). BUN will be elevated due to the low glomerular filtration rate and further increased due to the high antidiuretic hormone levels in this low volume state. The ratio of BUN to creatinine is expected to be high; because P_{CR} is three times normal, BUN will be significantly more elevated than this.

61—B. $Paco_2$ is very elevated, defining respiratory acidosis. pH is acidic. No metabolic compensation is present.

62—D. The patient has low plasma $[HCO_3^-]$ (metabolic acidosis) and low $Paco_2$ (respiratory alkalosis). The pH is acidic, indicating primary metabolic acidosis. The expected compensation is a 1.3 mm Hg decrease in $Paco_2$ for every 1 mEq/L decrease in plasma HCO_3^-.

63—E. VIP is a potent secretagogue in small intestine. The other choices (i.e., gastrin, cholecystokinin, motilin, and glucose-dependent insulinotropic polypeptide) have little effect on fluid secretion.

64—D. The contractions described are the migrating motor complex. Motilin stimulates this pattern of motility, under the direction of the enteric nervous system.

65—E. Somatostatin is a potent inhibitor in the gastrointestinal system. Other substances listed are either stimulatory for secretion in the stomach (acetylcholine and gastrin) or pancreas (secretin and cholecystokinin).

66—E. At point Y, salivation has been stimulated. The primary control of salivation is via parasympathetic tone. Sleep and dehydration reduce salivation. Sympathetic tone has minor effects on salivation. Aldosterone slightly increases Na^+ absorption from saliva.

67—B. The pyloric sphincter only allows small particles to pass during the fed state. It is only during the fasting state that the migrating motor complex flushes residual stomach contents into the duodenum.

68—A. Cholecystokinin is the most important agonist that stimulates pancreatic acinar cells to release zymogen granules by exocytosis. Acetylcholine is a weak agonist (not listed here).

69—A. The duodenum is the main site of iron and Ca^{2+} uptake, particularly iron uptake. Other ions are extensively reabsorbed along the small intestine; Na^+ is also reabsorbed in large intestine.

70—B. Iron overload is caused by excessive intestinal uptake because no regulated excretion pathway exists for iron. In hereditary hemochromatosis, there is a failure of negative feedback control of intestinal uptake through the hepcidin pathway.

71—B. Galactose and glucose have equal affinity at the same Na-linked cotransport protein (SGLT1). Equimolar galactose would compete for binding to the transporter, reducing the rate of glucose uptake.

72—C. A fecal osmolar gap indicates the presence of organic molecules that are measured as part of the total osmolarity but are present in addition to electrolytes such as Na^+ and K^+. Lactase deficiency would cause undigested lactose in the feces, resulting in osmotic diarrhea.

73—C. Fat-soluble vitamins rely on normal fat reabsorption for their assimilation. A high proportion of dietary fat-soluble vitamins remain in fecal fat in patients with steatorrhea (excess fecal fat excretion). Vitamins A and D are fat soluble; vitamins B_1 and C are water soluble.

74—C. The presence of food in the stomach and duodenum stimulates the gastrocolic reflex. This is a feed-forward reflex in which mass movement contractions occur in the colon to propel feces into the rectum. The response is particularly well developed in young children in whom reflex defecation follows.

75—E. Enterogastrones cause feedback inhibition of gastric emptying. Low pH, high osmolarity, and high nutrient content of chyme all stimulate enterogastrones.

76—B. A cholesterol derivative is most likely to behave like a steroid hormone. Steroids are usually bound to carrier proteins in blood. Classic steroid effects are long lasting; they are mediated by diffusion into cells, binding to intracellular receptors and changes in gene transcription.

77—B. Reading the standard curve across from the y-axis, a value of 50% ^{125}I-ANP displacement corresponds to a serum ANP concentration of about 25 pg/mL.

78—D. The signs and symptoms noted in this patient are classic manifestations of growth hormone excess after puberty (acromegaly). Growth hormone has diabetogenic actions that result in an increase in blood glucose concentration, including increased gluconeogenesis in the liver and inhibition of glucose uptake by muscle.

79—E. Symptoms suggest loss of antidiuretic hormone (ADH) action (diabetes insipidus). Acquired central diabetes insipidus may be caused by a head injury. ADH is produced mainly in the supraoptic nucleus so damage here would compromise ADH secretion.

80—E. Ninety percent of secreted thyroid hormone is T_4. T_3 is the most potent form, but is produced in the tissues by the action of 5'/3' deiodinase.

81—C. The symptoms describing this patient indicate hyperthyroidism. Ophthalmopathy suggests Graves' disease, in which thyroid-stimulating immunoglobulins (TSI) act as TSH agonists, driving high levels of T_4 secretion. Negative feedback suppresses endogenous TSH secretion to produce low TSH levels.

82—A. The zona glomerulosa is the sole source of aldosterone because it is the only region of gland to express aldosterone synthase.

83—A. Glucocorticoids mobilize glucose, amino acids, and fatty acids.

84—D. 11β-Hydroxysteroid dehydrogenase modifies cortisol to prevent it from acting at the mineralocorticoid receptor. This is necessary because it is an agonist at the receptor, and it circulates at much higher concentration than aldosterone. Inhibition of 11β-hydroxysteroid dehydrogenase by licorice allows cortisol to activate the mineralocorticoid receptor, causing salt retention.

85—B. The patient's clinical signs are characteristic of glucocorticoid excess. However, there is low cortisol and low ACTH, so physical signs can only be explained by exogenous glucocorticoid medication.

86—D. Pheochromocytoma is a secretory tumor of adrenal medullary chromaffin cells. High levels of the catecholamines epinephrine and norepinephrine are excreted in the urine. Metabolism of catecholamines via catechol-O-methyltransferase (COMT) and monoamine oxidase (MAO) enzymes produce high levels of metanephrine and VMA, which are excreted in urine.

87—E. The resident is likely to be hypoglycemic due to prolonged fasting. Insulin secretion is stimulated by hyperglycemia and suppressed by hypoglycemia. All the other listed hormones are stimulated by hypoglycemia.

88—A. Insulin increases net protein synthesis, and insulin secretion is stimulated by increased plasma amino acid concentration. To prevent hypoglycemia from developing, glucagon secretion is also stimulated by increased plasma amino acid concentration.

89—D. Enteroendocrine cells release glucose-dependent insulinotropic polypeptide (GIP) and glucagon-like peptide-1 in response to a carbohydrate-rich meal. These incretins stimulate insulin release by pancreatic β cells as an "anticipatory" response to an impending glucose load.

90—C. The patient has type 1 diabetes mellitus. Lack of insulin prevents proper oxidation of fatty acids. High levels of glucagon direct hepatic formation of ketones from acetyl CoA instead.

91—D. Glucagon and epinephrine stimulate gluconeogenesis by the liver and increase the supply of glucose precursors from muscle to the liver. Other effects include increased release of fatty acids from adipose tissue and the increased rate of glycogen breakdown in liver and muscle.

92—C. Urine phosphate excretion is controlled by parathyroid hormone, which inhibits tubular phosphate reabsorption.

93—F. The patient has humoral hypocalcemia of malignancy due to PTH-rp secretion, whose action is similar to endogenous PTH. Ca^{2+} retention and phosphate excretion occur. Hypercalcemia suppresses PTH secretion.

94—A. The patient has complete androgen insensitivity (testicular feminization). Androgen-induced development of the mesonephric duct fails. Sertoli cells continue to secrete müllerian-inhibiting substance, so female internal reproductive organs also fail to develop.

95—D. High concentrations of estrogen, progesterone, and inhibin, all at the same time, indicate peak secretion from the corpus luteum around days 18–24. Negative feedback produces low LH and FSH.

96—A. Changes in renal function that increase plasma volume in pregnancy are due to up-regulation of the renin-angiotensin II-aldosterone axis. High levels of progesterone and estrogen bring about this up-regulation, but do not act directly themselves to increase plasma volume.

97—A. Alveolar ventilation increases in pregnancy due to higher tidal volumes. CO_2 levels decrease as a primary result. Renal compensation brings about a decrease in $[HCO_3^-]$ to compensate the pH.

98—C. The lactation reflex occurs in response to a baby suckling, which produces a surge of oxytocin secretion and milk ejection. This reflex can be conditioned by stimuli such as the sound of a baby crying.

99—D. Oxytocin secretion increases in a positive feedback fashion as the cervix dilates, resulting in high concentrations about the time of birth, which produce powerful uterine contractions.

100—A. Human chorionic gonadotropin is a pregnancy-specific hormone secreted by the early embryonic trophoblast. Trace amounts can be detected in urine as early as 7–10 days after ovulation.

101—E. The syncytiotrophoblast persists in the mature placenta as a multinucleated cell layer outermost in chorionic villi, and is bathed in maternal blood within the intervillous space.

102—A. A sustained high estrogen concentration produces positive feedback stimulation of luteinizing hormone secretion by sensitizing gonadotropes to gonadotropin-releasing hormone.

103—C. Ferning of cervical mucus indicates the most receptive time for passage of sperm. This thinner mucus is produced during estrogen dominance about midcycle.

104—A. The vas deferens carries sperm from the epididymis to the ejaculatory duct. Severing the vas prevents sperm from being added to seminal plasma.

105—D. In this child, there is failure of male external genitalia to develop correctly with a normal XY karyotype. External genitalia require dihydrotestosterone for development, which is synthesized in the tissues from testosterone via the enzyme 5α-reductase. Testosterone is produced normally by the testes, allowing masculinization at puberty.

106—B. Estrogens are produced in a two-cell system of granulosa and theca cells. Theca cells provide androgen precursors under the influence of LH. Granulosa cells use androgens to synthesize estrogens, which is accomplished via FSH-stimulated aromatase activity.

107—A. Blood in the umbilical artery is returning from fetal tissues to the placenta for oxygenation and removal of CO_2.

108—A. This is a case of true precocious puberty in which normal puberty has occurred, but too early. A pubertal growth spurt caused the patient to be tall as a child. Early production of sex steroids caused early closure of epiphyseal growth plates, resulting in short adult height.

INDEX

Note: Page numbers followed by f indicate figures; those followed by t indicate tables.

CPSIA information can be obtained
at www.ICGtesting.com
Printed in the USA
FSHW01n0950280718
50903FS

9 780071 485678